WILLIAM BARRY INMAN

INFECTION CONTROL

&

Emerging Infectious Diseases

THIRD EDITION

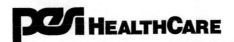

PESI HEALTHCARE, LLC
PO Box 1000
200 Spring Street
Eau Claire, Wisconsin 54702

ISBN: 1-55957-998-6

Printed in the United States

PESI HealthCare strives to obtain knowledgeable authors and faculty for its publications and seminars. The clinical recommendations contained herein are the result of extensive author research and review. Obviously, any recommendations for patient care must be held up against individual circumstances at hand. To the best of our knowledge any recommendations included by the author or faculty reflect currently accepted practice. However, these recommendations cannot be considered universal and complete. The authors and publisher repudiate any responsibility for unfavorable effects that result from information, recommendations, undetected omissions or errors. Professionals using this publication should research other original sources of authority as well.

For information on this and other PESI HealthCare manuals and audiocassettes, please call

800-843-7763

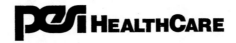

MATERIALS PROVIDED BY

WILLIAM BARRY INMAN is certified in infection control and the Epidemiologist for the Brevard County Health Department in Merritt Island, Fl. He is responsible for development/implementation of surveillance and investigation of communicable disease in Brevard County. Mr. Inman received his BA/BS from the University of Florida with a major in Public Administration/Health. He has completed over 15 credits toward his Master in Public Health. He has received vast training in HIV/AIDS, various communicable diseases, and disease outbreak investigations. Currently he has completed advanced training in Bio-terrorism through the Department of Health in Florida, Center for Disease Control and Prevention, and the United States Army Institute of Research for Infectious Diseases. He is a registered Health Educator by The Association of Professional Health Educator and is a CDC-certified HIV/AIDS Trainer. He was past president of the Association of Professionals in Infection Control (chapter 45) in Orlando, Florida. He was Vice President of the AIDS Consortium in area 7 of Florida and Past President of the American Cancer Society in Brevard County Florida. He also is a Board Member for Comprehensive Health Care (AIDS service providers). Mr. Inman has investigated many outbreaks, including those in long-term care facilities, hospitals, day-care and various food outbreaks. Recently he has experience and training with suspicious substances from letters and packages. He has published many papers on outbreaks and writes a quarterly article for the local AMA journal. Mr. Inman's work experience has been supervisory over the HIV/AIDS and Communicable Disease programs, Project AIDS Care Case Manager and Director of the HIV Counseling and Testing Program at the Brevard County Health Department. He also worked in the Infection Control Departments at the Orlando Regional Medical Center and the Holmes Regional Medical Center. Mr. Inman provides Infection Control Consulting services for Health First, Inc., Pediatrics of Brevard, Circles of Care, Inc., Wuesthoff Health Care Systems, Inc., and is and Infection Control/HIV/AIDS/ TB/OSHA adjunct faculty member for Brevard Community College and the University of Central Florida. Mr. Inman is the recipient of the PESI HealthCare's Excellence in Education award.

INFECTION CONTROL AND EMERGING INFECTION DISEASES

Table of Contents

By William Barry Inman

Foreword

This book is the result of numerous seminar attendees at my public seminars saying they wish there was a reference text that contained, in one place, all the CDC guidelines for infection control, summaries of emerging infectious diseases and discussions on noscomial infections. This work is the result of those requests. It is our hope that this book will provide you with the necessary ammunition to carry out effective and competent infection control programs in your place of work.

Barry Inman

This book is dedicated to the prevention, control, and understanding of Infectious Disease. The book is comprised of three sections. The first will discuss the control of Nosocomial Infections within health care facilities. The second will address the Emerging Infectious Disease problems facing the United States and the World. The last section will provide guidelines for the control of Nosocomial Infections within health care facilities. These CDC guidelines will provide prevention and control measures for appropriate isolation-precautions, immunization of children, adults, and health care workers. Also, appropriate precautions/isolation for disease specific conditions, compliance monitoring form, etc. Specific guidelines are provided for the control and prevention of Nosocomial Surgical Site Infections, Nosocomial Pneumonia, Bactermias related to Intravascular Devices, and the control of antibiotic resistant microorganisms such as Methicillin Resistant Staphylococcus Aureus and Vancomycin Resistant Enterococcus.

My belief is that if you and your facility can provided effective **education**, surveillance, policy and procedures, precautions, handwashing, immunizations, disinfection, etc. you should have the ability to control nosocomial infections in your health care facility.

Unfortunately, nosocomial infections have been increasing in the past years (see chart below). This is primarily due to the increase prevalence of chronically ill patients in our facilities and in the community. This trend will **not change.** Therefore, our ability to control or prevent nosocomial infections is becoming more difficult.

Year	Admissions $(x10^6)$	Patient days[a] $(x10^6)$	Length of stay (days)	Nosocomial infection $(x10^6)$	Nosocomial infections (/1000 patient days)
1975	38	299	7.9	2.1	7.2
1995	36	190	5.3	1.9	9.8

[a]Patient days = total inpatientdays

The control of infections in the United States and in the world will also be very challenging due to dramatic increase in population in the next fifty years, inadequate health care delivery within indigent countries, etc. The slides and technical notes will discuss the situation we will face in our infection control endeavors.

I sincerely hope you find this book helpful in your efforts to understand and assist with Infection Control and the control of Communicable Diseases in your facility and in your community.

The slides and narratives on the following pages can be viewed and printed out from the web at the following URL:

http://www.pesihealthcare.com/ppt/infection.pps

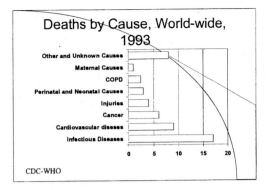

Deaths by Cause, World-wide, 1993

CDC-WHO

Most individuals in the world expire from infectious diseases. It is estimate that 19 million died of infectious diseases in 2001. In the United States most may expire from Cardiovascular disease or cancer. However, most cancer patients die of complications from infection, such as MRSA, VRE, Candidiasis, etc. Some experts believe that a co-factor to atherosolerosis may be prior infection with chlamydia tachomatis infection. Therefore the actually estimates deaths due to direct and indirect causes may be underestimated.

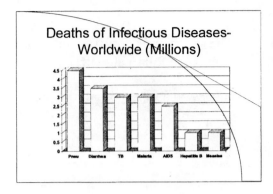

Deaths of Infectious Diseases- Worldwide (Millions)

Of those who expire from infectious diseases most expire from pneumonia. The underlying disease for pneumonia is usually influenza. Some experts have argued that diarrhea illnesses may actually cause more deaths than any other disease. Most deaths are due to Typhoid Fever (Salmonella Typhi), Cholera, and E-Coli. However, another 2-3 million children may die due to Rotavirus. Another 600,000 individuals may expire from shigella. Usually because they are born in the indigent countries and do not have assess to appropriate re- hydration.

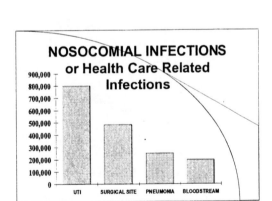

NOSOCOMIAL INFECTIONS or Health Care Related Infections

Approximately 2 million patients acquire nosocomial infections each year in the United States. Urinary Infections comprise 800 thousand, surgical site infections reporting 500,000, pneumonias 200 to 300 thousand and bloodstream estimated at 100 to 200 thousand patients each year. These are the most reported nosocomial infections from acute care and VA hospitals. Other infections which occur such as upper respiratory, Gastro-intestinal, skin, etc. Infections acquired from same-day surgery center, physicians and dental offices, etc are usually not reported. Therefore, the actual occurrence of nosocomial infections is not know from these various other potential sources.

The Institutes of Medicine in Washington, D.C. reported that nearly 100,000 expire from sentinel events in hospitals each year. At least 20,000 may have died as a direct result of nosocomial infections.

Nosocomial Infections may be renamed to Health Care Related Infections due that we have a continuum of health care

Health care has vastly changed in the past years. More and more patients may be transferred between facilities. Therefore, a continuum of care exist among those seen above. The Joint Commission requires facilities share information concerning infections among one another.

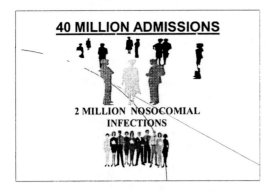

Approximately 2 million patients acquire nosocomial infections each year in the United States, or about 5% of those admitted at acute or VA hospitals. Nursing Home rates will be discussed later. However, the rate of infection from other facilities such as same day surgery center, rehabilitation hospital, etc are at this time difficult to estimate.

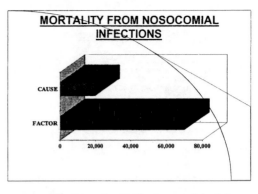

An estimated 60 to 80 thousands patients die each year has a direct or indirect result of nosocomial infection. Other risk factors such as neutropenia due to cancer, etc, may have dire consequences should those patients acquire infections. This is three to four times the death rate from HIV/AIDS. For some patients this is the direct result of death due to nosocomial microorganism. However, in many it's the result of immuno-compromised secondary diagnosis or treatment which suppress the immune system and therefore make them patient more vulnerable to infection.

5

6

Consequences of Nosocomial Infections
Extra Hospital Stay
Antibiotics
Diagnostic Procedures
Extra Medical Supplies
Infection Control program

Site	Days	Costs		Fee for Service	Captivation
SSI	7.3	1838			
Pneumonia	5.9	1500	Infection	Charge Insurance	Subtract from Amount
BSI	7.4	1000			
UTI	1	180			
Other	5	569	No Infection	No Benefit-Penality	Profit

Consequences of nosocomial infections can be extremely costly. Most patients who acquire pneumonia, bactermias, and surgical site infection will usually have extended hospitalizations which in itself will increase cost dramatically. Since capitation, HMOs will generally deduct any payment of nosocomial infections occurs. This provides the health care industry more incentive to try everything possible (within scientific reason) to control nosocomial infections.

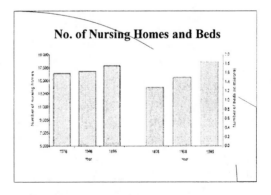

Nursing home growth has expanded greatly in the past decade. There are some 6 to 7 thousand long term care facilities in the United States. Patients may be a risk for nosocomial infections. Nursing homes are admitting more and more patients with more risks for infections, extreme age, various chronic medical conditions, IV therapy, central lines, ventilators, etc.

NOSOCOMIAL INFECTIONS IN NURSING HOMES

- ▷ **1.5 MILLION RESIDENTS ACQUIRE NOSOCOMIAL INFECTIONS**
- ▷ **7.1 INFECTIONS PER 1,000 DAYS OF CARE**
- ▷ **25% SKIN INFECTIONS**
- ▷ **47% RESPIRATORY TRACT & PNEUMONIAS**
- ▷ **18% UTI's**
- ▷ **2% BLOOD STREAM**
- ▷ **SPENDING $60,000 FOR IC PROGRAMS USUALLY SAVES $260,000 ANNUALLY IN ACUTE CARE HOSPITALS, NURSING HOME UNKNOWN?**

SOURCE: ICP Report July 97 Vol 2, No 7

We now have some data from the nursing home industry which now reports 1.5 million residents acquiring nosocomial infections each year. They report that about 7 infections occurs per 1,000 days of care on average (mean). The formula for determining these rates works this way: For example, if in a 30-day month an Long Term Care Facility (LTCF) with an average census of 200 has 15 new nosocomial infections: Infection (incidence) rate =Number of new nosocomial infections '1,000 =

Number of resident days in the month

$\frac{15 \times 1,000}{(30)(200)=6000}$ = 2.5 infections per 1,000 resident days

The preferred rate is infections per 1,000 resident days. Infection control data, including rates, then need to be displayed and distributed to appropriate committees and personnel (including administration) and used in planning infection control efforts. The data should lead to specific educational and control programs. To compare

rates within a facility or to other facilities, the method of calculation must be identical (including the denominator). Even when calculation methods are consistent, infection rates may vary between facilities because of differences in resident risk factors and

9

Infection Control Rates

- ➤ **Facility wide-surveillance**
- ➤ **Patient days X No. of Infections**
  - 70 patients census X days in month (30 days)
  - D=2100 days divided by N=10 infections
  - 10/2100=0.0047
  - 0.0047 x 1000=4.7
- ➤ **Procedure Surveillance (Central line days, Vent days)**
  - D=500 hysterectomy with N=20 infections
  - 20/500=0.04 X 100= 4%

Facility-wide surveillance is useful for establishing an infection control "presence" in the LTCF and may be required as a part of local or state regulatory programs. To establish base-line infection rates, track progress, determine trends, and detect outbreaks, site-specific rates should be calculated. Routine analysis should try to explain the variation in site-specific rates. For example, a change in the rate might be related to a change in the resident population. Focused or high-risk resident surveillance may permit conservation of resources. Published studies of LTCF infections have yet to describe adequately the specific risk factors (eg, device use) for site-specific infections. When such data become available, appropriate risk stratification of infection rates might be a worthwhile objective for this field of practice. This also could lead to focusing resources on those residents at highest risk for developing infections. Also needed are methods that are simple and appropriate for the comparison of site-specific data within an LTCF over time, to establish endemic levels of infection and to recognize potential outbreaks. The statistics used in analysis of data need not be complex. Computerization for sorting and analysis of data may be time-saving for larger pro-grams, and software for use on a personal computer is available. Graphs and charts facilitate presentation and understanding of infection control data and also may be facilitated by computer programs. The commercially available programs may help with analysis of surveillance data, but manual data collection is still necessary.

10

Special Cause 1-3
For Detecting Shifts in the Middle Value

By tracking rates each month, we establish a threshold of infection within our facilities. If our threshold is 4.7%, (may take 6-12 months data to determine) this demonstrates our prevalence of infections. Should rate stay consistently above (as is demonstrated in the above slide) this could provide evidence of a special cause, such as an increase due to a "hidden outbreak" or lack of adherence to infection control practices. It could also mean a change in the patient population with more debilitating illnesses which could make them more susceptible to infections.

Reducing UTIs: Nursing Homes

- ❖ **Hydration**
- ❖ **Keeping Perianal area clean**
  - → **Reduce drying**
  - → **Hormone Replacement-Women?**
- ❖ **Remind residents to use restroom (Every2-3 hours)**
- ❖ **Limit catheter use**
- ❖ **Colonization vs Infection**
  - ❖ **(JCAHO) & State health surveyors**

Urinary tract infections are a major concern for Nursing Homes. Remember to have patients drink plenty of water, 8-10 glasses of water if possible. Keep the perianal area clean as possible. Whether hormone replacement actually might reduce risk is still uncertain? Try and remind patients to use the restroom frequently.

In my experience I have seen some facilities may actually over reported or not correctly diagnose nosocomial urinary tract infection. The patient may only be colonized. Such as a positive culture but no evidence of infection (urine analysis with on evidence of infection, no or few white cells, no symptoms). This could cause concern with the Joint Commission or your state surveyors. Please review the criteria for nosocomial infections in section II.

12

"CHAIN OF INFECTION"

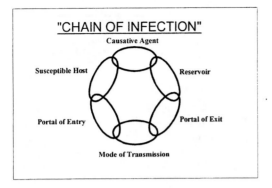

We are all responsible for prevention of cross-contamination of microorganisms. The best way to accomplish is the "breaking" the chain of infections. The above steps "must" happen for infection to occur to the susceptible host.

•Causative Agents: Bacteria, virus, parasites, fungi, etc

•Reservoir: Contaminated air, food or water,etc,. or an individual or groups of people, etc.

•Portal of Exit: from the source; expelling microorganisms in the environment or direct exposure by coughing, ingestion, sexual, blood, draining wound, etc.

•Mode of Transmission: Skin to skin contact, sexual, airborne, bloodborne, foodborne, etc.

•Portal of Entry: By ingestion of contaminated food, breathing in contaminated air (TB), unprotected sex, etc.

•Susceptible Host: All the above have occurred with no protection: prior antibodies by way of vaccine or prior exposure.

It is our responsibility to prevent infections from incurring to protect our patients. The following slides will give you some procedures to reduce the risk of infections to our patients.

VECTORS FOR COLONIZATION-INFECTION

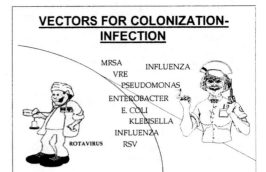

Unfortunately, Healthcare Workers (HCWs) can act as "vectors" in the transmission of microorganisms. The most common reason is due to lack of handwashing. HCWs may go from patient A to patient B without washing hands, or may go from site to site with the same patient and be the vector for transfer or microorganisms.

All to often healthcare workers come to work ill and/or brings organisms from home without washing hands. Beyond popular belief, most organisms are transmitted through touch not through the air.

Physical Barriers Against Infection

- Skin barriers
  – Fatty acids
- Normal bacterial Microflora

Before we discuss why you or the patients acquire various infections, lets discuss the physical barriers we have in place. First is skin, no organism will soak through skin with short duration of contact (< 20 minutes). Also the fatty acids will help control the numbers of microorganism on our skin. Second the the endogenous bacteria we have especially in the respiratory, GI, uro-genital tract which acts as a lining and barrier to prevent the colonization of organisms foreign to us. Third is the respiratory tract; here we have cilia (may caught organism), rinsing-lavage (wash them away), an other secretions which reduce or eliminate passage. Last is the GI tract which we have acidity which destroys many organism but not all such as E-Coli, Hepatitis A, and other foodborne illnesses.

Probability of Infection

$$P_i = \frac{(V)(n)}{HD} \times (k)(t)$$

Where: P_i=Probability of infection
V=Virulence of microbes
n= Number of microbes
HD=Host defenses
k=Constant (transmissibility/route)
t=Time of exposure

The probability we acquire infections has a good bit to do with:

•The virulence of the microbe. Some organisms are very likely to result in disease with appropriate exposure, such as Anthrax, Shigella, E-Coli, and Cholera.

•Numbers: Some organism such as salmonella usually requires great numbers for infection to occur compared to malaria which usually only takes a very few organism to result in infection. Pathogenic E. Coli and Shigella only require 10-100 organisms for infection when ingested.

•Host defense: are you susceptible or not? Some organisms are certainly more easily transmitted that other. We know that measles or smallpox are very contagious. AS we mature (age 7-60) and have been exposed to some organisms, we are less likely to become infected if we are not immuno-compromised>

•Time of exposure: The longer you are exposed, the more likely infection will occur. Such as living with or taking a long car ride with some coughing Tuberculoisis. If we ingest more of the contaminated food the more likely for foodborne illness.

HANDWASHING

- **When to wash hands:**
  - Prolonged contact with patients, mucous membrane, body secretions
  - When ever touching immunocompromised patients, newborns, before and after wound care, fecal contact (very important)
  - When performing invasive procedures
  - Whenever gloves are used
  - Intensive areas are very important!
  - Before and after work , Food preparation, after restroom, sneezing/coughing
- **How to wash hands:**
  - For ≥ 15 seconds
  - Friction is important!
    - Lathering, rubbing all areas of the skin
    - Followed by rinsing

• Now as of September 2002 there is a recommendation change in handwashing from the CDC. Hand rinses have demonstrated they may eliminate more bacteria and virus than traditional handwashing technique. Studies in Europe demonstrated more gram negative organism are killed by handrinse vs traditional handwashing. Also Health Care Workers are more likely to utilize hand rinses. Therefore, you may have a increase in hand hygiene activities if hand rinses are encouraged.

• CDC now states that when health Care workers utilized handrinses they do not need to also wash hands with soap and water. For the reason stated above. Also please see the recommendation for hand hygiene in the back section of this book for your information

• Handwashing is the single most important procedure for preventing nosocomial (facility-acquired) infections.

• Just from contact with body secretions, health-care workers' hands can carry bacteria, viruses, and fungi that may be potentially infectious to themselves and others.

• Handwashing is recommended when there is prolonged and intense contact with any patient.

• Handwashing is necessary *before* and *after* situations in which hands are likely to become contaminated, especially when hands have had contact with mucous membranes, blood and body fluids, and secretions or excretions, and *after* touching contaminated items such as urine-measuring devices.

• As a general rule, when in doubt health-care workers should wash their hands.

• The generally accepted correct handwashing time and method is a 10- to 15-second vigorous rubbing together of all lathered surfaces followed by rinsing in a flowing stream of water. If hands are visibly soiled, more time may be required.

• The choice of plain or antiseptic soap, or of alcohol-based hand rinses should depend on whether it is important to reduce and maintain minimal counts of colonizing flora as well as to mechanically remove the contaminating flora. *Consult your infection control department if you*

Hand Wash Antiseptics

- ➢ **Alcohols**
- ➢ **Chlorhexidine 4%**
- ➢ **Iodine compounds**
- ➢ **Iodophors**
- ➢ **PCMX**
- ➢ **Triclosan**

Various handwashing antiseptics are available to healthcare workers. See the document on Recommendation for handwashing in section II. Remember it usually does not matter was antiseptic or non-antiseptic soaps you may use, but how and when you wash your hands. Alcohols are probably the most effect in destroying and quickly reducing bacteria counts on hands, however may cause severe drying. Chlorhexidene rare causes reactions, it is more appropriate in the intensive care, surgery areas. Iodine like chlorhexidine is every effect, however there are reports of reactions with over use. PCMX and Triclosan are good antiseptics for general handwashing in the usually medical/surgery floors and are also good in facilities outside the hospital setting.

Hand rinse-does it work?

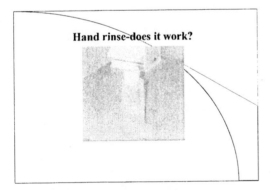

Hand rinses work very well. However, OSHA mandates that once you use these items you should wash your hands with a sink, soap and water as soon as available. A recent study demonstrated that participants could used the hand rinse 5 to 6 times before needing to use a sink. Remember that sinks are still more effects due to the fact that use a scrubbing, rinsing, etc. When using these hand rinses it is usually recommended use those which are impregnated with foam or lubricants to reduce the drying effect.

DID NOT WASH HANDS!!!

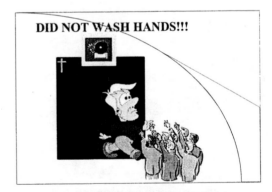

Many studies have identified the lack of handwashing. Some restaurants have installed various monitoring device such as mini-cameras, various scanners to identify food handlers who wash there hands at least 10-15 times a day. Those who do not may receive disciplinary action. This same monitoring could be done in healthcare, however I believe education is the key to increased compliance.

Nearly everyone including our children in school should wash hands 10-15 times a day. If someone is not doing anything, go wash your hands!

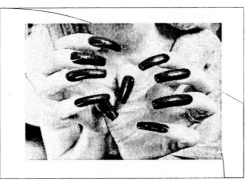

Acrylic nails have been in question in healthcare. Now CDC strongly recommendation that acrylic nail not be allowed for health Care Workers whom perform invasive type procedures. Acrylic nails when damaged with cracks have been implicated as source to outbreak particularly in the neonatal setting. Various studies have identified higher bacteria counts than with natural nails. The CDC also does not recommended scrub brush for scrubbing before surgery and the time is recommended to be 3-5 minutes. Please see the hand hygiene recommendations in the back of this book.

Disinfectants

- **Low level**
  - Alcohol
  - Chlorine
  - Iodophors
  - Phenolics
  - Quaternary Ammonium Compounds (Quats)
- **Intermediate Level**
  - Glutaraldehyde (Gluts)
  - Hydrogen Peroxide
  - Peracetic Acid

Proper disinfections is paramount to appropriate infection control procedures. **BEFORE ANY ITEM IS TO BE PROPERLY DISINFECTED, IT MUST BE CLEANED OF ORGANIC / SOIL MATERIAL AS POSSIBLE!**

Low Level Disinfectants: are primary used for general disinfection of rooms and other inanimate objects and/or when spill occurs with bodily secretions and excretions. When spills occur the secretion or excretion should be flooded with chlorine (usually one to ten dilution bleach and water), phenolic or quats (Iodophors are rarely used due staining and corrosiveness). Then, as much soiled or organic material must be removed with paper towels, sponges, mops, etc. as possible! Make sure you wear to appropriate personal protective equipment (gloves are usually enough). Then once this is accomplished, a final terminal disinfection is required (see next slide).

Alcohol should only be used to disinfect thermometers or occasionally stethoscopes. Alcohols cause drying and any device which is subject to alcohol should be inspected for cracks, crevices, etc. They should not be used for general room or equipment disinfecting due of inadequate contact time.

High Level Disinfectants: Are used for endoscopes. Any above may be used. Glutaralydehyde may cause skin, URI irritation. Newer formulations have reduced the risk for toxic exposure to glutaralydehydes. Efforts should be made to reduce exposure to fumes. Placing containers up wind, always covered and minimizing any splashing or shaking.

Endoscopes should be pre-cleaned with scrubbing or enzymes. Place in the intermediated level disinfectant, usually for 20 minutes, rinsed with **sterile** water and forced air dry. If sterile water is not available this wipe down with alcohol.

Cleaning-Decontaminating of spills of blood/other bodily fluids

- Most disinfectants are adequate
- Flood with germicide or soap & water
- Then Remove bio-burden
- Then decontaminate, allowing ≥ 30-60 seconds to dry
- Wear gloves while cleaning/decontaminating

Appropriate disinfection procedure is necessary for the environment to safe from an over burdening of microorganisms. First gloves need to donned. The area should first be flood or with an appropriate disinfectant "spilled kits" are often used. Allow approximately 30-60 seconds for the disinfectant to kill as many surface organism as possible. Once this has been done, use paper towels, mops or other materials and congregate the area together, careful not to expand the contaminated site. Once as much of the contaminted bio-burden can be collected an disposed of, then flood area again with appropriate disinfectant allowing it to try for about 30-60 seconds. Most bodily fluids do not need to be placed in a red bag unless they are caked, dripping, or soaked with bloody material (when compressed blood components are released). Most materials can be placed in hoppers or toilets if it will not physical damage drainage system and if connected to a city sewer system.

Descending Order of Resistance to Germicidal Chemicals

1. **Bacterial spores.**
   - B. Subtilis.
2. **Mycobacteria.**
   - M. Tuberculosis.
3. **Nonlipid or small virus.**
   - Polio.
   - Hepatitis A.
4. **Fungi.**
   - Trichsphyton spp.
5. **Vegative bacteria**
   - P. Aeruginosa.
   - S. Aureus
   - Streptococcus
6. **Lipid or medium size viruses**
   - HSV
   - HBV
   - HIV

This is a list of resistance to germicidal chemicals by organisms. As is clearly shown, bloodborne pathogens are generally every easy to destroy. OSHA in their original Bloodborne Pathogen Standard in 1991 stated that when cleaning spills, use a disinfect which can destroy TB. Since that time OSHA has rescinded that rule. Try and use the disinfectant for situations they where designed for. See Guidelines for disinfection in section II.

Appropriate Precautions

- **Standard:** Combines Universal (Blood, semen, vaginal secretions, etc) with all body secretions
- **Airborne**
  - TB, Measles
- **Droplet**
  - Meningococcal Disease, Rubella, Influenza
- **Contact**
  - MRSA?, VRE?, Herpes, CD, Ebola & Lassa Fever

Appropriate precautions again are essential in the control of nosocomial infections. Standard precautions replace Universal in that standard applies to all bodily fluids (sweat is not considered potentially infectious). Thin secretions and excretions may transmitted various harmful microorganisms. Therefore, Standard precautions are needed for *all patients*!

See at the back of this section appropriate policies and procedures for these policies and CDC recommendation for appropriate disease specific precautions.

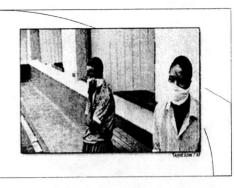

This photo was taken during and Ebola outbreak in Zaire 2000. Ebola is a hemorrhagic fever. Symptoms include flu-like syndrome, and bleeding from the mucous membranes. Transmission usually occurs when individuals expire and other tribe member touch them to show proper respect. Usually when the CDC and the WHO(World Health Organization) give out gloves the epidemic resolves. During this last outbreak, the death rate was about 45% compared to other outbreaks in the past which experienced death rates of 85%. The reduction in deaths was due to prompt administration of I.V. therapies to control hydration.

Illness and the HCW

- ➢ **Do not come to work with fever, diarrhea, infectious skin rash!!**
- ➢ **If you must come to work; no patient contact!!**
- ➢ **Frequent handwashing**
- ➢ **URI-may be! Wash hands frequently**
  - ➢ **May wish to use hand- rinse**

It is very important for Health Care Workers who have patient contact not to come to work with fever, rash, or diarrhea. Health Care Workers can bring infections in from the community and unfortunately infected patients. This type of exposure happens all too frequently. Many outbreaks from various bacteria (staph, strep, etc) to Influenza have the source related to a previously ill Health Care Worker.

The reality is Health Care Workers may come to work ill due to unnecessary job pressure. If this occurs, patients contact should not occur and frequent handwashing should be accomplished. Some facilities may have a "zero tolerance policy" to Health Care Workers showing to work with fever, rash, and/or diarrhea.

Upper Respiratory Infections are frequent among Health Care Workers. If at all possible Health Care Workers should not have contact with patients. However, if this is unavoidable frequently handwashing must occur. Hand-rinses may be provided to encourage handwashing and reduce risk for transmission.

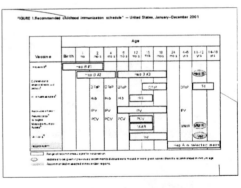

Immunization are very important in protecting the public health. Some experts believe our population would be much less if we did not have the immunizations available to us. The above immunizations are recommended for children and in nearly all states will require most of these before admission in public school or day care. Below is a brief discussion of each. Please refer to your health department or www.immunize.org for more detailed information.

- •Hepatitis B: If given at birth will greatly reduce hepatitis B in the next generations. Usually will prevent perinatal transmission and the younger they receive this vaccine the more likely for lifelong immunity.

- •Diphtheria, Tetanus, and Pertussis (Whooping Cough): Of these the only disease still somewhat prevalent is Pertussis. Due to non completion of DTP and immigration.

- •Hamophilus: This has virtually eliminated this form of meningitis, bacteremia, epiglottitis, and cellulitis.

- •Inject-able Polio: We administer inject-able due to no wide outbreaks in the United States. The child who receives the oral vaccine could spread the virus in feces, which cause a vaccine associated polio is someone immuno-compromised (HIV, Cancer, etc.).

- •Pneumococcal: Designed from elimination and/or reducing meningitis, bacteremia, and pneumonia. (following slides)

- •Measles, Mumps, and Rubella: Children and many adults need two injections to be near 99-100% protected.

- •Varicella: See slide no.39

- •Hepatitis A: usually only recommended for child with immuno-suppression

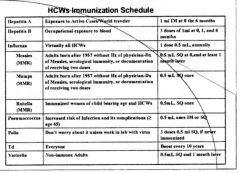

HCWs Immunization Schedule

Hepatitis A	Exposure to Active Cases/World traveler	1 ml IM at 0 the 6 months
Hepatitis B	Occupational exposure to blood	3 doses of 1ml at 0, 1, and 6 months
Influenza	Virtually all HCWs	1 dose 0.5 mL, annually
Measles (MMR)	Adults born after 1957 without Hx of physician-Dx of Measles, serological immunity, or documentation of receiving two doses	0.5 mL SQ at 0,and at least 1 month later
Mumps (MMR)	Adults born after 1957 without Hx of physician-Dx of Measles, serological immunity, or documentation of receiving two doses	0.5 mL SQ once
Rubella (MMR)	Immunized women of child bearing age and HCWs	0.5mL, SQ once
Pneumococcus	Increased risk of infection and its complications (≥ age 65)	0.5 ml, once IM or SQ
Polio	Don't worry about it unless work in lab with virus	3 doses 0.5 ml SQ, if never immunized
Td	Everyone	Boost every 10 years
Varicella	Non-immune Adults	0.5mL SQ and 1 month later

These vaccines are recommended for healthcare workers in the United States. Most will be discussed in later slides. Please refer to the document of Immunization of Health Care Workers in section II>

•MMR: Healthcare workers need to 2 if born after 1956 to be 99-100% immunized and not spread measles, mumps, and rubella to other employees and patients.

•Hepatitis A is only recommended if you work with patients with increased endemicity (children-adults with active, endemic cases)or you travel a great deal to foreign countries.

•Influenza: see the following slides!

•Pneumococcal: Over 65 years of age or chronic illness at any age (diabetes, Chronic Hepatitis B & C). See following slides.

•Polio: Rarely indicated

•Tetanus/Diphtheria: Tetanus shot every 10 years. If > 5 years and receive injury. obtain booster. Whenever you receive tetanus, diphtheria is given as a co-vaccine to reduce risk and eliminate diphtheria.

Recommended Schedule for use of 7-valent Pneumococcal Vaccine

Age at First dose (mos)	Primary Series	Additional dose
2-8	3 doses, 2 mos apart	1 dose at 12-15 mos
7-11	2 doses, 2 mos apart	1 dose at 12-15 mos
12-23	2 doses, 2 mos apart	–
24-59 (health children) Children with Immuno suppression	1 dose 2 doses, 2 mos apart	–

Above is the recommended dose schedule of administration of the 7-valent Pneumococcal vaccine. The vaccine is not needed for child > 5 years of age.

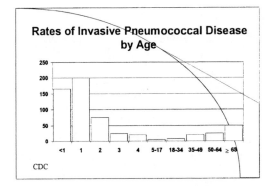

Rates of Invasive Pneumococcal Disease by Age

CDC

Most cases of Invasive Pneumococcal disease occur among the very young vs the very old. The vaccine was designed to to greatly reduce pneumonia, bacteremia, and meningitis. The vaccine may reduce the otitis media by 20%. If administered after first episode of otitis, this may reduce the incidence by 50%. Most bacteria which result in otitis are pneumococcal or haemophilus.

Influenza

- 25,000 to 30,000 die each year to Influenza
- 20,000 to 200,000 are hospitalized
- Influenza and Pneumococcal pneumonia are the 5th leading cause of death for those ≥ 65
- Cost the nation $12 billion each year
- 10% to 20% of the population become infected each year
- Nursing homes can experience an attach rate of 60% with a death rate of 30%

- Vaccine: For nearly everyone,
- Do not receive if severe reaction in past or allergic to eggs
  - Those age ≥50 and those with chronic medical conditions
  - pregnant females in 2nd 3rd trimester,
  - HCWs so not to infect patients, teachers, day care workers, kids
  - If we are around chronically ill individuals at home work, etc.

Influenza is probably one of the least respect diseases through the world. Yet it will kill at least 25,000 to 30,000 in a "mild" flu year. Unfortunately, we may have healthcare workers contribute to the spread by coming to work ill. Below is a letter from Dr. Atkinson of the CDC on the importance of Influenza immunization among healthcare workers.

Dear Colleagues,

If you're like most people who work in medicine, your patients' well-being is of primary concern to you. Yet every year more than 200,000 MDs and RNs needlessly expose their patients to the influenza virus. Are you one of them? According to CDC, only 34% of MDs and RNs get vaccinated annually against influenza. This means that over 2.3 million MDs and RNs are unvaccinated and at risk not only for contracting influenza but also for passing it on to others. On average, 20,000 people die annually in the U.S. from influenza or its complications. Some of these cases are unwittingly passed from health professionals to their patients. Why are so many of us unvaccinated? According to surveys, here are some reasons:

1. I don't get sick and I never get influenza.

About 10–25% of people get influenza each year, and health professionals are not exempt. Many of us develop only mild symptoms of the disease, so we often don't get a florid influenza syndrome. But even with minimal symptoms, we can still transmit the full-blown illness to our patients.

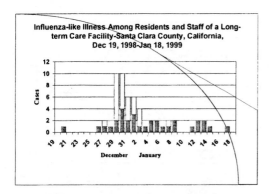

Influenza-like Illness Among Residents and Staff of a Long-term Care Facility-Santa Clara County, California, Dec 19, 1998-Jan 18, 1999

This slide demonstrates an Influenza outbreak in a nursing home which began with a nurse (index case) coming to work ill. The finally result was 24 patients with three deaths and nurses and other healthcare workers became infected. Influenza vaccine compliance was only 25% among healthcare workers at this nursing home. Unfortunately, the utilization of influenza vaccine among healthcare workers is low.

Classes and Names of Influenza Antivirals

Drug Class	Resistance	Drug Name
Neuraminidase Inhibitors	Uncommon	Zanamivir Oseltamirvir
M2 Inhibitors	Common	Amantadine Rimantadine

These are medications which reduce the productions of influenza in patients. These can be administered to patients to reduce illness and contagion to other individuals. Sometimes these medications are used to control an outbreak of influenza in a heathcare facility along with cohorting (staff and patients) and strict attention to handwashing, etc.

Composition of the 2002-2003 Influenza Vaccine

- A/New Caledonia/20/99-like H1N1
- A/Moscow/10/99 like H3N2
- B/Hong Kong/330/01 like virus

This is the Influenza composition for 2001-2002. How does the WHO and CDC usually know. Surveillance is other countries, usually in the lower hemisphere (but not always, like this year Moscow). Surveillance among Flu-Epidemiologist take samples from patients with flu-like illness, if a particular type of Influenza is evident in many individuals (like those above) a vaccine can be produced to help protect others. The tract record for the World Health Organization in predicting Flu-types has been very successful.

Flu Symptoms vs Cold Symptoms

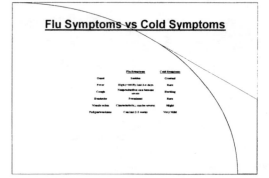

Symptoms of Influenza usually occur suddenly. Many individuals can pin point the day and time when symptom abruptly occurred. Symptoms are listed above, however adults are contagious for 3-4 days while children are contagious for 4-6 days (another reason to immunize children for Flu). Many patients will have a lasting fatigue/weakness for 2-3 weeks. This is very common with influenza.

Varicella Vaccine

- ◆ 4 million infected each year in USA
- ◆ 100-200 hundred thousand with complication: may be at increase risk to GAS (skin necrotitis strept)
- ◆ 10 thousand hospitalized
- ◆ 100-200 die each year
- ◆ Vaccine recommendations for HCWs
  - ♦ Receive if no prior exposure; No HX or titers
  - ♦ No titers drawn after vaccine
  - ♦ If exposed to varicella; Check for titers immediately after exposure, if antibody appear-go back to work, if no antibody, repeat titers 5 to 6 days after exposure, if antibody appears, go to work, if not-no contact with patients or report to employee health to monitor for signs and symptoms from 10-21 day after initial exposure

Varicella is a serious disease. Along with the information above, may communities have at least 5-20 children diagnosised with Encephalitis due to chickenpox.

Below are some other reason to vaccinate yourself (if you never had chickenpox) or your child:

•You reduce your Childs risk for skin necrosissing streptococcus

•They are not as likely to suffer from shingles as they age!

•They will not become infected or have mild illness without complications

•They are very unlikely to infects others which chickenpox.

•Much less likely to miss school or day care and that will make it less likely you miss work or other activities

Healthcare workers who have never had chickenpox should receive the Varicella Vaccine. All should be screened who do not remember prior infection with chickenpox. Those who do remember do not need to be screened. Screen for IgG to Varicella; if positive or reactive the healthcare worker is immune and does not need vaccine. If not, administer vaccine (two does at least one month apart). Do not do antibody screens unless the following occurs.

•Varicella vaccine recipent report exposure (at work or home)

♦If exposed to varicella; Check for titers immediately after exposure, if antibody appear-go back to work, if no antibody, repeat titers 5 to 6 days after exposure, if antibody appears, go to work, if not-no contact with patients or report to employee health to monitor for signs and symptoms from 10-21 day after initial exposure

Pneumococcal Vaccine: Algorithm for vaccinating persons aged 65 years

Usually most individuals will receive pneumococcal vaccine at 65 years of age or greater. However if some received the vaccine earlier than at 65. A one time revaccination should be considered for adults at highest risk for serious pneumococcal infection and persons likely to have a rapid decline antibody levels, provided at **least five years** have passed since receipt of the first dose. Someone could receive the vaccine at age 50, however most (unless severely immunocompromised-see next slide) will not need a second dose until they reach age 65.

Recommendation for the Use of Pneumococcal Vaccine

Groups for which Vaccination is recommended	Revaccination
Persons Aged ≥ 65	Second dose of vaccine if patient received vaccine 5 years previously and were aged< 65 years at time of vaccination
Persons aged 2-64 years with COPD, chronic cardiovascular disease, diabetes melitus	Not Recommended
Persons aged 2-64 years with alcoholism, chronic liver disease, cerebrospinal fluid leaks	Not Recommended
Persons aged 2-64 years with functional or anatomic asplenia	If person is aged ≥ 10 years, single revaccination ≥ 5 years after previous dose. If patient ≤ 10 years, consider revaccination 3 years after previous dose
Persons aged 2-64 years living in special environments or social settings	Not recommended
Immunocompromised persons Immunocompromised persons aged ≥ 2 years, including those with HIV, leukemia, lymphoma, Hodgkins disease, multiple myeloma, generalized malignancy, chronic renal failure, or nephrotic syndrome; those receiving immunosuppressive therapy, chemo/corticosteroids; and those who have received an organ or bone marrow transplant	Single revaccination of ≥5 years have elapsed since receipt of first dose. If patient is aged ≤10 years: consider revaccination 3 years after previous dose

A=strong evidence and substantial clinical benefit support recommendation of vaccine B=Moderate evidence supports the recommendation for vaccine use C=Effectiveness of vaccination is not proven, but increased risk for disease and the potential benefits and safety of the vaccine justify vaccination

Rule of Immunization

- ● No Vaccine should be started over!
  - – Pick up where you-employee left off
  - – Should employee not return for scheduled immunization, continue schedule as usual then they return
  - – They received 1st HBV vaccine but forgot to return for second dose until 6 months later. Administer 2nd and 3rd dose at usual schedule

No vaccine should be started over. Should someone forget an appointment just start where you left off. This includes the Hepatitis B vaccine for healthcare workers.

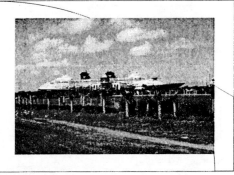

Rubella-Cruise Ship

- Incubation: 14-17 days-range 14-23 days
- Transmission: Contact with nasopharyngeal secretions-droplet spread
- Communicability: 1 week before and at least 5 days after onset of rash
- Symptoms: None to febrile viral disease with diffuse maculopapular rash. Adults may have 1-5 days of prodromal fever, H/A, malaise, coryza, conjunctivitis, occipital and posterior cervical lymphadenopathy, red eyes, joint pain (mostly females).
- Complications:Produce abnormalities in developing fetus. CRS occurs in 90% of infants born to women infected with Rubella in 1st Trimister. Risk for intrauterine death, spon abortion, malformation of major organs, deafness, cataracts, glaucoma, microcephalic, meningoencephalitis, mental retardation, heptosplenomegally, radiolucent bone disease
- 5 confirmed cases
- 4 Cases in the USA for 2001

Cruise ships unfortunately have been the source for influenza and chickenpox outbreaks. Many of the employees who work on these ships are from countries where the "childhood illness" are endemic. In our local area employees of these ships have been diagnosed with rubella, measles, and mumps. Other diseases such as Tuberculosis and leprosy have also occurred. My recommendation for anyone considering a cruise is that you and your family be well immunized for the childhood illness, influenza and chickenpox. The incidence of foodborne illness is low. The CDC is responsible for monitoring these ships and do an excellent job with the lack of personnel they have available.

Recently both Disney cruise ships have experienced a Rubella and Norwalk viral (Gastroenteritis). In August of 2002 5 cases of Rubella were found to be infected with Rubella. The entire crews of both ships where administered MMR vaccine to increase herd immunity and prevent further Rubella cases. In November of 2002 a Norwalk virus outbreak on two cruises had about 4% of passengers ill and about .5% of crew members. Handwashing was increased along with disinfection of ship. The Cruise ship Magic canceled a cruise to break the chain of infection. See next two slides for more information on Rubella and Norwalk virus,

Rubella-Cruise Ship

- Contact investigation of confirmed and suspect cases
- Blood drawn of IgM & IgG antibodies for Rubella on all contacts-or active surveillance, 130 Blood Draws
- Suspect/Confirmed cases isolated in Medical unit or in state rooms, until deemed not infectious
- Active surveillance-Retro and Prospective
- Notification by letter for everyone boarding ship and Retro-Prospective notification
- All pregnant females counseled about risks-particularly those from other countries-TORCH TITERS

Microbiology of SSIs

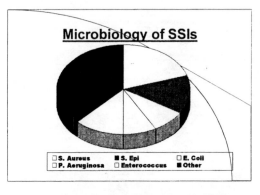

| □ S. Aureus | ■ S. Epi | □ E. Coli |
| □ P. Aeruginosa | □ Enterococcus | ■ Other |

As demonstrated in a pervious slide, the CDC has estimated that 500,000 Surgical Site Infections (SSIs) occur each year. Surgeries are usually classified as clean, clean contaminated, contaminated, and dirty. Those with endogenous bacteria (GI, respiratory tract) are more likely to develop infections. Above, the most common organisms associated with SSI. Most are Staphylococcus infections, however organism such as E.Coli and Enterococcus, which are found in fecal matter, comprise a significant percentage associated with SSIs.

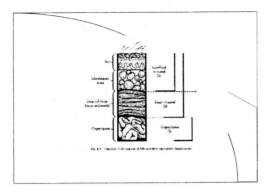

Fig. 3-1 Schematic of the cross section of SSIs and their appropriate classifications.

When an infection occurs, the infection should be classified using the above schematic. Those infection in deep soft tissue and organ/space are of most concern to increase risk of severe outcomes and may be more likely for organisms to spread via hands of healthcare personnel.

Methods for Reducing Risk of Surgical Site Infections

- Preoperative treatment of remote infection
- Control of diabetes, wt reduction by obese patients, discontinuation or decrease steroid use
- Expeditions surgery
- Gentle handling of tissue
- Reduction of blood loss and hematoma
- Elimination of dead space
- Debridement of devitalized tissue, removal of material by irrigation and suction and removal of foreign matter
- Avoidance of unnecessary surgical drains
- Placement of drain beside primary incision
- Use close suction drains
- Surgical skill for clean procedures

The above guidelines from the CDC are available to reduce the risk of surgical site infections. 1) Treat or remove any other infectious process if possible (e.g. UTI, abscess, etc.). The organism will break off and try to find a weakened area-opportunistic, where it is more likely to cause infection. 2) If possible control diabetes, wt reduction and/or control steroids which can suppress the immune system. 3) Quicker the surgery the less time and less opportunities for organism to invade the site. 4) Trying to to dramatize-abrade issue will reduce risk. 5-7) Reduction in blood loss, elimination of dead space, and debridement of devitalized tissue, and remove of foreign matter further reduce the risk. 8) Should should be avoided, however if necessary should be placed through another area and not the original insertion site. 9) Closed drain are always associated with reduce risk of infection 10) The more experience a surgeon has the less likelihood of infections. New residents in teaching medical centers may be associated with higher rates of infection, but this varies greatly

45

46

Intervention to reduce Microbial Contamination

- Preoperative bathing of patient with antiseptic soap
- Improved air filtration
- Traffic control in the OR
- Preoperative antiseptic hand scrub of surgical team
- Barrier protection with gloves, gown, masks, drapes and hoods
- Antiseptic scrubbing of skin at surgical site
- Limiting postoperative stay
- Wounds
  - Closed: Incisions are resistant to penetration of exogenous bacteria shortly after surgery. II/W before dressing avoiding direct contact and wear appropriate gowns
  - Open: Sterile technique for burn wounds, second intention healing sites, and incision being prepared for delayed primary closure

Reduction microbial contamination on your skin and hands also is likely to reduce the risk of surgical site infections. 1) Having a patient bath with chlorexidine will reduce endogenous bacteria. 2) Improved air filtration, particularly where large numbers of implant surgeries are preformed. 3) Limiting the operation room only to necessary personnel will reduce the amount of microbes (where people go, so does microbes). 4) Appropriate barriers (masks, gloves, gowns, etc.) are very important reduce the patients exposure to health care workers organisms. 5) Scrubbing the site of where surgery will occur will reduce risk, have the area pre-cleaned (free of obvious dirt, debris), use a circular rotation motion. 6) Patients should be discharged as soon as possible, if medically appropriate. The longer patients are in hospitals after surgery the more likely they could be exposed to microorganisms. 7) Once wounds are closed, it is usually unlikely for organisms to invade. If infections occurs the organisms where usually introduced during surgery when the patient is "open" and when organisms could have been directed or indirectly introduced. Health care workers should wash hands and use non-sterile gloves when caring for closed wounds (usually 1-2 days post-Op). Sterile gloves with aseptic technique should always be used to care for open wounds

Preoperative Hair Removal

- Method of Hair Removal — SSI Rate

Method of Hair Removal	SSI Rate
– Razor	5.6%
– Depiltory	0.6%
– No Hair removal	0.6%

- Timing of hair removal

Timing of hair removal	
– Shaving immediately before	3.1%
– Shaving ≤ 24 hours before	7.1%
– Shaving ≥ 24 hours before	>20%
– Clipping immediately before operation associated with lower SSI risk than shaving or clipping the night before operation	

Hair remove is an important aspect of controlling surgical site infections. Hair should be removed as close to the time of surgery as possible. If feasible, do not remove hair; if hair is very low level and few fibers are evident, no hair removal may be needed. See Section II for further information to reduce risk for SSIs.

48

Antimicrobial Prophylaxis (AMP)

- 1st and 2nd generation cephalosporins most commonly used AMP agents
- Administration of AMP agent ≤ 2 hours before incision reduced SSI risk (0.59 vs ≥ 3.3%)
- General consensus: Administer AMP no more than 30 min before incision
  - Except C-SEC, immediately after cord clamping
  - Except vancomycin, about 1 hour before incision
- **Require patients to shower or bathe with an antiseptic agent on at least the night before the operation day**

Antibiotic prophylaxis can decrease the incidence of infection, particularly wound infection, after operations, but this benefit must be weighed against the risks of toxic and allergic reactions, emergence of resistant bacteria, drug interactions and superinfections. Some experts believe antimicrobial prophylaxis only for procedures with high infection rates, those involving implantation of prosthetic devices and those in which the consequences of infections are high.

An effective prophylactic regimen should be directed against the most likely infecting organisms, but need no eradicate every potential pathogen. For most procedures, cefazolin (Ancef, and others), which has a moderately long serum half life, has been effective. In institutions which MRSA are important post-operative pathogens, vancomycin can be used, but not routinely because of potential emergence of resistance organism to vancomycin.. For colorectal surgery and appendectomy, cefaxitin (Mefoxin) or cefetetan (Cefotan) is preferred because they are more active than cefazolin against bowel anaerobes, including bacteroides. Third and fourth generations antibiotic should be discouraged.

With most antibiotics, a single dose given 30 minutes or less before the skin incision provides adequate tissue concentrations through the operation. As stated above, there are some exceptions.

Risk for Nosocomial Pneumonia (NP)
Risk and Mechanism of Infection

- Altered swallowing & cough reflux
- Coma or depressed consciousness
- Seizures
- Dysphagia
- Endotracheal tube
- Orenteral nasoenteral tube
- Immunospressed, granulocytopenia, both from disease or therapy
- Airway obstruction-tumors, mucosal edema etc.
- Altered orophargngeal flora and or gastric colonization

The patients in the above and next slide are at increased risk for for nosocomial infections. Most of these patients are unable to clear secretions which will attract microorganisms. Patient which are ventilated for more than 14 days have a risk of up to 50% for nosocomial pneumonia. These patients maybe the one of the most frustrating in trying to prevent infections.

Risk for NP
Risk and Mechanism of Infection

- **Antimicrobial therapy-local or systemic, H² Blockers antacids,**
  - **Growth and multiplication of gastric juices**
- **Trauma penetrating wounds, unintentional surgical procedure**
  - **Introduce organism directly**
- **Burns, adult respiratory distress syndrom. Post thoriac or upper abdominal surgery**
  - **Can not clear secretions!**
  - **Pooling of secretions**
- **URI, COPD, Musculoskeletal disorders, extreme age, diabetes**
  - **Can not clear secretions!**
  - **Pooling of secretions**

Patients who are administered H² blockers may have bacterial over growth and if reflux occurs, this may damage the upper respiratory tract, therefore increase risk for infection. Patients which are not ambulatory, mainly because they have difficulty in clearing secretions.

Procedure/devices With Increased Risk of NP
With Intervention to decrease such risk

- **Gloving: Contact with Resp. secretions**
- **Semicritical devices/Equipment:**
  - **Resp., anesthesia, diagnostic, breathing circuits**
- **Breathing circuits**
- **Hydroscopic-condenser humidifiers**
- **Mechanical ventilation bags**
- **Nebulizers**
- **Budding humidifiers**

Above are some basic steps to pneumonia:

•Glove-up before coming in contact with respiratory sections and of course wash hands

•All equipment which has been used on other patients needs to be adequately disinfected before use again.

•Breathing circuits should not be replaced until 48 hours have passed since insertion. Many hospitals change circuits every 10-14 days without increased risk for nosocomial pneumonia.

•All other equipment needs to be disinfected appropriately (follow manufacture recommendations).

Other Situations Associated with Increased Risk of NP

> Antibiotic Administration
>> Do not routinely prophylaxis for NP
> Winter
>> Vaccinate HCWs against Influenza
>> Prophylaxis and treated exposed (not vaccinated or ill)
>> Cohort
>> Don't work it you have the Flu!
> RSV Season
>> Cohort
>> Standard Precautions
> Hospital Construction

As previously stated, healthcare workers should be vaccinated against influenza along with patient at risk. If an outbreak occurs, patients maybe cohorted along with healthcare worker. When and if cohorting is implemented to control influenza, RSV, or other illnesses other healthcare workers such as physicians, PT, OT, RT should visit the cohorted patients last before leaving the facility or the floor/department. This is done to reduce further spread of of these diseases to other facilities or within a facility. Patients and employees who have not been vaccinated should be encouraged to receive influenza vaccination during an outbreak. Also prophylaxis can be implemented with anti-influenza medications (see previous slides) to reduce severe outcomes and infectiousness.

The Joint Commission takes construction very seriously due to previous outbreaks among immuno-compromised patients. Patients must be separated from work areas, this includes the ventilation systems. Wall used for separation must be hard-sheet rock type which must extend to the floor above or ceiling. Construction workers must have designed traffic routes to work areas and must not travel through patient care areas. Please review the guidelines for prevention and control of nosocomial pneumonia in section II.

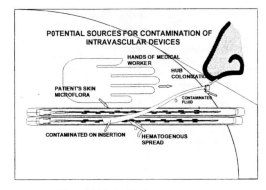

POTENTIAL SOURCES FOR CONTAMINATION OF INTRAVASCULAR DEVICES

Some of the most serious infections patients may acquire are from intravascular devices particularly those related to central lines. Microorganism may be introduced in several ways:

•Recent studies have found that up to 30-40% of the organisms related to central lines are found in the anterior nares (nose). There has been much discussion about treating the nares with antimicrobial ointments. Most experts do not believe this to be useful because the ointments will only be effected for time treated (a few days). However may be useful when catheter is placed for only short duration?

•Microorganism may be introduced by hands of medical worker, and the patients own microflora.

•Contaminated fluids are also possible but fairly rare.

•Many times organisms may be introduced during inappropriate insertion technique. This is the most common reason for infection related to central lines.

•Often infection may occur from other infection sites. Such as a abscess which microorganisms migrate from into the bloodstream and find the line insertion, causing infection.

Intravascular Catheter-related Infections

- 15 million CVC days occur is ICUs each year
- ~ 80,000 BSI occur each year
- Up to 35% mortality
- Cost per infection=$34,000-$56000
- Cost for patients with CVC, BSI range from $300 million to $2.3 billion-USA

Nosocomial Bloodstream Infections

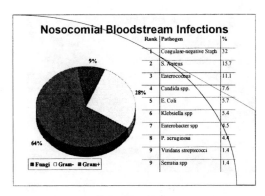

Rank	Pathogen	%
1	Coagulase-negative Staph	32
2	S. Aureus	15.7
3	Enterococcus	11.1
4	Candida spp.	7.6
5	E. Coli	5.7
6	Klebsiella spp	5.4
7	Enterobacter spp	4.5
8	P. aeruginosa	4.1
9	Viridans streptococci	1.4
9	Serratia spp	1.4

9% 28% 64%

■ Fungi □ Gram- ■ Gram+

The most common organisms associated with central lines are usually Staphylococcus. However E-Coli and Enterococcus which are found in the GI tract are also common. The other organisms listed such as klebisella or pseudomonas are usually "water" bugs, although healthcare workers can easily be the "vector" for transmission with any other the organisms listed above.

Intravascular-Device Guidelines

> Insertion technique is most important! Good aseptic technique
> Use single-lumen vs multi (unless necessary)
> If use multi-lumen designate one line for nutrition and blood. May want to acquire multi-lumen which are impregnated with chlorhexidine or silver sulfadiazine
> Replace IV tubing & add-ons device on more frequent than 72 hours. Blood & Lipid in 24 hours
> Place subclavian; if possible
> Wipe cath hub with alcohol or saline
> Flush with saline; if possible
> Do not apply antimicrobial ointments to insertion sites (increase risk for Candida)
> Catheter dressing; either transparent (7 days) or gauze (2 days) is ok!
> Catheter teams have less infections

A recent study found that up to 20 to 30% of patients who had a central line inserted could have received therapy through peripheral lines, PIC lines, and mid lines. Which have a much lower rate of infection. Proper insertion technique is the most common reason central line infection occur. Try and use only single lumen if possible. When triple lumens are used this gives microorganism two more portals of entry into the bloodstream. If multi-lumens must be used, designate one line for blood products and one or nutrition (these products can attract microorganism and the media these organisms utilize for food-reproduce).

Multi-lumen lines should be impregnated with chlorhexidine or silver sulfadiazine, these impregnated lines has demonstrated lower incidences of infections. If possible lines should be place in the subclavian area vs femoral or jugular (much closer to endogenous organisms in upper respiratory and GI tract). Flush with saline, or other anticoagultants with anti-microbial activities. Transducers should not be reused, however if disinfection is to occur this should be done by persons in central supply. Antimicrobal ointments at insertion site may increase risk for Candida infections by destroying the resident bacteria. Catheter dressing are your choice. Many patients and healthcare nursing personnel prefer transparent dress vs gauze due that they can monitor more effectively and it is convenient for patients when bathing and doing other activities of daily living. However recent CDC guidelines changing transparent dressing every 7 days and gauze every 2 days. Of course if dressing become loose or patient is diaphoretic, changing will be more often

Major Factors Contributing to the Emergence of Infectious Diseases: I

1. Human demographics and behavior
2. Technology and industry
3. Economic development and land use

Institute of Medicine Report, 1992

CDC

Many factors, or combinations of factors, contribute to disease emergence. Human demographics and behavior play a critical role. For example, changing sexual mores and other high-risk behavior associated with injecting drug use contributed to the spread of the human immunodeficiency virus (HIV) and the AIDS epidemic. Lyme disease was able to spread because as farming was discontinued in the Northeast, forests grew back and deer multiplied. Ticks, who lived off the deer, increased also, and ticks infected with the bacteria *Borrelia burgdorferi* transmitted Lyme disease to people who were exposed through outdoor activities or because they lived in new suburbs built next to the forests. Changes in technology and industry also cause infectious disease to emerge. Organ transplants, made possible by advanced edicaltechnology, require immunosuppression, and immunosuppressed patients are more vulnerable to numerous infectious organisms found in hospitals. Economic development and land use affect not only ecology, but the public's health. For instance, land development near watershed areas may lead to the contamination of public water supplies, illustrated by the 1993 Milwaukee outbreak of *Cryptosporidium* infection that affected more than 400,000 people. Human ehrlichioses, virtually unknown a decade ago, have become increasingly recognized as people use land areas where infected ticks are found. Hantavirus has been endemic or many years particularly in the western United States

Major Factors Contributing to the Emergence of Infectious Diseases: II

4. International travel and commerce
5. Microbial adaptation and change
6. Breakdown of public health measures

Institute of Medicine Report, 1992

CDC

International travel and commerce have made it possible for pathogens to be quickly

transported from one side of the country or globe to the other. New, more virulent,

pathogens may appear, such as *Escherichia coli* O157:H7, which in one multi-state

outbreak in 1993, was transmitted by contaminated hamburger meat used by a fast-food

restaurant chain, causing 700 to become ill and four children to die of kidney

disease. Infectious diseases also emerge when existing organisms mutate (change or

evolve). Many strains of some bacteria (such as *Streptococcus pneumoniae* and

enterococci) are now drug-resistant, and for some infectious agents, only one effec-tive

antibiotic is left. The breakdown of public health measures also has contributed

to the reemergence of infectious diseases. When mosquito control efforts were dis-continued

in Latin America, the mosquito vectors of dengue fever increased, and the

disease has reappeared in countries where it was believed to have been eliminated.

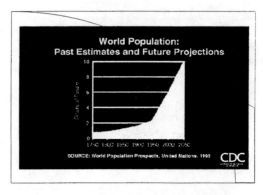

World Population:
Past Estimates and Future Projections

SOURCE: World Population Prospects, United Nations. 1995

CDC

A growing population and increasing urbanization contribute to emerging infectious

disease problems. In many parts of the world, urban population growth has been

accompanied by overcrowding, poor hygiene, inadequate sanitation, and unclean

drinking water. Urban development has also caused ecologic damage. In these cir-cumstances, certain disease-causing organisms and some of the vectors that transmit

them have thrived, making it more likely that people will be infected with new or

reemerging pathogens. The existing public health infrastructure is already overtaxed

and ill-prepared to deal with new health threats.

Creutzfelt-Jakob Disease

- **Infectious Agent: Prion (only Protein-no DNA or RNA)**
- **Three Forms of CJD**
  - Genetic
  - Infectious
  - Sporadic
- **Incubation: 2 to 35 years**
- **Transmission**
  - Corneal Transplant, Dura Mater Graft, Pericardial Homograft
  - Human Gonadotropin, Human Neurosurgical
  - Instrumentation, Depth Electrodes
  - Blood Transfusion-not confirmed
    - Blood Bank system will not except donor who have liked in UK for > 6 months during 1986-1993

Creutzfeldt-Jakob disease (CJD) is a rapidly progressive, invariably fatal neurodegenerative disorder believed to be caused by an abnormal isoform of a cellular glycoprotein known as the prion protein. CJD occurs worldwide and the estimated annual incidence in many countries, including the United States, has been reported to be about one case per million population. The vast majority of CJD patients usually die within 1 year of illness onset. CJD is classified as a transmissible spongiform encephalopathy (TSE) along with other prion diseases that occur in humans and animals. In about 85% of patients, CJD occurs as a sporadic disease with no recognizable pattern of transmission. A smaller proportion of patients (5 to 15%) develop CJD because of inherited mutations of the prion protein gene. These inherited forms include Gerstmann-Straussler-Scheinker syndrome and fatal familial insomnia.

Physicians suspect a diagnosis of CJD on the basis of the typical signs and symptoms and progression of the disease. In most CJD patients, the presence of 14-3-3 protein in the cerebrospinal fluid and/or a typical electroencephalogram (EEG) pattern, both of which are believed to be diagnostic for CJD, have been reported. However, a confirmatory diagnosis of CJD requires neuropathologic and/or immunodiagnostic testing of brain tissue obtained either at biopsy or autopsy.

What is bovine spongiform encephalopathy? Bovine spongiform encephalopathy (BSE) is a progressive neurological disorder of cattle that results from infection by an unconventional transmissible agent. As of November 2000, more than 177,500 cases of BSE were confirmed in the United Kingdom alone in more than 35,000 herds. The BSE epidemic in the United Kingdom peaked in January 1993 at almost 1,000 new cases per week. The outbreak may have resulted from the feeding of scrapie-containing sheep meat-and-bone meal to cattle. There is strong evidence and general agreement that the outbreak was amplified by feeding rendered bovine meat-and-bone meal to young calves. The nature of the transmissible agent is unknown. Currently, the most accepted theory is that the agent is a modified form of a normal cell surface component known as prion protein, a pathogenic form of the protein that is both less soluble and more resistant to enzyme degradation than the normal form.

CJD variant and BSE
(Are they associated?)

- **BSE exposure began in UK 1984-1986**
  - Use of ruminant tissue in ruminant feed-feeding of scrapie containing sheep meat and bone meal to cattle-then feeding to young cattle)
  - **Onset of CJD variant began 1993**
    - (Mostly young adults-median age 28)
    - Symptoms similar in cows as humans
    - Western Blot similar in CJD and BSE
    - Infecting mice with both also seems similar
- **A relationship? Probably yes**
- **Risk in USA? Little to none**

BSE:Bovine Spongiform Encephalopathy CJD:Creutzfeldt Jacob Disease

Is BSE occurring in the United States? According to the Animal and Plant Health Inspection Service of the U.S. Department of Agriculture, BSE has not been detected in the United States, despite active surveillance efforts since May 1990. As of October 31, 2000, 11,700 bovine brain specimens had been examined by an ongoing BSE surveillance system in the United States, and no evidence of BSE was seen. Further, to prevent BSE from entering the United States, severe restrictions were placed on the importation of live ruminants and certain ruminant products from countries where BSE was known to exist. These restrictions were later extended to include importation of ruminants and certain ruminant products from all European countries.

Is BSE a foodborne hazard in the United States? As indicated above, BSE has not been shown to exist in the United States. Thus, it is extremely unlikely that BSE would be a foodborne hazard in this country. Because the use of ruminant tissue in ruminant feed was probably a necessary factor responsible for the BSE outbreak in the United Kingdom and because of the current evidence for possible transmission of BSE to humans, the U.S. Food and Drug Administration instituted a ruminant feed ban in June 1997 that became fully effective as of October 1997. Therefore if the U.S. public has benn exposed to no or very minimal levels of ruminant feed beef

Is there any monitoring of the incidence of Creutzfeldt-Jakob disease in the United States? Yes. The possibility that BSE can spread to humans has focused increased attention on the desirability of national Creutzfeldt-Jakob disease (CJD) surveillance. The Centers for Disease Control and Prevention (CDC) monitors the trends and current incidence of CJD in the United States by analyzing death certificate information from U.S. multiple cause-of-death data, compiled by the National Center for Health Statistics, CDC. By 4-year periods from 1987 through 1998, the average annual death rates have remained relatively constant, ranging from 0.98 cases per 1 million in 1987-1990 to 1.03 cases per 1 million in 1995-1998. In addition, CJD deaths in persons aged <30 years in the United States remain extremely rare (<5 cases per 1 billion per year). In contrast, in the United Kingdom, over half of the patients who died with new variant CJD were in this young age group.

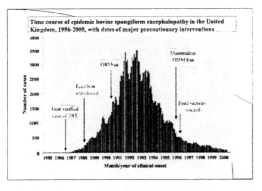

Time course of epidemic bovine spongiform encephalopathy in the United Kingdom, 1986-2000, with dates of major precautionary interventions

Is there any monitoring of the incidence of Creutzfeldt-Jakob disease in the United States? Yes. The possibility that BSE can spread to humans has focused increased attention on the desirability of national Creutzfeldt-Jakob disease (CJD) surveillance. The Centers for Disease Control and Prevention (CDC) monitors the trends and current incidence of CJD in the United States by analyzing death certificate information from U.S. multiple cause-of-death data, compiled by the National Center for Health Statistics, CDC. By 4-year periods from 1987 through 1998, the average annual death rates have remained relatively constant, ranging from 0.98 cases per 1 million in 1987-1990 to 1.03 cases per 1 million in 1995-1998. In addition, CJD deaths in persons aged <30 years in the United States remain extremely rare (<5 cases per 1 billion per year). In contrast, in the United Kingdom, over half of the patients who died with new variant CJD were in this young age group.

What is the new variant form of CJD that the experts in the United Kingdom believe might be related to the BSE outbreak in cattle? In contrast to the classic form of CJD, the new variant form in the United Kingdom predominantly affects younger persons (median age at death: 27.5 years as of October 2000), has atypical clinical features, with prominent psychiatric or sensory symptoms at the time of clinical presentation and delayed onset of neurologic abnormalities, including ataxia within weeks or months, dementia and myoclonus late in the illness, a duration of illness of at least 6 months, and a diffuse abnormal nondiagnostic electroencephalogram. The characteristic neuropathologic profile of new variant CJD includes, in both the cerebellum and cerebrum, numerous kuru-type amyloid plaques surrounded by vacuoles and prion protein (PrP) accumulation at high concentration indicated by immunohistochemical analysis. Recently published data show an increasing trend for the epidemic of new variant CJD in the United Kingdom.

Is there evidence directly linking this newly recognized variant of CJD to BSE exposure? There is strong epidemiologic and laboratory evidence for a causal association between new variant CJD and BSE. The absence of confirmed cases of new variant CJD in other geographic areas free of BSE supports a causal association

Chronology of vCJD disease in United Kingdom and other European Countries as of December 2000

Year of Onset	United Kingdom	France	Ireland
1994	8	1	
1995	10		
1996	11		
1997	14		
1998	17		
1999	20+4	1+1	1
2000	1+2		

CDC-EID

In addition, the interval between the most likely period for the initial extended exposure of the population to potentially BSE-contaminated food (1984-1986) and onset of new variant CJD cases (1994-1996) is consistent with known incubation periods for CJD. An experimental study reported in June 1996 showed that three cynomolgus macaque monkeys inoculated with brain tissue obtained from cattle with BSE had clinical and neuropathological features strikingly similar to those of new variant CJD. A study published in 1996 indicated that Western blot analysis of infecting prions obtained from 10 new variant CJD patients and BSE-infected animals had similar molecular characteristics that were distinct from prions obtained from patients with other types of CJD. Interim results of an ongoing experimental study involving inoculation of a panel of inbred mice with the agents causing BSE and new variant CJD substantially increased the strength of the scientific evidence for a causal association between new variant CJD and BSE. Two additional groups of inbred mice and a group of cross-bred mice inoculated with brain homogenates from new variant CJD cases were also reported to have had latency periods and lesion profiles consistent with the BSE pattern (Bruce, pers. comm. 2000). The latency period, neuropathology, and disease-causing PrP isoforms in transgenic mice expressing bovine PrP that were inoculated with new variant CJD, BSE, and scrapie brain extracts provided additional evidence supporting the link between BSE and new variant CJD.

Has CDC initiated increased surveillance efforts to determine whether the newly recognized variant of CJD occurs in the United States? Yes. In addition to the ongoing review of national CJD mortality data, CDC conducted active CJD surveillance in its four established Emerging Infections Program areas (Minnesota, Oregon, Connecticut, and the San Francisco Bay area, California) and in a metropolitan Atlanta site during April and May 1996. In 1996, with the support of the Council of State and Territorial Epidemiologists, CDC initiated an ongoing follow-up review of clinical and neuropathological records of CJD decedents aged <55 years who are identified through the national mortality data analysis. Also in 1996, the American Association of Neuropathologists (AANP), in collaboration with CDC, alerted its members about the new variant CJD neuropathology and requested reports of any such cases, regardless of the clinical diagnosis or age of the patient. These surveillance efforts have not detected evidence of the occurrence of new variant CJD in the United States.

Meningococcal Disease

- Incidence USA 1.1/100,000-College freshman in dorm 3.1/100,000, increase in late winter, early spring. Subtypes A-B-C-W135
- Increase incidence among children usually < 2. Mortality 10-19%
- In USA increases in Texas, Florida, Oregon
- Symptoms-H/A, Nuchal Ridigity, Fever, Vomiting, Abd Pain, Lethargy, Malaise
- Seizure occur in 20%, petechial rash usually early in symptoms
- 20% of population carriers N. Meningitidis-non encapsulated
- Rx = Rocephin ASAP
- N. Meningitidis produces great amounts of endotoxins
- Prophylaxis: close secretion contact; share food, kissing, family members
  - HCWs: Intubations, extubation: none after RX has begun!

Between 2500-3000 cases of Meningococcal Disease are reported each year in the United States. Some states have had increases in the past years, particularly Oregon, Texas, and Florida. Most cases probably occur among children, however all may acquire this infection. Symptoms are stated above, however anyone with stiff neck, headache, and fever should be immediately evaluated. 20% of the population may carry Nesseria Meningitidis (causative agent) in the anterior nares (nose). This organism we may carry is usually non-encapsulated, however should it encapsulated this is more likely to result in illness because the organism can become more pathogenic. About 20% of patients diagnosised will have a petechial rash or purpura. There is a slightly higher incidence among college students as stated above. The question is often asked should they be administered the vaccine. Below are some things to consider:

•The vaccine is available for subtypes A,C, and W135

•The vaccine needs to re-boosted in three to five years, however most college students would be outside the dormitory at that time.

•The vaccine does not provide a "herd" immunity as others are able to provide. There still would be some risk for the disease even if administered this vaccine.

•I believe it is hard to justify the vaccine, however this should be an individual decision among the family and there physician.

•Most colleges require this vaccine before admission.

Diagnosis is usually accomplished by remove some spinal fluid or blood. A culture is usually performed to determine infection. There are quick antigen-antibody assay which are also available. Some cases do not have meningitis

65

TABLE. Schedule for administering chemoprophylaxis against meningococcal disease

Drug	Age group	Dosage	Duration and route of administration*
Rifampin	Children <1 mo	5 mg/kg every 12 hrs	2 days
	Children ≥1 mo	10 mg/kg every 12 hrs	2 days
	Adults	600 mg every 12 hrs	2 days
Ciprofloxacin	Adults	500 mg	Single dose
Ceftriaxone	Children <15 yrs	125 mg	Single IM† dose
Ceftriaxone	Adults	250 mg	Single IM dose

*Oral administration unless indicated otherwise.
†Intramuscular.

The above table describes the prophylaxis for meningococcal disease. These antibiotics will eliminate the carriers state of N. meningiditis (causative organism) in the Upper Respiratory Tract.

66

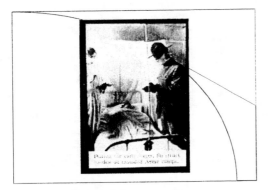

Picture in early stages, flu attack noticed in crowded Army camps.

Natural History of Human Influenza

Antigenic shift occurs only occasionally. When it does occur, large numbers of people, and sometimes the entire population, have no antibody protection against the virus. If the new virus is capable of being spread easily from person to person, a worldwide epidemic, called a pandemic, can occur. During this century, pandemics occurred in 1918, 1957, and 1968, each of which resulted in large numbers of deaths, as noted below.
Mortality associated with pandemics:

•1918-19 "Spanish flu" A(H1N1) -- Caused the highest known influenza-related mortality: approximately 500,000 deaths occurred in the United States, 20 million worldwide.

1957-58 "Asian flu" A(H2N2) -- 70,000 deaths in the United States.

•1968-69 "Hong-Kong flu" A(H3N2) -- 34,000 deaths in the United States.

The emergence of the "Hong Kong flu" in 1968-69 marked the beginning of the type A(H3N2) era. When this virus first emerged, it was associated with fewer deaths than that caused by the two previous pandemic viruses. There are several possible reasons for this. First, only the hemagglutinin changed from the "Asian" strain [type A(H2N2)]; the neuraminidase(N2) stayed the same, and therefore, people previously infected with H2N2 viruses may have had some protection against the H3N2 virus.

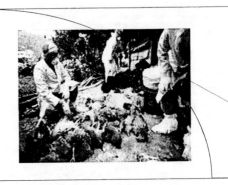

A strain of influenza virus that previously was known to infect only birds has been associated with infection and illness in humans in Hong Kong. The first known human case of influenza type A(H5N1) occurred in a 3-year-old child who died from respiratory failure in May 1997. In Hong Kong, the virus initially was identified as influenza type A, but the subtype could not be determined using standard reagents. By August, CDC; the National Influenza Center, Rotterdam, the Netherlands; and the National Institute for Medical Research, London, United Kingdom, had independently identified the virus as influenza A(H5N1). An investigation conducted during August-September by the Hong Kong Department of Health and CDC excluded the possibility of laboratory contamination. Since this initial case was identified, six additional persons in Hong Kong have been confirmed to have influenza A(H5N1) infection, and two possible cases have been identified. This report summarizes the nine cases identified thus far and describes preliminary findings from the ongoing investigation, which indicate that multiple influenza A(H5N1) infections have occurred and that both the source and mode of transmission are uncertain at this time.

The cases described in this report represent the first documented human infections with avian influenza A(H5N1) virus. One of the most important aspects of the investigation is to determine the source of infection and mode of transmission. However, this effort is complicated by the high prevalence of exposure to live poultry among residents of Hong Kong.

68

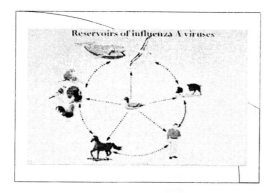

Reservoirs of influenza A viruses

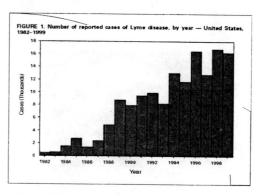

FIGURE 1. Number of reported cases of Lyme disease, by year — United States, 1982–1999

The 1918 Influenza pandemic probably occurred with a bird carrying a strain of influenza came in contact with a pig carrying another type of strain. The two combined together to create a new virulent stain. This is called an anteginic shift, which has the capability to create a new virulent virus which could lead to a pandemic. This came close in 1997 with the discovery of the Hong-Kong Flu. By destroying the chickens we may have diverted a pandemic. Pandemics occur about every 100 years in the world.

Infection with this influenza strain that is new to humans prompts consideration about whether this virus has the potential to spread globally and cause a pandemic. For an influenza pandemic to occur, a novel human influenza strain against which all or most of the human population has no antibody must be capable of sustained person-to-person transmission, causing widespread illness (1). As of December 17, acute respiratory illness among the population of Hong Kong apparently had not increased.

Although the potential for widespread transmission of this strain is presently unknown, as a precautionary measure, laboratory studies have been initiated to identify a candidate A(H5N1) vaccine strain. At this time, there are no plans for commercial vaccine production.

Two antiviral drugs, amantadine and rimantadine, inhibit replication of virtually all naturally occurring human and animal strains of influenza type A and therefore can be useful for prophylaxis and treatment of influenza A infections (2-4). Influenza A viruses resistant to amantadine and rimantadine can emerge during treatment, but drug-resistant influenza viruses have only rarely been isolated from specimens collected as part of routine influenza surveillance (5,6). Influenza

69

Reported cases of Lyme disease have greatly increased over the past years. Partly due the increase in forestation in the Northeast and the North Mid-West. The deer population become more numerous and with the white footed mouse as the additional reservoir gave the right opportunity for the disease to increase rather rapidly. The number of annually reported cases of Lyme disease in the United States has increased about 25-fold since national surveillance began in 1982, and a mean of approximately 12,500 cases annually were reported by states to the Centers for Disease Control and Prevention (CDC) from 1993-1997. In the United States, the disease is mostly localized to states in the northeastern, mid-Atlantic, and upper north-central regions, and to several counties in northwestern California.

National Lyme disease risk map with four categories of risk. Most B. burgdorferi infections are thought to result from periresidential exposure to infected ticks during property maintenance, recreation, and leisure activities. Thus, individuals who live or work in residential areas surrounded by woods or overgrown brush infested by vector ticks are at risk of getting Lyme disease. In addition, persons who participate in recreational activities away from home such as hiking, camping, fishing and hunting in tick habitat, and persons who engage in outdoor occupations, such as landscaping, brush clearing, forestry, and wildlife and parks management in endemic areas may also be at risk of getting Lyme disease.

70

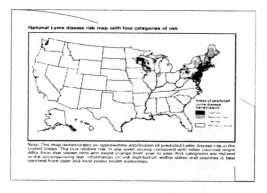

National Lyme disease risk map with four categories of risk

Note: This map demonstrates an approximate distribution of predicted Lyme disease risk in the United States. The true relative risk in any given county compared with other counties might differ from that shown here and might change from year to year. Risk categories are defined in the accompanying text. Information on risk distribution within states and counties is best obtained from state and local public health authorities.

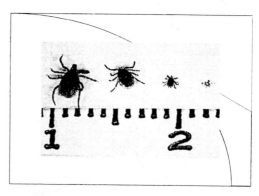

Lyme disease is an infection caused by the corkscrew-shaped bacteria Borrelia burgdorferi that are transmitted by the bite of deer ticks (Ixodes scapularis) and western black-legged ticks (Ixodes pacificus). The deer tick, which normally feeds on the white-footed mouse, the white-tailed deer, other mammals, and birds, is responsible for transmitting Lyme disease bacteria to humans in the northeastern and north-central United States. On the Pacific Coast, the bacteria are transmitted to humans by the western black-legged tick.

Life cycle of the deer tick: For Lyme disease to exist in an area, at least three closely interrelated elements must be present in nature: (1) the Lyme disease bacteria, (2) ticks that can transmit the bacteria, and (3) mammals (such as mice and deer) to provide food for the ticks in their various life stages. Ticks that transmit Lyme disease can be found in temperate regions that may have periods of very low or high temperature and a constant high relative humidity at ground level. Knowing the complex life cycle of the ticks that transmit Lyme disease is important in understanding the risk of acquiring the disease and in finding ways to prevent it: The life cycle of these ticks requires 2 years to complete. Adult ticks feed and mate on large animals, especially deer, in the fall and early spring. Female ticks then drop off these animals to lay eggs on the ground. By summer, eggs hatch into larvae. Larvae feed on mice and other small mammals and birds in the summer and early fall and then are inactive until the next spring when they molt into nymph.

19

Tick larvae are smaller than the nymphs, but they rarely carry the infection at the time of feeding and are probably not important in the transmission of Lyme disease to humans. Adult ticks can transmit the disease, but since they are larger and more likely to be removed from a person's body within a few hours, they are less likely than the nymphs to have sufficient time to transmit the infection. Moreover, adult Ixodes ticks are most active during the cooler months of the year, when outdoor activity is limited. Ticks search for host animals from the tips of grasses and shrubs (not from trees) and transfer to animals or persons that brush against vegetation. Ticks only crawl; they do not fly or jump. Ticks found on the scalp usually have crawled there from lower parts of the body. Ticks feed on blood by inserting their mouth parts (not their whole bodies) into the skin of a host animal. They are slow feeders: a complete blood meal can take several days. As they feed, their bodies slowly enlarge. Although in theory Lyme disease could spread through blood transfusions or other contact with infected blood or urine, no such transmission has been documented. There is no evidence that a person can get Lyme disease from the air, food or water, from sexual contact, or directly from wild or domestic animals. There is no convincing evidence that Lyme disease can be transmitted by insects such as mosquitoes, flies, or fleas. Campers, hikers, outdoor workers, and others who frequent wooded, brushy, and grassy places are commonly exposed to ticks, and this may be important in the transmission of Lyme disease in some areas.

72

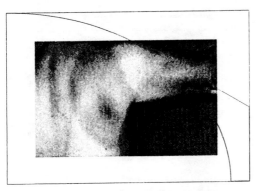

Lyme disease most often presents with a characteristic "bull's-eye" rash, erythema migrans, accompanied by nonspecific symptoms such as fever, malaise, fatigue, headache, muscle aches (myalgia), and joint aches (arthralgia). The incubation period from infection to onset of erythema migrans is typically 7 to 14 days but may be as short as 3 days and as long as 30 days. Some infected individuals have no recognized illness (asymptomatic infection determined by serologic testing), or manifest only non-specific symptoms such as fever, headache, fatigue, and myalgia. Lyme disease spirochetes disseminate from the site of the tick bite by cutaneous, lymphatic and blood borne routes. The signs of early disseminated infection usually occur days to weeks after the appearance of a solitary erythema migrans lesion. In addition to multiple (secondary) erythema migrans lesions, early disseminated infection may be manifest as disease of the nervous system, the musculoskeletal system, or the heart. Early neurologic manifestations include lymphocytic meningitis, cranial neuropathy (especially facial nerve palsy), and radiculoneuritis. Musculoskeletal manifestations may include migratory joint and muscle pains with or without objective signs of joint swelling. Cardiac manifestations are rare but may include myocarditis and transient atrioventricular blocks of varying degree. *B. burgdorferi* infection in the untreated or inadequately treated patient may progress to late disseminated disease weeks to months after infection. The most common objective manifestation of late disseminated Lyme disease is intermittent swelling and pain of one or a few joints, usually large, weight-bearing joints such as the knee. Some patients develop chronic axonal polyneuropathy, or encephalopathy, the latter usually manifested by cognitive disorders, sleep disturbance,

73

Symptoms of Hantavirus
Incubation: Few days-6 weeks-usually 2 weeks

Most Frequent	Frequent	Other
fever	headaches	shortness of breath
chills	nausea, vomiting	dizziness
myalgias	**abdominal pain**	arthralgia
	diarrhea	back or chest pain
	cough	sweats
	malaise	

How Is Hantavirus Transmitted?
The Rodent Connection

So just how do people get hantavirus pulmonary syndrome (HPS)? It all starts with rodents, like the deer mouse and cotton rat, which carry hantaviruses.

The Basic Transmission Cycle

The short story is that some rodents are infected with a type of hantavirus that causes HPS. In the United States, deer mice (plus cotton rats and rice rats in the southeastern states and the white-footed mouse in the Northeast) are the rodents carrying hantaviruses that cause hantavirus pulmonary syndrome.

Click here to meet the rodents and learn to identify them!

These rodents shed the virus in their urine, droppings and saliva. The virus is mainly transmitted to people when they breathe in air contaminated with the virus.

This happens when fresh rodent urine, droppings or nesting materials are stirred up. When tiny droplets containing the virus get into the air, this process is known as "aerosolization."

Watch how mice transmit hantavirus!

There are several other ways rodents may spread hantavirus to people:

• If a rodent with the virus bites someone, the virus may be spread to that person—but this is very rare.

74

Hantavirus Pulmonary Syndrome, United States Descriptive Demographic Statistics, January 30, 2002

Characteristics		Total
	N	289 (100%)
Gender		
	Male	174 (60%)
	Female	115 (40%)
Race		
	White	224 (78%)
	American Indian	56 (19%)
	Black	6 (2%)
	Asian	3 (1%)
Ethnicity		
	Hispanic	34 (12%)
Case Fatality		
	Dead	109 (38%)
Age (years)		Mean=37 [10-75]

Hantavirus Pulmonary Syndrome Cases by State of Residence United States – January 30, 2002

Total Cases (N=289 in 31 States)

0 Cases
1-4 Cases
5-9 Cases
>=10 Cases

Most cases occur in the western United States. These states usually have the particular house or farm mice which can carry the hanta virus in their stool and urine. Probably most cases in the eastern United States have occurred through travel to the west. However some cases are reported with no travel to the west.

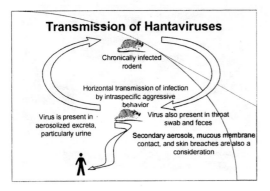

Transmission of Hantaviruses

Chronically infected rodent

Horizontal transmission of infection by intraspecific aggressive behavior

Virus is present in aerosolized excreta, particularly urine

Virus also present in throat swab and feces

Secondary aerosols, mucous membrane contact, and skin breaches are also a consideration

---

The Geographic Distribution of the Japanese Encephalitis Serocomplex of the Family Flaviridae, 2000.

St. Louis encephalitis
Rocio and St. Louis (Brazil)
West Nile virus
Japanese encephalitis
West Nile and Japanese encephalitis
Japanese and Murray Valley encephalitis
Murray Valley and Kunjin

Mosquito control is very important in reducing the risk for various diseases. Particularly with encephalitis which now has more implication due to the discovery of the West Nile Virus which has now been found as far south as Florida. No is completely sure how the virus made it way to the United States, but was probably introduced by a mosquito or bird on an airplane from the above (blue color) endemic areas. Other species of Encephalitis have been found in the United States particularly St. Louis, Eastern & Western Equine.

Blood-feeding *Anopheles gambiae* mosquito-Malaria

Various mosquitoes may transmit disease. Not all mosquitoes transmit disease. The above mosquito is known to transmit Malaria. A human can become a reservoir for transmission of Malaria, Yellow Fever, and Denque Fever. This is not the case with Encephalitis. Human are the "dead end host" with regards to encephalitis. Mosquitoes become infected when they feed on infected birds, which may circulate the virus in their blood for a few days. Infected mosquitoes can then transmit West Nile virus to humans and animals while biting to take blood. The virus is located in the mosquito's salivary glands. During blood feeding, the virus may be injected into the animal or human, where it may multiply, possibly causing illness.

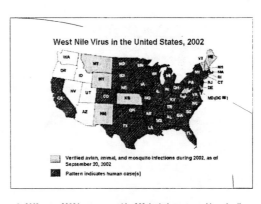

West Nile Virus in the United States, 2002

Verified avian, animal, and mosquito infections during 2002, as of September 20, 2002

Pattern indicates human case(s)

In 2002 over ~ 3000 human cases with ~300 deaths have occurred in early all states.

Centers for Disease Control and Prevention
West Nile Virus (WNV) Infection
Information for Clinicians

Clinical Features

Mild Infection

Most WNV infections are mild and often clinically unapparent.

o   Approximately 20% of those infected develop a mild illness (West Nile fever).

o   The incubation period is thought to range from 3 to 14 days.

o   Symptoms generally last 3 to 6 days.

Reports from earlier outbreaks describe the mild form of WNV infection as a febrile illness of sudden onset often accompanied by

<   malaise

<   anorexia

<   nausea

<   vomiting

Culex pipiens-West Nile

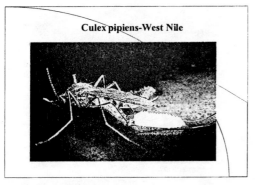

The above mosquito has been identify as the vector for transmission of West Nile in the North East. Mosquitoes become infected when they feed on infected birds, which may circulate the virus in their blood for a few days. Infected mosquitoes can then transmit West Nile virus to humans and animals while biting to take blood. The virus is located in the mosquito's salivary glands. During blood feeding, the virus may be injected into the animal or human, where it may multiply, possibly causing illness.

In other areas of the country the mosquito could be a different species. Among those with severe illness due to West Nile virus, case-fatality rates range from 3% to 15% and are highest among the elderly. Less than 1% of those infected with West Nile virus will develop severe illness.

To prevent Transmission:

•Stay indoors at dawn, dusk, and in the early evening.

•Wear long-sleeved shirts and long pants whenever you are outdoors.

•Spray clothing with repellents containing permethrin or DEET since mosquitoes may bite through thin clothing.

•Apply insect repellent sparingly to exposed skin. An effective repellent will contain 35% DEET (N,N-diethyl-meta-toluamide). DEET in high concentrations (greater than 35%) provides no additional protection.

•Repellents may irritate the eyes and mouth, so avoid applying repellent to the hands of children.

•Whenever you use an insecticide or insect repellent, be sure to read and follow the manufacturer's DIRECTIONS FOR USE, as printed on the product.

•Note: Vitamin B and "ultrasonic" devices are NOT effective in preventing mosquito bites.

The Expanding Epizootic of Raccoon Rabies, Eastern United States, 1977-1996

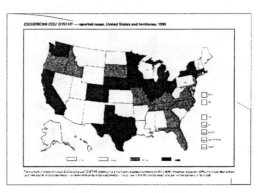

Rabies has expanded greatly via the Raccoon. The expansion is probably due to hunter in Florida took raccoon to the Virginia to hunter and where found to be infected with rabies. Bats are another great reservoir. Should someone wake-up at home or in a cave and find evidence of bats, they should report this to their local health department because they are a good candidate for prophylaxis:

Postexposure prophylaxis regimen

In the United States, PEP consists of a regimen of one dose of immune globulin and five doses of rabies vaccine over a 28-day period. Rabies immune globulin and the first dose of rabies vaccine should be given as soon as possible after exposure. Additional doses of rabies vaccine should be given on days 3, 7, 14, and 28 after the first vaccination. Current vaccines are relatively painless and are given in your arm, like a flu or tetanus vaccine.

What to do after a possible exposure

If you are exposed to a potentially rabid animal, wash the wound thoroughly with soap and water, and seek medical attention immediately. Most experts believe this could reduce the risk 75%, however plese still report the exposure! A health care provider will care for the wound and will assess the risk for rabies exposure. The following information will help your health care provider assess your risk:

•the geographic location of the incident

•the type of animal that was involved

•how the exposure occurred (provoked or unprovoked)

•the vaccination status of animal

E. Coli O157-H7

- 1982-First recognized as pathogen
- 1985-Associated with Hemolyic Uremic Syndrome (HUS)
- Outbreaks have occurred with drinking water, apple juice-cider, raw milk, fast food hamburgers, fresh produce, petting zoos, cheese curds, swimming pools?
- Incubation: 2-8 days, median 3-4 days
- Transmission: fecal-animal or human through beef (mostly hamburger), person to person
- Communicability: 1week adults, up to 3 weeks children
- Treatment: Supportive fluid electrolyte replacement
- Antibiotics may precipitate complications with HUS!

This disease has been of particular concern in the past two decades. An estimated 73,000 cases occur annually in the United States. Uncommonly reported in patients in less industrialized countries.

Hemolytic uremic syndrome (HUS): Persons with this illness have kidney failure and often require dialysis and transfusions. Some develop chronic kidney failure or neurologic impairment (e.g., seizures or stroke). Some have surgery to remove part of the bowel. Estimated 61 fatal cases annually; 3-5% with HUS die.

Estimated 2,100 hospitalizations annually in the United States. The illness is often misdiagnosed; therefore, expensive and invasive diagnostic procedures may be performed. Patients who develop HUS often require prolonged hospitalization, dialysis, and long-term follow-up.

Major source is ground beef; other sources include consumption of unpasteurized milk and juice, sprouts, lettuce, and salami, and contact with cattle. Waterborne transmission occurs through swimming in contaminated lakes, pools, or drinking inadequately chlorinated water. Organism is easily transmitted from person to person and has been difficult to control in child day-care centers.

All persons. Children <5 years old and the elderly are more likely to develop serious complications.

E. coli O157:H7 infection is nationally reportable and is reportable in most U.S. states. HUS is also reportable in most states.

ESCHERICHIA COLI O157:H7 — reported cases, United States and territories, 1999

A total of 42 confirmed outbreaks of E. coli O157:H7 infection were reported to CDC in 1998;in contrast, an average of 31 outbreaks were reported annually between 1994 and 1997. The reason for this increase is unclear, but may be related to the widespread use of pulsed-field gel electrophoresis (PFGE) by health departments to subtype E. coli O157:H7 strains. PFGE can link both widely dispersed cases in different states and small clusters within states that might not previously have been recognized as related. In 1998, E. coli O157:H7 outbreaks were reported from 25 states and affected 777 persons. One-hundred fifty-three (20%) persons were hospitalized, 29 (4%) developed HUS and 3 (0.4%) died. Almost half of these illnesses occurred in four large outbreaks in North Carolina, Wisconsin (2outbreaks), and Wyoming. Sixteen (38%) of the 42 outbreaks involved fewer than 5 persons, compared with 5 (23%) of 22 outbreaks in 1997. Cole slaw emerged as a new vehicle for E. coli O157:H7 infection and was responsible for outbreaks in Indiana and North Carolina. Contaminated drinking water was responsible for a large community outbreak in Wyoming, and a contaminated pool at a water park led to one death. Six

(14%) outbreaks were attributed to person-to-person transmission in day care centers, and no vehicle was identified in 10 (24%) of outbreaks.

Ten outbreaks occurred in a community setting, including two multistate outbreaks resulting inrecalls of contaminated ground beef, and four outbreaks in which ground beef was the suspected vehicle. Seven outbreaks occurred in restaurants, delis, or settings with catered food. In contrast, only one outbreak was associated with these locations 1997.

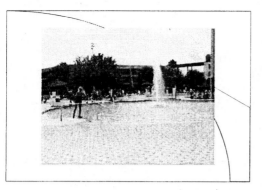

Swimming is one of the most popular activities in the country. Millions of people swim safely each year. However, transmission of illness can occur while swimming. Some may by accident defecate into the pool and before the chlorine can destroy the bacteria someone else may swalow adjacent water and become ill

When in these areas try not to swallow water and wash hands frequently particularly after the restroom or if you changed your child's diaper

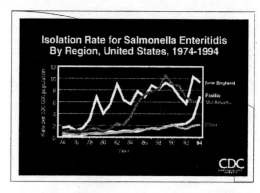

Salmonellosis is an infection with a bacteria called Salmonella. Most persons infected with Salmonella develop diarrhea, fever, and abdominal cramps 12 to 72 hours after infection. The illness usually lasts 4 to 7 days, and most persons recover without treatment. However, in some persons the diarrhea may be so severe that the patient needs to be hospitalized. In these patients, the Salmonella infection may spread from the intestines to the blood stream, and then to other body sites and can cause death unless the person is treated promptly with antibiotics. The elderly, infants, and those with impaired immune systems are more likely to have a severe illness.

The Salmonella germ is actually a group of bacteria that can cause diarrheal illness in humans. They are microscopic living creatures that pass from the feces of people or animals, to other people or other animals. There are many different kinds of Salmonella bacteria. Salmonella serotype Typhimurium and Salmonella serotype Enteritidis are the most common in the United States. Salmonella has been known to cause illness for over 100 years. They were discovered by a American scientist named Salmon, for whom they are named.

Salmonella infections usually resolve in 5-7 days and often do not require treatment unless the patient becomes severely dehydrated or the infection spreads from the intestines. Persons with severe diarrhea may require rehydration, often with intravenous fluids. Antibiotics are not usually necessary unless the infection spreads from the intestines, then it can be treated with ampicillin, gentamicin, trimethoprim/sulfamethoxazole, or ciprofloxacin. Unfortunately, some Salmonella bacteria have become resistant to antibiotics, largely as a result of the use of antibiotics to promote the growth of feed animals.

Salmonella live in the intestinal tracts of humans and other animals, including

Cryptosporidiosis

- 1976-First human case diagnosed
- 1984-First well-water outbreak
- 1987-First river water outbreak
- 1992-Multi-municipal water supply outbreak
- 1993-Largest water outbreak in US history (Milwaukee, WI)
- 1993-Fresh press apple cider outbreak (Central Maine)
- 1994-First outbreak in community with state-of-the-art water treatment system (Las Vegas)

Often we believe our municipal water supply to be safe and usually that is the case. However the above organism made it way into the drinking water in Milwaukee and over 400,000 people became ill. Some of the immuno-compromised patients (AIDS/HIV) died during this outbreak. Another outbreak similar to the Milwaukee outbreak occurred in Las Vegas where more than 100,000 people became ill. No one is quite sure what happened for these outbreaks to occur and both cities had good water management controls to prevent such occurrences.

Risk of Foodborne Ilness

- 50-75 million individuals suffer foodborne illness with 5 thousand deaths
- Over $5 billion in medical and social costs
- 1 in 5 meals of fish (not including shellfish) results in an illness compared to:
  - 1 to 200,000 meals of beef
  - 1 in 20,000 poultry meals
  - 1 in 250 meals of shellfish
- Rice in Chinese food with soil contamination
  - Bacillus cereus
- Ingestion of raw foods; sushi, raw oysters, steak tartar and ready to eat meals
- Common foodborne organisms: Salmonella, Campylobacter, Staph, E-Coli, Shigella

An estimated 76 million cases of foodborne disease occur each year in the United States. The great majority of these cases are mild and cause symptoms for only a day or two. Some cases are more serious, and CDC estimates that there are 325,000 hospitalizations and 5,000 deaths related to foodborne diseases each year. The most severe cases tend to occur in the very old, the very young, those who have an illness already that reduces their immune system function, and in healthy people exposed to a very high dose of an organism. Over 5 million become infected with Salmonella each year in the United States

Raw foods of animal origin are the most likely to be contaminated; that is, raw meat and poultry, raw eggs, unpasteurized milk, and raw shellfish. Because filter-feeding shellfish strain microbes from the sea over many months, they are particularly likely to be contaminated if there are any pathogens in the seawater. Foods that mingle the products of many individual animals, such as bulk raw milk, pooled raw eggs, or ground beef, are particularly hazardous because a pathogen present in any one of the animals may contaminate the whole batch. A single hamburger may contain meat from hundreds of animals. A single restaurant omelet may contain eggs from hundreds of chickens. A glass of raw milk may contain milk from hundreds of cows. A broiler chicken carcass can be exposed to the drippings and juices of many thousands of other birds that went through the same cold water tank after slaughter.

Medical Management of Biological Casualties

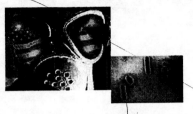

Aerosol Delivery

- Simple technology but weather dependent
- Industrial sprayers with modified nozzles delivered from plane or boat upwind
- Missile dispensing bomblets with BW
- Weather : Stable, 5-10 mph wind with temperature inversion
- Nighttime and early morning hours best

The technology is rather simple to disperse the right microbe (if someone has the knowledge). Usually little to no wind is required for dispersion to be effect. Also you need a temperature inversion particularly at the evening or early morning. Cruise type missiles, bomblets, airplanes and jets can disperse these microbes, over large population area. If these microbes are dispersed correctly a fatality (particularly with Anthrax) of > 80%. Some radical political groups have tried to obtain these microbes by mail or by breaking into military bases and the CDC in Alabama!

The Four Rights of Aerosol Delivery

- Right **organism**: Anthrax, plague, botulinin toxin, smallpox.
- Right **Size**: 1 -5 microns
- Right **method**: Crops dusters, AC system, bomblets.
- Right **weather** conditions: Calm wind, thermal inversion, darkness.

The organism must be the right size, small enough to pass through the upper respiratory tract and into the lungs. The perfect size need to be 1-5 microns which is the size of Tuberculosis. The small micron can easily be easily infiltrate the upper and lower respiratory tracts. Where they can (dependant to the organism) can infective the air sacs (alveoli) or the lymphatic systems, germinate and spread to other areas of the body via the blood stream or the lymphatic network.

Gen. Jeffery Amherst   Catapults

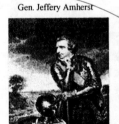 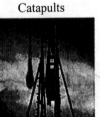

Nations at war would hurled dead bodies at their enemies. They knew that they spread disease and of course this practice was extremely intimidating to the enemy! General Amherst of the British Army was given permission by the King of England to take scabs from individuals with Smallpox, place the scabs on and in blankets and give them the American Indians. The result was 2-3 million American Indians became infected and many died. These blankets also where made for the revolutionary American soldiers and several outbreaks occurred from these blankets. General George Washington was ready to attack the British at Toronto, however to many of his troops where infected with smallpox.

History of Biological Warfare

- 6th c BC - Assyrians poisoned enemy wells with rye ergot.
- 1346 - Tartars hurled plague infected corpses over city walls to force surrender.
- 1710 - Russians use the same plague infected corpse tactic against Sweden
- 15th c & 1754 - Smallpox contaminated clothing causing epidemic casualties

The use of germ warfare is nothing new. It probably has been practiced since man inhabited the earth. The Assyrians poisoned enemy wells with a rye ergot which is crude form of LSD. In the medical ages during the crusades, the crusaders attacked the city of Azores where the inhabitants hurled bodies infested with plague at the crusaders. They (crusaders) apparently became infected with the plague and sailed back to Italy, where the first outbreak of the plague occurred ultimately killing some 35 million Europeans over a three century period.

Biological Warfare in WWI

- WWI - German agents infected horses in the US with glanders before they were shipped to France.
- Germans infected large numbers of   Russian horses and mules with glanders on the Eastern Front to affect troop & supply convoys & artillery movement
- Influenza thought to be a BW-probably prevented Germany from continuing WWI

During WWI Germany sent agents into Russia and the united States and infected horses and mules with a disease call Glanders (Burkholders). Mules and horses of course where use to hall equipment, supplies and troops for the war effort.

As was mentioned yearly, WWI was ended actually by Influenza A outbreak of 1918. Germany of course was using mustard gas against it enemies. American troops infected Germany troops with influenza. Germany actually believed American where able to weaponize the flu due to the devastating impact this disease made on the German war effort! Of course this was not true, mother nature was the responsible one!

BW in WWII

- "Unit 731" 1937-45. Japan's ambitious BW program in Harbin Manchuria. - experiments conducted on Chinese POW's; anthrax & plague. 3,000 deaths from the   experiments!
- Camp (Fort) Detrick 1943-69. US BW research b/o perceived German threat.   - anthrax, botulinin, tularemia, brucella, VEE/SEB

Japan had a very ambitious program. With many experiments on prisoners of war where infected with Plague and Anthrax. Most studies where made with Bubonic Plague and cutaneous Anthrax. Many thousand of prisoners died during these experiments. Japan had planned to expose the west coast of the United States for Anthrax however this plan never materialized.

Gulf War

- UN has established that Iraq conducted R&D on:
  - - anthrax (8,500) concentrated liters)
  - - botulinun (19,000 liters)
  - - ricin
  - - aflatoxin (2,200 liters)
- All were weaponized and loaded in R400 bombs, SCUDS, spray tanks & rockets

Saddam Hussein had weaponized anthrax and botulism which had been load on various weapons. There is concerned he got this expertise from defectors from the former Soviet Union. He used chemical weapons on the Kurds in the 1980s.

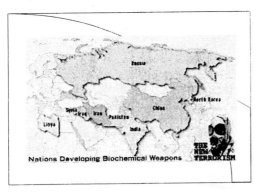

Nations Developing Biochemical Weapons

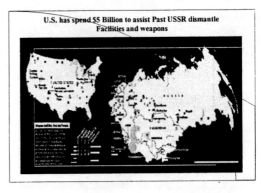

U.S. has spend $5 Billion to assist Past USSR dismantle Facilities and weapons

Many counties have apparently have biological weapons or trying to develop. On e of the major concerns is the former Soviet Union which in an aggrement with other countries and the United states signed a treated to ban the use of biological weapons and destroy any of the weaponized microbes. Russia however, starts a massive effort to increase it biolgoical weapons program. Since the world signed this agreement and the world stop immunization of Smallpox. Russian had Smallpox missiles which may have had a weaponized from of Smallpox with a shorter incubation period and a more virluent strain which may have had a death rate of 50-60%. Some of the scientist employed are now without employment and could be working from some rogue nations to develop these weapons.

This map demonstrates areas where the former Soviet union and the United States had research facilities and weapons plants for nuclear, biological, and chemical weapons. The United States has spend >$5 billion to assist the former Soviet Union to dismantle these sites. However apparently more $ is needed to complete this task

97

98

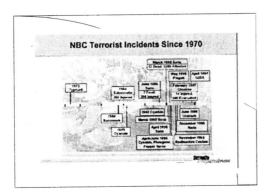

NBC Terrorist Incidents Since 1970

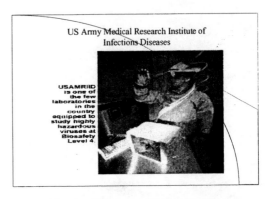

US Army Medical Research Institute of Infections Diseases

There have been events in recent times where some political or religious groups tried to use chemical, biological, and nuclear terrorism. The Aum Chrimco religious cult had place sarin gas in the subways in Tokyo, which effected >5000 and 12 expired. They also tried to disseminate inhaled Anthrax, but fortunately was unsuccessful due that they laced the expertise.

The united States Army Medical research Institute of Infectious Diseases is working to develop more efficient vaccines and other medication which could hopefully neutralize these horror able weapons. They where very much involved with the letter events on the east coast of the United States, fall of 2001.

26

100

Epidemiological Clues

- Massive point source outbreak
- Apparent aerosol route of infection
- High morbidity/mortality rates
- Illness limited to localized geographical areas
- Low attack rates in personnel with closed or filtered air supplies
- Unusual disease entity
- Dead animals of multiple species

A massive exposure over a large population could result in high death and mortality rates. Of course it could be over a specific area such as a city, event (sports event) or school or college. This could be accomplished with an aerolized substance such has botulism or anthrax. Could be dispensed by plane, bomblet, truck, or a boat on nearby river passing by target area. The optimum result would usually be when the wind is only about 5-10 MPH and usually in the morning or evening when you have more temperature conversion. We may see animals becoming ill and dieing before humans.

Biological Diseases by Category

- Category A: high mortality, spread easily, panic & social disruption, special efforts to control

Anthrax	Smallpox
Botulism	Tularemia
Plague	Viral Hemorrhagic fevers

- Category B: somewhat easy to disseminate, moderate mortality, special surveillance, labs

Brucellosis	Q Fever
Clostrudium perfringens	Ricin Toxin
Glanders	Staph enterotoxin B

- Category C: available, easy to produce & disseminate, possible high mortality and morbidity, major public health impact

Hantavirus	Tickborne encephalitis
MDR-TB	Tickborne Hemorrhagic fevers
Nipah virus	Yellow Fever

Above are category of disease by effectiveness. Category A are the most dangerous and Category B would be more like to cause some death but high morbidity. Category A & B have been weaponized by some countries particularly the former Soviet Union. Category B could be weaponized but experts are unsure if this has occurred.

The Four Rights of Aerosol Delivery

- Right **organism**: Anthrax, plague, botulinin toxin, smallpox. (Not CW)
- Right Size: 1 -5 microns
- Right **method**: Crops dusters, AC system, bomblets.
- Right **weather** conditions: Calm wind, thermal inversion, darkness.

The right organism is one that can be easily breath in the upper respiratory tract. So small organism that are less than 5 microns would be able to accomplish this invasion of our URT and would and countries have the ability to disseminate these organism through various aerolized methods.

ANTHRAX:
"A likely agent"

- Bacillus anthracis, gram + spore
- Easy to cultivate spores - stable
- Good for aerosalization -- 1-5 microns
- High mortality - >95% fatal if inhaled
  - Experience with recent letter attacks: 40-50% fatal
- Delayed diagnosis
- Fear and panic
- During 2 month period in 1998, FBI reported 7 hoaxes re: anthrax

Anthrax would be readily transmitted through the air or in a fine power which demonstrated in the fall of 2001. The organism is easily cultivated, but a biological weapons expert needs to be able to mill this organism down and incorporate a negative static charge so the organism will not clump together. If it clumps the organism will become too large to attack the upper respiratory tract. If effective weaponized the death rate is high. However with last years events the death rate was reduced by appropriate and quick treatment.

ANTHRAX
Clinical Features

- Cutaneous: Carbuncles and swelling on hand and forearms. Scabs over lesions are black as coal. (Anthrax=Greek for coal). Mortality up to 25% (untreated)
- Inhalation of spores: (Woolsorters disease). Case fatality almost 100%
  - Manchester, NH
- Intestinal: Rare in man. 20%-60% fatal.

There are three types of anthrax mentioned above; Cutaneous is usually easily treated and death should not occur in the United States with appropriate treatment. Intestinal is rare and there is not a lot of experience with this type. There was an outbreak in Africa and the death rate was approximately 25-30%, due to lack of antibiotic therapy.

ANTHRAX:
Symptoms

- Incubation is 1-7 days, late as 60 days, longer?
- Nonspecific flu-like illness
- Fever, headache, non-productive cough, myalgia
- Short period of improvement, hours to 3 days
  - Not seen with recent experience
- Abrupt crash, resp distress, cyanosis
- Shock and death in 24-36 hrs

Incubation for anthrax is usually 1-7 days, however spores where found in monkey studies to exist in the air sacks for ≥ 60 days. Symptoms may start as non-specific type of symptoms and there are differences between Influenza and Anthrax. Patients will usually move immediately from non-specific symptoms to severe symptoms such as meningitis, respiratory distress, and cyanosis. Death is likely unless appropriate antibiotics and other support therapy is provided. Even with appropriate therapy death rate still may be 40-50%.

Clinical Features

- Inhalational
  - Fulminant Phase
    - Correlates with high-grade bacteremia/toxemia
    - Critically Ill
      - Fever, diaphoresis
      - Respiratory distress/failure, cyanosis
      - Septic shock, multiorgan failure, DIC
    - 50% develop hemorrhagic meningitis
      - Headache, meningismus, delirium, coma
      - May be most prominent finding
    - Usually progresses to death in <36 hrs
      - Mean time from symptom onset to death ~3 days

Many patients will suffer from high fever with diaphoresis, respiratory failure, septic shock, multi organ failure, and disseminated intra-vascular coagluase. Meningitis is the leading cause of death, or lungs that are over burden with blood (edema). Death will usually occur in one to two days due to massive hemorrhaging unless aggressive treatment has been implemented very early in the clinical course.

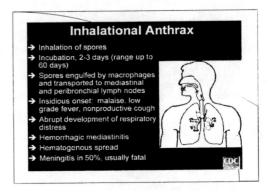

Inhalational Anthrax

- Inhalation of spores
- Incubation, 2-3 days (range up to 60 days)
- Spores engulfed by macrophages and transported to mediastinal and peribronchial lymph nodes
- Insidious onset: malaise, low grade fever, nonproductive cough
- Abrupt development of respiratory distress
- Hemorrhagic mediastinitis
- Hematogenous spread
- Meningitis in 50%, usually fatal

CDC

Inhalation Anthrax is inhaled into the upper respiratory tract and moves to the alveoli. Spores are engulfed by macrophages and taken to the mediastinal and peribronchial lymph notes where the bacterial germinate and then start to release toxins which bring about cell and tissue destruction. The bacterial will spread through the system, including the cerebrospinal system. Cells and tissue may be destroyed.

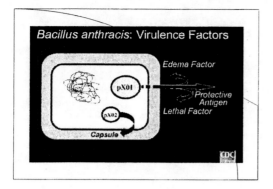

Bacillus anthracis: Virulence Factors

•Protective Antigen

    Binds Edema Factor to form Edema Toxin

    Facilitates entry of Edema Toxin into cells

•Edema Factor

    Massive edema by increasing intracellular cAMP

    Also inhibits neutrophil function

•Lethal Factor

    Stimulates macrophage release of TNF-α, IL-1β

    Initiates cascade of events leading to sepsis

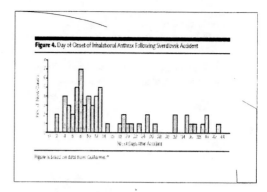

Figure 4. Day of Onset of Inhalational Anthrax Following Sverdlovsk Accident

In the former Soviet Union in 1978 an accident occurred with a weapons plant that produced anthrax. Apparently a pipe had a crack which created a flume which in turn created a cloud which moved over the city of Sverdlovsk and resulted in 66 death. No children died. As you can see the incubation extended beyond the 1-7 days. The reason why the spores can persist is not totally understood.

Pathogenesis

• Inhalational
- Phagocytosed by alveolar macrophages
  - Not all spores killed:innoculum 2500>
- Migration to mediastinal/hilar lymph nodes
- Germination into vegetative bacilli
  • Triggered by nutrient-rich environment
  • May be delayed up to 60 days
    - Factors not completely understood
    - Dose, host factors likely play a role
    - Antibiotic exposure may contribute
      » Delayed germination after antibiotic suppression

Many spores may be killed by our alveolar macrophages, however some or many, depending on the inoculums, will not be killed resulting in infection of the host (Human).

Microbiology

● Environmental Survival
- Spores are hardy
  • Resistant to drying, boiling <10 minutes
  • Survive for years in soil
  • Still viable for decades in perma-frost
- Favorable soil factors for spore viability
  • High moisture
  • Organic content
  • Alkaline pH
  • High calcium concentration

Spores can live in the environment for many years if the soil has the right factors for viability. Cattle can carry anthrax and it not unusual for cutaneous anthrax to occur among cattle and other mammals. We find soil anthrax in states that had old cattle trail in the 19th century. Spores can resist changes in temperature and other types of changes in the environment. They can lay in the spore state until they find a host to infect which has blood, tissue and other bodily substances to germinate.

Pathogenesis

- Disease requires entry of spores into body
- Exposure does not always cause disease
  - Inoculation dose
  - Route of entry
  - Host immune status
  - May depend on pathogen strain characteristics

As stated in the first slides about Infection Control, the reason some individuals become infected and others not, may have to do with the amount of the exposing dose, route of entry, how healthy or unhealthy the host is and depend on the pathogen strain which may be highly weaponized which was apparent with a least three letter during the events of fall 2001

Pathogenesis

- Inhalational
  - Spores on particles 1-5 μm
  - Inhaled and deposited into alveoli
  - Estimated LD50% = 2500 – 55,000 spores
    - Dose required for lethal infection in 50% exposed
    - Contained in imperceptibly small volume
    - Most believe this to still dose/inoculums despite experience with recent letters

Most experts believe the appropriate exposure dose would need to be as small as 2,500 spores up to 55,000 spores. Between these ranges you have estimated a lethal dose of up to 50%

ANTHRAX:
Diagnosis

- PE non specific
- Gram + blood cultures
- WBC, usually + when symptoms begin, Bacteremia occurs early
- Chest x-ray, widened mediastinum with pleural effusion (common), patchy infilitrates (spores concentrated in mediastinal lymph nodes)
- Confirmation by blood cultures

Diagnosis of anthrax should be fairly straight forward. Most labs have the ability to identify the gram positive spore forming rods which are not motile. White cell counts may be leveled during the non-specific symptoms and the CXR may reveal a widening mediastinum with or without pleural effusion (most common syndrome noticed on patients during the fall 2001 events).

Diagnosis

- Presumptive diagnosis
  - History of possible exposure
    - Epidemiology
  - Typical signs & symptoms
  - Rapidly progressing nonspecific illness
  - Widened mediastinum on CXR
  - Large Gram+ bacilli from specimens
    - Can be seen on Gram stain if hi-grade bacteremia
  - Appropriate colonial morphology
  - Necrotizing mediastinitis, meningitis at autopsy

When determining when and whom to treat, clinicians should not under estimate the epidemiology. During the events of 2001, those at risk for exposure where:

•Postal workers

•Media building and selective personnel

•Government workers and select officials

We should of course determine the clinical presentation along with the epidemiology to determine treatments.

TABLE 1. Symptoms and signs of inhalational anthrax, laboratory-confirmed influenza, and influenza-like illness (ILI) from other causes

Symptom/Sign	Inhalational anthrax (n=10)	Laboratory-confirmed influenza	ILI from other causes
Elevated temperature	70%	68%–77%	40%–73%
Fever or chills	100%	83%–90%	75%–89%
Fatigue/malaise	100%	75%–94%	62%–94%
Cough (minimal or nonproductive)	90%	84%–93%	72%–86%
Shortness of breath	80%	6%	0%
Chest discomfort or pleuritic chest pain	60%	35%	23%
Headache	50%	84%–91%	74%–89%
Myalgias	50%	67%–94%	73%–94%
Sore throat	20%	64%–84%	64%–84%
Rhinorrhea	10%	79%	68%
Nausea or vomiting	80%	12%	12%
Abdominal pain	30%	22%	22%

As stated before, there are difference between influenza and anthrax. Usually with anthrax you will have gastro intestinal involvement, however not usually with influenza. Influenza usually has rhinorrhea, but rare in the inhalational anthrax cases. Also with anthrax you will have shortness of breath while with influenza not usually.

ANTHRAX
Presumptive and Confirmatory identification Criteria
(Level A Laboratory)

- Presumptive
  - From clinical samples, such as blood, CSF, or skin lesions (vesicular fluid or eschar) material: encapsulated Gram + rods
  - From growth on sheep blood agar: large Gram + rods, non motile and non-hemolytic

- Confirmatory
  - Capsule production (visualization of capsule), and
  - Lysis by gamma-phage, or
  - Direct fluorescent antibody assays (DFA)
  - Lab levels B and C may also use **PCR** or other nucleic acid signatures assays

Presumptive diagnosis has been discussed in previous slides. Confirmation usually will be accomplished by state laboratories or the CDC. The mostly widely used confirmatory test is the PCR (Polmerse Chain Reaction) assay. Special precautions are need for gathering specimens and submitting to CDC or lab level B-C lab at your state. For more information on collecting and submitting specimens go to this web site at the CDC:

www.bt.cdc.gov

Anthrax

- Mediastinitis <u>not pneumonia</u>
  - Recent experience pleural effusion -most common
- Macrophage will take spores to mediastinal nodes
- Cat Scan should be done, not just CXR
- If meningitis occurs death is nearly 100%
  - Hemorrhage
- Children have <reactivity to Inhaled anthrax

If CXR reveals pneumonia, this is not anthrax. As stated before patients usually have a widening mediastinum usually with pleural effusion which chest tubes will need to be inserted ASAP. Please review the next two slides for illustration of mediastinitis and pleural effusion. The pleural effusion chest x-ray was taken from an individual with inhalational anthrax that occurred in the fall of 2001

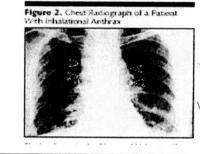

Figure 2. Chest Radiograph of a Patient With Inhalational Anthrax

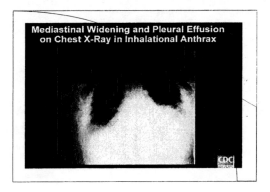

Mediastinal Widening and Pleural Effusion on Chest X-Ray in Inhalational Anthrax

CDC

ANTHRAX
Medical Management

- Tx of choice: IV Cipro, 400mg q 8-12 hrs, Doxy 100mg q 12hr (200 initial) + two other antibiotics
- Almost all sensitive to penicillin, however, penicillin resistant strains exist naturally and can be laboratory produced.
- Most cases of inhalation anthrax fatal if tx started 48 hrs after sx
- Standard precautions -person to person *not* reported

Treatment of of inhalational anthrax is aggressive IV therapy with Cipro or doxycycline. If meningitis is suspected Ciproflaxin must be utilized. Also other antibiotics should be utilized to be more effects (see next slide).

Remember: Anthrax is not transmitted from person to person!

Treatment

- Empiric Therapy
  - Until susceptibility patterns known
  - Adults
    - Ciprofloxacin 400 mg IV q12°
      OR
    Doxycycline 100mg IV q12°
      AND (for inhalational)
    One or two other antibiotics
    *Rif, *Vanco, Imp, *Clinda, Clarithromycin,
    no cephalosporins

Other antibiotics should be utilized with cipro or doxy. No cephalsporins due to lack of concentration in tissue and does not move past the blood brain barrier. Additional antibiotics are listed above, however clindamycin has gained favor due to it anti-toxin effects which has been demonstrated in the treatment of Toxic Shock Syndrome.

Children will need the same treatment even though cipro and doxy may have undesirable side effects. Once patient has had effective treatment they must still take cipro or doxy for 60 days due that spores could be lingering in the alveoli and could germinate.

TABLE 1 Inhalational anthrax treatment protocol for cases associated with this bioterrorism attack

---

Clinical Features

- Cutaneous – progression of <u>painless</u> lesions –
- Incubation 1-12 days

Papule – pruritic

↓ 24-36 hrs

Vesicle/bulla

↓

Ulcer – contains organisms, sig. edema

↓ 3-4 days

Eschar – black, rarely scars

Cutaneous form of anthrax is the most common. It may have a death rate up to 25% without appropriate antibiotics. Death should not occur in the U.S. due to availability of antibiotics. The spore must find a portal of entry so it may invade, germinate and produce signs and symptoms of infection. General first symptoms are described as a "spider bite" with a papule which is painless, then a vesicle/bulla, then ulcer and lastly a black eschar occurs.

Diagnosis is usually by culture with blood agar and the PCR, which is usually done by the CDC.

Incubation is usually 3-5 days, range is 1-12 days.

Clinical Features

- Cutaneous
  - Systemic disease may develop
    - Lymphangitis and lymphadenopathy
    - If untreated, can progress to sepsis, death

Usually you will find lympthgitis and lymphadenoathy in the adjacent lymphnodes.

Clinical Features

- Cutaneous
  - Most common areas of exposure
    - Hands/arms
    - Neck/head
  - Incubation period
    - 3-5 days typical
    - 12 days maximum

Cutaneous anthrax is usually found in areas of the body that have been previously abraded such as the face, neck, and upper extremities.

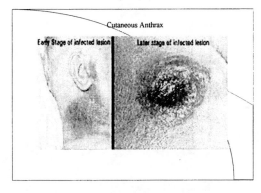

Cutaneous Anthrax

Early Stage of infected lesion | Later stage of infected lesion

Illustration of a typical cutaneous anthrax lesion from early stages to later stages. Cutaneous anthrax is usually easily treated and may not be as severe as streptococcus infections (necrosising facitious).

TABLE 2. Cutaneous anthrax treatment protocol* for cases associated with this bioterrorism attack

Category	Initial therapy (oral)†	Duration
Adults*	Ciprofloxacin 500 mg BID	60 days†
	or	
	Doxycycline 100 mg BID	
Children*	Ciprofloxacin 10–15 mg/kg every 12 hrs	60 days†
	(not to exceed 1 g/day)†	
	or	
	Doxycycline:*	
	>8 yrs and >45 kg: 100 mg every 12 hrs	
	>8 yrs and ≤45 kg: 2.2 mg/kg every 12 hrs	
	≤8 yrs: 2.2 mg/kg every 12 hrs	
Pregnant women ***	Ciprofloxacin 500 mg BID	60 days†
	or	
	Doxycycline 100 mg BID	
Immunocompromised persons*	Same for nonimmunocompromised persons and children	60 days†

* Cutaneous anthrax with signs of systemic involvement, extensive edema, or lesions on the head or neck require intravenous therapy, and a multidrug approach is recommended. Table 1.
Ciprofloxacin or doxycycline should be considered first line therapy. Amoxicillin 500 mg po TID for adults or 80 mg/kg/day divided every 8 hours for children is an option for completion of therapy after clinical improvement. Oral amoxicillin dose is based on the need to achieve appropriate minimum inhibitory concentrations levels.
† Previous guidelines have suggested treating cutaneous anthrax for 7-10 days, but 60 days is recommended in the setting of this attack, given the likelihood of exposure to aerosolized B. anthracis (8).
‡ The American Academy of Pediatrics recommends treatment of young children with tetracyclines for serious infections (e.g., Rocky Mountain spotted fever).
** Although tetracyclines or ciprofloxacin are not recommended during pregnancy, their use may be indicated for life-threatening illness. Adverse effects on developing teeth and bones are dose related; therefore, doxycycline might be used for a short time (7-14 days) before 6 months of gestation.

This slides gives the protocol for appropriate treatment for cutaneous anthrax. Please note that children should also be treated with Cipro or Doxy despite risk for side effects.

Also those whom acquired cutaneous anthrax from deliberate, intentional exposure must be prophylaxis with 60 days of cipro or doxy. This is need due to the risk for possible potential exposure to inhalational anthrax.

ANTHRAX
*
Laboratory Testing

- Nasal swab and serology are not used for clinical Dx or screening for anthrax!
  - Define area of exposure
  - Only + after 3-7 days
  - Negative swab, still need prophylaxis
- Currently there is no reliable screening test for anthrax
- Cutaneous Anthrax: Bacterial cultures of vesicular fluid or ulcer margins. A gram stain of fluid or ulcer margins and blood cultures may be helpful
- Gastrointestinal: blood and stool culture
- Inhalation: Blood, CSF, (if meningeal signs are present), CXR that may show evidence of thoracic edema and a widened mediastinum and sputum culture

Nasal swabs maybe utilized to determine a area of exposure to confirmed anthrax. This was implemented in areas where anthrax intentional exposure occurred. If swabs are positive for person or persons in a designed area, this will give information among who needs to be prophylaxis with antibiotics. Even if only one or two individuals test positive probably persons in the entire area will need prophylaxis. Nasal swabs are still somewhat investigational concerning their specific use. Actually only persons who have acute and convalescent titers (drawn 3 weeks after acute) drawn (blood sample) can be determined to have a true exposure to anthrax. Though nasal swabs which test positive is **probably** an exposure to anthrax.

Postexposure Prophylaxis

- Avoid unnecessary antibiotic usage
  - Potential shortages of those who need them
  - Potential adverse effects
    - Hypersensitivity
    - Neurological side effects, especially elderly
    - Bone/cartilage disease in children
    - Oral contraceptive failure
  - Future antibiotic resistance
    - Individual's own flora
    - Community resistance patterns
  - Gas masks-NO!!!

No individual should take antibiotics for a possible exposure to anthrax. Someone may need antibiotics and if you pervious took them you now could be resistant, an the antibiotics may not be effects in protection someone. Antibiotics can have adverse effects (see above).

Gas masks are not effect for the general public. Individuals would have to have available masks specific for biological or chemical attacks, with appropriate "fit testing" and would need to wear them at all times.

One of the main factors in the therapy of inhalational anthrax is the

"...persistence of spores in the tissues and their germination after the blood-penicillin level has fallen..."

J. M. Barnes
J. Path. Bact. 59 113 (1947)

Prophylaxis is a critical component of protecting other individuals whom have confirmed to intentional anthrax exposure. Antibiotic are need for at least 60 days because spores can persist in tissues and germinated. As stated before primate studies have found spores still viable ≥ 60 days in their air sacks.

Postexposure Prophylaxis

- Antibiotic therapy
  - Treat ASAP
  - Prompt therapy can improve survival
  - Continue for 60 days
    - 30-45 days if vaccine administered
  - Cutaneous cases also needs prophylaxis if bio-attack victim for 60 days also

For those individuals whom have confirmed exposure to anthrax, prophylaxis treatment needs to be as soon as possible to improve survival.

Prophylaxis indicated for 60 days

1. Boca Raton, FL---prophylaxis is recommended for employees and visitors who spent >1 hour during August 1--October 6 in the American Media, Inc., building.
2. New York City, NY---prophylaxis is recommended for all employees who worked during October 9--26 on the second and third floors of the south section of the Morgan Central Postal Facility in Manhattan.
3. Hamilton Township, NJ---prophylaxis is recommended for all employees and business visitors (i.e., temporary postal workers, vendors, contractors, and anyone in nonpublic work sites) who were in the U.S. Postal Service Route 130 Processing and Distribution Center during September 18--October 18.
4. Washington, DC (Capitol Hill)---prophylaxis is recommended for persons who were on the fifth and sixth floors of the southeast wing of the Senate Hart Building on October 15, from 9 a.m. to 7 p.m.
5. Washington, DC---prophylaxis is recommended for all employees and business visitors to the nonpublic mail room of the U.S. Postal Service Processing and Distribution Center at 900 Brentwood Road during October 12--21.
5. Sterling, VA---prophylaxis is recommended for all mail room employees and business visitors who were at the Department of State Annex 32 mail room facility during October 12--22.
6. **~10,000 prophylaxis for 60 days**

~10,000 persons in the United States where prophylaxis for 60 days due to their determined confirmed exposure to anthrax. Retrospective studies have determined that many individuals did not complete to recommended prophylaxis! However, no cases occurred among those whom where determined at risk and received antibiotics.

Postexposure Prophylaxis

- Antibiotic therapy
  - Same regimen as active treatment
    - Substituting oral equivalent for IV
    - Ciprofloxacin 500 mg po bid empirically
    - Alternatives
      - Doxycycline 100 mg po bid
      - Amoxicillin 500 mg po tid-option for children

Appropriate prophylaxis is with cipro or doxy for 60 days as stated previously. Children should also receive the same antibiotics. Amoxicillin may be used if it is confirmed that the anthrax they where exposed to is sensitive to penicillin! Clinicians will have to deal with the side effects. Usually with the lower dosage, side effects should be less. See next slide.

TABLE 1. Interim recommendations for postexposure prophylaxis for prevention of inhalational anthrax after intentional exposure to *Bacillus anthracis*

Category	Initial therapy	Duration
Adults (including pregnant women and immunocompromised persons)	Ciprofloxacin 500 mg po BID or Doxycycline 100 mg po BID	60 days
Children	Ciprofloxacin 10-15 mg/kg po Q12 hrs* or Doxycycline: >8 yrs and >45 kg: 100 mg po BID >8 yrs and ≤45 kg: 2.2 mg/kg po BID ≤8 yrs: 2.2 mg/kg po BID	60 days

*Ciprofloxacin dose should not exceed 1 gram per day in children.

ANTHRAX
Vaccine and Prophylaxis

- Vaccine is FDA licensed (1970)
- Primary series: 6 doses: 0-2-4 weeks, 6-12-18 months
- Booster: Yearly
- For known or imminent exposure vaccinate the unvaccinated and tx
- Cipro 500 mg bid, or Doxy 100 mg bid, for 4 weeks. Continue for 8 wks if vaccine not available
- New Rx and prophy: Clindamycin has anti-toxin effect I.G., better Vaccine, and Toxin inhibitors

A vaccine has been available for years against anthrax. Experts are not certain of its effective to inhalational anthrax. It is though very effect against cutaneous anthrax. Side effects are similar to placebo.

Concerning prophylaxis: Should someone receive the first three dosage of the anthrax vaccine, they would only need 4 weeks of appropriate antibiotics. This was considered for postal workers to reduce risk of exposure and potential side effects of antibiotics. This was not implemented because the letters stopped occurring in the mail and there was concern about side effects for this vaccine among postal workers and others.

Preventing Anthrax After Exposure: Options

- Initial recommendation:
  Antibiotics for 60 days
- New Option 1:
  Antibiotics for 100 days
- New Option 2:
  40 more days antibiotics plus vaccine (3 doses over 4 weeks): Investigational

In the winter of 2002, the CDC asked those individuals who had significant exposure to these letters to participate in a study and also possibly reduce risk for inhalational anthrax. Very few postal workers or others in the exposed buildings participated in this proposal

Senator Daschle & Leahy
Envelopes: Postmarked 10/9/01

The above two letter where captured. Both letter contained high grade, weaponized powered for of anthrax. Senator Leavy was intercepted in the mail once it was stopped. Therefore no one was exposed. However the letter which went to the Hart building, Senator Daschle did exposure many individuals to a very dangerous anthrax power. There probably would have been many more deaths had not prophylaxis been implemented immediately.

Outbreak Investigations 2001

- Washington, D.C.
  - Letter sent to Senator Daschle
    - Originated from Trenton, NJ
    - 28 Senate staff confirmed exposure
      - Acute/Convalscent serum-not nasal swabs!
    - Evacuation of Senate then House

Studies where done to determined to risk for acquiring anthrax from these letters. It was later determined that a 500 to 3,000 percent increase of a lethal dose of 50% would have occurred in a standard size office of 10x10x18 feet. In other words this power was extremely dangerous!!

Decontamination

- Opened envelope with suspicious substance
  - Gently cover, avoid all contact
  - Leave room and isolate from others
  - Thoroughly wash hands with soap and water
  - Notify local security / law enforcement
  - Carefully remove outer clothing, put in plastic
  - Shower with soap and water
  - List all persons in area

Opened envelope or packages with suspicious substance, should be covered with care, if possible. All persons in the adjacent area should warned of the situation hand should leave the building immediately but in a orderly manner. Just in the suspected area should meet somewhere outside. If you are the "lucky" one who handled the suspicious envelope or packages you should wash or hands with soap and water. Hand rinses or toweletts are not effective. Whom ever is responsible should have the ventilation system shut down for the building and all fans or separate ventilation systems should also be shut off. Call 911 ASAP. Obtain the name and locating information for all those whom may have been exposed.

TABLE 1. Number of cases of anthrax, by site — September-October 2001

Site	Florida	New York City	District of Columbia	New Jersey*	Total
Inhalational					
Confirmed	2	1	5	2	10
Suspected	0	0	0	0	0
Total	2	1	5	2	10
Cutaneous					
Confirmed	0	4	0	3	7
Suspected	0	3	0	2	5
Total	0	7	0	5	12

*Includes one case each from Pennsylvania and Delaware.

Above are the diagnosed cases of last year. Of interest 6 individuals, mostly postal workers survived inhalational anthrax due to prompt and appropriate therapy and insertion of chest tubes to drain the pleural effusion.

Two "outlier" cases occurred. One was a hospital worker, 66 year old female in New York city and the other was 95 year old female in Connecticut. Both individuals expired. Definitive source was not found on these cases, however it was believe to cross-contamination of the mail.

Environmental Issues

- Environmental samples
  - Suspicious powders
    - Must be sent to reference laboratories as part of epidemiologic/criminal investigation
    - Assessed using cultures, stains, PCR
  - Air sampling
  - First responders
    - Handheld immunoassays
      - Not validated, NOW NOT RECOMMENDED!
      - Useful for detecting massive contamination, > 10,000 spores

Any suspicious powders which are suspect should be collected by the emergency management in our area usually the Bomb squad. They should be sent to state laboratories for analyst. The hand held immunossays (Smart Ticket™) are not recommended due to their high incidence of false positive and false negative. Air sampling is usually not indicated unless the CDC initiate and performs such actions.

Decontamination

- Skin, clothing
  - Thorough washing with soap and water
  - Avoid bleach on skin
- Instruments for invasive procedures
  - Sterilize, e.g. 5% hypochlorite solution
- Sporicidal agents
  - Sodium or calcium hypochlorite (bleach)

Decontamination efforts are:

Environment-

One to ten dilution bleach and water will inactive spores of anthrax. When aerosolized anthrax has occurred the building will be shut down and only those entering with level A and B protective gear will be allowed in at least for the few days. After this period, it is believed that the spores will settle to the ground, carpet, and/or floor and there they will lose the static charge and will attach to soil, dust, etc. If this occurs the spores will probably be too large to be inhaled. However, cutaneous anthrax could occur as the situation in the media building in New York city. However, this is not known for sure and re- aerosolized could occur, however most experts believe this to be very unlikely.

Individuals exposed to suspicious substance-

As stated before hand and other exposure body areas must be washed with soap and water. A bath/shower may be necessary. Cloths should be removed and placed in sealed bags and washed in automatic washer and drier

PLAGUE: History

- 1346 Tartars laid siege to the Port of Azov (Asia) using plague killed bodies as weapons tossed over the ramparts. Fleeing, but infected(not by dead bodies) survivors carried plague to Italy
- Plague burned across Europe for 4 centuries, killing 25,000,000.
- 17th Century understanding that rats were associated with plague.

Many believe the plague outbreak of the middle ages occurred when fleeing crusaders returning from the middle east, came to Italy and infected others in which the Plague or Black Death killed over 35,000 for 4 centuries.

PLAGUE:

- 1920 Plague outbreak in Pensacola, 10 cases 6 deaths. Cause: rats from ships.
- 1996 U.S. 5 cases, 2 deaths. Diagnosis after deaths. Cause: Prairie dog fleas
- Zoonotic disease caused by *Yersinia pestis*. Humans become infected from contact with infected rodents and their fleas (bites).
- BW?- contaminated fleas (bubonic) or aerosolized plague bacillus (pneumonic)

Plague in certain parts of the country is not unusual particularly in the south west where the prairie dogs carry fleas infected with bubonic plague bacterial. However should patient/patients be diagnosed with plague in New York or Florida this would be a concern particularly if they have not traveled to endemic areas of plague. The disease is caused by Yersenia pestis bacteria. Those who acquired bubonic plague about 10-15% will develop pneumonic plague which is airborne transmitted.

PLAGUE: Three Types
Bubonic, Primary septicemic, Pneumonic

- Transmission: Rodent fleas (cat and dog fleas can contract and transmit to humans).
- Incubation 1-10 days.
- Clinical features: Onset acute, often fulminant. Malaise, fever, inguinal lymphaddenitis (bubo). Bubonic may progress septicemic and pneumonic.
- Pneumonic-Highly transmissible person to person?

There are three types of plague as show above. Incubation is 1-10 days after exposure. Symptoms are fairly similar to Tuberculosis,

h**emoptysis** is common. The disease is transmitted from person to person. However this is a larger droplet than other respiratory diseases and is no where near has contagious has smallpox

Bubonic Plague

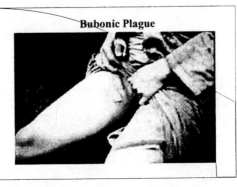

This slides demonstrates an inguinal lymphaddenitis (bubo) which is characteristic for the bubonic plague.

There recently been some interesting finding concerning survivors of the black death in the middle ages and HIV/AIDS in our century. It has been recently learned that some individuals whom do not have a receptor site called the CCR5 usually do not become infected with HIV. Apparently this mutation of T-cells was initiated during the middle ages to protect some population of the middle ages from becoming infected with the plague. It seems those particular descents of English families have the mutation/defect that greatly lowers their risk for acquiring HIV today. If you are interested in this, go to the following website for more information:

http://www.pbs.org/wnet/secrets/case_plague/background_pop_8.html

PLAGUE: Therapy and Prevention

- Droplet & Contact isolation, good surgical mask (filters about <1 micron), N-95 masks ?, antibiotics, supportive management of critical cases.
- D/C isolation after 48-72 hours of appropriate antibiotics
- Environmental decontamination-usually not needed
- Prevention: No vaccine available to the public at this time

Should a patient appear with pneumonic plague, they would need isolation. Negative pressure room are not needed. This bacteria is a large droplet and will drop to the ground after 3 feet. Those entering the room would need to wear N-95 TB masks. Once the patients has been appropriately treated for 2-3 days the patient can be discharged from isolation.

The environment plays no risk for exposure.

* Plague

Disease	Vaccine	Chemotherapy	Prophylaxis	Comments
PLAGUE	No longer available Was so until 1998, only effective for bubonic not effective against pneumonic plague	Streptomycin 30mg/kg/d IM in 2 divided doses x 10 days Doxy 200 mg IV Then 100 IV bid x 10-14 days	In past 6 days & within 3 feet: Doxy 100 mg PO bid x 7 d or duration of exposure Cipro 500 mg PO Bid x 7 days	

Transport	Incubation	Symptoms
Fleas? Bubonic or aerosolized Pneumonic	1-10 days	Initial: Chest pain, cough, dyspnea, within 24 hours of prodrome onset. Fulminate, fever, inguinal lymphaddentis, Cyanosis, Septic, Pneumonia

The Plague can be aerosolized or someone could become infected with a Pneumonic Plague and subsequently infect many other particularly in a crowded area. Treatment and prophylaxis is presented above in the slide.

Diagnosis-Plague

- Clinical features
- Staining-gram-negative coccobacillus
- Growth from culture
- ELISA, DFA, PCR
- Serological: detection of anti-capsular antibodies or ≥ 4 fold rise-acute to convalescent titers

Diagnosis could be somewhat difficult. Clinical features could be confused with other infectious agents, tuberculosis. Usually state laboratories or the CDC has the expertise to definitely diagnosis plague. A PCR is available at some state laboratories and definitely at the CDC in Atlanta.

Biological Toxins

- Any toxic substance of natural origin produced by animal, plant or microbe.
- Usually *not* dermally active
- Tend to be more toxic than chemical agents
- Most toxic: Botulinum toxins (7 related toxins)
- Effects most severe when inhaled

Aerosolized Botulism may be one of the most devastating biological weapons. Botulism is usually much more lethal than chemical weapons. Counties such as Iraq and Russia and probably other counties had botulism weaponized with it loaded on missiles, tanks, planes, etc.

Toxins on the Battlefield

- Enemy would have to present toxins to target populations in the form of aerosols, foodborne bot (worse) unlikely.
- Protective mask, *worn properly*, is effective against toxin aerosols.
- Use of TW can cause "terror effect"
- Better educated troops decreases panic among military personnel

Botulism also comes in food. There a sporadic cases in the United States when food is not processed or stored correctly. Early in 2002 an individual and his son in Maine developed food botulism due improper canning procedures. Both had to be placed on ventilators for 1 to 2 weeks.

Botulinum Toxins
"Most toxic compound"

- 15k x more toxic than vx. 100k x than sarin
- Iraq filled and deployed 100 munitions with bot.
- "1/3 weight of penny of Botulism could kill ~1 million!"
- Botulinum neurotoxins kills by "slow" onset (24-74 hrs). Respiratory failure follows visual disturbance and muscle weakness (1st seen as droopy eyelids)
- "Very tired, very weak, stop breathing".

Botulism is much more toxic than sarin gas. As stated above only a very small amount could kill million unless they are donning the proper chemical mask protection. Botulism can cause permanent nerve damage by binding to synapses and interferes with release of acetylcholine. Without the release of acetylcholine we lose our ability to manipulate fine motor skills. Individuals may present with a "Guilliam Barre" type syndrome. They are lose ability to walk but they can talk cause the toxin does not go past the brain barrier. Eyes will start to droop and they become very tired and stop breathing. They need ventilation to survive.

Botulism

- Another spore-forming bacillus
  - Clostridium botulism
  - Most potent neurotoxin known to man
- Three types
  - Wound
  - Food
  - Inhalation
- Cause permanent nerve damage by binding to synapses and interferes with release of acetylcholine
- Cannot cross blood-brain barrier

"Botulism"
The clinical syndrome

- Clinical diagnosis. No routine labs
- Treatment: Intubation & vent assistance. Administer botulinum antitoxin (decreases progression and hastens recovery)
- Prophylaxis: only for those with exposure and illness-severe shortage
- Decom: Not dermally active, no secondary aerosols from patients, remove cloths wash and bath person. Surfaces can be decom with 1:10 bleach/water solution.
- Gastro: killed easily by cooking

Diagnosis will usually be by clinical presentation. CDC can provide diagnostic laboratory test such as the PCR. Should a massive exposure occur an anti-toxin in available however there would probably not be adequate supplies. Therefore if a massive exposure occurs over a large city for event we could have thousands upon thousands who need ventilation which are probably not able to attend to at this point in time.

Areas are are exposed can the flushed with large amounts of water and small areas such as office building can be decontaminated with one to ten dilution bleach and water

Botulism

Disease	Vaccine	Chemotherapy	Prophylaxis	Comments
Botulism	DOD pentavelent toxiod For serotypes A-E: 0.5 ml deep SC @ 0, 2 & 12 Wk, then yearly booster	CDC trivalent equine antitoxin for serotypes A,B,E DOD heptavelent equine despeciated anti-Toxin-serotypes A-G: 1vial (10mL) IV	None? CDC trivalent equine antitoxin for serotypes A,B,E-only if Sy begins	
Transport	**Incubation**	**Symptoms** **Inoculums: LD50=.001 ug/kg**		
Aerosols-Food	12 hrs to 5 days usually	Initial: slow onset, Gillain-Barre like-Syndrome, respiratory failure, visual disturbance, muscle weakness, dry mouth, sensory system intact but flaccid paralysis, Pt remains alert		

Incubation is usually short for hours to a few days. Botulism can be aerosolized or could be placed in food which could have a devastating effect among large populations. There is not an effect antibiotic, however an anti-Toxin is available only through the CDC. The onset of illness is very slow and insidious, however when neurological symptoms occurs, demise of the infected person is imminent.

157

Variola
Smallpox virus

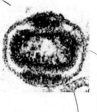

- Large DNA virus
- Dumbbell-shaped core
- Complex membranes
- Two types: Major-death rate >30%
  - Minor-death rate <1%

Smallpox is a most formidable biomedical weapon. Due to its high risk of death and the ease of transmissibility from person to person. A above is a picture of the electron microscopy view of the smallpox virus. This virus is somewhat fragile and easy to destroy in the environment.

158

SMALLPOX:
"The most terrifying BW threat"

- Unique to humans – Variola virus
- Highly infectious – person to person
  - Secondary attack rate 25-40% in unvaccinated adults
- High mortality – 30% unvaccinated, >40% infants and elderly
- Limited vaccine – 15 million doses
- 300 million doses maybe available 12/02
- Virtually no one is immune
  - <20% of U.S. with substantial immunity
  - Immunity wanes with time, some may have partial immunity with less severe disease

As of 11/02 the United States has the ability to vaccinate the entire population. Due to the success with dilution results of prior stored vaccines. Some public health, emergency management, police and other law enforcement, and various health care workers will be offered the vaccine in very late 2002 or 2003. There are many different things to consider where to take the vaccine or not. Some individuals with poor immune systems and dermatitis will not be able to receive the vaccine. This will be discussed later.

SMALLPOX: History and Significance

- 1350 BC Hittite warriors acquire disease from Egyptian Prisoners-King infected-Hittite empire falls
- 180 AD 5 to 7 million die in Roman Empire
- 1017 First Immunization in China
- 1520 Cortes goes to Mexico-brings Smallpox, kills millions of the Aztecs
- 1796 First Vaccination of boy using Cow Pox
- Vaccinations ceased in 1972 (US) 1980 (World) and for the US military in 1989
- Last Case of Smallpox in World 1976-Somalia-Variola minor
- Two WHO approved repositories exist: CDC Atlanta & VECTOR Novizbersk, Russia.
- Russia-Smallpox missiles, 1980s
- All stocks of smallpox to be destroyed in 1999. Extended to ?
- Russia has two other "known" producing labs with one able to produce tons q month

The history of smallpox is devastating for many cultures and civilizations. The Hittite empire was destroyed by Smallpox when Egyptians where taken prisoners and had Smallpox. An outbreak began among the Hittites and ultimately the King became infected and then their civilization crumbled. Smallpox greatly affected the Roman empire and brought one of the greatest civilization nearly to its knees! The first immunization was in China however western civilization gives credit to Dr. Genner who in the 18 century noticed that children whom lived and worked around cows did not become infected with Smallpox. By taking scrapping of Cowpox and injecting them into children and others he developed one of the first vaccinations for smallpox. Cortez when came and conquered Mexico did with the help of Smallpox which his troops where infected with. The Hawaiian culture was nearly devastated by Smallpox and Syphilis which Captain Cook and his sailors brought to the Islands.

Vaccination stopped in the USA, due to the lack of cases in the USA and the World. The last case of Smallpox (Variola Minor) was in Somalia in 1976. As stated in early slides President Nixon brought many countries together to seize the production and destroy any stockpiles of biological weapons. The former Soviet Union signed this agreement, however decided to continue production and produced Smallpox missiles which had the ability the devastate large urban areas. Russian still may have some labs which could produce tons of Smallpox and other biological weapons. The USA as given the former Soviet Union some $5 billion to clean and destroy these facilities.

160

SMALLPOX: Clinical Features

- Spread by droplet, aerosol, exudate
- Incubation: 7-17 days, median 12 days post exposure
- Sx: fever, malaise, prostration, aches
- 2-3 days of prodrome with high fever, malaise, prostration, severe H/A, backache
- Signs: rash 1-2 days later-pre eruption stage
- Febrile throughout course
- Death in second week – 30% mortality
- Environment plays small role in transmission
  - Seems to like dry less humid climate, Fall-Winter

Smallpox is a very contagious disease usually only 10-100 virions are needed for transmission. The incubation is usually a short time span with the a range of 7 to 17 days, though the average is usually 12 days after exposure. Smallpox usually begin with a prodromal period of patients presenting with prostration, fever (>101°), malaise, headache and severe body aches. They particularly complain of lower back pain. After a few days of the prodromal period patients will develop a rash which may present as macular but moves into a papular presentation. Through this course the patient is very febrile. Death is much more likely in the second week when there is a second viremia which invades reticuloendothelial organs.

Two rare forms of smallpox that can be difficult to recognize are hemorrhagic and malignant or flat-type. Both are characterized by a somewhat shorter incubation period and severely prostrating prodromal illness with fever, headache, and backache. Hemorrhagic smallpox is uniformly fatal; pregnant women appear to be unusually susceptible. Death usually occurs on the fifth or sixth day after the onset of rash. Malignant smallpox is frequently fatal. Constitutional symptoms are similar, but lesions develop slowly and do not progress to the pustular stage, remaining soft, flat, and velvety to the touch. If the patient survives, the lesions disappear without forming scabs, or, in severe cases, large amounts of skin may peel away.

The environment plays minor role in the transmission of smallpox. The virus is fragile and is easily destroyed with most any disinfectant. Building will not need to be burned or go through special fumigation processes.

161

Clinical Features

- Rash stages of development
  - All lesions in one region at same stage
  - Starts macular, then papular
  - Deep, tense vesicles by Day 2 of rash
  - Turns to round, tense, deep pustules
  - Pustules dry to scabs by Day 9 (least infectious)
  - Scabs separate
- Patients are > contagious when oral mucosa lesions ulcerate-release large amounts of virus into saliva

Patients are contagious when the oral mucosa has lesions that are ulcerated and release large amount of the virus into saliva. When a patient is coughing, this will propel the virus for up to six feet. Patients are considered contagious unless all lesions have separated (see following slides). The pustules will also shed virus and may be problematic for laundry and cloths. Although hot water will bleach will certainly destroy the virus.

162

Clinical Features

- Complications
  - Sepsis/toxemia
    - Usual cause of death
    - Associated with multiorgan failure
    - Usually occurs during 2nd week of illness
  - Encephalitis
    - Occasional
    - Similar to demylination of measles, varicella
- Other complications
  - Secondary bacterial infections uncommon
    - Staphylococcus aureus cellulitis
      - Responds to appropriate antibiotics
    - Corneal ulcers
      - A leading cause of blindness before 20th Century
  - Conjunctivitis rare
    - During 1st week of illness

Many patients (≥ 30%) will develop sepsis, with multi-organ failure. On occasion encephalitis does are with demylination which also occurs with measles and varicella. Lesions may become infected with secondary staphlococcus infection. We will experience secondary infections due to MRSA, possible VRE, and necrotizing fasciitis due to streptococcus.

Some patient will develop cornea ulcers which may lead in blindness.

Diagnosis

- Clinical Dx-sufficient, >90% have classical syndrome
- Traditional confirmatory methods
  - Electron microscopy of vesicle fluid
    - Rapidly confirms if orthopoxvirus
  - Culture on chick membrane or cell culture
    - Slow, specific for variola
- Newer rapid tests
  - Available only at reference labs (e.g. CDC)
  - PCR, RFLP

- Laboratory confirmation of the diagnosis is important. Visualization of an orthopoxvirus particle, to suggest a diagnosis of smallpox infection, can be quickly accomplished by electron microscopic examination of vesicular or pustular fluid or scabs.

- Specimen collection should be done by personnel who are knowledgeable and who have been vaccinated. Contact precautions should be observed, with the additional use of a facemask. Guidance for proper specimen collection procedures can be obtained from the CDC.

- State and local health department labs should be immediately contacted, as examination requires high-containment facilities and should be undertaken only by those with appropriate training and equipment. Definitive lab identification and characterization of the virus involves growing the virus in cell culture or on chorioallantoic egg membrane and performing various biologic assays, including PCR (polymerase chain reaction) technique and restriction fragment-length polymorphisms. PCR studies can be completed within a few hours at CDC.

164

Pathogenesis

- Virus lands on respiratory/oral mucosa
- Macrophages carry to regional nodes
- Primary viremia on Day 3
- Invades reticuloendothelial organs
- Secondary viremia on Day 8
  - deadly

One reason Smallpox can be very contagious is because the virus is a small micron (1-5), which is easily inhaled into the respiratory and oral mucosa. The macrophages will engulf the virus and will carry virus to the regional lymphnodes. Smallpox will infect white cells including macrophages and utilize the DNA structure to replicate more virus. See next slide.

Transmission:

Persons with smallpox are most infectious during the first week of illness, because that is when the largest amount of virus is present in saliva. Coughing > increases spread. However, some risk of transmission lasts until all scabs have fallen off.

Pathogenesis

- White Blood Cells infected
  - WBCs migrate capillaries, invade dermis
  - Infects dermal cells
  - Influx of WBCs, mediators cause vesicle
- Systemic inflammatory response
  - Triggered by viremia
  - Sepsis, multiorgan failure, often DIC

The virus also invades the dermal cells which produces the various rash formations with the influx of white cells will assist in production of the vesicles. Smallpox produces a huge inflammatory response, which may lead to sepsis, organ failure and often dissemination intravascular coagulase which is produced by other bacterial.

Pathogenesis

- **Severity of disease**
  - **Not influenced by severity of source case**
  - **Probably related to degree of viremia**
    - **Inoculation dose**
      - **Longer exposure, higher concentration at release 1infective dose 10-100**
    - **Virulence of variola**
      - **strain, engineered resistance**
    - **Host immune status**
  - **Type of rash predictive of outcome**
    - **More severe rashes = poorer outcomes**

As with most infectious diseases the amount of the inoculums, close and longer exposure may produce more severe disease presentation. Also some strain are more virulent than others. The former Soviet Union may have produced a specific weaponized-engineered type which would have been more lethal and possibility a short incubation of 3-5 days! Certainly the host immune status would play a significant role in severity of disease although most persons infected without any previous immunization for smallpox would become febrile with death occurring from 30 to 50%.

The rash is the malignant-flat type death is common and almost 100% with hemorrhagic form.

Smallpox

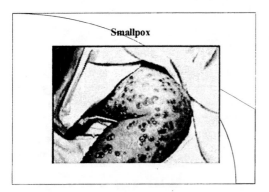

Above is a presentation a typical measles rash which is disfiguring. Also the lesion will in internal. Many patients are unable the drink or eat because ulcerative lesion will be evident in the oral mucosa. Patients may need medication to assist with pain management such as morphine.

Smallpox

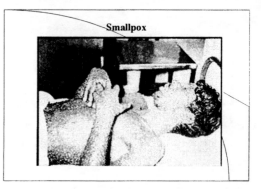

Above the a presentation of the malignant-flat Smallpox.

Differential Diagnosis

	Smallpox	Chickenpox
Incubation	7-17 days	14-21 days
Prodromal	2-4 days, "low back pain"	Same as rash
Rash	Face to extremities	Trunk/clusters
Rash formation	Firm-rash still evident 7-10 days	Collapse-resolves in 7-10 days
Soles/Palms	Yes	No

Although Smallpox and Chickenpox may be similar there are distinct difference is the symptom logy. As noted above the incubation is longer for Chickenpox. Smallpox has a prodromal period before the rash where Chickenpox has not prodromal period. The rash for Chickenpox starts in the trunk and is found in clusters where Smallpox starts in the face and spread to the extremities. Usually the rash for Smallpox is firm and will not collapse if pressure is applied where Chicken will easily collapse. Last but not least, Smallpox is found on the soles and palms where Chickenpox is almost always not found on soles and palms.

SMALLPOX : Prevention/Treatment

- Airborne-Contact-Standard precautions (negative pressure room) for 17 days, home is preferred – quarantined until all scabs separate highest infectivity from rash on
- Assign immune person for care
- Supportive care and prophylaxis
- Vaccinate close contacts as late as 7 (Preferred within 4 days) days post-exposure – intradermal – vesicle to scar denotes immunity-
- Household contact, vaccination contraindicated persons should be separated from other vaccinated persons until site scabs-prevent transmission of vaccinia virus
- Maybe able to dilute available vaccine from 15 to 300 million doses and be effective in prevention and prophylaxis.
- Also VIG – vaccinia immune globulin for high risk (immuno-deficient) exposures and reduce risk of severe side effects of vaccine-very short supply
  - VIG may increase with more HCWs receiving vaccine a donation of blood
- Vaccine side effects – viral sx, can cause death in ~ 1 in 1 million?
- No absolute contraindications

If we deem a suspicious cases be possible Smallpox the patient should be placed in airborne precautions (negative pressure room) for 17 days until all lesions have separated. A suspect patient can be kept at home if they only need minimal medical attention. All contacts within the past 7 days(preferred within 4 days) in the medical or home setting will be prophylaxis with vaccination, unless recently previously immunized for smallpox. Should someone be vaccinated and a contact person at home is at risk for complication (e.g. eczema, immune suppression) the contact must not stay/live with the vaccinated person until vaccine site has completely scabbed over (17 days). Those whom have severe reaction to the vaccine can be administered immune globulin which can reduce side effects. Currently however there is a short supply. As more persons are vaccinated (military, HCWs) they will be able to obtain blood donation to secure more vaccinia immune globulin.

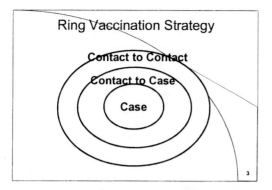

Ring Vaccination Strategy

Contact to Contact

Contact to Case

Case

3

If we have a case of smallpox all contact with six feet from time of diagnosis plus incubation will be prophylaxis with Smallpox vaccination. Also contact of the contact to a known case of Smallpox will also be vaccinated. This not usually done in public health. However, this ring strategy will be implemented to protect as many persons in the public as possible. This strategy was used in the 1950s & 1960s to eradicate Smallpox worldwide. This would be problematic due to vast mobility of our society today, which is why the government is moving towards vaccination of more person as soon as the feasibility is possible

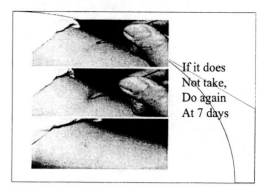

If it does
Not take,
Do again
At 7 days

Above is a picture of the bifurcated needle which will have a small drop of the vaccinia vaccine. A small spot on the arm will be identified and the needle will prick the skin ~ 15 times making the arm bleed to allow the vaccinia a portal of entry. individuals with risk for immunization should not be vaccinated if have diagnoses with eczema, immuno suppression, atopic dermatitis and other acute, chronic, or exfoliative skin conditions, high to moderated dosage of immunodeficiency or immunosuppression treatments, and pregnancy. Also infants < 1 year of age. If the vaccination does not take it should be given again. The next slide illustrates how the vaccine will progress. Those individuals whom have a direct exposure to confirmed Smallpox must be re-vaccinated if the first administration does not take. Those whom may be offered to be vaccinated as HCWs are not nearly as urgent to have the vaccine re-administered if first administration does not take.

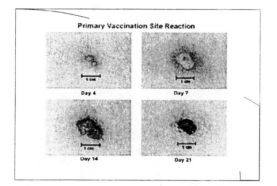

Primary Vaccination Site Reaction

Day 4

Day 7

Day 14

Day 21

As I am writing this information, hospitals, health departments and emergency services personnel (first responders) are being asked to be on a "Smallpox Team". Once the vaccine becomes available probably some time at the end of January-February 2003 you will be offered the vaccine for pre-exposure.

Above is what can be the expect reaction for those HCWs whom will take the vaccine for the first time. Those whom have had prior vaccination/s will have a modified response which may not appear somewhat less blister like with a scab forming soon (see next slide). The site should be kept covered for up to 17 days. HCWs will be able to work with patients at risk but must have the site covered with gauze first and then with transparent dressing. Those HCWs whom have little to no contact may have site covered with only gauze. The site will probably produce pruritic reactions. It will be very important for the site not to be touched and if the site is touched, hands must be washed effectively and immediately after contact.

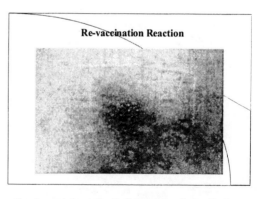

Re-vaccination Reaction

Above is re-vaccination reaction. Usually less pustule and heals quicker than initial vaccination with Smallpox.

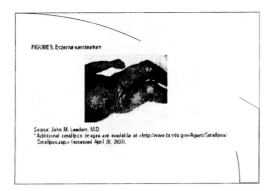

FIGURE 5. Eczema vaccinatum

Source: John M. Leedom, M.D.
* Additional smallpox images are available at <http://www.bt.cdc.gov/Agent/Smallpox/
Smallpox.asp.> (accessed April 20, 2001).

Individuals with Eczema must not be vaccinated. Dermal reactions seem to be the most common complication of Smallpox vaccination. Encephalitis occurs in about 2-3 in a million whom receive the vaccine.

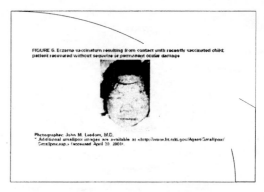

FIGURE 6. Eczema vaccinatum resulting from contact with recently vaccinated child; patient recovered without sequelae or permanent ocular damage

Photographer: John M. Leedom, M.D.
* Additional smallpox images are available at <http://www.bt.cdc.gov/Agent/Smallpox/
Smallpox.asp.> (accessed April 20, 2001).

This mother contracted Eczema Vaccinatum after her child had been vaccinated with smallpox. Lost vision in one eye.

177

178

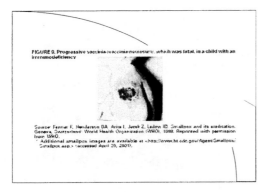

FIGURE 8. Progressive vaccinia or vaccinia necrosum, which was fatal, in a child with an immunodeficiency

Source: Fenner F, Henderson DA, Arita I, Jezek Z, Ladnyi ID. Smallpox and its eradication. Geneva, Switzerland: World Health Organization (WHO), 1988. Reprinted with permission from WHO.
* Additional smallpox images are available at <http://www.bt.cdc.gov/Agent/Smallpox/
Smallpox.asp.> (accessed April 20, 2001).

Above is a child which had a severe immunodeficiency and received the Smallpox vaccine and developed a fatal progressive vaccinia (vaccinia necrosum).

Smallpox Vaccine Reaction

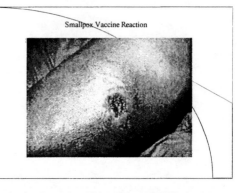

Another view of progressive vaccinia (vaccinia necrosum) lesion in patient with chronic granulocytic leukemia.

46

180

Isolation Guidelines

Isolation Facilities

- **Type C: Contagious facility**
  - hospital
- **Type X: Febrile contacts, no rash**
  - MASH units, hospitals
- **Type R: Asymptomatic contacts**

Patients whom are infected will need to be isolated. Those more severely ill will need hospitalization, or possibly other facilities (motels, hotels, mash units) may need to be utilized if more cases occur than the hospitals can accommodate.

Contacts whom develop fever will also need to be isolated. This could occur is various designated building and some could be isolated at home.

Asymptomatic contacts will need to evaluated daily form any suspicious symptoms. If symptoms occur appropriated medical test and isolation will be initiated.

High-Risk Groups for Vaccination

- Exposure to initial virus release
- Close contacts
- Public health, medical, and transportation personnel, morticians
- Laboratory personnel
- Laundry, housekeeping, and waste management staff
- Support of response: law, military, emergency workers
- Others at hospitals

5

As of 12/02 some hospital staff, public health, other medical facilities and law, military, and emergency workers are going to asked to be vaccinated for Smallpox. Those individuals with risk factors and if you live with someone with those risk previous discussed should not be vaccinated. Other probably can be vaccinated with little risk for complications particularly those whom where previously vaccinated without incident.

SMALLPOX:
Summary

- Acute infection - person to person
- S&S: Incubation 7-17days-median 12 days, rash is synchronous, febrile
- DX: Clinically, skin scrapings, PCR (CDC)
- TX: Supportive
- Prophylaxis: Vaccination
- Isolation: Droplet for 17 days following exposure for all contacts.

Clinical Features

- Modified variant
  - Previously vaccinated with partial immunity
  - Milder rash, better outcome, faster resolution

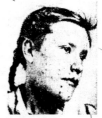

Photo: National Archives

Those of us whom have had previous vaccine may have a modified variant, milder rash, better outcome and resolve infection quickly. Some individuals will have a partial immunity particularly if vaccination occurred in the past 10-15 years (military).

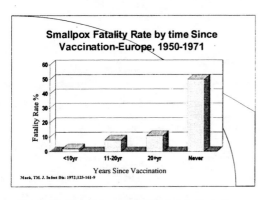

Smallpox Fatality Rate by time Since Vaccination-Europe, 1950-1971

Years Since Vaccination

Mack, TM. J. Infect Dis: 1972;125-161-9

However, even with previous vaccination the risk for death still exist. The above study was compiled in Europe and found those vaccinated some ≥ 20 years early could have a 10% chance of death. With the current vaccine protection only last about 3-5 years depend on host immunity, initial inoculums, virulent strains, etc. In outbreak setting the vaccine usually protects > 80% exposed. Some may still develop disease but with milder symptoms.

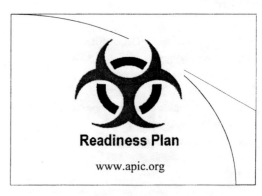

Readiness Plan

www.apic.org

All health care facilities need a plan to know whom to contact if a suspect case occurs. A free plan is available at the above website.

BIOTERRORISM

- Activate emergency response system
- Public Health authorities, epidemiology, decontamination and prophylaxis need
  - Syndromic surveillance
- FBI has jurisdiction, evidence collection
- Vaccine available through CDC, Push packs-8 in U.S.

Health care facilities should contact their local Health Departments first. Most Health Departments have a response team which will evaluate this situation and try to determine if the reported case is indeed valid. They would in turn contact the State Health Department and they would contact CDC. The FBI will have jurisdiction in most diagnosed cases of biological diseases. Should it be deemed that an attacked as occurred the CDC has 8 pushpacks in 8 U.S. cities which will come to the particular area and have supplies of vaccine, antibiotics, and other medical equipment to assist the area attacked.

Common Resistant Organisms

- **Streptococcus pneumonia**
- **Mycobacterium tuberculosis**
- **Salmonella-Shigella**
- **Candidasis**
- **MRSA-MRSE**
- **VRE**
- **Gonorrhea**

The following are the most common resistant microorganism, which are prevalent in hospital settings. MRSA and VRE will be discussed in detail in adjacent slides. Epidemiologists have noticed that approximately 10 to 15% of gonorrhea specimens are now resistant to Ciprofloxin. Salmonella resistance has been reported through feeding cattle antibiotics (TCN) which humans acquire through ingestion of beef (where's the beef?). Candidiasis is increasing with resistance to Mycolex™ and Diflucan™. Nearly 50% of a Streptococcus Pneumonia are resistant to penicillin and cephlosporins. The management of these organisms particularly in health care setting is ever important.

Patients at Risk for Antibiotic Resistance

- Immuno-compromised
- Prolonged drug therapy
- Age
- Nutritional Deficiency
- Increased gastric pH
- Risk for Pneumonia
- Patients with invasive procedures
- ICU Patients-Genius Patients
  - Receive Antibiotic Therapy

Patients with the above risk are too likely to receive antibiotics due to constant colonization and infection with microorganisms. If antibiotics are not used or dispensed appropriately, patients may have trace organisms, which may re-multiply if their condition changes. A good example would be cystic fibrosis patients who have prior infections with pseudomonas. When they acquire URI this usually results in a "super imposed" infection. The URI would increase a flow of secretions, which would provide the underlying pseudomonas with the proper media for the organism to multiply and result in an infection (pneumonia).

HOW BACTERIA OPERATIONALIZE RESISTANCE AGAINST ANTIBIOTICS

- ◇ Barrier to entry into the microbial organisms
  - ◇ Less pore size of transmembrane porin channels
- ◇ Prevention of antibiotic from reaching its target
  - ◇ Pump antibiotic out of microbe (E. Coli)
- ◇ Inactivation or modification of the antimicrobial drug by enzymes in the organism
  - ◇ B-lactam bond certain drugs such as penicillins or cephalosporins; makes them inactivated
- ◇ Alteration of the drug target
  - ◇ Bacteria may alter its target to the antibiotic
  - ◇ Move target, inactivate it (alteration of the a DNA enzyme)

Am. Journal of Infection Control Vol25 No1 2/97

Other microbes can form pores so small the antibiotic cannot invade and disrupt the cellular structure. Pathogenic E. Coli and other microbes have the ability to "pump out" the antibiotic before reaching the target (DNA, reproduction, etc). And others poses enzymes which can alter or neutralize antibiotics (beta-lactam).

PREEXISTING RESISTANCE

- ◇ Some microbes inherently possess genes that confers resistance
- ◇ Intrinsic Characteristic
  - ◇ Organisms without cell wall-resistance to B-lactam inhibitors
- ◇ Genetic Mutation:
  - ◇ Rapid mutation and recombination may give microbes opportunity for an antibiotic resistance mutant to emerge and then multiply
- ◇ Transfer of Genetic Material:
  - ◇ Transformation: acquire free DNA that contains resistance genes and incorporates DNA into their own genomes
  - ◇ Transduction: A bacteriophage infects the bacterium, transmitting resistance genes
  - ◇ Conjugation: Plasmids -extrachromosomal genetic elements (microbes communicate with each other)
    - ◇ Transposons -mobile segments of DNA
      - ◇ May be floating in body fluids with other organisms in a microbial "soup"
- ◇ Microbes past resistance among individual bacterial of the same or different bacteria
  - ◇ Nonpathogenic to Pathogenic

Am. Journal of Infection Control Vol25 No1 2/97

Resistance can be passed from one microorganism to another. The resistance pattern can be passed to their off-spring. Some organism poses genes, which can rapidly develop resistance when exposed to various antibiotics. Mycoplasma and Chylamdia have no cell wall so antibiotics such as penicillin or cephlosporins will have no effect except develop resistance. Other organisms may spread their DNA in a microbial "soup" (wounds) that integrate into the new bacteria. Some develop resistance through virus which is exposed to antibiotics and the virus infects the bacteria (phage).

Hospital-Acquired Infections

Most Frequent Site	Total	Staphylococcal
Primary bacteremia	260,000	122,000 (47%)
Surgical Site	320,000	100,000 (33%)
Pneumonia	320,000	70,000 (22%)
Other	460,000	150,000 (31%)

Staphylococcus comprises up to 50% of nosocomial microorganism in the hospital setting and other health care facilities. This has increased rapidly in the past 20 years and unfortunately has no end in site. More antibiotics are now being formulated that will assist with the treatment of these resistant microorganisms. However, up to 30% of patients may acquire their resistant organism through improper infection control technique. Most resistant organism is acquired through improper distribution or compliance of antibiotic usage.

MRSA-1996 (NNIS)

- Overall 35% of Staph Aureus are MRSA
- Hospital with >500 beds:
  - 41% for ICU vs 34% for nonICU pts
- Hospitals with <500 beds:
  - 30% for ICU vs 24% for nonICU pts
- Rate continues to rise for nonICU in smaller hospitals

Methicillin Resistant Staphylococcus Aureus (MRSA) is more prevalent in larger hospitals. However this organism is found in virtually all health care facilities. As stated in slide 92 often the patients will receive massive antibiotics in the ICU due to severe illness or injury. This may well result in the patient developing MRSA or other resistant microorganism. Through improper infection control practices by healthcare workers, this patient could be the "genius" individual with the spread of resistance microorganisms are transferred to other areas of the hospital, nursing homes, or rehabilitation facility.

MRSA

- Grows readily on skin & mucous membranes
- A variation Staph aureus which is resistant to beta-lactam antibiotics and possibly others as well
- Resistant to Methicillin, Oxacillin or Nafcillin
- Not-more infectious
- Not-more virulent
- Is-more difficult to treat
- Treatment of choice is Vancomycin

You find MRSA readily on you and your patients skin and mucous membranes (see next slide). MRSA is only a variation of Staphylococcus Aureus which is resistant to Methicillin, Oxacillin or Naficillin. This organism is definitely not more infectious or more virulent (likely to cause disease or death). However it is more difficult to treat due to the resistance to Methicilllin.

MRSA

- Colonization
  - Nares, axallae, chronic wounds, perineum, around g-tubes or Trach tubes, in sputum and urine
- Transmission occurs when contact with a person with purulent site of infections, Resp tract infection, UTI
- Hands of personnel are the most common mode of transmission

- Risk factors
  - Multi hospitalization
  - Medically complex
  - > 65 years of age
  - Multi invasive procedures
  - Severe underlying disease
  - Administration of broad spectrum antibiotics

This slides explains where you usually find MRSA. MRSA is usually transmitted from person to person when healthcare workers come in contact with purulent sites of infection or colonization, such as tracheotomies, wounds, or UTIs. It's less likely to occur when low levels of colonization's exist with the patient. The emphasize should be placed on purulent sites of infection, not on the areas of colonization.

Patients Should be placed in Contact Precautions who have purulent sites of infection. Those who have controllable sites (wounds, trach) can be placed in Standard Precautions. Patient with UTI and are catheterized can have a roommate if that patient does not have a catheter.

Use of Vancomycin

- ➤ Easier to use than other alternatives
- ➤ Must use for MRSA, allergic to penicillin
- ➤ Medicare-will pay for Vanco, but no for the other alternatives

Many physician prefer to prescribe Vancomycin because it produces few side effects, easy to administer, and is needed for those patients allergic to penicillin or cephalsporins. Many patients who have had prior experience with Vancomycin may ask to be placed of the antibiotic! HICFA-Medicare will pay for the use of Vancomycin but not for the other alternatives. This policy in itself encourages the use of the wrong antibiotics, which many of us are trying to discourage!

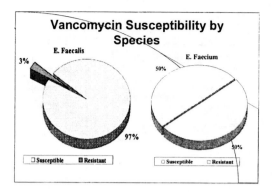

Vancomycin Susceptibility by Species

E. Faecalis

3%

97%

☐ Susceptible   ▩ Resistant

E. Faecium

50%

50%

☐ Susceptible   ☐ Resistant

Whenever Enterococcus organisms are cultured, we must know the species. As this slide demonstrates, faecalis species is rarely resistant to Vancomycin while up to 50% of faecium species are resistant to Vancomycin.

VRE
(Vancomycin Resistant Enterococcus)

- First reported in 1986-Europe
- Associated with nosocomial bacteremia, surgical site infection and UTI
- 20% increase 1989-1995 (.3 to 8%)
- 34x high in ICU
- Mostly seen in hospitals with >200 beds
- Like MRSA is not!
  - More infectious
  - More virulent
- Is much more difficult to treat

Vancomycin Resistant Enterococcus (VRE) was first reported in Europe. The spread of VRE in Europe may have been due to patients who where admitted but where colonized through the ingestion of beef. Back in the 1980s Europe feed their livestock Vancomycin to encourage growth. Since then, Europe no longer practices antibiotic feeding to their livestock. However, this practice still occurs in the United States.

VRE has increased rapidly in the United States, mostly in large hospitals. Cases have been reported in nursing homes and rehabilitation facilities.

Like MRSA, VRE is not more contagious than other Enterococcus organisms and it is not more virulent. However it is much more difficult to treat!

Transmission of VRE

- By direct contact via transient carriage on the hands of HCW
- By possible contact with contaminated environmental surfaces? & patient care equipment
- Reservoir
  - GI tract and female GU tract
  - Colonized LTC residents may be reservoirs for acute care setting
  - Acute care patients can reintroduce VRE to LTC

Transmission like MRSA is usually by direct contact via carriage on the hands of healthcare workers. The environment may play a role in transmission if **inadequate disinfection** has occurred (electronic thermometers, etc). The room of a VRE or MRSA, only needs to be disinfected as other patients rooms. The disinfectants available are very effect in destroying these resistant organisms. If spills occur they should (as with any patient) be cleaned immediately!

The reservoir for Enterococcus is usually the GI tract and the female genital-urinary tract. Patients have been admitted into hospitals from nursing homes whom are colonized, and should inadequate infection control practices occur, VRE is transmitted!

Risk Factors for VRE Colonization and Infection

- Extended Hospital stay
- Extended ICU stay
- Prior nosocomial infection
- Proximity to other patients with VRE
- Severe illness
- Hematologic malignancy
- Mucositis

- Nurse caring for another VRE patient
- Neutropenia
- Liver transplantation
- Vancomycin
- 3rd generation cephalosporins
- Ciprofloxacin
- Anti-anaerobic drugs

The above patients are at increased risk for acquiring VRE colonization for infection. See slide 92.

However, resistant can also occur to those patients who are on long term third generations cephalosporins, ciprofloxacin, and anti-anerobic (clindamycin) antibiotics.

Control Measures

- Infection Control Plan
  - Detect, prevent & control infection and colonization
  - Control antibiotic usage, antibiotic formulary
- Specific Guidelines for control of Vanco

To control these resistant microorganisms all health care facilities need a plan to identify these organisms, policies and procedures to prevent and control colonization and infection. The pharmacy in conjunction with the physician should have an antibiotic formulary so physicians can better treat patients empirically until results of the cultures are available. Many facilities such as nursing homes do not culture as frequently as hospitals therefore antibiotic formularies may be very useful in such setting.

Antibiotic Formulary

Disease	Likely Microorganisms	Therapy (IV unless noted otherwise)	Comments
Pneumonia			
Community Acquired	Unknown Mycoplasma/Chlamydia	Beta-lactam+/- Macrolide Or Quinolone	Bl=Ceftriaxone, Cefuroxime Macrolide= Erythromycin, Azithromycin
Hospital Acquired	E.Coli, Enterobacter, Pseudomonas, Klebsiella	Piperacillin/ tazobactam+ tobramycin	60% of nosocomial pneumonias are gram-negative in origin, 15% staph

The antibiotic formularies consist of prior cultures completed at a healthcare facility. As the above slide demonstrates, this hospital has data revealing that the most common microorganism associated with community and hospital acquired pneumonias. This data reveals, which antibiotics are cost and medically effective. Therefore, when a physician treats he can be reasonable assured he has used the most judicious course of antibiotics, which will assist the patient medically and reduce abuse of more costly antibiotics and probably reduce the emergency of resistant organisms.

Reasonable MRSA / VRE Precautions

- **Contact precautions:**
  - Wound heavily colonized or infected with uncontrollable exudates, VRE-Incontinent, medically complex patients
  - Trach with colonized or infected Resp. tract and unable to handle secretions.
  - Indwelling urinary catheter with MRSA or VRE.
  - All cases of MRSA or VRE when a cluster of nosocomial infections are found-outbreak.

- **Standard Precautions:**
  - Nasally or superficially colonized with MRSA (in sputum culture but without purulence)
  - Controllable wound exudate
  - VRE patient colonized in the GI tract, continent of stool and capable of maintaining hygiene practices (handwashing)

Isolate the Organism not the Patient!

Again, those MRSA patients with uncontrollable wound exudates, trachs and sometimes those with UTIs should be placed in contact precautions. VRE patients who are incontinent or medically complex patients should also be placed in contact precautions. Other patients with controllable wounds, trachs, continent of stool and capable of maintaining hygiene practices are placed in Standard precautions.

The idea is to isolate the organism not the patient. Many times patients are placed on isolation/precautions when the science does not warrant such a response. Sometimes this can have a negative psychological/emotional impact on the patient.

These precautions can be used if a facility understands handwashing and standard precautions. This usually can only be accomplished by aggressive education and re-education each year. I usually try to have this done during OSHA training which is required each year.

PREVENTING AND CONTROLLING VRE

- ◇ Notify I.C. staff immediately when VRE is detected
- ◇ Inform clinical staff of hospitals policies-isolate ASAP!
- ◇ Q.I. monitoring:
  - ◇ Compliance with isolation protocol
  - ◇ Time from VRE detection and isolation
  - ◇ Identifying other colonized or infected after first case
- ◇ Isolation Precautions:
  - ◇ Place in private room and cohorts others
  - ◇ Wear appropriate PPE's (Contact & Standard Precautions)
  - ◇ Remove all PPE's when leaving room-wash hands thoroughly
  - ◇ Minimize contact with environment

More specific polices for the control of VRE are found in section II of this book. The CDC has taken a rather aggressive approach requiring all patient with VRE to be placed in Contact precautions. The emphasizes is to monitor compliance with handwashing and use of personal protective equipment with appropriate disinfection practices. It is recommended that when a patient is found to have VRE, Infection Control should be notified as soon as possible! This is usually recommended to evaluate the patient and possibly change the type of precautions the patient was originally placed on. Patients which are discharged and are re-admitted should be flagged by the computer so again a re-assessment can be implemented.

PREVENTING AND CONTROLLING VRE

◇ Dedicate use of noncritical items (stethoscope, rectal thermometer, etc)
◇ Obtain stool cultures for roommates of VRE clients
◇ When can you d/c isolation?
  ◇ Negative stools x 3≥ 1 week apart?
◇ Policy to identify clients with VRE when readmitted to facility
◇ <u>Be careful with all fecal contact!!!!</u>

Patients who are usually colonized with VRE will probably keep this organism in their GI tract or life unless they improve dramatically. Usually they would need be off nearly all antibiotics for an extended period of time.

To summarize with respects to VRE; I believe we should be careful with all fecal contact. If we have one patient with VRE or MRSA it is very possible that we may well have 4 or 5 additional patients colonized or infection with resistant organisms!

Hospital With Endemic VRE or Continued VRE Transmission

◇ **Focus control efforts in ICU**
  ◇ **Can be reservoirs for VRE; may spread to other areas of hospital**
◇ **Cohort Staff**
◇ **Staff who are carriers are rarely implicated in transmission:**
  ◇ **However, examine staff for lesions, chronic skin problems, nail problems, etc**
  ◇ **Swab their <u>rear-ends</u> !**
  ◇ **If VRE positive; don't work with VRE - patients!**

Healthcare facilities which have endemic (part of the hospital microflora) VRE, may need additional measures, such as a strict enforcement of contact precautions. Also examine healthcare workers for rashes and lesions. Culturing these lesions may help identify potential source with regards to work restrictions until these lesions or rashes are resolved. However if healthcare workers understand and utilize effect standard precautions this should also control further spread.

Home Health/Hospice

• Contact/Standard Precautions with emphasis on preventing cross contamination
  - Clinical bag-leave in car? Bring In items (disposal)
  - Clothing-cover if likely to be soiled
  - Equipment should be cleaned or bagged prior to leaving home
  - Hands washed with waterless antiseptic before leaving home

Guidelines to assist home health agencies with infection control have been forth coming. Please see section II for more specific guidelines. Patients could acquire infections in the home and if/when this occurs it should be documented. As previously stated in the first part of this section, the Joint Commission requires that should an infections occurs as a result for prior medical treatment (surgery, IV site, wound drainage) at another facility this should be reported back to that particular facility (i.e. hospital, nursing home, rehab facility). Recommendations on whether to keep rates is rather unclear at this time, however infections should be logged into some kind of database (i.e. Epi Info, Excel, Lotus, etc.).

There should be policies and procedures for all aspects of Infection Control (Handwashing, precautions, immunizations, employee health, disinfections, IV therapy, etc).

There have been some guidelines concerning MRSA and VRE control with respect to home healthcare. Actually not that much differs from the discussion in the pervious slides although there is some attention to medical bags. Some would say leave it in the car and remove the items you need. I would recommend clean your bag regularly and all medical equipment should be adequately disinfected after use if feasible. Blood pressure cuffs usually only need to disinfected if soiled. They have rarely if ever implicated in transmission of microorganisms.

Community-Acquired MRSA: It's Here and probably in your area too!

➢ **Dallas, TX (1998) 2 day care center had index cases of MRSA infection: surveillance cultures of other children in the centers revealed colonization rates of 3% to 24%**
➢ **Chicago, Il (1993-95): colonization/infection rate in children without predisposing factors 26/10,000 admission**
➢ **MN, ND (1997-98): 4 children with severe invasive, fatal MRSA community-acquired infections**
➢ **VT (1993-94): 7/32 (22%) high school wrestling team members acquired MRSA (6 infected, 1 colonized)**

MRSA has now been found the in the community. We need to realize that this organism is somewhat different than what we seen in the healthcare setting, in that it has a different anti-biogram. Many patients may develop infections, particularly wounds with no known contact with nursing homes, hospitals, etc. The epidemiology of the community MRSA is still under investigation. At this time the CDC does not consider this to a major public health threat, however as demonstrated in the above slide cases have occurred and other will occur.

Pulse Field Electrophoresis

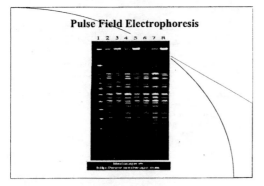

Should you have a cluster for MRSA or VRE or any other microorganism you should consider Pulse-Field Electrophoreses (DNA) assays for those you believe to be epidemiological relevant. Usually with this "finger printing" process, we can identify whether these organism are related. Usually all state laboratories can provide this free of charge. You must contact your local health department first to assist you with investigations and shipping of the specimens. Microorganism with different anti-biograms should not be pulse field tested because they are definitely not related.

Potential New Drugs for Resistant Gram-Positive Bacteria

- ➢ Quinupristin/dalfopristin
- ➢ Daptomycin
- ➢ Linezolid
- ➢ LY 333328
- ➢ Everninomicin
- ➢ Glycylcyclines

- ➢ **Ketolides**
- ➢ **Conventional**
  - ➢ VRE: TCN+Chloro+FQ
  - ➢ VISA, GISA, VRSA: Vanco+beta-lactam?
  - ➢ Pneumococcus: Some Beta-lactams-FQ-Vanco

New drugs have and are being developed to combat resistant microorganisms. New antibiotics have not been developed for over 25 years. Two are now approved Quinupristin/dafopristin (Synercide™) and Linezolid. They are only available in hospital pharmacies. This is to reduce the chance of over use and abuse. These new drugs have show to be effect from 50 to 80% for various infection sites (bacteremia, wounds, peumonia). Sometimes using existing drug combination, as demonstrated above **may** be effective.

What does the Joint want!(JCAHO)

5 Key Activities

- ➢ How do you <u>identify infections</u>
  - ➢ Total house
  - ➢ Priority-directed, targeted
  - ➢ Problem-outbreak response
  - ➢ What data is collected ?
    - ▪ Where does data come from?
    - ▪ CDC criteria for Nosocomial Infections, Cultures, Liasion, when antibiotics are dispensed
- ➢ <u>Analyzing infection data</u>
  - ➢ Internal or External

The Joint Commission takes infection control very seriously. Health care facilities who which to receive or keep accreditation should have an effect, up-to-date program. Before we get to the five key activities lets first discuss the process of Joint Commission surveys.

•They usually they want to know who is responsible for Infection Control (IC) and their qualifications and/or background. Who does IC coordinator, who they report too, and what is the table or organization.

•IC should be specific to your organization with regards to patient populations, services provided for clients and legitimate concerns/problems in respect to infection control.

•The joint commission wants to make sure IC has the proper resources to adequately do their jobs. Who is on the IC committee, who are the members and chairman, when and how often are meeting held and what issues are discussed. Do you address issues and resolve them, or continually monitor? Do not continually monitor, no action!

Five Key Issues:

•How do you identify infections and employee exposures? Total surveillance or target specific patients with increased risk, (central lines, ventilator, open heart patients, etc). Its up to you and what is best for your facility. How do you identify patient who may have nosocomial infections (cultures, antibiotic usage, CXR, CBC, liaison, etc).

What does the Joint want!(JCAHO)

- • <u>Guidelines for the prevention of infections</u>
  - – H/W, Standard precautions, Immunization, Food Prep, Compliance monitoring, Education
- • <u>Guidelines for the control of infections</u>
  - – Standard precautions, Transmission based precautions (contact, airborne), Education specific to audience, Biohazardous waste management
- • <u>Reporting of infections</u>
  - – Surveillance
  - – Nosocomial, Public Health, Employee exposures and illness
  - – Whom do you report them?

•You must have policy and procedures on infection control for each department. Policy and procedures to reduce infections (Precautions, UTIs, pneumonia, bacteremia, surgical site infections, etc). Education should be specific to audience, and how do you educate (lectures, tapes, innovation, games, etc). Compliance monitoring is important to identify problems and correct a situation if needed.

•Joint commission will ask if you report those communicable diseases required by state law and whom do you report them too. Remember health departments have different sections (AIDS, STDs, Epidemiology, TB)

JCAHO

- More time on inspections, less on interviews.
- Ask employees about disinfectants used, who is responsible for I.C., Sharing info about infections among facilities and professionals, etc.
- Does staff adhere to your policies on I.C.
- Interested in continuous quality improvement.
- Waterborne Pathogens/Construction
- Surveyors will ask the unexpected questions!

The surveyors are taking more time on inspections, asking employees who is responsible for infection control, where and what is disinfectants you utilize and how do you use it! They will themselves watch staff to see if the wash hands, practice standard precautions, etc. They may ask who received the Flu vaccine.

They will ask what have you improved on concerning infection control-continuous quality improvement (handwashing, red bag trash, precautions, etc).

They also will ask what do is done when construction occurs to help protect the clients from mold, fungi, etc. Also do you try and reduce the risk of waterborne pathogens (eliminating dead end water lines, flushing lines if feasible, test all patients with nosocomial pneumonia for legionella).

And they can ask the unexpected question that you can not answer?

Tell them what you are trying to accomplish concerning infection control, nothing more!

213

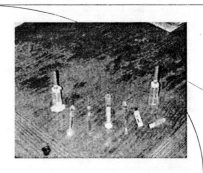

Above are some examples of safety devices for administering injections or drawing blood. The recent Needle Safety Act requires healthcare facilities to evaluate safety devices to reduce the risk of injury and therefore the risk for exposure to bloodborne pathogens. The new definition of Engineering controls as it applies to safety devices is: means controls (e.g., sharps disposal containers, self-sheathing needles, safer medical devices, such as sharps with engineered sharps injury protections and needleless systems) that isolate or remove the bloodborne pathogens hazard from the workplace."

 Identification, evaluation, and selection of engineering controls must select employees that are: Responsible for direct patient care, Representative sample of those with potential exposure (see section II).

•Your exposure control plan should "updated to include: changes in technology that reduce/eliminate exposure annual documentation of consideration and implementation of safer medical devices solicitation of input from non-managerial employees".

•Employers must <u>select</u> and <u>implement</u> appropriate engineering controls to reduce or eliminate employee exposure.

•Where engineering controls will reduce employee exposure either by removing, eliminating, or isolating the hazard, they <u>must</u> be used."

Also employee must be trained to utilized such devices

214

New BBP Directive from OSHA

- Review/Update BBP each year
- Must incorporate CDC Post-Exposure Protocol for Bloodborne Pathogens
- Evaluation of Safety Devices-Peer review
- SE on OSHA 300-301 log with info. On device
- Has fill-in BBP & Safety Device evaluation forms
- Nursing can except an inspection from OSHA in 2003-2003
  - The full text can be found at-
  - www.osha-slc.gov/OshDoc/Directive_data/CPL_2-2_44d.html

Also the employer must:

Review and update plan each year, must make sure that a provider who assists with the post exposure evaluation must follow the CDC guidelines(see section II), significant exposures must with documented on the OSHA 300 log which will ask about the device, type and brand of device involved, department or area of incident, and description of incident

Document evaluation and implementation in ECP

 •Review, update ECP at least annually

 •Review new devices and technologies annually

 •Implement *new* device use, as appropriate and available

There is at the above website at OSHA the compliance directive, which has available a "fill-in-the-blank" Bloodborne Pathogen plan and the evaluation form for safety devices.

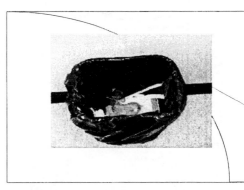

The only items that need to be red bagged are those things which are soaked, dripping, and/or caked with blood or other potentially infectious body fluids. State OSHA offices usually regulate red bagged trash. Red bag trash will cost a healthcare facility over .35 per pound, where as regular brown or white bag trash cost only about 1 to 2 cents per pound. As you can see above, nothing in this red bagged needed to be there.

Top Ten OSHA Violations

- Red Bag Usage-held to state regulations
- Hepatitis B Vaccine Availability
- Declination Statements-must have exact OSHA wordage
- Warning Labels on Waste Containers
- Implementation Schedule
- Locations and Use of Sharps Containers
- Physician letters of Written Opinion-in 15 days to patient & Employer
- Engineering Controls
- Mask, Eye Protection/Face Shields
- Use of PPEs-availability & use of
  - Compliance monitoring-what to do with noncompliance employees

---

DECLINATION OF HEPATITIS B VACCINATION

I understand that due to my occupational exposure to blood and other potentially infectious materials, I may be at risk of acquiring Hepatitis B virus (HBV) infection. I have been given the opportunity to be vaccinated with Hepatitis B vaccine at no charge to myself. However, I decline the hepatitis B vaccine at this time. I understand that by declining this vaccine, I continue to be at risk of acquiring Hepatitis B, a serious liver disease. If in the future I continue to have occupational exposure to blood or other potentially infectious materials and I want to be vaccinated with Hepatitis B vaccine, I can receive the vaccination series at no charge to me.

Employee Name (please print)

Employee Signature

Social Security Number

Signature of Witness

Date

Above are the 10 major violations of OSHA concerning bloodborne pathogens. OSHA receives funding through the levying of fines, not much funding through taxes!

•The number one violation is red bag usage. This is held to state regulations. In Florida once and item is placed in the red bag it must be removed within 30 days.

•You must offer the hepatitis B vaccine to category I (always exposed) and II (sometime-first aid, security, aggression control) employees. You only need to do titers on employees you vaccine and are category I (see section II).

•Those who do not wish to receive the hepatitis B vaccine and are determined by employer at risk must sign the declination form (next slide).

•Must have the St-Andrew cross on containers, storage areas, etc. (see slide no.84)

•Implementation schedule is when you implemented your plan and it must be updated/review each year. This must be documented on the outside cover of your plan.

•Sharp containers must be assessable to patient care cares where sharp devices are present and worked with.

•If a significant exposure occurs, in 15 days the employee should receive in writing what course of action is needed for follow-up (testing intervals, prophylaxis, etc) and a copy of your facilities bloodborne pathogen plan.

•Appropriate engineering controls should be available, such as hand washing sinks, autoclave, enough sharps containers, etc.

•Personal protective equipment which is available, how to use it, when to use.

"Slaying the Scared Cows"
Of Infection Control

- Disposable isolation trays
- Double-bagging isolation waste or linen
- Soak boats for disinfection instruments
- Using both alcohol and iodine as a skin prep
- Pregnant females I.C. polices
- Annual chest x-rays on PPD positive employees

- Sterile linen of neutropenic patients
- Routine cultures on disinfected endoscopes
- A dedicated scope for infected patients
- Environmental cultures
- Extra "Blood/Body Fluid precautions for known infected patients"
- Exempting pregnant women from PPD and Flu vaccine

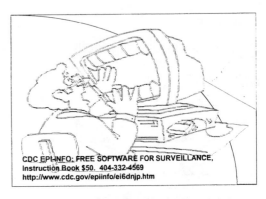

CDC EPI-INFO: FREE SOFTWARE FOR SURVEILLANCE, Instruction Book $50. 404-332-4569
http://www.cdc.gov/epiinfo/ei6dnjp.htm

Above are some practices we may have done or still doing that are not based in science. If you continue to practice these items you just cease. You'll probably washing time and money!

Disposable isolation trays: not need, not much you can acquire from isolation tray.

Double-bagging isolation waste or linen: single bagging is adequate

Soak boats for disinfection instruments: may contribute to nosocomial infections!

Using both alcohol and iodine as a skin prep: one is fine, no evidence that two is better than one.

Pregnant females I.C. polices: They need to do what we all need to do, Standard/Universal precautions, need to be well immunized (should not receive MMR)

Annual chest x-rays on PPD positive employees: only initial after PPD +.

Sterile linen of neutropenic patients: The idea of reserve isolation has long been stopped.

Routine cultures on disinfected endoscopes: Only if you have an outbreak, but not on a routine bases.

A dedicated scope for infected patients: NO, why? Disinfected each scope adequately after each patient.

Environmental cultures: On very rare occasion, such as outbreak from legionella(cooling towers), aspergilosis(construction, leasing).

You should keep you exposures and nosocomial infections (significant exposures, PPD +), in some kind of database. You can decide what you would like to use. Excel, lotus, d-base, its up to you. There are some database products made specifically for this purpose (AICE™). You can also use a free data base from the CDC called Epi-Info 6 (D-base program). This is free; call the above phone number or you can download it directly from the internet at: http: //www.cdc.gov/epiinfo/ei6dnjp.htm

There also a windows version now available at: ftp://ftp.cdc.gov/pub/Software/epi2000/ALL_IN_1.ZIP

The slides and narratives on the preceding pages can be viewed and printed out from the web at the following URL:

http://www.pesihealthcare.com/ppt/infection.pps

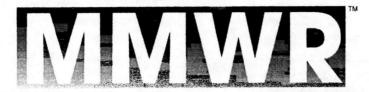

Morbidity and Mortality Weekly Report

Recommendations and Reports   October 25, 2002 / Vol. 51 / No. RR-16

Guideline for Hand Hygiene in Health-Care Settings

Recommendations of the Healthcare Infection Control Practices Advisory Committee and the HICPAC/SHEA/APIC/IDSA Hand Hygiene Task Force

INSIDE: Continuing Education Examination

CENTERS FOR DISEASE CONTROL AND PREVENTION
SAFER • HEALTHIER • PEOPLE™

The *MMWR* series of publications is published by the Epidemiology Program Office, Centers for Disease Control and Prevention (CDC), U.S. Department of Health and Human Services, Atlanta, GA 30333.

SUGGESTED CITATION

Centers for Disease Control and Prevention. Guideline for Hand Hygiene in Health-Care Settings: Recommendations of the Healthcare Infection Control Practices Advisory Committee and the HICPAC/SHEA/APIC/IDSA Hand Hygiene Task Force. MMWR 2002;51(No. RR-16):[inclusive page numbers].

Centers for Disease Control and Prevention

Julie L. Gerberding, M.D., M.P.H.
Director

David W. Fleming, M.D.
Deputy Director for Science and Public Health

Dixie E. Snider, Jr., M.D., M.P.H.
Associate Director for Science

Epidemiology Program Office

Stephen B. Thacker, M.D., M.Sc.
Director

Office of Scientific and Health Communications

John W. Ward, M.D.
Director
Editor, MMWR Series

Suzanne M. Hewitt, M.P.A.
Managing Editor

Rachel J. Wilson
Douglas W. Weatherwax
Project Editors

Malbea A. Heilman
Beverly J. Holland
Visual Information Specialists

Quang M. Doan
Erica R. Shaver
Information Technology Specialists

CONTENTS

Guideline for Hand Hygiene in Health-Care Settings

Recommendations of the Healthcare Infection Control Practices Advisory Committee and the HICPAC/SHEA/APIC/IDSA Hand Hygiene Task Force

Prepared by
John M. Boyce, M.D.[1]
Didier Pittet, M.D.[2]
[1]Hospital of Saint Raphael
New Haven, Connecticut
[2]University of Geneva
Geneva, Switzerland

Summary

The Guideline for Hand Hygiene in Health-Care Settings provides health-care workers (HCWs) with a review of data regarding handwashing and hand antisepsis in health-care settings. In addition, it provides specific recommendations to promote improved hand-hygiene practices and reduce transmission of pathogenic microorganisms to patients and personnel in health-care settings. This report reviews studies published since the 1985 CDC guideline (Garner JS, Favero MS. CDC guideline for handwashing and hospital environmental control, 1985. Infect Control 1986;7:231–43) *and the 1995 APIC guideline* (Larson EL, APIC Guidelines Committee. APIC guideline for handwashing and hand antisepsis in health care settings. Am J Infect Control 1995;23:251–69) *were issued and provides an in-depth review of hand-hygiene practices of HCWs, levels of adherence of personnel to recommended handwashing practices, and factors adversely affecting adherence. New studies of the in vivo efficacy of alcohol-based hand rubs and the low incidence of dermatitis associated with their use are reviewed. Recent studies demonstrating the value of multidisciplinary hand-hygiene promotion programs and the potential role of alcohol-based hand rubs in improving hand-hygiene practices are summarized. Recommendations concerning related issues (e.g., the use of surgical hand antiseptics, hand lotions or creams, and wearing of artificial fingernails) are also included.*

Part I. Review of the Scientific Data Regarding Hand Hygiene

Historical Perspective

For generations, handwashing with soap and water has been considered a measure of personal hygiene (*1*). The concept of cleansing hands with an antiseptic agent probably emerged in the early 19th century. As early as 1822, a French pharmacist demonstrated that solutions containing chlorides of lime or soda could eradicate the foul odors associated with human corpses and that such solutions could be used as disinfectants and antiseptics (*2*). In a paper published in 1825, this pharmacist stated that physicians and other persons attending patients with contagious diseases would benefit from moistening their hands with a liquid chloride solution (*2*).

In 1846, Ignaz Semmelweis observed that women whose babies were delivered by students and physicians in the First Clinic at the General Hospital of Vienna consistently had a higher mortality rate than those whose babies were delivered by midwives in the Second Clinic (*3*). He noted that physicians who went directly from the autopsy suite to the obstetrics ward had a disagreeable odor on their hands despite washing their hands with soap and water upon entering the obstetrics clinic. He postulated that the puerperal fever that affected so many parturient women was caused by "cadaverous particles" transmitted from the autopsy suite to the obstetrics ward via the hands of students and physicians. Perhaps because of the known deodorizing effect of chlorine compounds, as of May 1847, he insisted that students and physicians clean their hands with a chlorine solution between each patient in the clinic. The maternal mortality rate in the First Clinic subsequently dropped dramatically and remained low for years. This intervention by Semmelweis represents the first evidence indicating that cleansing heavily contaminated hands with an antiseptic agent between patient contacts may reduce health-care–associated transmission of contagious diseases more effectively than handwashing with plain soap and water.

In 1843, Oliver Wendell Holmes concluded independently that puerperal fever was spread by the hands of health personnel (*1*). Although he described measures that could be taken to limit its spread, his recommendations had little impact on

The material in this report originated in the National Center for Infectious Diseases, James M. Hughes, M.D., Director; and the Division of Healthcare Quality Promotion, Steve Solomon, M.D., Acting Director.

obstetric practices at the time. However, as a result of the seminal studies by Semmelweis and Holmes, handwashing gradually became accepted as one of the most important measures for preventing transmission of pathogens in health-care facilities.

In 1961, the U. S. Public Health Service produced a training film that demonstrated handwashing techniques recommended for use by health-care workers (HCWs) (4). At the time, recommendations directed that personnel wash their hands with soap and water for 1–2 minutes before and after patient contact. Rinsing hands with an antiseptic agent was believed to be less effective than handwashing and was recommended only in emergencies or in areas where sinks were unavailable.

In 1975 and 1985, formal written guidelines on handwashing practices in hospitals were published by CDC (5,6). These guidelines recommended handwashing with non-antimicrobial soap between the majority of patient contacts and washing with antimicrobial soap before and after performing invasive procedures or caring for patients at high risk. Use of waterless antiseptic agents (e.g., alcohol-based solutions) was recommended only in situations where sinks were not available.

In 1988 and 1995, guidelines for handwashing and hand antisepsis were published by the Association for Professionals in Infection Control (APIC) (7,8). Recommended indications for handwashing were similar to those listed in the CDC guidelines. The 1995 APIC guideline included more detailed discussion of alcohol-based hand rubs and supported their use in more clinical settings than had been recommended in earlier guidelines. In 1995 and 1996, the Healthcare Infection Control Practices Advisory Committee (HICPAC) recommended that either antimicrobial soap or a waterless antiseptic agent be used for cleaning hands upon leaving the rooms of patients with multidrug-resistant pathogens (e.g., vancomycin-resistant enterococci [VRE] and methicillin-resistant *Staphylococcus aureus* [MRSA]) (9,10). These guidelines also provided recommendations for handwashing and hand antisepsis in other clinical settings, including routine patient care. Although the APIC and HICPAC guidelines have been adopted by the majority of hospitals, adherence of HCWs to recommended handwashing practices has remained low (11,12).

Recent developments in the field have stimulated a review of the scientific data regarding hand hygiene and the development of new guidelines designed to improve hand-hygiene practices in health-care facilities. This literature review and accompanying recommendations have been prepared by a Hand Hygiene Task Force, comprising representatives from HICPAC, the Society for Healthcare Epidemiology of America (SHEA), APIC, and the Infectious Diseases Society of America (IDSA).

Normal Bacterial Skin Flora

To understand the objectives of different approaches to hand cleansing, a knowledge of normal bacterial skin flora is essential. Normal human skin is colonized with bacteria; different areas of the body have varied total aerobic bacterial counts (e.g., 1×10^6 colony forming units (CFUs)/cm^2 on the scalp, 5×10^5 CFUs/cm^2 in the axilla, 4×10^4 CFUs/cm^2 on the abdomen, and 1×10^4 CFUs/cm^2 on the forearm) (13). Total bacterial counts on the hands of medical personnel have ranged from 3.9×10^4 to 4.6×10^6 (14–17). In 1938, bacteria recovered from the hands were divided into two categories: transient and resident (14). Transient flora, which colonize the superficial layers of the skin, are more amenable to removal by routine handwashing. They are often acquired by HCWs during direct contact with patients or contact with contaminated environmental surfaces within close proximity of the patient. Transient flora are the organisms most frequently associated with health-care–associated infections. Resident flora, which are attached to deeper layers of the skin, are more resistant to removal. In addition, resident flora (e.g., coagulase-negative staphylococci and diphtheroids) are less likely to be associated with such infections. The hands of HCWs may become persistently colonized with pathogenic flora (e.g., *S. aureus*), gram-negative bacilli, or yeast. Investigators have documented that, although the number of transient and resident flora varies considerably from person to person, it is often relatively constant for any specific person (14,18).

Physiology of Normal Skin

The primary function of the skin is to reduce water loss, provide protection against abrasive action and microorganisms, and act as a permeability barrier to the environment. The basic structure of skin includes, from outer- to innermost layer, the superficial region (i.e., the stratum corneum or horny layer, which is 10- to 20-μm thick), the viable epidermis (50- to 100-μm thick), the dermis (1- to 2-mm thick), and the hypodermis (1- to 2-mm thick). The barrier to percutaneous absorption lies within the stratum corneum, the thinnest and smallest compartment of the skin. The stratum corneum contains the corneocytes (or horny cells), which are flat, polyhedral-shaped nonnucleated cells, remnants of the terminally differentiated keratinocytes located in the viable epidermis. Corneocytes are composed primarily of insoluble bundled keratins surrounded by a cell envelope stabilized by cross-linked proteins and covalently bound lipid. Interconnecting the corneocytes of the stratum corneum are polar structures (e.g., corneodesmosomes), which contribute to stratum corneum cohesion.

The intercellular region of the stratum corneum is composed of lipid primarily generated from the exocytosis of lamellar bodies during the terminal differentiation of the keratinocytes. The intercellular lipid is required for a competent skin barrier and forms the only continuous domain. Directly under the stratum corneum is a stratified epidermis, which is composed primarily of 10–20 layers of keratinizing epithelial cells that are responsible for the synthesis of the stratum corneum. This layer also contains melanocytes involved in skin pigmentation; Langerhans cells, which are important for antigen presentation and immune responses; and Merkel cells, whose precise role in sensory reception has yet to be fully delineated. As keratinocytes undergo terminal differentiation, they begin to flatten out and assume the dimensions characteristic of the corneocytes (i.e., their diameter changes from 10–12 μm to 20–30 μm, and their volume increases by 10- to 20-fold). The viable epidermis does not contain a vascular network, and the keratinocytes obtain their nutrients from below by passive diffusion through the interstitial fluid.

The skin is a dynamic structure. Barrier function does not simply arise from the dying, degeneration, and compaction of the underlying epidermis. Rather, the processes of cornification and desquamation are intimately linked; synthesis of the stratum corneum occurs at the same rate as loss. Substantial evidence now confirms that the formation of the skin barrier is under homeostatic control, which is illustrated by the epidermal response to barrier perturbation by skin stripping or solvent extraction. Circumstantial evidence indicates that the rate of keratinocyte proliferation directly influences the integrity of the skin barrier. A general increase in the rate of proliferation results in a decrease in the time available for 1) uptake of nutrients (e.g., essential fatty acids), 2) protein and lipid synthesis, and 3) processing of the precursor molecules required for skin-barrier function. Whether chronic but quantitatively smaller increases in rate of epidermal proliferation also lead to changes in skin-barrier function remains unclear. Thus, the extent to which the decreased barrier function caused by irritants is caused by an increased epidermal proliferation also is unknown.

The current understanding of the formation of the stratum corneum has come from studies of the epidermal responses to perturbation of the skin barrier. Experimental manipulations that disrupt the skin barrier include 1) extraction of skin lipids with apolar solvents, 2) physical stripping of the stratum corneum using adhesive tape, and 3) chemically induced irritation. All of these experimental manipulations lead to a decreased skin barrier as determined by transepidermal water loss (TEWL). The most studied experimental system is the treatment of mouse skin with acetone. This experiment results in a marked and immediate increase in TEWL, and therefore a decrease in skin-barrier function. Acetone treatment selectively removes glycerolipids and sterols from the skin, which indicates that these lipids are necessary, though perhaps not sufficient in themselves, for barrier function. Detergents act like acetone on the intercellular lipid domain. The return to normal barrier function is biphasic: 50%–60% of barrier recovery typically occurs within 6 hours, but complete normalization of barrier function requires 5–6 days.

Definition of Terms

Alcohol-based hand rub. An alcohol-containing preparation designed for application to the hands for reducing the number of viable microorganisms on the hands. In the United States, such preparations usually contain 60%–95% ethanol or isopropanol.

Antimicrobial soap. Soap (i.e., detergent) containing an antiseptic agent.

Antiseptic agent. Antimicrobial substances that are applied to the skin to reduce the number of microbial flora. Examples include alcohols, chlorhexidine, chlorine, hexachlorophene, iodine, chloroxylenol (PCMX), quaternary ammonium compounds, and triclosan.

Antiseptic handwash. Washing hands with water and soap or other detergents containing an antiseptic agent.

Antiseptic hand rub. Applying an antiseptic hand-rub product to all surfaces of the hands to reduce the number of microorganisms present.

Cumulative effect. A progressive decrease in the numbers of microorganisms recovered after repeated applications of a test material.

Decontaminate hands. To Reduce bacterial counts on hands by performing antiseptic hand rub or antiseptic handwash.

Detergent. Detergents (i.e., surfactants) are compounds that possess a cleaning action. They are composed of both hydrophilic and lipophilic parts and can be divided into four groups: anionic, cationic, amphoteric, and nonionic detergents. Although products used for handwashing or antiseptic handwash in health-care settings represent various types of detergents, the term "soap" is used to refer to such detergents in this guideline.

Hand antisepsis. Refers to either antiseptic handwash or antiseptic hand rub.

Hand hygiene. A general term that applies to either handwashing, antiseptic handwash, antiseptic hand rub, or surgical hand antisepsis.

Handwashing. Washing hands with plain (i.e., non-antimicrobial) soap and water.

Persistent activity. Persistent activity is defined as the prolonged or extended antimicrobial activity that prevents or inhibits the proliferation or survival of microorganisms after application of the product. This activity may be demonstrated by sampling a site several minutes or hours after application and demonstrating bacterial antimicrobial effectiveness when compared with a baseline level. This property also has been referred to as "residual activity." Both substantive and nonsubstantive active ingredients can show a persistent effect if they substantially lower the number of bacteria during the wash period.

Plain soap. Plain soap refers to detergents that do not contain antimicrobial agents or contain low concentrations of antimicrobial agents that are effective solely as preservatives.

Substantivity. Substantivity is an attribute of certain active ingredients that adhere to the stratum corneum (i.e., remain on the skin after rinsing or drying) to provide an inhibitory effect on the growth of bacteria remaining on the skin.

Surgical hand antisepsis. Antiseptic handwash or antiseptic hand rub performed preoperatively by surgical personnel to eliminate transient and reduce resident hand flora. Antiseptic detergent preparations often have persistent antimicrobial activity.

Visibly soiled hands. Hands showing visible dirt or visibly contaminated with proteinaceous material, blood, or other body fluids (e.g., fecal material or urine).

Waterless antiseptic agent. An antiseptic agent that does not require use of exogenous water. After applying such an agent, the hands are rubbed together until the agent has dried.

Food and Drug Administration (FDA) product categories. The 1994 FDA Tentative Final Monograph for Health-Care Antiseptic Drug Products divided products into three categories and defined them as follows (*19*):

- *Patient preoperative skin preparation.* A fast-acting, broad-spectrum, and persistent antiseptic-containing preparation that substantially reduces the number of microorganisms on intact skin.
- *Antiseptic handwash or HCW handwash.* An antiseptic-containing preparation designed for frequent use; it reduces the number of microorganisms on intact skin to an initial baseline level after adequate washing, rinsing, and drying; it is broad-spectrum, fast-acting, and if possible, persistent.
- *Surgical hand scrub.* An antiseptic-containing preparation that substantially reduces the number of microorganisms on intact skin; it is broad-spectrum, fast-acting, and persistent.

Evidence of Transmission of Pathogens on Hands

Transmission of health-care–associated pathogens from one patient to another via the hands of HCWs requires the following sequence of events:

- Organisms present on the patient's skin, or that have been shed onto inanimate objects in close proximity to the patient, must be transferred to the hands of HCWs.
- These organisms must then be capable of surviving for at least several minutes on the hands of personnel.
- Next, handwashing or hand antisepsis by the worker must be inadequate or omitted entirely, or the agent used for hand hygiene must be inappropriate.
- Finally, the contaminated hands of the caregiver must come in direct contact with another patient, or with an inanimate object that will come into direct contact with the patient.

Health-care–associated pathogens can be recovered not only from infected or draining wounds, but also from frequently colonized areas of normal, intact patient skin (*20– 31*). The perineal or inguinal areas are usually most heavily colonized, but the axillae, trunk, and upper extremities (including the hands) also are frequently colonized (*23,25,26,28,30–32*). The number of organisms (e.g., *S. aureus*, *Proteus mirabilis*, *Klebsiella* spp., and *Acinetobacter* spp.) present on intact areas of the skin of certain patients can vary from 100 to $10^6/cm^2$ (*25,29,31,33*). Persons with diabetes, patients undergoing dialysis for chronic renal failure, and those with chronic dermatitis are likely to have areas of intact skin that are colonized with *S. aureus* (*34–41*). Because approximately 10^6 skin squames containing viable microorganisms are shed daily from normal skin (*42*), patient gowns, bed linen, bedside furniture, and other objects in the patient's immediate environment can easily become contaminated with patient flora (*30,43–46*). Such contamination is particularly likely to be caused by staphylococci or enterococci, which are resistant to dessication.

Data are limited regarding the types of patient-care activities that result in transmission of patient flora to the hands of personnel (*26,45–51*). In the past, attempts have been made to stratify patient-care activities into those most likely to cause hand contamination (*52*), but such stratification schemes were never validated by quantifying the level of bacterial contamination that occurred. Nurses can contaminate their hands with 100–1,000 CFUs of *Klebsiella* spp. during "clean" activities (e.g., lifting a patient; taking a patient's pulse, blood pressure, or oral temperature; or touching a patient's hand, shoulder, or groin) (*48*). Similarly, in another study, hands were cultured of nurses who touched the groins of patients heavily colonized with *P. mirabilis* (*25*); 10–600 CFUs/mL of this organism were recovered from glove juice samples from the nurses' hands. Recently, other researchers studied contamination of HCWs' hands during activities that involved direct patient-contact wound care, intravascular catheter care, respiratory-tract care, and the handling of patient secretions (*51*). Agar fingertip impression plates were used to culture bacteria; the number of bacteria recovered from fingertips ranged from 0 to 300 CFUs. Data from this study indicated that direct patient contact and respiratory-tract care were most likely to contaminate the fingers of caregivers. Gram-negative bacilli accounted for 15% of isolates and *S. aureus* for 11%. Duration of patient-care activity was strongly associated with the intensity of bacterial contamination of HCWs' hands.

HCWs can contaminate their hands with gram-negative bacilli, *S. aureus*, enterococci, or *Clostridium difficile* by performing "clean procedures" or touching intact areas of the skin of hospitalized patients (*26,45,46,53*). Furthermore, personnel caring for infants with respiratory syncytial virus (RSV) infections have acquired RSV by performing certain activities (e.g., feeding infants, changing diapers, and playing with infants) (*49*). Personnel who had contact only with surfaces contaminated with the infants' secretions also acquired RSV by contaminating their hands with RSV and inoculating their oral or conjunctival mucosa. Other studies also have documented that HCWs may contaminate their hands (or gloves) merely by touching inanimate objects in patient rooms (*46,53–56*). None of the studies concerning hand contamination of hospital personnel were designed to determine if the contamination resulted in transmission of pathogens to susceptible patients.

Other studies have documented contamination of HCWs' hands with potential health-care–associated pathogens, but did not relate their findings to the specific type of preceding patient contact (*15,17,57–62*). For example, before glove use was common among HCWs, 15% of nurses working in an isolation unit carried a median of 1×10^4 CFUs of *S. aureus* on their hands (*61*). Of nurses working in a general hospital, 29% had *S. aureus* on their hands (median count: 3,800 CFUs), whereas 78% of those working in a hospital for dermatology patients had the organism on their hands (median count: 14.3 $\times 10^6$ CFUs). Similarly, 17%–30% of nurses carried gram-negative bacilli on their hands (median counts: 3,400–38,000 CFUs). One study found that *S. aureus* could be recovered from the hands of 21% of intensive-care–unit personnel and that 21% of physician and 5% of nurse carriers had >1,000 CFUs of the organism on their hands (*59*). Another study found lower levels of colonization on the hands of personnel working in a neurosurgery unit, with an average of 3 CFUs of *S. aureus* and 11 CFUs of gram-negative bacilli (*16*). Serial

cultures revealed that 100% of HCWs carried gram-negative bacilli at least once, and 64% carried *S. aureus* at least once.

Models of Hand Transmission

Several investigators have studied transmission of infectious agents by using different experimental models. In one study, nurses were asked to touch the groins of patients heavily colonized with gram-negative bacilli for 15 seconds — as though they were taking a femoral pulse (*25*). Nurses then cleaned their hands by washing with plain soap and water or by using an alcohol hand rinse. After cleaning their hands, they touched a piece of urinary catheter material with their fingers, and the catheter segment was cultured. The study revealed that touching intact areas of moist skin of the patient transferred enough organisms to the nurses' hands to result in subsequent transmission to catheter material, despite handwashing with plain soap and water.

The transmission of organisms from artificially contaminated "donor" fabrics to clean "recipient" fabrics via hand contact also has been studied. Results indicated that the number of organisms transmitted was greater if the donor fabric or the hands were wet upon contact (*63*). Overall, only 0.06% of the organisms obtained from the contaminated donor fabric were transferred to recipient fabric via hand contact. *Staphylococcus saprophyticus, Pseudomonas aeruginosa,* and *Serratia* spp. were also transferred in greater numbers than was *Escherichia coli* from contaminated fabric to clean fabric after hand contact (*64*). Organisms are transferred to various types of surfaces in much larger numbers (i.e., >10^4) from wet hands than from hands that are thoroughly dried (*65*).

Relation of Hand Hygiene and Acquisition of Health-Care–Associated Pathogens

Hand antisepsis reduces the incidence of health-care–associated infections (*66,67*). An intervention trial using historical controls demonstrated in 1847 that the mortality rate among mothers who delivered in the First Obstetrics Clinic at the General Hospital of Vienna was substantially lower when hospital staff cleaned their hands with an antiseptic agent than when they washed their hands with plain soap and water (*3*).

In the 1960s, a prospective, controlled trial sponsored by the National Institutes of Health and the Office of the Surgeon General demonstrated that infants cared for by nurses who did not wash their hands after handling an index infant colonized with *S. aureus* acquired the organism more often and more rapidly than did infants cared for by nurses who used hexachlorophene to clean their hands between infant contacts (68). This trial provided evidence that, when compared with no handwashing, washing hands with an antiseptic agent between patient contacts reduces transmission of health-care–associated pathogens.

Trials have studied the effects of handwashing with plain soap and water versus some form of hand antisepsis on health-care–associated infection rates (69,70). Health-care–associated infection rates were lower when antiseptic handwashing was performed by personnel (69). In another study, antiseptic handwashing was associated with lower health-care–associated infection rates in certain intensive-care units, but not in others (70).

Health-care–associated infection rates were lower after antiseptic handwashing using a chlorhexidine-containing detergent compared with handwashing with plain soap or use of an alcohol-based hand rinse (71). However, because only a minimal amount of the alcohol rinse was used during periods when the combination regimen also was in use and because adherence to policies was higher when chlorhexidine was available, determining which factor (i.e., the hand-hygiene regimen or differences in adherence) accounted for the lower infection rates was difficult. Investigators have determined also that health-care–associated acquisition of MRSA was reduced when the antimicrobial soap used for hygienic handwashing was changed (72,73).

Increased handwashing frequency among hospital staff has been associated with decreased transmission of *Klebsiella* spp. among patients (48); these studies, however, did not quantitate the level of handwashing among personnel. In a recent study, the acquisition of various health-care–associated pathogens was reduced when hand antisepsis was performed more frequently by hospital personnel (74); both this study and another (75) documented that the prevalence of health-care–associated infections decreased as adherence to recommended hand-hygiene measures improved.

Outbreak investigations have indicated an association between infections and understaffing or overcrowding; the association was consistently linked with poor adherence to hand hygiene. During an outbreak investigation of risk factors for central venous catheter-associated bloodstream infections (76), after adjustment for confounding factors, the patient-to-nurse ratio remained an independent risk factor for bloodstream infection, indicating that nursing staff reduction below a critical threshold may have contributed to this outbreak by jeopardizing adequate catheter care. The understaffing of nurses can facilitate the spread of MRSA in intensive-care settings (77) through relaxed attention to basic control measures (e.g., hand hygiene). In an outbreak of *Enterobacter cloacae* in a neonatal intensive-care unit (78), the daily number of

hospitalized children was above the maximum capacity of the unit, resulting in an available space per child below current recommendations. In parallel, the number of staff members on duty was substantially less than the number necessitated by the workload, which also resulted in relaxed attention to basic infection-control measures. Adherence to hand-hygiene practices before device contact was only 25% during the workload peak, but increased to 70% after the end of the understaffing and overcrowding period. Surveillance documented that being hospitalized during this period was associated with a fourfold increased risk of acquiring a health-care–associated infection. This study not only demonstrates the association between workload and infections, but it also highlights the intermediate cause of antimicrobial spread: poor adherence to hand-hygiene policies.

Methods Used To Evaluate the Efficacy of Hand-Hygiene Products

Current Methods

Investigators use different methods to study the in vivo efficacy of handwashing, antiseptic handwash, and surgical hand antisepsis protocols. Differences among the various studies include 1) whether hands are purposely contaminated with bacteria before use of test agents, 2) the method used to contaminate fingers or hands, 3) the volume of hand-hygiene product applied to the hands, 4) the time the product is in contact with the skin, 5) the method used to recover bacteria from the skin after the test solution has been used, and 6) the method of expressing the efficacy of the product (i.e., either percent reduction in bacteria recovered from the skin or log reduction of bacteria released from the skin). Despite these differences, the majority of studies can be placed into one of two major categories: studies focusing on products to remove transient flora and studies involving products that are used to remove resident flora from the hands. The majority of studies of products for removing transient flora from the hands of HCWs involve artificial contamination of the volunteer's skin with a defined inoculum of a test organism before the volunteer uses a plain soap, an antimicrobial soap, or a waterless antiseptic agent. In contrast, products tested for the preoperative cleansing of surgeons' hands (which must comply with surgical hand-antisepsis protocols) are tested for their ability to remove resident flora from without artificially contaminating the volunteers' hands.

In the United States, antiseptic handwash products intended for use by HCWs are regulated by FDA's Division of Over-the-Counter Drug Products (OTC). Requirements for in vitro and in vivo testing of HCW handwash products and surgical hand scrubs are outlined in the FDA Tentative Final Monograph for Healthcare Antiseptic Drug Products (TFM) (*19*). Products intended for use as HCW handwashes are evaluated by using a standardized method (*19*). Tests are performed in accordance with use directions for the test material. Before baseline bacterial sampling and before each wash with the test material, 5 mL of a standardized suspension of *Serratia marcescens* are applied to the hands and then rubbed over the surfaces of the hands. A specified volume of the test material is dispensed into the hands and is spread over the hands and lower one third of the forearms. A small amount of tap water is added to the hands, and hands are completely lathered for a specified time, covering all surfaces of the hands and the lower third of the forearms. Volunteers then rinse hands and forearms under 40°C tap water for 30 seconds. Ten washes with the test formulation are required. After the first, third, seventh, and tenth washes, rubber gloves or polyethylene bags used for sampling are placed on the right and left hands, and 75 mL of sampling solution is added to each glove; gloves are secured above the wrist. All surfaces of the hand are massaged for 1 minute, and samples are obtained aseptically for quantitative culture. No neutralizer of the antimicrobial is routinely added to the sampling solution, but if dilution of the antimicrobial in the sampling fluid does not result in demonstrable neutralization, a neutralizer specific for the test formulation is added to the sampling solution. For waterless formulations, a similar procedure is used. TFM criteria for efficacy are as follows: a 2-$\log_{10}$ reduction of the indicator organism on each hand within 5 minutes after the first use, and a 3-$\log_{10}$ reduction of the indicator organism on each hand within 5 minutes after the tenth use (*19*).

Products intended for use as surgical hand scrubs have been evaluated also by using a standardized method (*19*). Volunteers clean under fingernails with a nail stick and clip their fingernails. All jewelry is removed from hands and arms. Hands and two thirds of forearms are rinsed with tap water (38°C– 42°C) for 30 seconds, and then they are washed with a non-antimicrobial soap for 30 seconds and are rinsed for 30 seconds under tap water. Baseline microbial hand counts can then be determined. Next, a surgical scrub is performed with the test formulation using directions provided by the manufacturer. If no instructions are provided with the formulation, two 5-minute scrubs of hands and forearms followed by rinsing are performed. Reduction from baseline microbial hand counts is determined in a series of 11 scrubs conducted during 5 days. Hands are sampled at 1 minute, 3 hours, and 6 hours after the first scrubs on day 1, day 2, and day 5. After washing, volunteers wear rubber gloves; 75 mL of sampling solution are then added to one glove, and all surfaces of the hands are massaged

for 1 minute. Samples are then taken aseptically and cultured quantitatively. The other glove remains on the other hand for 6 hours and is sampled in the same manner. TFM requires that formulations reduce the number of bacteria 1 $\log_{10}$ on each hand within 1 minute of product application and that the bacterial cell count on each hand does not subsequently exceed baseline within 6 hours on day 1; the formulation must produce a 2-$\log_{10}$ reduction in microbial flora on each hand within 1 minute of product application by the end of the second day of enumeration and a 3-$\log_{10}$ reduction of microbial flora on each hand within 1 minute of product use by the end of the fifth day when compared with the established baseline (*19*).

The method most widely used in Europe to evaluate the efficacy of hand-hygiene agents is European Standard 1500– 1997 (EN 1500—Chemical disinfectants and antiseptics. Hygienic hand-rub test method and requirements) (*79*). This method requires 12–15 test volunteers and an 18- to 24-hour growth of broth culture of *E. coli* K12. Hands are washed with a soft soap, dried, and then immersed halfway to the metacarpals in the broth culture for 5 seconds. Hands are removed from the broth culture, excess fluid is drained off, and hands are dried in the air for 3 minutes. Bacterial recovery for the initial value is obtained by kneading the fingertips of each hand separately for 60 seconds in 10 mL of tryptic soy broth (TSB) without neutralizers. The hands are removed from the broth and disinfected with 3 mL of the hand-rub agent for 30 seconds in a set design. The same operation is repeated with total disinfection time not exceeding 60 seconds. Both hands are rinsed in running water for 5 seconds and water is drained off. Fingertips of each hand are kneaded separately in 10 mL of TSB with added neutralizers. These broths are used to obtain the final value. $\log_{10}$ dilutions of recovery medium are prepared and plated out. Within 3 hours, the same volunteers are tested with the reference disinfectant (60% 2- propanol [isopropanol]) and the test product. Colony counts are performed after 24 and 48 hours of incubation at 36°C. The average colony count of both left and right hand is used for evaluation. The log-reduction factor is calculated and compared with the initial and final values. The reduction factor of the test product should be superior or the same as the reference alcohol-based rub for acceptance. If a difference exists, then the results are analyzed statistically using the Wilcoxon test. Products that have log reductions substantially less than that observed with the reference alcohol-based hand rub (i.e., approximately 4 $\log_{10}$ reduction) are classified as not meeting the standard.

Because of different standards for efficacy, criteria cited in FDA TFM and the European EN 1500 document for establishing alcohol-based hand rubs vary (*1,19,79*). Alcohol-based hand rubs that meet TFM criteria for efficacy may not necessarily meet the EN 1500 criteria for efficacy (80). In addition, scientific studies have not established the extent to which counts of bacteria or other microorganisms on the hands need to be reduced to minimize transmission of pathogens in health-care facilities (1,8); whether bacterial counts on the hands must be reduced by 1 $\log_{10}$ (90% reduction), 2 $\log_{10}$ (99%), 3 $\log_{10}$ (99.9%), or 4 $\log_{10}$ (99.99%) is unknown. Several other methods also have been used to measure the efficacy of antiseptic agents against various viral pathogens (81–83).

Shortcomings of Traditional Methodologies

Accepted methods of evaluating hand-hygiene products intended for use by HCWs require that test volunteers wash their hands with a plain or antimicrobial soap for 30 seconds or 1 minute, despite the observation in the majority of studies that the average duration of handwashing by hospital personnel is <15 seconds (52,84–89). A limited number of investigators have used 15-second handwashing or hygienic hand-wash protocols (90–94). Therefore, almost no data exist regarding the efficacy of plain or antimicrobial soaps under conditions in which they are actually used by HCWs. Similarly, certain accepted methods for evaluating waterless antiseptic agents for use as antiseptic hand rubs require that 3 mL of alcohol be rubbed into the hands for 30 seconds, followed by a repeat application for the same duration. This type of protocol also does not reflect actual usage patterns among HCWs. Furthermore, volunteers used in evaluations of products are usually surrogates for HCWs, and their hand flora may not reflect flora found on the hands of personnel working in health-care settings. Further studies should be conducted among practicing HCWs using standardized protocols to obtain more realistic views of microbial colonization and risk of bacterial transfer and cross-transmission (51).

Review of Preparations Used for Hand Hygiene

Plain (Non-Antimicrobial) Soap

Soaps are detergent-based products that contain esterified fatty acids and sodium or potassium hydroxide. They are available in various forms including bar soap, tissue, leaflet, and liquid preparations. Their cleaning activity can be attributed to their detergent properties, which result in removal of dirt, soil, and various organic substances from the hands. Plain soaps have minimal, if any, antimicrobial activity. However, handwashing with plain soap can remove loosely adherent transient flora. For example, handwashing with plain soap and water for 15 seconds reduces bacterial counts on the skin by 0.6–1.1 $\log_{10}$, whereas washing for 30 seconds reduces counts

by 1.8–2.8 $\log_{10}$ (1). However, in several studies, handwashing with plain soap failed to remove pathogens from the hands of hospital personnel (25,45). Handwashing with plain soap can result in paradoxical increases in bacterial counts on the skin (92,95–97). Non-antimicrobial soaps may be associated with considerable skin irritation and dryness (92,96,98), although adding emollients to soap preparations may reduce their propensity to cause irritation. Occasionally, plain soaps have become contaminated, which may lead to colonization of hands of personnel with gram-negative bacilli (99).

Alcohols

The majority of alcohol-based hand antiseptics contain either isopropanol, ethanol, n-propanol, or a combination of two of these products. Although n-propanol has been used in alcohol-based hand rubs in parts of Europe for many years, it is not listed in TFM as an approved active agent for HCW handwashes or surgical hand-scrub preparations in the United States. The majority of studies of alcohols have evaluated individual alcohols in varying concentrations. Other studies have focused on combinations of two alcohols or alcohol solutions containing limited amounts of hexachlorophene, quaternary ammonium compounds, povidone-iodine, triclosan, or chlorhexidine gluconate (61,93,100–119).

The antimicrobial activity of alcohols can be attributed to their ability to denature proteins (120). Alcohol solutions containing 60%–95% alcohol are most effective, and higher concentrations are less potent (120–122) because proteins are not denatured easily in the absence of water (120). The alcohol content of solutions may be expressed as percent by weight (w/w), which is not affected by temperature or other variables, or as percent by volume (vol/vol), which can be affected by temperature, specific gravity, and reaction concentration (123). For example, 70% alcohol by weight is equivalent to 76.8% by volume if prepared at 15°C, or 80.5% if prepared at 25°C (123). Alcohol concentrations in antiseptic hand rubs are often expressed as percent by volume (19).

Alcohols have excellent in vitro germicidal activity against gram-positive and gram-negative vegetative bacteria, including multidrug-resistant pathogens (e.g., MRSA and VRE), *Mycobacterium tuberculosis*, and various fungi (120–122,124–129). Certain enveloped (lipophilic) viruses (e.g., herpes simplex virus, human immunodeficiency virus [HIV], influenza virus, respiratory syncytial virus, and vaccinia virus) are susceptible to alcohols when tested in vitro (120,130,131) (Table 1). Hepatitis B virus is an enveloped virus that is somewhat less susceptible but is killed by 60%–70% alcohol; hepatitis C virus also is likely killed by this percentage of alcohol (132). In a porcine tissue carrier model used to study antiseptic activity, 70% ethanol and 70% isopropanol were found to

TABLE 1. Virucidal activity of antiseptic agents against enveloped viruses

Ref. no.	Test method	Viruses	Agent	Results
(379)	Suspension	HIV	19% EA	LR = 2.0 in 5 minutes
(380)	Suspension	HIV	50% EA 35% IPA	LR > 3.5 LR > 3.7
(381)	Suspension	HIV	70% EA	LR = 7.0 in 1 minute
(382)	Suspension	HIV	70% EA	LR = 3.2B 5.5 in 30 seconds
(383)	Suspension	HIV	70% IPA/0.5% CHG 4% CHG	LR = 6.0 in 15 seconds LR = 6.0 in 15 seconds
(384)	Suspension	HIV	Chloroxylenol Benzalkonium chloride	Inactivated in 1 minute Inactivated in 1 minute
(385)	Suspension	HIV	Povidone-iodine Chlorhexidine	Inactivated Inactivated
(386)	Suspension	HIV	Detergent/0.5% PCMX	Inactivated in 30 seconds
(387)	Suspension/dried plasma chimpanzee challenge	HBV	70% IPA	LR = 6.0 in 10 minutes
(388)	Suspension/plasma chimpanzee challenge	HBV	80% EA	LR = 7.0 in 2 minutes
(389)	Suspension	HSV	95% EA 75% EA 95% IPA 70% EA + 0.5% CHG	LR > 5.0 in 1 minute LR > 5.0 LR > 5.0 LR > 5.0
(130)	Suspension	RSV	35% IPA 4% CHG	LR > 4.3 in 1 minute LR > 3.3
(141)	Suspension	Influenza Vaccinia	95% EA 95% EA	Undetectable in 30 seconds Undetectable in 30 seconds
(141)	Hand test	Influenza Vaccinia	95% EA 95% EA	LR > 2.5 LR > 2.5

Note: HIV = human immunodeficiency virus, EA = ethanol, LR = Log_{10} reduction, IPA = isopropanol, CHG = chlorhexidine gluconate, HBV = hepatitis B virus, RSV = respiratory syncitial virus, HSV = herpes simplex virus, HAV = hepatitis A virus, and PCMX = chloroxylenol.

reduce titers of an enveloped bacteriophage more effectively than an antimicrobial soap containing 4% chlorhexidine gluconate (133). Despite its effectiveness against these organisms, alcohols have very poor activity against bacterial spores, protozoan oocysts, and certain nonenveloped (nonlipophilic) viruses.

Numerous studies have documented the *in vivo* antimicrobial activity of alcohols. Alcohols effectively reduce bacterial counts on the hands (14,121,125,134). Typically, log reductions of the release of test bacteria from artificially contaminated hands average 3.5 $\log_{10}$ after a 30-second application and 4.0–5.0 $\log_{10}$ after a 1-minute application (1). In 1994, the FDA TFM classified ethanol 60%–95% as a Category I agent (i.e., generally safe and effective for use in antiseptic handwash or HCW hand-wash products) (19). Although TFM placed isopropanol 70%–91.3% in category IIIE (i.e., insufficient data to classify as effective), 60% isopropanol has subse-

quently been adopted in Europe as the reference standard against which alcohol-based hand-rub products are compared (79). Alcohols are rapidly germicidal when applied to the skin, but they have no appreciable persistent (i.e., residual) activity. However, regrowth of bacteria on the skin occurs slowly after use of alcohol-based hand antiseptics, presumably because of the sublethal effect alcohols have on some of the skin bacteria (135,136). Addition of chlorhexidine, quaternary ammonium compounds, octenidine, or triclosan to alcohol-based solutions can result in persistent activity (1).

Alcohols, when used in concentrations present in alcohol-based hand rubs, also have in vivo activity against several nonenveloped viruses (Table 2). For example, 70% isopropanol and 70% ethanol are more effective than medicated soap or nonmedicated soap in reducing rotavirus titers on fingerpads (137,138). A more recent study using the same test methods evaluated a commercially available product containing 60%

TABLE 2. Virucidal activity of antiseptic agents against nonenveloped viruses

Ref. no.	Test method	Viruses	Antiseptic	Result
(390)	Suspension	Rotavirus	4% CHG	LR < 3.0 in 1 minute
			10% Povidone-Iodine	LR > 3.0
			70% IPA/0.1% HCP	LR > 3.0
(141)	Hand test	Adenovirus	95% EA	LR > 1.4
		Poliovirus	95% EA	LR = 0.2–1.0
		Coxsackie	95% EA	LR = 1.1–1.3
	Finger test	Adenovirus	95% EA	LR > 2.3
		Poliovirus	95% EA	LR = 0.7–2.5
		Coxsackie	95% EA	LR = 2.9
(389)	Suspension	ECHO virus	95% EA	LR > 3.0 in 1 minute
			75% EA	LR ≤ 1.0
			95% IPA	LR = 0
			70% IPA + 0.5% CHG	LR = 0
(140)	Finger pad	HAV	70% EA	87.4% reduction
			62% EA foam	89.3% reduction
			plain soap	78.0% reduction
			4% CHG	89.6% reduction
			0.3% Triclosan	92.0% reduction
(105)	Finger tips	Bovine	n-propanol + IPA	LR = 3.8 in 30 seconds
		Rotavirus	70% IPA	LR = 3.1
			70% EA	LR = 2.9
			2% triclosan	LR = 2.1
			water (control)	LR = 1.3
			7.5% povidone-iodine	LR = 1.3
			plain soap	LR = 1.2
			4% CHG	LR = 0.5
(137)	Finger pad	Human	70% IPA	98.9% decrease in 10 seconds
		Rotavirus	plain soap	77.1%
(138)	Finger pad	Human	70% IPA	99.6% decrease in 10 seconds
		Rotavirus	2% CHG	80.3%
			plain soap	72.5%
(81)	Finger pad	Rotavirus	60% EA gel	LR > 3.0 in 10 seconds
		Rhinovirus	60% EA gel	LR > 3.0
		Adenovirus	60% EA gel	LR > 3.0
(139)	Finger pad	Poliovirus	70% EA	LR = 1.6 in 10 seconds
			70% IPA	LR = 0.8
(200)	Finger tips	Poliovirus	Plain soap	LR = 2.1
			80% EA	LR = 0.4

Note: HIV = human immunodeficiency virus, EA = ethanol, LR = Log$_{10}$ reduction, IPA = isopropanol, CHG = chlorhexidine gluconate, HBV = hepatitis B virus, RSV = respiratory syncitial virus, HSV = herpes simplex virus, and HAV = hepatitis A virus.

ethanol and found that the product reduced the infectivity titers of three nonenveloped viruses (i.e., rotavirus, adenovirus, and rhinovirus) by >3 logs (81). Other nonenveloped viruses such as hepatitis A and enteroviruses (e.g., poliovirus) may require 70%–80% alcohol to be reliably inactivated (82,139). However, both 70% ethanol and a 62% ethanol foam product with emollients reduced hepatitis A virus titers on whole hands or fingertips more than nonmedicated soap; both were equally as effective as antimicrobial soap containing 4% chlorhexidine gluconate in reducing reduced viral counts on hands (140). In the same study, both 70% ethanol and the 62% ethanol foam product demonstrated greater virucidal activity against poliovirus than either non-antimicrobial soap or a 4% chlorhexidine gluconate-containing soap (140). However, depending on the alcohol concentration, the amount of time that hands are exposed to the alcohol, and viral variant, alcohol may not be effective against hepatitis A and other nonlipophilic viruses. The inactivation of nonenveloped viruses is influenced by temperature, disinfectant-virus volume ratio, and protein load (141). Ethanol has greater activity against viruses than isopropanol. Further in vitro and in vivo studies of both alcohol-based formulations and antimicrobial soaps are warranted to establish the minimal level of virucidal activity that is required to interrupt direct contact transmission of viruses in health-care settings.

Alcohols are not appropriate for use when hands are visibly dirty or contaminated with proteinaceous materials. However, when relatively small amounts of proteinaceous material (e.g., blood) are present, ethanol and isopropanol may reduce viable bacterial counts on hands more than plain soap or antimicrobial soap (*142*).

Alcohol can prevent the transfer of health-care–associated pathogens (*25,63,64*). In one study, gram-negative bacilli were transferred from a colonized patient's skin to a piece of catheter material via the hands of nurses in only 17% of experiments after antiseptic hand rub with an alcohol-based hand rinse (*25*). In contrast, transfer of the organisms occurred in 92% of experiments after handwashing with plain soap and water. This experimental model indicates that when the hands of HCWs are heavily contaminated, an antiseptic hand rub using an alcohol-based rinse can prevent pathogen transmission more effectively than can handwashing with plain soap and water.

Alcohol-based products are more effective for standard handwashing or hand antisepsis by HCWs than soap or antimicrobial soaps (Table 3) (*25,53,61,93,106–112,119,143–152*). In all but two of the trials that compared alcohol-based solutions with antimicrobial soaps or detergents, alcohol reduced bacterial counts on hands more than washing hands with soaps or detergents containing hexachlorophene, povidone-iodine, 4% chlorhexidine, or triclosan. In studies examining antimicrobial-resistant organisms, alcohol-based products reduced the number of multidrug-resistant pathogens recovered from the hands of HCWs more effectively than did handwashing with soap and water (*153–155*).

Alcohols are effective for preoperative cleaning of the hands of surgical personnel (*1,101,104,113–119,135,143,147,156–159*) (Tables 4 and 5). In multiple studies, bacterial counts on the hands were determined immediately after using the product and again 1–3 hours later; the delayed testing was performed to determine if regrowth of bacteria on the hands is inhibited during operative procedures. Alcohol-based solutions were more effective than washing hands with plain soap in all studies, and they reduced bacterial counts on the hands more than antimicrobial soaps or detergents in the majority of experiments (*101,104,113–119,135,143,147,157–159*). In addition, the majority of alcohol-based preparations were more effective than povidone-iodine or chlorhexidine.

The efficacy of alcohol-based hand-hygiene products is affected by several factors, including the type of alcohol used, concentration of alcohol, contact time, volume of alcohol used, and whether the hands are wet when the alcohol is applied. Applying small volumes (i.e., 0.2–0.5 mL) of alcohol to the hands is not more effective than washing hands with plain soap and water (*63,64*). One study documented that 1 mL of alcohol was substantially less effective than 3 mL (*91*). The ideal volume of product to apply to the hands is not known

TABLE 3. Studies comparing the relative efficacy (based on log₁₀ reductions achieved) of plain soap or antimicrobial soaps versus alcohol-based antiseptics in reducing counts of viable bacteria on hands

Ref. no.	Year	Skin contamination	Assay method	Time (sec)	Relative efficacy
(*143*)	1965	Existing hand flora	Finger-tip agar culture	60	Plain soap < HCP < 50% EA foam
(*119*)	1975	Existing hand flora	Hand-rub broth culture	—	Plain soap < 95% EA
(*106*)	1978	Artificial contamination	Finger-tip broth culture	30	Plain soap < 4% CHG < P-I < 70% EA = alc. CHG
(*144*)	1978	Artificial contamination	Finger-tip broth culture	30	Plain soap < 4% CHG < 70% EA
(*107*)	1979	Existing hand flora	Hand-rub broth culture	120	Plain soap < 0.5% aq. CHG < 70% EA < 4% CHG < alc.CHG
(*145*)	1980	Artificial contamination	Finger-tip broth culture	60–120	4% CHG < P-I < 60% IPA
(*53*)	1980	Artificial contamination	Finger-tip broth culture	15	Plain soap < 3% HCP < P-I < 4% CHG < 70% EA
(*108*)	1982	Artificial contamination	Glove juice test	15	P-I < alc. CHG
(*109*)	1983	Artificial contamination	Finger-tip broth culture	120	0.3–2% triclosan = 60% IPA = alc. CHG < alc. triclosan
(*146*)	1984	Artificial contamination	Finger-tip agar culture	60	Phenolic < 4% CHG < P-I < EA < IPA < n-P
(*147*)	1985	Existing hand flora	Finger-tip agar culture	60	Plain soap < 70% EA < 95% EA
(*110*)	1986	Artificial contamination	Finger-tip broth culture	60	Phenolic = P-I < alc. CHG < n-P
(*93*)	1986	Existing hand flora	Sterile-broth bag technique	15	Plain soap < IPA < 4% CHG = IPA-E = alc. CHG
(*61*)	1988	Artificial contamination	Finger-tip broth culture	30	Plain soap < triclosan < P-I < IPA < alc. CHG < n-P
(*25*)	1991	Patient contact	Glove-juice test	15	Plain soap < IPA-E
(*148*)	1991	Existing hand flora	Agar-plate/image analysis	30	Plain soap < 1% triclosan < P-I < 4% CHG < IPA
(*111*)	1992	Artificial contamination	Finger-tip agar culture	60	Plain soap < IPA < EA < alc. CHG
(*149*)	1992	Artificial contamination	Finger-tip broth culture	60	Plain soap < 60% n-P
(*112*)	1994	Existing hand flora	Agar-plate/image analysis	30	Plain soap < alc. CHG
(*150*)	1999	Existing hand flora	Agar-plate culture	N.S.	Plain soap < commercial alcohol mixture
(*151*)	1999	Artificial contamination	Glove-juice test	20	Plain soap < 0.6% PCMX < 65% EA
(*152*)	1999	Artificial contamination	Finger-tip broth culture	30	4% CHG < plain soap < P-I < 70% EA

Note: Existing hand flora = without artificially contaminatiing hands with bacteria, alc. CHG = alcoholic chlorhexidine gluconate, aq. CHG = aqueous chlorhexidine gluconate, 4% CHG = chlorhexidine gluconate detergent, EA = ethanol, HCP = hexachlorophene soap/detergent, IPA = isopropanol, IPA-E = isopropanol + emollients, n-P = n-propanol, PCMX = chloroxylenol detergent, P-I = povidone-iodine detergent, and N.S. = not stated.

TABLE 4. Studies comparing the relative efficacy of plain soap or antimicrobial soap versus alcohol-containing products in reducing counts of bacteria recovered from hands immediately after use of products for pre-operative cleansing of hands

Ref. no.	Year	Assay method	Relative efficacy
(143)	1965	Finger-tip agar culture	HCP < 50% EA foam + QAC
(157)	1969	Finger-tip agar culture	HCP < P-I < 50% EA foam + QAC
(101)	1973	Finger-tip agar culture	HCP soap < EA foam + 0.23% HCP
(135)	1974	Broth culture	Plain soap < 0.5% CHG < 4% CHG < alc. CHG
(119)	1975	Hand-broth test	Plain soap < 0.5% CHG < 4% CHG < alc. CHG
(118)	1976	Glove-juice test	0.5% CHG < 4% CHG < alc. CHG
(114)	1977	Glove-juice test	P-I < CHG < alc. CHG
(117)	1978	Finger-tip agar culture	P-I = 46% EA + 0.23% HCP
(113)	1979	Broth culture of hands	Plain soap < P-I < alc. CHG < alc. P-I
(116)	1979	Glove-juice test	70% IPA = alc. CHG
(147)	1985	Finger-tip agar culture	Plain soap < 70% - 90% EA
(115)	1990	Glove-juice test, modified	Plain soap < triclosan < CHG < P-I < alc. CHG
(104)	1991	Glove-juice test	Plain soap < 2% triclosan < P-I < 70% IPA
(158)	1998	Finger-tip broth culture	70% IPA < 90% IPA = 60% n-P
(159)	1998	Glove-juice test	P-I < CHG < 70% EA

Note: QAC = quaternary ammonium compound, alc. CHG = alcoholic chlorhexidine gluconate, CHG = chlorhexidine gluconate detergent, EA = ethanol, HCP = hexachlorophene detergent, IPA = isopropanol, and P-I = povidone-iodine detergent.

TABLE 5. Efficacy of surgical hand-rub solutions in reducing the release of resident skin flora from clean hands

Study	Rub	Concentration* (%)	Time (min)	Mean log reduction	
				Immediate	Sustained (3 hr)
1	n-Propanol	60	5	2.9[†]	1.6[†]
2			5	2.7[†]	NA
3			5	2.5[†]	1.8[†]
4			5	2.3[†]	1.6[†]
5			3	2.9[§]	NA
4			3	2.0[†]	1.0[†]
4			1	1.1[†]	0.5[†]
6	Isopropanol	90	3	2.4[§]	1.4[§]
6		80	3	2.3[§]	1.2[§]
7		70	5	2.4[†]	2.1[†]
4			5	2.1[†]	1.0[†]
6			3	2.0[§]	0.7[§]
5			3	1.7[c]	NA
4			3	1.5[†]	0.8[†]
8			2	1.2	0.8
4			1	0.7[†]	0.2
9			1	0.8	NA
10		60	5	1.7	1.0
7	Isopropanol + chlorhexidine gluc. (w/v)	70 + 0.5	5	2.5[†]	2.7[†]
8			2	1.0	1.5
11	Ethanol	95	2	2.1	NA
5		85	3	2.4[§]	NA
12		80	2	1.5	NA
8		70	2	1.0	0.6
13	Ethanol + chlorhexidine gluc. (w/v)	95 + 0.5	2	1.7	NA
14		77 + 0.5	5	2.0	1.5[¶]
8		70 + 0.5	2	0.7	1.4
8	Chlorhexidine gluc. (aq. Sol., w/v)	0.5	2	0.4	1.2
15	Povidone-iodine (aq. Sol., w/v)	1.0	5	1.9[†]	0.8[†]
16	Peracetic acid (w/v)	0.5	5	1.9	NA

Note: NA = not available.

Source: Rotter M. Hand washing and hand disinfection [Chapter 87]. In: Mayhall CG, ed. Hospital epidemiology and infection control. 2nd ed. Philadelphia, PA: Lippincott Williams & Wilkins, 1999. Table 5 is copyrighted by Lippincott Williams & Wilkins; it is reprinted here with their permission and permission from Manfred Rotter, M.D., Professor of Hygiene and Microbiology, Klinisches Institute für Hygiene der Universitat Wien, Germany.

* Volume/volume unless otherwise stated.

[†] Tested according to Deutsche Gesellschaft fur Hygiene, and Mikrobiologic (DGHM)-German Society of Hygiene and Microbiology method.

[§] Tested according to European Standard prEN.

[¶] After 4 hours.

and may vary for different formulations. However, if hands feel dry after rubbing hands together for 10–15 seconds, an insufficient volume of product likely was applied. Because alcohol-impregnated towelettes contain a limited amount of alcohol, their effectiveness is comparable to that of soap and water (63,160,161).

Alcohol-based hand rubs intended for use in hospitals are available as low viscosity rinses, gels, and foams. Limited data are available regarding the relative efficacy of various formulations. One field trial demonstrated that an ethanol gel was slightly more effective than a comparable ethanol solution at reducing bacterial counts on the hands of HCWs (162). However, a more recent study indicated that rinses reduced bacterial counts on the hands more than the gels tested (80). Further studies are warranted to determine the relative efficacy of alcohol-based rinses and gels in reducing transmission of health-care–associated pathogens.

Frequent use of alcohol-based formulations for hand antisepsis can cause drying of the skin unless emollients, humectants, or other skin-conditioning agents are added to the formulations. The drying effect of alcohol can be reduced or eliminated by adding 1%–3% glycerol or other skin-conditioning agents (90,93,100,101,106,135,143,163,164). Moreover, in several recent prospective trials, alcohol-based rinses or gels containing emollients caused substantially less skin irritation and dryness than the soaps or antimicrobial detergents tested (96,98,165,166). These studies, which were conducted in clinical settings, used various subjective and objective methods for assessing skin irritation and dryness. Further studies are warranted to establish whether products with different formulations yield similar results.

Even well-tolerated alcohol hand rubs containing emollients may cause a transient stinging sensation at the site of any broken skin (e.g., cuts and abrasions). Alcohol-based hand-rub preparations with strong fragrances may be poorly tolerated by HCWs with respiratory allergies. Allergic contact dermatitis or contact urticaria syndrome caused by hypersensitivity to alcohol or to various additives present in certain alcohol hand rubs occurs only rarely (167,168).

Alcohols are flammable. Flash points of alcohol-based hand rubs range from 21°C to 24°C, depending on the type and concentration of alcohol present (169). As a result, alcohol-based hand rubs should be stored away from high temperatures or flames in accordance with National Fire Protection Agency recommendations. In Europe, where alcohol-based hand rubs have been used extensively for years, the incidence of fires associated with such products has been low (169). One recent U.S. report described a flash fire that occurred as a result of an unusual series of events, which included an HCW applying an alcohol gel to her hands, immediately removing a polyester isolation gown, and then touching a metal door before the alcohol had evaporated (170). Removing the polyester gown created a substantial amount of static electricity that generated an audible static spark when the HCW touched the metal door, igniting the unevaporated alcohol on her hands (170). This incident emphasizes the need to rub hands together after application of alcohol-based products until all the alcohol has evaporated.

Because alcohols are volatile, containers should be designed to minimize evaporation. Contamination of alcohol-based solutions has seldom been reported. One report documented a cluster of pseudoinfections caused by contamination of ethyl alcohol by *Bacillus cereus* spores (171).

Chlorhexidine

Chlorhexidine gluconate, a cationic bisbiguanide, was developed in England in the early 1950s and was introduced into the United States in the 1970s (8,172). Chlorhexidine base is only minimally soluble in water, but the digluconate form is water-soluble. The antimicrobial activity of chlorhexidine is likely attributable to attachment to, and subsequent disruption of, cytoplasmic membranes, resulting in precipitation of cellular contents (1,8). Chlorhexidine's immediate antimicrobial activity occurs more slowly than that of alcohols. Chlorhexidine has good activity against gram-positive bacteria, somewhat less activity against gram-negative bacteria and fungi, and only minimal activity against tubercle bacilli (1,8,172). Chlorhexidine is not sporicidal (1,172). It has in vitro activity against enveloped viruses (e.g., herpes simplex virus, HIV, cytomegalovirus, influenza, and RSV) but substantially less activity against nonenveloped viruses (e.g., rotavirus, adenovirus, and enteroviruses) (130,131,173). The antimicrobial activity of chlorhexidine is only minimally affected by the presence of organic material, including blood. Because chlorhexidine is a cationic molecule, its activity can be reduced by natural soaps, various inorganic anions, nonionic surfactants, and hand creams containing anionic emulsifying agents (8,172,174). Chlorhexidine gluconate has been incorporated into a number of hand-hygiene preparations. Aqueous or detergent formulations containing 0.5% or 0.75% chlorhexidine are more effective than plain soap, but they are less effective than antiseptic detergent preparations containing 4% chlorhexidine gluconate (135,175). Preparations with 2% chlorhexidine gluconate are slightly less effective than those containing 4% chlorhexidine (176).

Chlorhexidine has substantial residual activity (106,114–116,118,135,146,175). Addition of low concentrations (0.5%–1.0%) of chlorhexidine to alcohol-based preparations results in greater residual activity than alcohol alone (116,135). When used as recommended, chlorhexidine has a good safety record (172). Minimal, if any, absorption of the compound occurs through the skin. Care must be taken to avoid contact with the eyes when using preparations with ≥1% chlorhexidine, because the agent can cause conjunctivitis and severe corneal damage. Ototoxicity precludes its use in surgery involving the inner or middle ear. Direct contact with brain tissue and the meninges should be avoided. The frequency of skin irritation is concentration-dependent, with products containing 4% most likely to cause dermatitis when used frequently for antiseptic handwashing (177); allergic reactions to chlorhexidine gluconate are uncommon (118,172). Occasional outbreaks of nosocomial infections have been traced to contaminated solutions of chlorhexidine (178–181).

Chloroxylenol

Chloroxylenol, also known as parachlorometaxylenol (PCMX), is a halogen-substituted phenolic compound that has been used as a preservative in cosmetics and other products and as an active agent in antimicrobial soaps. It was developed in Europe in the late 1920s and has been used in the United States since the 1950s (182).

The antimicrobial activity of PCMX likely is attributable to inactivation of bacterial enzymes and alteration of cell walls (1). It has good in vitro activity against gram-positive organisms and fair activity against gram-negative bacteria, mycobacteria, and certain viruses (1,7,182). PCMX is less active against P. aeruginosa, but addition of ethylenediaminetetraacetic acid (EDTA) increases its activity against Pseudomonas spp. and other pathogens.

A limited number of articles focusing on the efficacy of PCMX-containing preparations intended for use by HCWs have been published in the last 25 years, and the results of studies have sometimes been contradictory. For example, in studies in which antiseptics were applied to abdominal skin, PCMX had the weakest immediate and residual activity of any of the agents studied (183). However, when 30-second handwashes were performed using 0.6% PCMX, 2% chlorhexidine gluconate, or 0.3% triclosan, the immediate effect of PCMX was similar to that of the other agents. When used 18 times per day for 5 consecutive days, PCMX had less cumulative activity than did chlorhexidine gluconate (184). When PCMX was used as a surgical scrub, one report indicated that 3% PCMX had immediate and residual activity comparable to 4% chlorhexidine gluconate (185), whereas two other studies demonstrated that the immediate and residual activity of PCMX was inferior to both chlorhexidine gluconate and povidone-iodine (176,186). The disparity between published studies may be associated with the various concentrations of PCMX included in the preparations evaluated and with other aspects of the formulations tested, including the

presence or absence of EDTA (7,182). PCMX is not as rapidly active as chlorhexidine gluconate or iodophors, and its residual activity is less pronounced than that observed with chlorhexidine gluconate (7,182). In 1994, FDA TFM tentatively classified PCMX as a Category IIISE active agent (i.e., insufficient data are available to classify this agent as safe and effective) (19). Further evaluation of this agent by the FDA is ongoing.

The antimicrobial activity of PCMX is minimally affected by the presence of organic matter, but it is neutralized by nonionic surfactants. PCMX, which is absorbed through the skin (7,182), is usually well-tolerated, and allergic reactions associated with its use are uncommon. PCMX is available in concentrations of 0.3%–3.75%. In-use contamination of a PCMX-containing preparation has been reported (187).

Hexachlorophene

Hexachlorophene is a bisphenol composed of two phenolic groups and three chlorine moieties. In the 1950s and early 1960s, emulsions containing 3% hexachlorophene were widely used for hygienic handwashing, as surgical scrubs, and for routine bathing of infants in hospital nurseries. The antimicrobial activity of hexachlorophene results from its ability to inactivate essential enzyme systems in microorganisms. Hexachlorophene is bacteriostatic, with good activity against S. aureus and relatively weak activity against gram-negative bacteria, fungi, and mycobacteria (7).

Studies of hexachlorophene as a hygienic handwash and surgical scrub demonstrated only modest efficacy after a single handwash (53,143,188). Hexachlorophene has residual activity for several hours after use and gradually reduces bacterial counts on hands after multiple uses (i.e., it has a cumulative effect) (1,101,188,189). With repeated use of 3% hexachlorophene preparations, the drug is absorbed through the skin. Infants bathed with hexachlorophene and personnel regularly using a 3% hexachlorophene preparation for handwashing have blood levels of 0.1–0.6 ppm hexachlorophene (190). In the early 1970s, certain infants bathed with hexachlorophene developed neurotoxicity (vacuolar degeneration) (191). As a result, in 1972, the FDA warned that hexachlorophene should no longer be used routinely for bathing infants. However, after routine use of hexachlorophene for bathing infants in nurseries was discontinued, investigators noted that the incidence of health-care–associated S. aureus infections in hospital nurseries increased substantially (192,193). In several instances, the frequency of infections decreased when hexachlorophene bathing of infants was reinstituted. However, current guidelines still recommend against the routine bathing of neonates with hexachlorophene because of its potential neurotoxic effects (194). The agent is classified by FDA TFM as not generally recognized as safe and effective for use as an antiseptic handwash (19). Hexachlorophene should not be used to bathe patients with burns or extensive areas of susceptible, sensitive skin. Soaps containing 3% hexachlorophene are available by prescription only (7).

Iodine and Iodophors

Iodine has been recognized as an effective antiseptic since the 1800s. However, because iodine often causes irritation and discoloring of skin, iodophors have largely replaced iodine as the active ingredient in antiseptics.

Iodine molecules rapidly penetrate the cell wall of microorganisms and inactivate cells by forming complexes with amino acids and unsaturated fatty acids, resulting in impaired protein synthesis and alteration of cell membranes (195). Iodophors are composed of elemental iodine, iodide or triiodide, and a polymer carrier (i.e., the complexing agent) of high molecular weight. The amount of molecular iodine present (so-called "free" iodine) determines the level of antimicrobial activity of iodophors. "Available" iodine refers to the total amount of iodine that can be titrated with sodium thiosulfate (196). Typical 10% povidone-iodine formulations contain 1% available iodine and yield free iodine concentrations of 1 ppm (196). Combining iodine with various polymers increases the solubility of iodine, promotes sustained release of iodine, and reduces skin irritation. The most common polymers incorporated into iodophors are polyvinyl pyrrolidone (i.e., povidone) and ethoxylated nonionic detergents (i.e., poloxamers) (195,196). The antimicrobial activity of iodophors also can be affected by pH, temperature, exposure time, concentration of total available iodine, and the amount and type of organic and inorganic compounds present (e.g., alcohols and detergents).

Iodine and iodophors have bactericidal activity against gram-positive, gram-negative, and certain spore-forming bacteria (e.g., clostridia and *Bacillus* spp.) and are active against mycobacteria, viruses, and fungi (8,195,197–200). However, in concentrations used in antiseptics, iodophors are not usually sporicidal (201). In vivo studies have demonstrated that iodophors reduce the number of viable organisms that are recovered from the hands of personnel (113,145,148,152,155). Povidone-iodine 5%–10% has been tentatively classified by FDA TFM as a Category I agent (i.e., a safe and effective agent for use as an antiseptic handwash and an HCW handwash) (19). The extent to which iodophors exhibit persistent antimicrobial activity after they have been washed off the skin is unclear. In one study, persistent activity was noted for 6 hours (176); however, several other studies demonstrated persistent activity for only 30–60 minutes after washing hands with an iodophor (61,117,202). In studies in which bacterial counts

were obtained after gloves were worn for 1–4 hours after washing, iodophors have demonstrated poor persistent activity (1,104,115,189,203–208). The in vivo antimicrobial activity of iodophors is substantially reduced in the presence of organic substances (e.g., blood or sputum) (8).

The majority of iodophor preparations used for hand hygiene contain 7.5%–10% povidone-iodine. Formulations with lower concentrations also have good antimicrobial activity because dilution can increase free iodine concentrations (209). However, as the amount of free iodine increases, the degree of skin irritation also may increase (209). Iodophors cause less skin irritation and fewer allergic reactions than iodine, but more irritant contact dermatitis than other antiseptics commonly used for hand hygiene (92). Occasionally, iodophor antiseptics have become contaminated with gram-negative bacilli as a result of poor manufacturing processes and have caused outbreaks or pseudo-outbreaks of infection (196).

Quaternary Ammonium Compounds

Quaternary ammonium compounds are composed of a nitrogen atom linked directly to four alkyl groups, which may vary in their structure and complexity (210). Of this large group of compounds, alkyl benzalkonium chlorides are the most widely used as antiseptics. Other compounds that have been used as antiseptics include benzethonium chloride, cetrimide, and cetylpyridium chloride (1). The antimicrobial activity of these compounds was first studied in the early 1900s, and a quaternary ammonium compound for preoperative cleaning of surgeons' hands was used as early as 1935 (210). The antimicrobial activity of this group of compounds likely is attributable to adsorption to the cytoplasmic membrane, with subsequent leakage of low molecular weight cytoplasmic constituents (210).

Quaternary ammonium compounds are primarily bacteriostatic and fungistatic, although they are microbicidal against certain organisms at high concentrations (1); they are more active against gram-positive bacteria than against gram-negative bacilli. Quaternary ammonium compounds have relatively weak activity against mycobacteria and fungi and have greater activity against lipophilic viruses. Their antimicrobial activity is adversely affected by the presence of organic material, and they are not compatible with anionic detergents (1,210). In 1994, FDA TFM tentatively classified benzalkonium chloride and benzethonium chloride as Category IIISE active agents (i.e., insufficient data exists to classify them as safe and effective for use as an antiseptic handwash) (19). Further evaluation of these agents by FDA is in progress.

Quaternary ammonium compounds are usually well tolerated. However, because of weak activity against gram-negative bacteria, benzalkonium chloride is prone to contamination by these organisms. Several outbreaks of infection or pseudoinfection have been traced to quaternary ammonium compounds contaminated with gram-negative bacilli (211–213). For this reason, in the United States, these compounds have been seldom used for hand antisepsis during the last 15–20 years. However, newer handwashing products containing benzalkonium chloride or benzethonium chloride have recently been introduced for use by HCWs. A recent study of surgical intensive-care unit personnel found that cleaning hands with antimicrobial wipes containing a quaternary ammonium compound was about as effective as using plain soap and water for handwashing; both were less effective than decontaminating hands with an alcohol-based hand rub (214). One laboratory-based study reported that an alcohol-free hand-rub product containing a quaternary ammonium compound was efficacious in reducing microbial counts on the hands of volunteers (215). Further studies of such products are needed to determine if newer formulations are effective in health-care settings.

Triclosan

Triclosan (chemical name: 2,4,4' –trichloro-2'-hydroxydiphenyl ether) is a nonionic, colorless substance that was developed in the 1960s. It has been incorporated into soaps for use by HCWs and the public and into other consumer products. Concentrations of 0.2%–2% have antimicrobial activity. Triclosan enters bacterial cells and affects the cytoplasmic membrane and synthesis of RNA, fatty acids, and proteins (216). Recent studies indicate this agent's antibacterial activity is attributable to binding to the active site of enoyl-acyl carrier protein reductase (217,218).

Triclosan has a broad range of antimicrobial activity, but it is often bacteriostatic (1). Minimum inhibitory concentrations (MICs) range from 0.1 to 10 ug/mL, whereas minimum bactericidal concentrations are 25–500 ug/mL. Triclosan's activity against gram-positive organisms (including MRSA) is greater than against gram-negative bacilli, particularly P. aeruginosa (1,216). The agent possesses reasonable activity against mycobacterial and Candida spp., but it has limited activity against filamentous fungi. Triclosan (0.1%) reduces bacterial counts on hands by 2.8 $\log_{10}$ after a 1-minute hygienic handwash (1). In several studies, log reductions have been lower after triclosan is used than when chlorhexidine, iodophors, or alcohol-based products are applied (1,61,149,184,219). In 1994, FDA TFM tentatively classified triclosan $\leq$1.0% as a Category IIISE active agent (i.e., insufficient data exist to classify this agent as safe and effective for use as an antiseptic handwash) (19). Further evaluation of this agent by the FDA is underway. Like chlorhexidine, triclosan has persistent activity on the skin. Its activity in hand-care products is affected by pH, the presence of surfactants, emollients, or humectants and by the ionic nature of the particular formulation (1,216). Triclosan's activity is not substantially affected by organic matter, but it can be inhibited by sequestration of the agent in micelle structures formed by surfactants present in certain formulations. The majority of formulations containing <2% triclosan are well-tolerated and seldom cause allergic reactions. Certain reports indicate that providing hospital personnel with a triclosan-containing preparation for hand antisepsis has led to decreased MRSA infections (72,73). Triclosan's lack of potent activity against gram-negative bacilli has resulted in occasional reports of contamination (220).

Other Agents

Approximately 150 years after puerperal-fever–related maternal mortality rates were demonstrated by Semmelweis to be reduced by use of a hypochlorite hand rinse, the efficacy of rubbing hands for 30 seconds with an aqueous hypochlorite solution was studied once again (221). The solution was demonstrated to be no more effective than distilled water. The regimen used by Semmelweis, which called for rubbing hands with a 4% [w/w] hypochlorite solution until the hands were slippery (approximately 5 minutes), has been revisited by other researchers (222). This more current study indicated that the regimen was 30 times more effective than a 1-minute rub using 60% isopropanol. However, because hypochlorite solutions are often irritating to the skin when used repeatedly and have a strong odor, they are seldom used for hand hygiene.

Certain other agents are being evaluated by FDA for use in health-care-related antiseptics (19). However, the efficacy of these agents has not been evaluated adequately for use in handwashing preparations intended for use by HCWs. Further evaluation of these agents is warranted. Products that use different concentrations of traditional antiseptics (e.g., low concentrations of iodophor) or contain novel compounds with antiseptic properties are likely to be introduced for use by HCWs. For example, preliminary studies have demonstrated that adding silver-containing polymers to an ethanol carrier (i.e., Surfacine®) results in a preparation that has persistent antimicrobial activity on animal and human skin (223). New compounds with good in vitro activity must be tested in vivo to determine their abilities to reduce transient and resident skin flora on the hands of HCWs.

Activity of Antiseptic Agents Against Spore-Forming Bacteria

The widespread prevalence of health-care–associated diarrhea caused by Clostridium difficile and the recent occurrence in the United States of human *Bacillus anthracis* infections associated with contaminated items sent through the postal system has raised concern regarding the activity of antiseptic agents against spore-forming bacteria. None of the agents (including alcohols, chlorhexidine, hexachlorophene, iodophors, PCMX, and triclosan) used in antiseptic handwash or antiseptic hand-rub preparations are reliably sporicidal against *Clostridium* spp. or *Bacillus* spp. (*120,172,224,225*). Washing hands with non-antimicrobial or antimicrobial soap and water may help to physically remove spores from the surface of contaminated hands. HCWs should be encouraged to wear gloves when caring for patients with *C. difficile*-associated diarrhea (*226*). After gloves are removed, hands should be washed with a non-antimicrobial or an antimicrobial soap and water or disinfected with an alcohol-based hand rub. During outbreaks of *C. difficile*-related infections, washing hands with a non-antimicrobial or antimicrobial soap and water after removing gloves is prudent. HCWs with suspected or documented exposure to *B. anthracis*-contaminated items also should be encouraged to wash their hands with a non-antimicrobial or antimicrobial soap and water.

Reduced Susceptibility of Bacteria to Antiseptics

Reduced susceptibility of bacteria to antiseptic agents can either be an intrinsic characteristic of a species or can be an acquired trait (*227*). Several reports have described strains of bacteria that appear to have acquired reduced susceptibility (when defined by MICs established in vitro) to certain antiseptics (e.g., chlorhexidine, quaternary ammonium compounds, and triclosan) (*227–230*). However, because the antiseptic concentrations that are actually used by HCWs are often substantially higher than the MICs of strains with reduced antiseptic susceptibility, the clinical relevance of the in vitro findings is questionable. For example, certain strains of MRSA have chlorhexidine and quaternary ammonium compound MICs that are several-fold higher than methicillin-susceptible strains, and certain strains of *S. aureus* have elevated MICs to triclosan (*227,228*). However, such strains were readily inhibited by the concentrations of these antiseptics that are actually used by practicing HCWs (*227,228*). The description of a triclosan-resistant bacterial enzyme has raised the question of whether resistance to this agent may develop more readily than to other antiseptic agents (*218*). In addition, exposing *Pseudomonas* strains containing the MexAB-OprM efflux system to triclosan may select for mutants that are resistant to multiple antibiotics, including fluoroquinolones (*230*). Further studies are needed to determine whether reduced susceptibility to antiseptic agents is of epidemiologic significance and whether resistance to antiseptics has any influence on the prevalence of antibiotic-resistant strains (*227*).

Surgical Hand Antisepsis

Since the late 1800s, when Lister promoted the application of carbolic acid to the hands of surgeons before procedures, preoperative cleansing of hands and forearms with an antiseptic agent has been an accepted practice (*231*). Although no randomized, controlled trials have been conducted to indicate that surgical-site infection rates are substantially lower when preoperative scrubbing is performed with an antiseptic agent rather than a non-antimicrobial soap, certain other factors provide a strong rationale for this practice. Bacteria on the hands of surgeons can cause wound infections if introduced into the operative field during surgery (*232*); rapid multiplication of bacteria occurs under surgical gloves if hands are washed with a non-antimicrobial soap. However, bacterial growth is slowed after preoperative scrubbing with an antiseptic agent (*14,233*). Reducing resident skin flora on the hands of the surgical team for the duration of a procedure reduces the risk of bacteria being released into the surgical field if gloves become punctured or torn during surgery (*1,156,169*). Finally, at least one outbreak of surgical-site infections occurred when surgeons who normally used an antiseptic surgical scrub preparation began using a non-antimicrobial product (*234*).

Antiseptic preparations intended for use as surgical hand scrubs are evaluated for their ability to reduce the number of bacteria released from hands at different times, including 1) immediately after scrubbing, 2) after wearing surgical gloves for 6 hours (i.e., persistent activity), and 3) after multiple applications over 5 days (i.e., cumulative activity). Immediate and persistent activity are considered the most important in determining the efficacy of the product. U.S. guidelines recommend that agents used for surgical hand scrubs should substantially reduce microorganisms on intact skin, contain a nonirritating antimicrobial preparation, have broad-spectrum activity, and be fast-acting and persistent (*19,235*).

Studies have demonstrated that formulations containing 60%–95% alcohol alone or 50%–95% when combined with limited amounts of a quaternary ammonium compound, hexachlorophene, or chlorhexidine gluconate, lower bacterial counts on the skin immediately postscrub more effectively than do other agents (Table 4). The next most active agents (in order of decreasing activity) are chlorhexidine gluconate, iodophors, triclosan, and plain soap (*104,119,186,188, 203,204,206,208,236*). Because studies of PCMX as a surgical scrub have yielded contradictory results, further studies are needed to establish how the efficacy of this compound compares with the other agents (*176,185,186*).

Although alcohols are not considered to have persistent antimicrobial activity, bacteria appear to reproduce slowly on the hands after a surgical scrub with alcohol, and bacterial counts on hands after wearing gloves for 1–3 hours seldom exceed baseline (i.e., prescrub) values (*1*). However, a recent study demonstrated that a formulation containing 61% ethanol alone did not achieve adequate persistent activity at 6 hours postscrub (*237*). Alcohol-based preparations containing 0.5% or 1% chlorhexidine gluconate have persistent activity that, in certain studies, has equaled or exceeded that of chlorhexidine gluconate-containing detergents (*1,118,135,237*).*

Persistent antimicrobial activity of detergent-based surgical scrub formulations is greatest for those containing 2% or 4% chlorhexidine gluconate, followed by hexachlorophene, triclosan, and iodophors (*1,102,113–115,159,189,203, 204,206–208,236*). Because hexachlorophene is absorbed into the blood after repeated use, it is seldom used as a surgical scrub.

Surgical staff have been traditionally required to scrub their hands for 10 minutes preoperatively, which frequently leads to skin damage. Several studies have demonstrated that scrubbing for 5 minutes reduces bacterial counts as effectively as a 10-minute scrub (*117,238,239*). In other studies, scrubbing for 2 or 3 minutes reduced bacterial counts to acceptable levels (*156,205,207,240,241*).

Studies have indicated that a two-stage surgical scrub using an antiseptic detergent, followed by application of an alcohol-containing preparation, is effective. For example, an initial 1- or 2-minute scrub with 4% chlorhexidine gluconate or povidone-iodine followed by application of an alcohol-based product has been as effective as a 5-minute scrub with an antiseptic detergent (*114,242*).

Surgical hand-antisepsis protocols have required personnel to scrub with a brush. But this practice can damage the skin of personnel and result in increased shedding of bacteria from the hands (*95,243*). Scrubbing with a disposable sponge or combination sponge-brush has reduced bacterial counts on the hands as effectively as scrubbing with a brush (*244–246*). However, several studies indicate that neither a brush nor a sponge is necessary to reduce bacterial counts on the hands of surgical personnel to acceptable levels, especially when alcohol-based products are used (*102,117,159,165,233,237, 247,248*). Several of these studies performed cultures immediately or at 45–60 minutes postscrub (*102,117, 233,247,248*), whereas in other studies, cultures were obtained 3 and 6 hours postscrub (*159,237*). For example, a recent laboratory-based study using volunteers demonstrated that brushless application of a preparation containing 1% chlorhexidine gluconate plus 61% ethanol yielded lower bacterial counts on the hands of participants than using a sponge/brush to apply a 4% chlorhexidine-containing detergent preparation (*237*).

Relative Efficacy of Plain Soap, Antiseptic Soap/Detergent, and Alcohols

Comparing studies related to the in vivo efficacy of plain soap, antimicrobial soaps, and alcohol-based hand rubs is problematic, because certain studies express efficacy as the percentage reduction in bacterial counts achieved, whereas others give $\log_{10}$ reductions in counts achieved. However, summarizing the relative efficacy of agents tested in each study can provide an overview of the in vivo activity of various formulations intended for handwashing, hygienic handwash, antiseptic hand rub, or surgical hand antisepsis (Tables 2–4).

Irritant Contact Dermatitis Resulting from Hand-Hygiene Measures

Frequency and Pathophysiology of Irritant Contact Dermatitis

In certain surveys, approximately 25% of nurses report symptoms or signs of dermatitis involving their hands, and as many as 85% give a history of having skin problems (*249*). Frequent and repeated use of hand-hygiene products, particularly soaps and other detergents, is a primary cause of chronic irritant contact dermatitis among HCWs (*250*). The potential of detergents to cause skin irritation can vary considerably and can be ameliorated by the addition of emollients and humectants. Irritation associated with antimicrobial soaps may be caused by the antimicrobial agent or by other ingredients of the formulation. Affected persons often complain of a feeling of dryness or burning; skin that feels "rough;" and erythema, scaling, or fissures. Detergents damage the skin by causing denaturation of stratum corneum proteins, changes in intercellular lipids (either depletion or reorganization of lipid moieties), decreased corneocyte cohesion, and decreased stratum corneum water-binding capacity (*250,251*). Damage

---

* In a recent randomized clinical trial, surgical site infection rates were monitored among patients who were operated on by surgical personnel who cleaned their hands preoperatively either by performing a traditional 5-minute surgical hand scrub using 4% povidone-iodine or 4% antisepsis antimicrobial soap, or by washing their hands for 1 minute with a non-antimicrobial soap followed by a 5-minute hand-rubbing technique using an alcohol-based hand rinse containing 0.2% mecetronium etilsulfate. The incidence of surgical site infections was virtually identical in the two groups of patients. (Source: Parienti JJ, Thibon P, Heller R, et al. for Members of the Antisepsie Chirurgicale des Mains Study Group. Hand-rubbing with an aqueous alcoholic solution vs traditional surgical hand-scrubbing and 30-day surgical site infection rates: a randomized equivalence study. JAMA 2002;288:722–7).

to the skin also changes skin flora, resulting in more frequent colonization by staphylococci and gram-negative bacilli (17,90). Although alcohols are among the safest antiseptics available, they can cause dryness and irritation of the skin (1,252). Ethanol is usually less irritating than n-propanol or isopropanol (252).

Irritant contact dermatitis is more commonly reported with iodophors (92). Other antiseptic agents that can cause irritant contact dermatitis (in order of decreasing frequency) include chlorhexidine, PCMX, triclosan, and alcohol-based products. Skin that is damaged by repeated exposure to detergents may be more susceptible to irritation by alcohol-based preparations (253). The irritancy potential of commercially prepared hand-hygiene products, which is often determined by measuring transepidermal water loss, may be available from the manufacturer. Other factors that can contribute to dermatitis associated with frequent handwashing include using hot water for handwashing, low relative humidity (most common in winter months), failure to use supplementary hand lotion or cream, and the quality of paper towels (254,255). Shear forces associated with wearing or removing gloves and allergy to latex proteins may also contribute to dermatitis of the hands of HCWs.

Allergic Contact Dermatitis Associated with Hand-Hygiene Products

Allergic reactions to products applied to the skin (i.e., contact allergies) may present as delayed type reactions (i.e., allergic contact dermatitis) or less commonly as immediate reactions (i.e., contact urticaria). The most common causes of contact allergies are fragrances and preservatives; emulsifiers are less common causes (256–259). Liquid soaps, hand lotions or creams, and "udder ointments" may contain ingredients that cause contact allergies among HCWs (257,258).

Allergic reactions to antiseptic agents, including quaternary ammonium compounds, iodine or iodophors, chlorhexidine, triclosan, PCMX, and alcohols have been reported (118,167,172,256,260–265). Allergic contact dermatitis associated with alcohol-based hand rubs is uncommon. Surveillance at a large hospital in Switzerland, where a commercial alcohol hand rub has been used for >10 years, failed to identify a single case of documented allergy to the product (169). In late 2001, a Freedom of Information Request for data in the FDA's Adverse Event Reporting System regarding adverse reactions to popular alcohol hand rubs in the United States yielded only one reported case of an erythematous rash reaction attributed to such a product (John M. Boyce, M.D., Hospital of St. Raphael, New Haven, Connecticut, personal communication, 2001). However, with increasing use of such products by HCWs, true allergic reactions to such products likely will be encountered.

Allergic reactions to alcohol-based products may represent true allergy to alcohol, allergy to an impurity or aldehyde metabolite, or allergy to another constituent of the product (167). Allergic contact dermatitis or immediate contact urticarial reactions may be caused by ethanol or isopropanol (167). Allergic reactions can be caused by compounds that may be present as inactive ingredients in alcohol-based hand rubs, including fragrances, benzyl alcohol, stearyl or isostearyl alcohol, phenoxyethanol, myristyl alcohol, propylene glycol, parabens, and benzalkonium chloride (167,256,266–270).

Proposed Methods for Reducing Adverse Effects of Agents

Potential strategies for minimizing hand-hygiene–related irritant contact dermatitis among HCWs include reducing the frequency of exposure to irritating agents (particularly anionic detergents), replacing products with high irritation potential with preparations that cause less damage to the skin, educating personnel regarding the risks of irritant contact dermatitis, and providing caregivers with moisturizing skin-care products or barrier creams (96,98,251,271–273). Reducing the frequency of exposure of HCWs to hand-hygiene products would prove difficult and is not desirable because of the low levels of adherence to hand-hygiene policies in the majority of institutions. Although hospitals have provided personnel with non-antimicrobial soaps in hopes of minimizing dermatitis, frequent use of such products may cause greater skin damage, dryness, and irritation than antiseptic preparations (92,96,98). One strategy for reducing the exposure of personnel to irritating soaps and detergents is to promote the use of alcohol-based hand rubs containing various emollients. Several recent prospective, randomized trials have demonstrated that alcohol-based hand rubs containing emollients were better tolerated by HCWs than washing hands with non-antimicrobial soaps or antimicrobial soaps (96,98,166). Routinely washing hands with soap and water immediately after using an alcohol hand rub may lead to dermatitis. Therefore, personnel should be reminded that it is neither necessary nor recommended to routinely wash hands after each application of an alcohol hand rub.

Hand lotions and creams often contain humectants and various fats and oils that can increase skin hydration and replace altered or depleted skin lipids that contribute to the barrier function of normal skin (251,271). Several controlled trials have demonstrated that regular use (e.g., twice a day) of such products can help prevent and treat irritant contact dermatitis caused by hand-hygiene products (272,273). In one study, frequent and scheduled use of an oil-containing lotion improved skin condition, and thus led to a 50% increase in handwashing frequency among HCWs (273). Reports from these studies emphasize the need to educate personnel regarding the value of regular, frequent use of hand-care products.

Recently, barrier creams have been marketed for the prevention of hand-hygiene–related irritant contact dermatitis. Such products are absorbed to the superficial layers of the epidermis and are designed to form a protective layer that is not removed by standard handwashing. Two recent randomized, controlled trials that evaluated the skin condition of caregivers demonstrated that barrier creams did not yield better results than did the control lotion or vehicle used (272,273). As a result, whether barrier creams are effective in preventing irritant contact dermatitis among HCWs remains unknown.

In addition to evaluating the efficacy and acceptability of hand-care products, product-selection committees should inquire about the potential deleterious effects that oil-containing products may have on the integrity of rubber gloves and on the efficacy of antiseptic agents used in the facility (8,236).

Factors To Consider When Selecting Hand-Hygiene Products

When evaluating hand-hygiene products for potential use in health-care facilities, administrators or product-selection committees must consider factors that can affect the overall efficacy of such products, including the relative efficacy of antiseptic agents against various pathogens (Appendix) and acceptance of hand-hygiene products by personnel (274,275). Soap products that are not well-accepted by HCWs can be a deterrent to frequent handwashing (276). Characteristics of a product (either soap or alcohol-based hand rub) that can affect acceptance by personnel include its smell, consistency (i.e., "feel"), and color (92,277,278). For soaps, ease of lathering also may affect user preference.

Because HCWs may wash their hands from a limited number of times per shift to as many as 30 times per shift, the tendency of products to cause skin irritation and dryness is a substantial factor that influences acceptance, and ultimate usage (61,98,274,275,277,279). For example, concern regarding the drying effects of alcohol was a primary cause of poor acceptance of alcohol-based hand-hygiene products in hospitals in the United States (5,143). However, several studies have demonstrated that alcohol-based hand rubs containing emollients are acceptable to HCWs (90,93,98,100,101,106, 143,163,164,166). With alcohol-based products, the time required for drying may also affect user acceptance.

Studies indicate that the frequency of handwashing or antiseptic handwashing by personnel is affected by the accessibility of hand-hygiene facilities (280–283). In certain health-care facilities, only one sink is available in rooms housing several patients, or sinks are located far away from the door of the room, which may discourage handwashing by personnel leaving the room. In intensive-care units, access to sinks may be blocked by bedside equipment (e.g., ventilators or intravenous infusion pumps). In contrast to sinks used for handwashing or antiseptic handwash, dispensers for alcohol-based hand rubs do not require plumbing and can be made available adjacent to each patient's bed and at many other locations in patient-care areas. Pocket carriage of alcohol-based hand-rub solutions, combined with availability of bedside dispensers, has been associated with substantial improvement in adherence to hand-hygiene protocols (74,284). To avoid any confusion between soap and alcohol hand rubs, alcohol hand-rub dispensers should not be placed adjacent to sinks. HCWs should be informed that washing hands with soap and water after each use of an alcohol hand rub is not necessary and is not recommended, because it may lead to dermatitis. However, because personnel feel a "build-up" of emollients on their hands after repeated use of alcohol hand gels, washing hands with soap and water after 5–10 applications of a gel has been recommended by certain manufacturers.

Automated handwashing machines have not been demonstrated to improve the quality or frequency of handwashing (88,285). Although technologically advanced automated handwashing devices and monitoring systems have been developed recently, only a minimal number of studies have been published that demonstrate that use of such devices results in enduring improvements in hand-hygiene adherence among HCWs. Further evaluation of automated handwashing facilities and monitoring systems is warranted.

Dispenser systems provided by manufacturers or vendors also must be considered when evaluating hand-hygiene products. Dispensers may discourage use by HCWs when they 1) become blocked or partially blocked and do not deliver the product when accessed by personnel, and 2) do not deliver the product appropriately onto the hands. In one hospital where a viscous alcohol-based hand rinse was available, only 65% of functioning dispensers delivered product onto the caregivers' hands with one press of the dispenser lever, and 9% of dispensers were totally occluded (286). In addition, the volume delivered was often suboptimal, and the product was sometimes squirted onto the wall instead of the caregiver's hand.

Only limited information is available regarding the cost of hand-hygiene products used in health-care facilities (165,287). These costs were evaluated in patient-care areas at a 450-bed community teaching hospital (287); the hospital spent $22,000 ($0.72 per patient-day) on 2% chlorhexidine-containing preparations, plain soap, and an alcohol hand rinse. (287) When hand-hygiene supplies for clinics and nonpatient care areas were included, the total annual budget for soaps and hand antiseptic agents was $30,000 (approximately $1 per patient-day). Annual hand-hygiene product budgets at other institutions vary considerably because of differences in usage patterns and varying product prices. One researcher (*287*) determined that if non-antimicrobial liquid soap were assigned an arbitrary relative cost of 1.0, the cost per liter would be 1.7 times as much for 2% chlorhexidine gluconate detergent, 1.6–2.0 times higher for alcohol-based hand-rub products, and 4.5 times higher for an alcohol-based foam product. A recent cost comparison of surgical scrubbing with an antimicrobial soap versus brushless scrubbing with an alcohol-based hand rub revealed that costs and time required for preoperative scrubbing were less with the alcohol-based product (*165*). In a trial conducted in two critical-care units, the cost of using an alcohol hand rub was half as much as using an antimicrobial soap for handwashing ($0.025 versus $0.05 per application, respectively) (*166*).

To put expenditures for hand-hygiene products into perspective, health-care facilities should consider comparing their budget for hand-hygiene products to estimated excess hospital costs resulting from health-care–associated infections. The excess hospital costs associated with only four or five health-care–associated infections of average severity may equal the entire annual budget for hand-hygiene products used in inpatient-care areas. Just one severe surgical site infection, lower respiratory tract infection, or bloodstream infection may cost the hospital more than the entire annual budget for antiseptic agents used for hand hygiene (*287*). Two studies provided certain quantitative estimates of the benefit of hand-hygiene–promotion programs (*72,74*). One study demonstrated a cost saving of approximately $17,000 resulting from reduced use of vancomycin after the observed decrease in MRSA incidence in a 7-month period (*72*). In another study that examined both direct costs associated with the hand-hygiene promotion program (increased use of hand-rub solution and poster production) and indirect costs associated with health-care–personnel time (*74*), costs of the program were an estimated $57,000 or less per year (an average of $1.42 per patient admitted). Supplementary costs associated with the increased use of alcohol-based hand-rub solution averaged $6.07 per 100 patient-days. Based on conservative estimates of $2,100 saved per infection averted and on the assumption that only 25% of the observed reduction in the infection rate was associated with improved hand-hygiene practice, the program was substantially cost-effective. Thus, hospital administrators must consider that by purchasing more effective or more acceptable hand-hygiene products to improve hand-hygiene practices, they

will avoid the occurrence of nosocomial infections; preventing only a limited number of additional health-care–associated infections per year will lead to savings that will exceed any incremental costs of improved hand-hygiene products.

Hand-Hygiene Practices Among HCWs

In observational studies conducted in hospitals, HCWs washed their hands an average of five times per shift to as many as 30 times per shift (Table 6) (*17,61,90,98,274,288*); certain nurses washed their hands ≤100 times per shift (*90*). Hospitalwide surveillance of hand hygiene reveals that the average number of handwashing opportunities varies markedly between hospital wards. For example, nurses in pediatric wards had an average of eight opportunities for hand hygiene per hour of patient care compared with an average of 20 for nurses in intensive-care units (*11*). The duration of handwashing or hygienic handwash episodes by HCWs has averaged 6.6–24.0 seconds in observational studies (Table 7) (*17,52,59,84–87,89,249,279*). In addition to washing their

TABLE 6. Handwashing frequency among health-care workers

Ref. no.	Year	Avg. no./ time period	Range	Avg. no./hr
(*61*)	1988	5/8 hour	N.S.	
(*89*)	1984	5–10/shift	N.S.	
(*96*)	2000	10/shift	N.S.	
(*273*)	2000	12–18/day	2–60	
(*98*)	2000	13–15/8 hours	5–27	1.6–1.8/hr
(*90*)	1977	20–42/8 hours	10–100	
(*391*)	2000	21/12 hours	N.S.	
(*272*)	2000	22/day	0–70	
(*88*)	1991			1.7–2.1/hr
(*17*)	1998			2.1/hr
(*279*)	1978			3/hr
(*303*)	1994			3.3/hr

Note: N.S. = Not Stated.

TABLE 7. Average duration of handwashing by health-care workers

Ref. no.	Year	Mean/median time
(*392*)	1997	4.7–5.3 seconds
(*303*)	1994	6.6 seconds
(*52*)	1974	8–9.3 seconds
(*85*)	1984	8.6 seconds
(*86*)	1994	<9 seconds
(*87*)	1994	9.5 seconds
(*88*)	1991	<10 seconds
(*294*)	1990	10 seconds
(*89*)	1984	11.6 seconds
(*300*)	1992	12.5 seconds
(*59*)	1988	15.6–24.4 seconds
(*17*)	1998	20.6 seconds
(*279*)	1978	21 seconds
(*293*)	1989	24 seconds

hands for limited time periods, personnel often fail to cover all surfaces of their hands and fingers (288).

Adherence of HCWs to Recommended Hand-Hygiene Practices

Observational Studies of Hand-Hygiene Adherence. Adherence of HCWs to recommended hand-hygiene procedures has been poor, with mean baseline rates of 5%–81% (overall average: 40%) (Table 8) (71,74,86,87,276,280,281,283,285, 289–313). The methods used for defining adherence (or nonadherence) and those used for conducting observations vary considerably among studies, and reports do not provide detailed information concerning the methods and criteria used. The majority of studies were conducted with hand-hygiene adherence as the major outcome measure, whereas a limited number measured adherence as part of a broader investigation. Several investigators reported improved adherence after implementing various interventions, but the majority of studies had short follow-up periods and did not confirm whether behavioral improvements were long-lasting. Other studies established that sustained improvements in handwashing behavior occurred during a long-term program to improve adherence to hand-hygiene policies (74,75).

TABLE 8. Hand-hygiene adherence by health-care workers (1981–2000)

Ref. no.	Year	Setting	Before/ after	Adherence baseline	Adherence after intervention	Invervention
(280)	1981	ICU	A	16%	30%	More convenient sink locations
(289)	1981	ICU	A	41%	—	
		ICU	A	28%	—	
(290)	1983	All wards	A	45%	—	
(281)	1986	SICU	A	51%	—	
		MICU	A	76%	—	
(276)	1986	ICU	A	63%	92%	Performance feedback
(291)	1987	PICU	A	31%	30%	Wearing overgown
(292)	1989	MICU	B/A	14%/28%*	73%/81%	Feedback, policy reviews, memo, and posters
		MICU	B/A	26%/23%	38%/60%	
(293)	1989	NICU	A/B	75%/50%	—	
(294)	1990	ICU	A	32%	45%	Alcohol rub introduced
(295)	1990	ICU	A	81%	92%	Inservices first, then group feedback
(296)	1990	ICU	B/A	22%	30%	
(297)	1991	SICU	A	51%	—	
(298)	1991	Pedi OPDs	B	49%	49%	Signs, feedback, and verbal reminders to physicians
(299)	1991	Nursery and NICU	B/A†	28%	63%	Feedback, dissemination of literature, and results of environmental cultures
(300)	1992	NICU/others	A	29%	—	
(71)	1992	ICU	N.S.	40%	—	
(301)	1993	ICUs	A	40%	—	
(87)	1994	Emergency Room	A	32%	—	
(86)	1994	All wards	A	32%	—	
(285)	1994	SICU	A	22%	38%	Automated handwashing machines available
(302)	1994	NICU	A	62%	60%	No gowning required
(303)	1994	ICU Wards	AA	30%29%	—	
(304)	1995	ICU Oncol Ward	A	56%	—	
(305)	1995	ICU	N.S.	5%	63%	Lectures, feedback, and demonstrations
(306)	1996	PICU	B/A	12%/11%	68%/65%	Overt observation, followed by feedback
(307)	1996	MICU	A	41%	58%	Routine wearing of gowns and gloves
(308)	1996	Emergency Dept	A	54%	64%	Signs/distributed review paper
(309)	1998	All wards	A	30%	—	
(310)	1998	Pediatric wards	B/A	52%/49%	74%/69%	Feedback, movies, posters, and brochures
(311)	1999	MICU	B/A	12%/55%	—	
(74)	2000	All wards	B/A	48%	67%	Posters, feedback, administrative support, and alcohol rub
(312)	2000	MICU	A	42%	61%	Alcohol hand rub made available
(283)	2000	MICU	B/A	10%/22%	23%/48%	Education, feedback, and alcohol gel made available
		CTICU	B/A	4%/13%	7%/14%	
(313)	2000	Medical wards	A	60%	52%	Education, reminders, and alcohol gel made available

Note: ICU = intensive care unit, SICU = surgical ICU, MICU = medical ICU, PICU = pediatric ICU, NICU = neonatal ICU, Emerg = emergency, Oncol = oncology, CTICU = cardiothoracic ICU, and N.S. = not stated.
* Percentage compliance before/after patient contact.
† After contact with inanimate objects.

Factors Affecting Adherence. Factors that may influence hand hygiene include those identified in epidemiologic studies and factors reported by HCWs as being reasons for lack of adherence to hand-hygiene recommendations. Risk factors for poor adherence to hand hygiene have been determined objectively in several observational studies or interventions to improve adherence (11,12,274,292,295,314–317). Among these, being a physician or a nursing assistant, rather than a nurse, was consistently associated with reduced adherence (Box 1).

In the largest hospitalwide survey of hand-hygiene practices among HCWs (11), predictors of poor adherence to recommended hand-hygiene measures were identified. Predictor variables included professional category, hospital ward, time of day/week, and type and intensity of patient care, defined as the number of opportunities for hand hygiene per hour of patient care. In 2,834 observed opportunities for hand hygiene, average adherence was 48%. In multivariate analysis, nonadherence was lowest among nurses and during weekends

BOX 1. Factors influencing adherence to hand-hygiene practices*

Observed risk factors for poor adherence to recommended hand-hygiene practices
- Physician status (rather than a nurse)
- Nursing assistant status (rather than a nurse)
- Male sex
- Working in an intensive-care unit
- Working during the week (versus the weekend)
- Wearing gowns/gloves
- Automated sink
- Activities with high risk of cross-transmission
- High number of opportunities for hand hygiene per hour of patient care

Self-reported factors for poor adherence with hand hygiene
- Handwashing agents cause irritation and dryness
- Sinks are inconveniently located/shortage of sinks
- Lack of soap and paper towels
- Often too busy/insufficient time
- Understaffing/overcrowding
- Patient needs take priority
- Hand hygiene interferes with health-care worker relationships with patients
- Low risk of acquiring infection from patients
- Wearing of gloves/beliefs that glove use obviates the need for hand hygiene
- Lack of knowledge of guidelines/protocols
- Not thinking about it/forgetfulness
- No role model from colleagues or superiors
- Skepticism regarding the value of hand hygiene
- Disagreement with the recommendations
- Lack of scientific information of definitive impact of improved hand hygiene on health-care–associated infection rates

Additional perceived barriers to appropriate hand hygiene
- Lack of active participation in hand-hygiene promotion at individual or institutional level
- Lack of role model for hand hygiene
- Lack of institutional priority for hand hygiene
- Lack of administrative sanction of noncompliers/rewarding compliers
- Lack of institutional safety climate

---

* **Source:** Adapted from Pittet D. Improving compliance with hand hygiene in hospitals. Infect Control Hosp Epidemiol 2000;21:381–6.

(Odds Ratio [OR]: 0.6; 95% confidence interval [CI] = 0.4–0.8). Nonadherence was higher in intensive-care units compared with internal medicine wards (OR: 2.0; 95% CI = 1.3–3.1), during procedures that carried a high risk of bacterial contamination (OR: 1.8; 95% CI = 1.4–2.4), and when intensity of patient care was high (21–40 handwashing opportunities — OR: 1.3; 95% CI = 1.0-1.7; 41–60 opportunities — OR: 2.1; 95% CI = 1.5-2.9; >60 opportunities — OR: 2.1; 95% CI = 1.3–3.5). The higher the demand for hand hygiene, the lower the adherence; on average, adherence decreased by 5% (± 2%) for each increase of 10 opportunities per hour when the intensity of patient care exceeded 10 opportunities per hour. Similarly, the lowest adherence rate (36%) was found in intensive-care units, where indications for hand hygiene were typically more frequent (on average, 20 opportunities per patient-hour). The highest adherence rate (59%) was observed in pediatrics wards, where the average intensity of patient care was lower than in other hospital areas (an average of eight opportunities per patient-hour). The results of this study indicate that full adherence to previous guidelines may be unrealistic, and that facilitated access to hand hygiene could help improve adherence (11,12,318).

Perceived barriers to adherence with hand-hygiene practice recommendations include skin irritation caused by hand-hygiene agents, inaccessible hand-hygiene supplies, interference with HCW-patient relationships, priority of care (i.e., the patients' needs are given priority over hand hygiene), wearing of gloves, forgetfulness, lack of knowledge of the guidelines, insufficient time for hand hygiene, high workload and understaffing, and the lack of scientific information indicating a definitive impact of improved hand hygiene on health-care–associated infection rates (11,274,292,295,315–317). Certain perceived barriers to adherence with hand-hygiene guidelines have been assessed or quantified in observational studies (12,274,292,295,314–317) (Box 1).

Skin irritation by hand-hygiene agents constitutes a substantial barrier to appropriate adherence (319). Because soaps and detergents can damage skin when applied on a regular basis, HCWs must be better informed regarding the possible adverse effects associated with hand-hygiene agents. Lack of knowledge and education regarding this subject is a barrier to motivation. In several studies, alcohol-based hand rubs containing emollients (either isopropanol, ethanol, or n-propanol in 60%–90% vol/vol) were less irritating to the skin than the soaps or detergents tested. In addition, the alcohol-based products containing emollients that were tested were at least as tolerable and efficacious as the detergents tested. Also, studies demonstrate that several hand lotions have reduced skin scaling and cracking, which may reduce microbial shedding from the hands (67,272,273).

Easy access to hand-hygiene supplies, whether sink, soap, medicated detergent, or alcohol-based hand-rub solution, is essential for optimal adherence to hand-hygiene recommendations. The time required for nurses to leave a patient's bedside, go to a sink, and wash and dry their hands before attending the next patient is a deterrent to frequent handwashing or hand antisepsis (11,318). Engineering controls could facilitate adherence, but careful monitoring of hand-hygiene behavior should be conducted to exclude the possible negative effect of newly introduced handwashing devices (88).

The impact of wearing gloves on adherence to hand-hygiene policies has not been definitively established, because published studies have yielded contradictory results (87,290,301,320). Hand hygiene is required regardless of whether gloves are used or changed. Failure to remove gloves after patient contact or between "dirty" and "clean" body-site care on the same patient must be regarded as nonadherence to hand-hygiene recommendations (11). In a study in which experimental conditions approximated those occurring in clinical practice (321), washing and reusing gloves between patient contacts resulted in observed bacterial counts of 0–4.7 log on the hands after glove removal. Therefore, this practice should be discouraged; handwashing or disinfection should be performed after glove removal.

Lack of 1) knowledge of guidelines for hand hygiene, 2) recognition of hand-hygiene opportunities during patient care, and 3) awareness of the risk of cross-transmission of pathogens are barriers to good hand-hygiene practices. Furthermore, certain HCWs believe they have washed their hands when necessary, even when observations indicate they have not (89,92,295,296,322).

Perceived barriers to hand-hygiene behavior are linked not only to the institution, but also to HCWs' colleagues. Therefore, both institutional and small-group dynamics need to be considered when implementing a system change to secure an improvement in HCWs' hand-hygiene practice.

Possible Targets for Hand-Hygiene Promotion

Targets for the promotion of hand hygiene are derived from studies assessing risk factors for nonadherence, reported reasons for the lack of adherence to recommendations, and additional factors perceived as being important to facilitate appropriate HCW behavior. Although certain factors cannot be modified (Box 1), others can be changed.

One factor that must be addressed is the time required for HCWs to clean their hands. The time required for traditional handwashing may render full adherence to previous guidelines unrealistic (11,12,318) and more rapid access to hand-hygiene materials could help improve adherence. One study conducted in an intensive-care unit demonstrated that it took nurses an average of 62 seconds to leave a patient's bedside, walk to a sink, wash their hands, and return to patient care (*318*). In contrast, an estimated one fourth as much time is required when using alcohol-based hand rub placed at each patient's bedside. Providing easy access to hand-hygiene materials is mandatory for appropriate hand-hygiene behavior and is achievable in the majority of health-care facilities (*323*). In particular, in high-demand situations (e.g., the majority of critical-care units), under hectic working conditions, and at times of overcrowding or understaffing, HCWs may be more likely to use an alcohol-based hand rub than to wash their hands (*323*). Further, using alcohol-based hand rubs may be a better option than traditional handwashing with plain soap and water or antiseptic handwash, because they not only require less time (*166,318*) but act faster (*1*) and irritate hands less often (*1,67,96,98,166*). They also were used in the only program that reported a sustained improvement in hand-hygiene adherence associated with decreased infection rates (*74*). However, making an alcohol-based hand rub available to personnel without providing ongoing educational and motivational activities may not result in long-lasting improvement in hand-hygiene practices (*313*). Because increased use of hand-hygiene agents might be associated with skin dryness, the availability of free skin-care lotion is recommended.

Education is a cornerstone for improvement with hand-hygiene practices. Topics that must be addressed by educational programs include the lack of 1) scientific information for the definitive impact of improved hand hygiene on health-care–associated infection and resistant organism transmission rates; 2) awareness of guidelines for hand hygiene and insufficient knowledge concerning indications for hand hygiene during daily patient care; 3) knowledge concerning the low average adherence rate to hand hygiene by the majority of HCWs; and 4) knowledge concerning the appropriateness, efficacy, and understanding of the use of hand-hygiene and skin-care–protection agents.

HCWs necessarily evolve within a group that functions within an institution. Possible targets for improvement in hand-hygiene behavior not only include factors linked to individual HCWs, but also those related to the group(s) and the institution as a whole (*317,323*). Examples of possible targets for hand-hygiene promotion at the group level include education and performance feedback on hand-hygiene adherence; efforts to prevent high workload, downsizing, and understaffing; and encouragement and provision of role models from key members in the work unit. At the institutional level, targets for improvement include 1) written guidelines, hand-hygiene agents, skin-care promotions and agents, or hand-hygiene facilities; 2) culture or tradition of adherence; and 3)

administrative leadership, sanction, support, and rewards. Several studies, conducted in various types of institutions, reported modest and even low levels of adherence to recommended hand-hygiene practices, indicating that such adherence varied by hospital ward and by type of HCW. These results indicate educational sessions may need to be designed specifically for certain types of personnel (*11,289,290,294,317,323*).

Lessons Learned from Behavioral Theories

In 1998, the prevailing behavioral theories and their applications with regard to the health professions were reviewed by researchers in an attempt to better understand how to target more successful interventions (*317*). The researchers proposed a hypothetical framework to enhance hand-hygiene practices and stressed the importance of considering the complexity of individual and institutional factors when designing behavioral interventions.

Although behavioral theories and secondary interventions have primarily targeted individual workers, this practice might be insufficient to produce sustained change (*317,324,325*). Interventions aimed at improving hand-hygiene practices must account for different levels of behavior interaction (*12,317,326*). Thus, the interdependence of individual factors, environmental constraints, and the institutional climate must be taken into account in the strategic planning and development of hand-hygiene campaigns. Interventions to promote hand hygiene in hospitals should consider variables at all these levels. Various factors involved in hand-hygiene behavior include intention, attitude towards the behavior, perceived social norm, perceived behavioral control, perceived risk for infection, hand-hygiene practices, perceived role model, perceived knowledge, and motivation (*317*). The factors necessary for change include 1) dissatisfaction with the current situation, 2) perception of alternatives, and 3) recognition, both at the individual and institutional level, of the ability and potential to change. Although the latter implies education and motivation, the former two necessitate a system change.

Among the reported reasons for poor adherence with hand-hygiene recommendations (Box 1), certain ones are clearly associated with the institution or system (e.g., lack of institutional priority for hand hygiene, administrative sanctions, and a safety climate). Although all of these reasons would require a system change in the majority of institutions, the third requires management commitment, visible safety programs, an acceptable level of work stress, a tolerant and supportive attitude toward reported problems, and belief in the efficacy of preventive strategies (*12,317,325,327*). Most importantly, an improvement in infection-control practices requires 1) questioning basic beliefs, 2) continuous assessment of the group (or individual) stage of behavioral change, 3) intervention(s) with an appropriate process of change, and 4) supporting individual and group creativity (*317*). Because of the complexity of the process of change, single interventions often fail. Thus, a multimodal, multidisciplinary strategy is likely necessary (*74,75,317,323,326*).

Methods Used To Promote Improved Hand Hygiene

Hand-hygiene promotion has been challenging for >150 years. In-service education, information leaflets, workshops and lectures, automated dispensers, and performance feedback on hand-hygiene adherence rates have been associated with transient improvement (*291,294–296,306,314*).

Several strategies for promotion of hand hygiene in hospitals have been published (Table 9). These strategies require education, motivation, or system change. Certain strategies are based on epidemiologic evidence, others on the authors' and other investigators' experience and review of current knowledge. Some strategies may be unnecessary in certain circumstances, but may be helpful in others. In particular, changing the hand-hygiene agent could be beneficial in institutions or hospital wards with a high workload and a high demand for hand hygiene when alcohol-based hand rubs are not available (*11,73,78,328*). However, a change in the recommended hand-hygiene agent could be deleterious if introduced during winter, at a time of higher hand-skin irritability, and if not accompanied by the provision of skin-care products (e.g., protective creams and lotions). Additional specific elements should be considered for inclusion in educational and motivational programs (Box 2).

Several strategies that could potentially be associated with successful promotion of hand hygiene require a system change (Box 1). Hand-hygiene adherence and promotion involve factors at both the individual and system level. Enhancing individual and institutional attitudes regarding the feasibility of making changes (self-efficacy), obtaining active participation of personnel at both levels, and promoting an institutional safety climate represent challenges that exceed the current perception of the role of infection-control professionals.

Whether increased education, individual reinforcement technique, appropriate rewarding, administrative sanction, enhanced self-participation, active involvement of a larger number of organizational leaders, enhanced perception of health threat, self-efficacy, and perceived social pressure (*12,317,329,330*), or combinations of these factors can improve HCWs' adherence with hand hygiene needs further investigation. Ultimately, adherence to recommended hand-hygiene practices should become part of a culture of patient safety where a set of interdependent quality elements interact to achieve a shared objective (*331*).

On the basis of both these hypothetical considerations and successful, actual experiences in certain institutions, strategies to improve adherence to hand-hygiene practices should be both multimodal and multidisciplinary. However, strategies must be further researched before they are implemented.

TABLE 9. Stategies for successful promotion of hand hygiene in hospitals

Strategy	Tool for change*	Selected references[†]
Education	E (M, S)	(*74,295,306,326,393*)
Routine observation and feedback	S (E, M)	(*74,294,306,326,393*)
Engineering control		
Make hand hygiene possible, easy, and convenient	S	(*74,281,326,393*)
Make alcohol-based hand rub available	S	(*74*)
(at least in high-demand situations)	S	(*74,283,312*)
Patient education	S (M)	(*283,394*)
Reminders in the workplace	S	(*74,395*)
Administrative sanction/rewarding	S	(*12,317*)
Change in hand-hygiene agent	S (E)	(*11,67,71,283,312*)
Promote/facilitate skin care for health-care–workers' hands	S (E)	(*67,74,274,275*)
Obtain active participation at individual and institutional level	E, M, S	(*74,75,317*)
Improve institutional safety climate	S (M)	(*74,75,317*)
Enhance individual and instituitional self-efficacy	S (E, M)	(*74,75,317*)
Avoid overcrowding, understaffing, and excessive workload	S	(*11,74,78,297,396*)
Combine several of above strategies	E, M, S	(*74,75,295,306,317,326*)

* The dynamic of behavioral change is complex and involves a combination of education (E), motivation (M), and system change (S).
[†] Only selected references have been listed; readers should refer to more extensive reviews for exhaustive reference lists (*1,8,317,323,397*).

BOX 2. Elements of health-care worker educational and motivational programs

Rationale for hand hygiene
- Potential risks of transmission of microorganisms to patients
- Potential risks of health-care worker colonization or infection caused by organisms acquired from the patient
- Morbidity, mortality, and costs associated with health-care–associated infections

Indications for hand hygiene
- Contact with a patient's intact skin (e.g., taking a pulse or blood pressure, performing physical examinations, lifting the patient in bed) (*25,26,45,48,51,53*)
- Contact with environmental surfaces in the immediate vicinity of patients (*46,51,53,54*)
- After glove removal (*50,58,71*)

Techniques for hand hygiene
- Amount of hand-hygiene solution
- Duration of hand-hygiene procedure
- Selection of hand-hygiene agents
  - Alcohol-based hand rubs are the most efficacious agents for reducing the number of bacteria on the hands of personnel. Antiseptic soaps and detergents are the next most effective, and non-antimicrobial soaps are the least effective (*1,398*).
  - Soap and water are recommended for visibly soil hands.
  - Alcohol-based hand rubs are recommended for routine decontamination of hands for all clinical indications (except when hands are visibly soiled) and as one of the options for surgical hand hygiene.

Methods to maintain hand skin health
- Lotions and creams can prevent or minimize skin dryness and irritation caused by irritant contact dermatitis
- Acceptable lotions or creams to use
- Recommended schedule for applying lotions or creams

Expectations of patient care managers/administrators
- Written statements regarding the value of, and support for, adherence to recommended hand-hygiene practices
- Role models demonstrating adherence to recommended hand hygiene practices (*399*)

Indications for, and limitations of, glove use
- Hand contamination may occur as a result of small, undetected holes in examination gloves (*321,361*)
- Contamination may occur during glove removal (*50*)
- Wearing gloves does not replace the need for hand hygiene (*58*)
- Failure to remove gloves after caring for a patient may lead to transmission of microorganizations from one patient to another (*373*).

Efficacy of Promotion and Impact of Improved Hand Hygiene

The lack of scientific information of the definitive impact of improved hand hygiene on health-care–associated infection rates is a possible barrier to appropriate adherence with hand-hygiene recommendations (Box 1). However, evidence supports the belief that improved hand hygiene can reduce health-care–associated infection rates. Failure to perform appropriate hand hygiene is considered the leading cause of health-care–associated infections and spread of multiresistant organisms and has been recognized as a substantial contributor to outbreaks.

Of nine hospital-based studies of the impact of hand hygiene on the risk of health-care–associated infections (Table 10) (*48,69–75,296*), the majority demonstrated a temporal relationship between improved hand-hygiene practices and reduced infection rates.

In one of these studies, endemic MRSA in a neonatal intensive-care unit was eliminated 7 months after introduction of a new

TABLE 10. Association between improved adherence with hand-hygiene practice and health-care–associated infection rates

Year	Ref. no.	Hospital setting	Results	Duration of follow-up
1977	(48)	Adult ICU	Reduction in health-care–associated infections caused by endemic *Klebsiella* spp.	2 years
1982	(69)	Adult ICU	Reduction in health-care-associated infection rates	N.S.
1984	(70)	Adult ICU	Reduction in health-care–associated infection rates	N.S.
1990	(296)	Adult ICU	No effect (average hand hygiene adherence improvement did not reach statistical significance)	11 months
1992	(71)	Adult ICU	Substantial difference between rates of health-care–associated infection between two different hand-hygiene agents	8 months
1994	(72)	NICU	Elimination of MRSA, when combined with multiple other infection-control measures. Reduction of vancomycin use	9 months
1995	(73)	Newborn nursery	Elimination of MRSA, when combined with multiple other infection-control measures	3.5 years
2000	(75)	MICU/NICU	85% relative reduction of VRE rate in the intervention hospital; 44% relative reduction in control hospital; no change in MRSA	8 months
2000	(74)	Hospitalwide	Substantial reduction in the annual overall prevalence of health-care–associated infections and MRSA cross-transmission rates. Active surveillance cultures and contact precautions were implemented during same period	5 years

Note: ICU = intensive care unit, NICU = neonatal ICU, MRSA = methicillin-resistant *Staphylococcus aureus*, MICU = medical ICU, and N.S. = not stated.

hand antiseptic (1% triclosan); all other infection-control measures remained in place, including the practice of conducting weekly active surveillance by obtaining cultures (72). Another study reported an MRSA outbreak involving 22 infants in a neonatal unit (73). Despite intensive efforts, the outbreak could not be controlled until a new antiseptic was added (i.e., 0.3% triclosan); all previously used control measures remained in place, including gloves and gowns, cohorting, and obtaining cultures for active surveillance.

The effectiveness of a longstanding, hospitalwide program to promote hand hygiene at the University of Geneva hospitals was recently reported (74). Overall adherence to hand-hygiene guidelines during routine patient care was monitored during hospitalwide observational surveys. These surveys were conducted biannually during December 1994–December 1997, before and during implementation of a hand-hygiene campaign that specifically emphasized the practice of bedside, alcohol-based hand disinfection. Individual-sized bottles of hand-rub solution were distributed to all wards, and custom-made holders were mounted on all beds to facilitate access to hand disinfection. HCWs were also encouraged to carry bottles in their pockets, and in 1996, a newly designed flat (instead of round) bottle was made available to further facilitate pocket carriage. The promotional strategy was multimodal and involved a multidisciplinary team of HCWs, the use of wall posters, the promotion of antiseptic hand rubs located at bedsides throughout the institution, and regular performance feedback to all HCWs (see http://www.hopisafe.ch for further

details on methodology). Health-care–associated infection rates, attack rates of MRSA cross-transmission, and consumption of hand-rub disinfectant were measured. Adherence to recommended hand-hygiene practices improved progressively from 48% in 1994 to 66% in 1997 ($p < 0.001$). Whereas recourse to handwashing with soap and water remained stable, frequency of hand disinfection markedly increased during the study period ($p < 0.001$), and the consumption of alcohol-based hand-rub solution increased from 3.5 to 15.4 liters per 1,000 patient-days during 1993–1998 ($p < 0.001$). The increased frequency of hand disinfection was unchanged after adjustment for known risk factors of poor adherence. During the same period, both overall health-care–associated infection and MRSA transmission rates decreased (both $p < 0.05$). The observed reduction in MRSA transmission may have been affected by both improved hand-hygiene adherence and the simultaneous implementation of active surveillance cultures for detecting and isolating patients colonized with MRSA (332). The experience from the University of Geneva hospitals constitutes the first report of a hand-hygiene campaign with a sustained improvement over several years. An additional multimodal program also yielded sustained improvements in hand-hygiene practices over an extended period (75); the majority of studies have been limited to a 6- to 9-month observation period.

Although these studies were not designed to assess the independent contribution of hand hygiene on the prevention of health-care–associated infections, the results indicate that improved hand-hygiene practices reduce the risk of transmission of pathogenic microorganisms. The beneficial effects of hand-hygiene promotion on the risk of cross-transmission also have been reported in surveys conducted in schools and day care centers (*333–338*), as well as in a community setting (*339–341*).

Other Policies Related to Hand Hygiene

Fingernails and Artificial Nails

Studies have documented that subungual areas of the hand harbor high concentrations of bacteria, most frequently coagulase-negative staphylococci, gram-negative rods (including *Pseudomonas* spp.), Corynebacteria, and yeasts (*14,342,343*). Freshly applied nail polish does not increase the number of bacteria recovered from periungual skin, but chipped nail polish may support the growth of larger numbers of organisms on fingernails (*344,345*). Even after careful handwashing or the use of surgical scrubs, personnel often harbor substantial numbers of potential pathogens in the subungual spaces (*346–348*).

Whether artificial nails contribute to transmission of health-care–associated infections is unknown. However, HCWs who wear artificial nails are more likely to harbor gram-negative pathogens on their fingertips than are those who have natural nails, both before and after handwashing (*347–349*). Whether the length of natural or artificial nails is a substantial risk factor is unknown, because the majority of bacterial growth occurs along the proximal 1 mm of the nail adjacent to subungual skin (*345,347,348*). Recently, an outbreak of *P. aeruginosa* in a neonatal intensive care unit was attributed to two nurses (one with long natural nails and one with long artificial nails) who carried the implicated strains of *Pseudomonas* spp. on their hands (*350*). Patients were substantially more likely than controls to have been cared for by the two nurses during the exposure period, indicating that colonization of long or artificial nails with *Pseudomonas* spp. may have contributed to causing the outbreak. Personnel wearing artificial nails also have been epidemiologically implicated in several other outbreaks of infection caused by gram-negative bacilli and yeast (*351–353*). Although these studies provide evidence that wearing artificial nails poses an infection hazard, additional studies are warranted.

Gloving Policies

CDC has recommended that HCWs wear gloves to 1) reduce the risk of personnel acquiring infections from patients, 2) prevent health-care worker flora from being transmitted to patients, and 3) reduce transient contamination of the hands of personnel by flora that can be transmitted from one patient to another (*354*). Before the emergence of the acquired immunodeficiency syndrome (AIDS) epidemic, gloves were worn primarily by personnel caring for patients colonized or infected with certain pathogens or by personnel exposed to patients with a high risk of hepatitis B. Since 1987, a dramatic increase in glove use has occurred in an effort to prevent transmission of HIV and other bloodborne pathogens from patients to HCWs (*355*). The Occupational Safety and Health Administration (OSHA) mandates that gloves be worn during all patient-care activities that may involve exposure to blood or body fluids that may be contaminated with blood (*356*).

The effectiveness of gloves in preventing contamination of HCWs' hands has been confirmed in several clinical studies (*45,51,58*). One study found that HCWs who wore gloves during patient contact contaminated their hands with an average of only 3 CFUs per minute of patient care, compared with 16 CFUs per minute for those not wearing gloves (*51*). Two other studies, involving personnel caring for patients with *C. difficile* or VRE, revealed that wearing gloves prevented hand contamination among the majority of personnel having direct contact with patients (*45,58*). Wearing gloves also prevented personnel from acquiring VRE on their hands when touching contaminated environmental surfaces (*58*). Preventing heavy contamination of the hands is considered important, because handwashing or hand antisepsis may not remove all potential pathogens when hands are heavily contaminated (*25,111*).

Several studies provide evidence that wearing gloves can help reduce transmission of pathogens in health-care settings. In a prospective controlled trial that required personnel to routinely wear vinyl gloves when handling any body substances, the incidence of *C. difficile* diarrhea among patients decreased from 7.7 cases/1,000 patient discharges before the intervention to 1.5 cases/1,000 discharges during the intervention (*226*). The prevalence of asymptomatic *C. difficile* carriage also decreased substantially on "glove" wards, but not on control wards. In intensive-care units where VRE or MRSA have been epidemic, requiring all HCWs to wear gloves to care for all patients in the unit (i.e., universal glove use) likely has helped control outbreaks (*357,358*).

The influence of glove use on the hand-hygiene habits of personnel is not clear. Several studies found that personnel who wore gloves were less likely to wash their hands upon leaving a patient's room (*290,320*). In contrast, two other studies found that personnel who wore gloves were substantially more likely to wash their hands after patient care (*87,301*).

The following caveats regarding use of gloves by HCWs must be considered. Personnel should be informed that gloves do not provide complete protection against hand contamination. Bacterial flora colonizing patients may be recovered from the hands of $\leq$30% of HCWs who wear gloves during patient contact (50,58). Further, wearing gloves does not provide complete protection against acquisition of infections caused by hepatitis B virus and herpes simplex virus (359,360). In such instances, pathogens presumably gain access to the caregiver's hands via small defects in gloves or by contamination of the hands during glove removal (50,321,359,361).

Gloves used by HCWs are usually made of natural rubber latex and synthetic nonlatex materials (e.g., vinyl, nitrile, and neoprene [polymers and copolymers of chloroprene]). Because of the increasing prevalence of latex sensitivity among HCWs and patients, FDA has approved several powdered and powder-free latex gloves with reduced protein contents, as well as synthetic gloves that can be made available by health-care institutions for use by latex-sensitive employees. In published studies, the barrier integrity of gloves varies on the basis of type and quality of glove material, intensity of use, length of time used, manufacturer, whether gloves were tested before or after use, and method used to detect glove leaks (359,361–366). In published studies, vinyl gloves have had defects more frequently than latex gloves, the difference in defect frequency being greatest after use (359,361,364,367). However, intact vinyl gloves provide protection comparable to that of latex gloves (359). Limited studies indicate that nitrile gloves have leakage rates that approximate those of latex gloves (368–371). Having more than one type of glove available is desirable, because it allows personnel to select the type that best suits their patient-care activities. Although recent studies indicate that improvements have been made in the quality of gloves (366), hands should be decontaminated or washed after removing gloves (8,50,58,321,361). Gloves should not be washed or reused (321,361). Use of petroleum-based hand lotions or creams may adversely affect the integrity of latex gloves (372). After use of powdered gloves, certain alcohol hand rubs may interact with residual powder on the hands of personnel, resulting in a gritty feeling on the hands. In facilities where powdered gloves are commonly used, various alcohol-based hand rubs should be tested after removal of powdered gloves to avoid selecting a product that causes this undesirable reaction. Personnel should be reminded that failure to remove gloves between patients may contribute to transmission of organisms (358,373).

Jewelry

Several studies have demonstrated that skin underneath rings is more heavily colonized than comparable areas of skin on fingers without rings (374–376). One study found that 40% of nurses harbored gram-negative bacilli (e.g., *E. cloacae, Klebsiella*, and *Acinetobacter*) on skin under rings and that certain nurses carried the same organism under their rings for several months (375). In a more recent study involving >60 intensive care unit nurses, multivariable analysis revealed that rings were the only substantial risk factor for carriage of gram-negative bacilli and *S. aureus* and that the concentration of organisms recovered correlated with the number of rings worn (377). Whether the wearing of rings results in greater transmission of pathogens is unknown. Two studies determined that mean bacterial colony counts on hands after handwashing were similar among persons wearing rings and those not wearing rings (376,378). Further studies are needed to establish if wearing rings results in greater transmission of pathogens in health-care settings.

Hand-Hygiene Research Agenda

Although the number of published studies concerning hand hygiene has increased considerably in recent years, many questions regarding hand-hygiene products and strategies for improving adherence of personnel to recommended policies remain unanswered. Several concerns must still be addressed by researchers in industry and by clinical investigators (Box 3).

Web-Based Hand-Hygiene Resources

Additional information regarding improving hand hygiene is available at http://www.hopisafe.ch
University of Geneva Hospitals, Geneva, Switzerland
http://www.cdc.gov/ncidod/hip
CDC, Atlanta, Georgia
http://www.jr2.ox.ac.uk/bandolier/band88/b88-8.html
Bandolier journal, United Kingdom
http://www.med.upenn.edu
University of Pennsylvania, Philadelphia, Pennsylvania

BOX 3. Hand-hygiene research agenda

Education and promotion
- Provide health-care workers (HCWs) with better education regarding the types of patient care activities that can result in hand contamination and cross-transmission of microorganisms.
- Develop and implement promotion hand-hygiene programs in pregraduate courses.
- Study the impact of population-based education on hand-hygiene behavior.
- Design and conduct studies to determine if frequent glove use should be encouraged or discouraged.
- Determine evidence-based indications for hand cleansing (considering that it might be unrealistic to expect HCWs to clean their hands after every contact with the patient).
- Assess the key determinants of hand-hygiene behavior and promotion among the different populations of HCWs.
- Develop methods to obtain management support.
- Implement and evaluate the impact of the different components of multimodal programs to promote hand hygiene.

Hand-hygiene agents and hand care
- Determine the most suitable formulations for hand-hygiene products.
- Determine if preparations with persistent antimicrobial activity reduce infection rates more effectively than do preparations whose activity is limited to an immediate effect.
- Study the systematic replacement of conventional handwashing by the use of hand disinfection.
- Develop devices to facilitate the use and optimal application of hand-hygiene agents.
- Develop hand-hygiene agents with low irritancy potential.
- Study the possible advantages and eventual interaction of hand-care lotions, creams, and other barriers to help minimize the potential irritation associated with hand-hygiene agents.

Laboratory-based and epidemiologic research and development
- Develop experimental models for the study of cross-contamination from patient to patient and from environment to patient.
- Develop new protocols for evaluating the in vivo efficacy of agents, considering in particular short application times and volumes that reflect actual use in health-care facilities.
- Monitor hand-hygiene adherence by using new devices or adequate surrogate markers, allowing frequent individual feedback on performance.
- Determine the percentage increase in hand-hygiene adherence required to achieve a predictable risk reduction in infection rates.
- Generate more definitive evidence for the impact on infection rates of improved adherence to recommended hand-hygiene practices.
- Provide cost-effectiveness evaluation of successful and unsuccessful promotion campaigns.

Part II. Recommendations

Categories

These recommendations are designed to improve hand-hygiene practices of HCWs and to reduce transmission of pathogenic microorganisms to patients and personnel in health-care settings. This guideline and its recommendations are not intended for use in food processing or food-service establishments, and are not meant to replace guidance provided by FDA's Model Food Code.

As in previous CDC/HICPAC guidelines, each recommendation is categorized on the basis of existing scientific data, theoretical rationale, applicability, and economic impact. The CDC/HICPAC system for categorizing recommendations is as follows:

Category IA. Strongly recommended for implementation and strongly supported by well-designed experimental, clinical, or epidemiologic studies.

Category IB. Strongly recommended for implementation and supported by certain experimental, clinical, or epidemiologic studies and a strong theoretical rationale.

Category IC. Required for implementation, as mandated by federal or state regulation or standard.

Category II. Suggested for implementation and supported by suggestive clinical or epidemiologic studies or a theoretical rationale.

No recommendation. Unresolved issue. Practices for which insufficient evidence or no consensus regarding efficacy exist.

Recommendations

1. Indications for handwashing and hand antisepsis
   A. When hands are visibly dirty or contaminated with proteinaceous material or are visibly soiled with blood or other body fluids, wash hands with either a non-antimicrobial soap and water or an antimicrobial soap and water (IA) (*66*).
   B. If hands are not visibly soiled, use an alcohol-based hand rub for routinely decontaminating hands in all other clinical situations described in items 1C–J (IA) (*74,93,166,169,283,294,312,398*). Alternatively, wash hands with an antimicrobial soap and water in all clinical situations described in items 1C–J (IB) (*69-71,74*).
   C. Decontaminate hands before having direct contact with patients (IB) (*68,400*).
   D. Decontaminate hands before donning sterile gloves when inserting a central intravascular catheter (IB) (*401,402*).
   E. Decontaminate hands before inserting indwelling urinary catheters, peripheral vascular catheters, or other invasive devices that do not require a surgical procedure (IB) (*25,403*).
   F. Decontaminate hands after contact with a patient's intact skin (e.g., when taking a pulse or blood pressure, and lifting a patient) (IB) (*25,45,48,68*).
   G. Decontaminate hands after contact with body fluids or excretions, mucous membranes, nonintact skin, and wound dressings if hands are not visibly soiled (IA) (*400*).
   H. Decontaminate hands if moving from a contaminated-body site to a clean-body site during patient care (II) (*25,53*).
   I. Decontaminate hands after contact with inanimate objects (including medical equipment) in the immediate vicinity of the patient (II) (*46,53,54*).
   J. Decontaminate hands after removing gloves (IB) (*50,58,321*).
   K. Before eating and after using a restroom, wash hands with a non-antimicrobial soap and water or with an antimicrobial soap and water (IB) (*404-409*).
   L. Antimicrobial-impregnated wipes (i.e., towelettes) may be considered as an alternative to washing hands with non-antimicrobial soap and water. Because they are not as effective as alcohol-based hand rubs or washing hands with an antimicrobial soap and water for reducing bacterial counts on the hands of HCWs, they are not a substitute for using an alcohol-based hand rub or antimicrobial soap (IB) (*160,161*).
   M. Wash hands with non-antimicrobial soap and water or with antimicrobial soap and water if exposure to *Bacillus anthracis* is suspected or proven. The physical action of washing and rinsing hands under such circumstances is recommended because alcohols, chlorhexidine, iodophors, and other antiseptic agents have poor activity against spores (II) (*120,172, 224,225*).
   N. No recommendation can be made regarding the routine use of nonalcohol-based hand rubs for hand hygiene in health-care settings. Unresolved issue.
2. Hand-hygiene technique
   A. When decontaminating hands with an alcohol-based hand rub, apply product to palm of one hand and rub hands together, covering all surfaces of hands and fingers, until hands are dry (IB) (*288,410*). Follow the manufacturer's recommendations regarding the volume of product to use.
   B. When washing hands with soap and water, wet hands first with water, apply an amount of product recommended by the manufacturer to hands, and rub hands together vigorously for at least 15 seconds, covering all surfaces of the hands and fingers. Rinse hands with water and dry thoroughly with a disposable towel. Use towel to turn off the faucet (IB) (*90-92,94,411*). Avoid using hot water, because repeated exposure to hot water may increase the risk of dermatitis (IB) (*254,255*).
   C. Liquid, bar, leaflet or powdered forms of plain soap are acceptable when washing hands with a non-antimicrobial soap and water. When bar soap is used, soap racks that facilitate drainage and small bars of soap should be used (II) (*412-415*).
   D. Multiple-use cloth towels of the hanging or roll type are not recommended for use in health-care settings (II) (*137,300*).
3. Surgical hand antisepsis
   A. Remove rings, watches, and bracelets before beginning the surgical hand scrub (II) (*375,378,416*).
   B. Remove debris from underneath fingernails using a nail cleaner under running water (II) (*14,417*).

C. Surgical hand antisepsis using either an antimicrobial soap or an alcohol-based hand rub with persistent activity is recommended before donning sterile gloves when performing surgical procedures (IB) (*115,159,232,234,237,418*).

D. When performing surgical hand antisepsis using an antimicrobial soap, scrub hands and forearms for the length of time recommended by the manufacturer, usually 2–6 minutes. Long scrub times (e.g., 10 minutes) are not necessary (IB) (*117,156,205, 207,238-241*).

E. When using an alcohol-based surgical hand-scrub product with persistent activity, follow the manufacturer's instructions. Before applying the alcohol solution, prewash hands and forearms with a non-antimicrobial soap and dry hands and forearms completely. After application of the alcohol-based product as recommended, allow hands and forearms to dry thoroughly before donning sterile gloves (IB) (*159,237*).

4. Selection of hand-hygiene agents

A. Provide personnel with efficacious hand-hygiene products that have low irritancy potential, particularly when these products are used multiple times per shift (IB) (*90,92,98,166,249*). This recommendation applies to products used for hand antisepsis before and after patient care in clinical areas and to products used for surgical hand antisepsis by surgical personnel.

B. To maximize acceptance of hand-hygiene products by HCWs, solicit input from these employees regarding the feel, fragrance, and skin tolerance of any products under consideration. The cost of hand-hygiene products should not be the primary factor influencing product selection (IB) (*92,93,166, 274,276-278*).

C. When selecting non-antimicrobial soaps, antimicrobial soaps, or alcohol-based hand rubs, solicit information from manufacturers regarding any known interactions between products used to clean hands, skin care products, and the types of gloves used in the institution (II) (*174,372*).

D. Before making purchasing decisions, evaluate the dispenser systems of various product manufacturers or distributors to ensure that dispensers function adequately and deliver an appropriate volume of product (II) (*286*).

E. Do not add soap to a partially empty soap dispenser. This practice of "topping off" dispensers can lead to bacterial contamination of soap (IA) (*187,419*).

5. Skin care

A. Provide HCWs with hand lotions or creams to minimize the occurrence of irritant contact dermatitis associated with hand antisepsis or handwashing (IA) (*272,273*).

B. Solicit information from manufacturers regarding any effects that hand lotions, creams, or alcohol-based hand antiseptics may have on the persistent effects of antimicrobial soaps being used in the institution (IB) (*174,420,421*).

6. Other Aspects of Hand Hygiene

A. Do not wear artificial fingernails or extenders when having direct contact with patients at high risk (e.g., those in intensive-care units or operating rooms) (IA) (*350–353*).

B. Keep natural nails tips less than 1/4-inch long (II) (*350*).

C. Wear gloves when contact with blood or other potentially infectious materials, mucous membranes, and nonintact skin could occur (IC) (*356*).

D. Remove gloves after caring for a patient. Do not wear the same pair of gloves for the care of more than one patient, and do not wash gloves between uses with different patients (IB) (*50,58,321,373*).

E. Change gloves during patient care if moving from a contaminated body site to a clean body site (II) (*50,51,58*).

F. No recommendation can be made regarding wearing rings in health-care settings. Unresolved issue.

7. Health-care worker educational and motivational programs

A. As part of an overall program to improve hand-hygiene practices of HCWs, educate personnel regarding the types of patient-care activities that can result in hand contamination and the advantages and disadvantages of various methods used to clean their hands (II) (*74,292,295,299*).

B. Monitor HCWs' adherence with recommended hand-hygiene practices and provide personnel with information regarding their performance (IA) (*74,276,292,295,299,306,310*).

C. Encourage patients and their families to remind HCWs to decontaminate their hands (II) (*394,422*).

8. Administrative measures

A. Make improved hand-hygiene adherence an institutional priority and provide appropriate administrative support and financial resources (IB) (*74,75*).

B. Implement a multidisciplinary program designed to improve adherence of health personnel to recommended hand-hygiene practices (IB) (*74,75*).

C. As part of a multidisciplinary program to improve hand-hygiene adherence, provide HCWs with a readily accessible alcohol-based hand-rub product (IA) (*74,166,283,294,312*).

D. To improve hand-hygiene adherence among personnel who work in areas in which high workloads and high intensity of patient care are anticipated, make an alcohol-based hand rub available at the entrance to the patient's room or at the bedside, in other convenient locations, and in individual pocket-sized containers to be carried by HCWs (IA) (*11,74,166,283,284,312,318,423*).

E. Store supplies of alcohol-based hand rubs in cabinets or areas approved for flammable materials (IC).

Part III. Performance Indicators

1. The following performance indicators are recommended for measuring improvements in HCWs' hand-hygiene adherence:

A. Periodically monitor and record adherence as the number of hand-hygiene episodes performed by personnel/number of hand-hygiene opportunities, by ward or by service. Provide feedback to personnel regarding their performance.

B. Monitor the volume of alcohol-based hand rub (or detergent used for handwashing or hand antisepsis) used per 1,000 patient-days.

C. Monitor adherence to policies dealing with wearing of artificial nails.

D. When outbreaks of infection occur, assess the adequacy of health-care worker hand hygiene.

References

1. Rotter M. Hand washing and hand disinfection [Chapter 87]. In: Mayhall CG, ed. Hospital epidemiology and infection control. 2nd ed. Philadelphia, PA: Lippincott Williams & Wilkins, 1999.
2. Labarraque AG. Instructions and observations regarding the use of the chlorides of soda and lime. Porter J, ed. [French] New Haven, CT: Baldwin and Treadway, 1829.
3. Semmelweis I. Etiology, concept, and prophylaxis of childbed fever. Carter KC, ed. 1st ed. Madison, WI: The University of Wisconsin Press, 1983.
4. Coppage CM. Hand washing in patient care [Motion picture]. Washington, DC: US Public Health Service, 1961.
5. Steere AC, Mallison GF. Handwashing practices for the prevention of nosocomial infections. Ann Intern Med 1975;83:683–90.
6. Garner JS, Favero MS. CDC guideline for handwashing and hospital environmental control, 1985. Infect Control 1986;7:231–43.
7. Larson E. Guideline for use of topical antimicrobial agents. Am J Infect Control 1988;16:253–66.
8. Larson EL, APIC Guidelines Committee. APIC guideline for handwashing and hand antisepsis in health care settings. Am J Infect Control 1995;23:251–69.
9. Hospital Infection Control Practices Advisory Committee (HICPAC). Recommendations for preventing the spread of vancomycin resistance. Infect Control Hosp Epidemiol 1995;16:105–13.
10. Garner JS, Hospital Infection Control Practices Advisory Committee. Guideline for isolation precautions in hospitals. Infect Control Hosp Epidemiol 1996;17:53–80.
11. Pittet D, Mourouga P, Perneger TV, Members of the Infection Control Program. Compliance with handwashing in a teaching hospital. Ann Intern Med 1999;130:126–30.
12. Boyce JM. It is time for action: improving hand hygiene in hospitals. Ann Intern Med 1999;130:153–5.
13. Selwyn S. Microbiology and ecology of human skin. Practitioner 1980;224:1059–62.
14. Price PB. Bacteriology of normal skin: a new quantitative test applied to a study of the bacterial flora and the disinfectant action of mechanical cleansing. J Infect Dis 1938;63:301–18.
15. Larson E. Effects of handwashing agent, handwashing frequency, and clinical area on hand flora. Am J Infect Control 1984;11:76–82.
16. Maki D. Control of colonization and transmission of pathogenic bacteria in the hospital. Ann Intern Med 1978;89(Pt 2):777–80.
17. Larson EL, Norton Hughes CA, Pyrak JD, Sparks SM, Cagatay EU, Bartkus JM. Changes in bacterial flora associated with skin damage on hands of health care personnel. Am J Infect Control 1998;26:513–21.
18. Sprunt K, Redman W, Leidy G. Antibacterial effectiveness of routine hand washing. Pediatrics 1973;52:264–71.
19. Food and Drug Administration. Tentative final monograph for healthcare antiseptic drug products; proposed rule. Federal Register 1994;59:31441–52.
20. Lowbury EJL. Gram-negative bacilli on the skin. Br J Dermatol 1969;81(suppl 1):55–61.
21. Noble WC. Distribution of the Micrococcaceae. Br J Dermatol 1969;81(suppl 1):27–31.
22. McBride ME, Duncan WC, Bodey GP, McBride CM. Microbial skin flora of selected cancer patients and hospital personnel. J Clin Microbiol 1976;3:14–20.
23. Casewell MW. Role of hands in nosocomial gram-negative infection. In: Maibach HI, Aly R, eds. Skin microbiology: relevance to clinical infection. New York, NY: Springer-Verlag, 1981.
24. Larson EL, McGinley KJ, Foglia AR, Talbot GH, Leyden JJ. Composition and antimicrobic resistance of skin flora in hospitalized and healthy adults. J Clin Microbiol 1986;23:604–8.
25. Ehrenkranz NJ, Alfonso BC. Failure of bland soap handwash to prevent hand transfer of patient bacteria to urethral catheters. Infect Control Hosp Epidemiol 1991;12:654–62.
26. Sanderson PJ, Weissler S. Recovery of coliforms from the hands of nurses and patients: activities leading to contamination. J Hosp Infect 1992;21:85–93.
27. Coello R, Jiménez J, García M, et al. Prospective study of infection, colonization and carriage of methicillin-resistant *Staphylococcus aureus* in an outbreak affecting 990 patients. Eur J Clin Microbiol Infect Dis 1994;13:74–81.

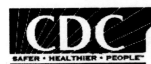

CDC Home | Search | Health Topics A-Z

Division of Healthcare Quality Promotion (DHQP)

Issues in Healthcare Settings

DHQP Home | Index

Antimicrobial Resistance

MRSA - Methicillin Resistant *Staphylococcus aureus*

About DHQP

Antimicrobial
Resistance

   -MRSA

      -For Patients

      -For Healthcare

      -Lab Detection

Bloodborne
Pathogens

Child Care

Dialysis

Guidelines and
Recommendations

Laboratory

Occupational Health

Outbreaks

Sterilization and Disinfection

Surveillance

Training

Information for Healthcare Personnel

Methicillin-resistant *Staphylococcus aureus* (MRSA) has become a prevalent nosocomial pathogen in the United States. In hospitals, the most important reservoirs of MRSA are infected or colonized patients. Although hospital personnel can serve as reservoirs for MRSA and may harbor the organism for many months, they have been more commonly identified as a link for transmission between colonized or infected patients. The main mode of transmission of MRSA is via hands (especially health care workers' hands) which may become contaminated by contact with a) colonized or infected patients, b) colonized or infected body sites of the personnel themselves, or c) devices, items, or environmental surfaces contaminated with body fluids containing MRSA. Standard Precautions, as described in the "Guideline for Isolation Precautions in Hospitals" (Infect Control Hosp Epidemiol 1996;17:53-80), should control the spread of MRSA in most instances.

Standard Precautions include:

1) Handwashing

Wash hands after touching blood, body fluids, secretions, excretions, and contaminated items, whether or not gloves are worn. Wash hands immediately after gloves are removed, between patient contacts, and when otherwise indicated to avoid transfer of microorganisms to other patients or environments. It may be necessary to wash hands between tasks and procedures on the same patient to prevent cross-contamination of different body sites.

Index

2) Gloving

Wear gloves (clean nonsterile gloves are adequate) when touching blood, body fluids, secretions, excretions, and contaminated items; put on clean gloves just before touching mucous membranes and nonintact skin. Remove gloves promptly after use, before touching noncontaminated items and environmental surfaces, and before going to another patient, and wash hands immediately to avoid transfer of microorganisms to other patients or environments.

Index

3) Masking

Wear a mask and eye protection or a face shield to protect mucous membranes of the eyes, nose, and mouth during procedures and patient-care activities that are likely to generate splashes or sprays of blood, body fluids, secretions, and excretions. Index

4) Gowning

Wear a gown (a clean nonsterile gown is adequate) to protect skin and prevent soiling of clothes during procedures and patient-care activities that are likely to generate splashes or sprays of blood, body fluids, secretions, and excretions or cause soiling of clothing.

Index

5) Appropriate device handling

Handle used patient-care equipment soiled with blood, body fluids, secretions, and excretions in a manner that prevents skin and mucous membrane exposures,

PAGE INDEX
▶ Standard Precautions
-Handwashing
-Gloving
-Masking
-Gowning
-Device handling
-Laundry handling
▶ Contact Precautions
▶ Culturing of Personnel
▶ Outbreak control

contamination of clothing, and transfer of microorganisms to other patients and environments. Ensure that reusable equipment is not used for the care of another patient until it has been appropriately cleaned and reprocessed and that single-use items are properly discarded. Index

6) Appropriate handling of laundry
Handle, transport, and process used linen soiled with blood, body fluids, secretions, and excretions in a manner that prevents skin and mucous membrane exposures, contamination of clothing, and transfer of microorganisms to other patients and environments. Index

If MRSA is judged by the hospital's infection control program to be of special clinical or epidemiologic significance, then Contact Precautions should be considered.

Contact Precautions consist of:

1) Placing a patient with MRSA in a private room. When a private room is not available, the patient may be placed in a room with a patient(s) who has active infection with MRSA, but with no other infection (cohorting).

2) Wearing gloves (clean nonsterile gloves are adequate) when entering the room. During the course of providing care for a patient, change gloves after having contact with infective material that may contain high concentrations of microorganisms (e.g., fecal material and wound drainage). Remove gloves before leaving the patient's room and wash hands immediately with an antimicrobial agent. After glove removal and handwashing, ensure that hands do not touch potentially contaminated environmental surfaces or items in the patient's room to avoid transfer of microorganisms to other patients and environments.

3) Wearing a gown when entering the room if you anticipate that your clothing will have substantial contact with the patient, environmental surfaces, or items in the patient's room, or if the patient is incontinent, or has diarrhea, an ileostomy, a colostomy, or wound drainage not contained by a dressing. Remove the gown before leaving the patient's room. After gown removal, ensure that clothing does not contact potentially contaminated environmental surfaces to avoid transfer of microorganisms to other patients and environments.

4) Limiting the movement and transport of the patient from the room to essential purposes only. If the patient is transported out of the room, ensure that precautions are maintained to minimize the risk of transmission of microorganisms to other patients and contamination of environmental surfaces or equipment.

5) Ensuring that patient-care items, bedside equipment, and frequently touched surfaces receive daily cleaning.

6) When possible, dedicating the use of noncritical patient-care equipment and items such as stethoscope, sphygmomanometer, bedside commode, or electronic rectal thermometer to a single patient (or cohort of patients infected or colonized with MRSA) to avoid sharing between patients. If use of common equipment or items is unavoidable, then adequately clean and disinfect them before use on another patient. Index

Culturing of Personnel and Management of Personnel Carriers of MRSA

Unless the objective of the hospital is to eradicate all MRSA carriage and treat all personnel who are MRSA carriers, whether or not they disseminate MRSA, it may be prudent to culture only personnel who are implicated in MRSA transmission based on epidemiologic data. MRSA-carrier personnel who are epidemiologically linked to transmission should be removed from direct patient care until treatment of the MRSA-carrier status is successful. If the hospital elects to culture all personnel to identify MRSA carriers, a) surveillance cultures need to be done frequently, and b) it is likely that personnel colonized by MRSA who are not linked to transmission and/or who may not be MRSA disseminators will be identified, subjected to treatment, and/or removed from patient contact unnecessarily. Because of the high cost attendant to repeated surveillance cultures and the potential of repeated culturing to result in serious consequences to health care workers, hospitals should weigh the advantages and the adverse effects of routinely culturing personnel before doing so. Index

Control of MRSA Outbreaks

When an outbreak of MRSA infection occurs, an epidemiologic assessment should be initiated to identify risk factors for MRSA acquisition in the institution; clinical isolates of MRSA should be saved and submitted for strain typing. Colonized or infected patients should be identified as quickly as possible, appropriate barrier precautions should be instituted, and handwashing by medical personnel before and after all patient contacts should be strictly adhered to.

All personnel should be reinstructed on appropriate precautions for patients colonized or infected with multiresistant microorganisms and on the importance of handwashing and barrier precautions in preventing contact transmission.

If additional help is needed by the hospital, a consultation with the local or state health department or CDC may be necessary. Index

---

DHQP Home | DHQP Index

NCID Home | CDC Home | CDC Search | CDC Health Topics A-Z

This page last reviewed August 27, 1999

Division of Healthcare Quality Promotion
National Center for Infectious Diseases
Centers for Disease Control and Prevention

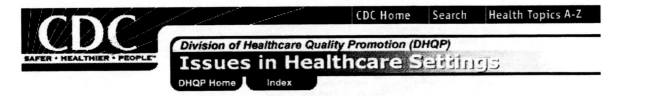

Part II. Recommendations for Isolation Precautions in Hospitals

Hospital Infection Control Practices Advisory Committee

RATIONALE FOR ISOLATION PRECAUTIONS IN HOSPITALS

Transmission of infection within a hospital requires three elements: a source of infecting microorganisms, a susceptible host, and a means of transmission for the microorganism.

Source

Human sources of the infecting microorganisms in hospitals may be patients, personnel, or, on occasion, visitors, and may include persons with acute disease, persons in the incubation period of a disease, persons who are colonized by an infectious agent but have no apparent disease, or persons who are chronic carriers of an infectious agent. Other sources of infecting microorganisms can be the patient's own endogenous flora, which may be difficult to control, and inanimate environmental objects that have become contaminated, including equipment and medications.

Host

Resistance among persons to pathogenic microorganisms varies greatly. Some persons may be immune to infection or may be able to resist colonization by an infectious agent; others exposed to the same agent may establish a commensal relationship with the infecting microorganism and become asymptomatic carriers; still others may develop clinical disease. Host factors such as age; underlying diseases; certain treatments with antimicrobials, corticosteroids, or other immunosuppressive agents; irradiation; and breaks in the first line of defense mechanisms caused by such factors as surgical operations, anesthesia, and indwelling catheters may render patients more susceptible to infection.

Transmission

Microorganisms are transmitted in hospitals by several routes, and the same microorganism may be transmitted by more than one route. There are five main routes of transmission: contact, droplet, airborne, common vehicle, and vectorborne. For the purpose of this guideline, common vehicle and vectorborne transmission will be discussed only briefly, because neither play a significant role in typical nosocomial infections.

(1) *Contact transmission*, the most important and frequent mode of transmission of nosocomial infections, is divided into two subgroups: direct-contact transmission and indirect-contact transmission.

    (a) Direct-contact transmission involves a direct body surface-to-body surface contact and physical ransfer of microorganisms between a susceptible host and an infected or colonized person, such as occurs when a person turns a patient, gives a patient a bath, or performs other patient-care activities that require direct personal contact. Direct-contact transmission also can occur between two patients, with one serving as the source of the infectious microorganisms and the other as a susceptible host.

    (b) Indirect-contact transmission involves contact of a susceptible host with a contaminated intermediate object, usually inanimate, such as contaminated instruments, needles, or dressings, or contaminated hands that are not washed and gloves that are not changed between patients.

(2) *Droplet transmission*, theoretically, is a form of contact transmission. However, the mechanism of transfer of the pathogen to the host is quite distinct from either direct- or indirect-contact transmission. Therefore, droplet transmission will be considered a separate route of transmission in this guideline. Droplets are generated from the source person primarily during coughing, sneezing, and talking, and during the performance of certain procedures such as suctioning and bronchoscopy. Transmission occurs when droplets containing microorganisms generated from the infected person are propelled a short distance through the air and deposited on the host's conjunctivae, nasal mucosa, or mouth. Because droplets do not remain suspended in the air, special air handling and ventilation are not required to prevent droplet transmission; that is, droplet transmission *must not* be confused with airborne transmission.

(3) *Airborne transmission* occurs by dissemination of either airborne droplet nuclei (small-particle residue [5 μm or smaller in size] of evaporated droplets containing microorganisms that remain suspended in the air for long periods of time) or dust particles containing the infectious agent. Microorganisms carried in this manner can be dispersed widely by air currents and may become inhaled by a

http://www.cdc.gov/ncidod/hip/ISOLAT/isopart2.htm

susceptible host within the same room or over a longer distance from the source patient, depending on environmental factors; therefore, special air handling and ventilation are required to prevent airborne transmission. Microorganisms transmitted by airborne transmission include Mycobacterium tuberculosis and the rubeola and varicella viruses.

(4) *Common vehicle transmission* applies to microorganisms transmitted by contaminated items such as food, water, medications, devices, and equipment.

(5) *Vectorborne transmission* occurs when vectors such as mosquitoes, flies, rats, and other vermin transmit microorganisms; this route of transmission is of less significance in hospitals in the United States than in other regions of the world.

Isolation precautions are designed to prevent transmission of microorganisms by these routes in hospitals. Because agent and host factors are more difficult to control, interruption of transfer of microorganisms is directed primarily at transmission. The recommendations presented in this guideline are based on this concept.

Placing a patient on isolation precautions, however, often presents certain disadvantages to the hospital, patients, personnel, and visitors. Isolation precautions may require specialized equipment and environmental modifications that add to the cost of hospitalization. Isolation precautions may make frequent visits by nurses, physicians, and other personnel inconvenient, and they may make it more difficult for personnel to give the prompt and frequent care that sometimes is required. The use of a multi-patient room for one patient uses valuable space that otherwise might accommodate several patients. Moreover, forced solitude deprives the patient of normal social relationships and may be psychologically harmful, especially to children. These disadvantages, however, must be weighed against the hospital's mission to prevent the spread of serious and epidemiologically important microorganisms in the hospital.

FUNDAMENTALS OF ISOLATION PRECAUTIONS

A variety of infection control measures are used for decreasing the risk of transmission of microorganisms in hospitals. These measures make up the fundamentals of isolation precautions.

Handwashing and Gloving

Handwashing frequently is called the single most important measure to reduce the risks of transmitting organisms from one person to another or from one site to another on the same patient. The scientific rationale, indications, methods, and products for handwashing have been delineated in other publications.(64-72)

Washing hands as promptly and thoroughly as possible between patient contacts and after contact with blood, body fluids, secretions, excretions, and equipment or articles contaminated by them is an important component of infection control and isolation precautions. In addition to handwashing, gloves play an important role in reducing the risks of transmission of microorganisms.

Gloves are worn for three important reasons in hospitals. First, gloves are worn to provide a protective barrier and to prevent gross contamination of the hands when touching blood, body fluids, secretions, excretions, mucous membranes, and nonintact skin (27-29); the wearing of gloves in specified circumstances to reduce the risk of exposures to bloodborne pathogens is mandated by the OSHA bloodborne pathogens final rule.(51) Second, gloves are worn to reduce the likelihood that microorganisms present on the hands of personnel will be transmitted to patients during invasive or other patient-care procedures that involve touching a patient's mucous membranes and nonintact skin. Third, gloves are worn to reduce the likelihood that hands of personnel contaminated with microorganisms from a patient or a fomite can transmit these microorganisms to another patient. In this situation, gloves must be changed between patient contacts and hands washed after gloves are removed.

Wearing gloves does not replace the need for handwashing, because gloves may have small, inapparent defects or may be torn during use, and hands can become contaminated during removal of gloves.(14,15,39,72-76) Failure to change gloves between patient contacts is an infection control hazard.(32)

Patient Placement

Appropriate patient placement is a significant component of isolation precautions. A private room is important to prevent direct- or indirect-contact transmission when the source patient has poor hygienic habits, contaminates the environment, or cannot be expected to assist in maintaining infection control precautions to limit transmission of microorganisms (i.e., infants, children, and patients with altered mental status). When possible, a patient with highly transmissible or epidemiologically important microorganisms is placed in a private room with handwashing and toilet facilities, to reduce opportunities for transmission of microorganisms.

When a private room is not available, an infected patient is placed with an appropriate roommate. Patients infected by the same microorganism usually can share a room, provided they are not infected with other potentially transmissible microorganisms and the likelihood of reinfection with the same organism is minimal. Such sharing of rooms, also referred to as cohorting patients, is useful especially during outbreaks or when there is a shortage of private rooms. When a private room is not available and cohorting is not achievable or recommended,(23) it is very important to consider the epidemiology and mode of transmission of the infecting pathogen and the patient population being served in determining patient placement. Under these circumstances, consultation with infection control professionals is advised before patient placement. Moreover, when an infected patient shares a room with a noninfected patient, it also is important that patients, personnel, and visitors take precautions to prevent the spread of infection and that roommates are selected carefully.

Guidelines for construction, equipment, air handling, and ventilation for isolation rooms have been delineated in other publications.(77-79) A private room with appropriate air handling and ventilation is particularly important for reducing the risk of transmission of microorganisms from a source patient to susceptible patients and other persons in hospitals when the microorganism is spread by airborne transmission. Some hospitals use an isolation room with an anteroom as an extra measure of precaution to prevent airborne transmission. Adequate data regarding the need for an anteroom, however, is not available. Ventilation recommendations for isolation rooms housing patients with pulmonary tuberculosis have been delineated in other CDC guidelines.(23)

Transport of Infected Patients

Limiting the movement and transport of patients infected with virulent or epidemiologically important microorganisms and ensuring that such patients leave their rooms only for essential purposes reduces opportunities for transmission of microorganisms in hospitals. When patient transport is necessary, it is important that 1) appropriate barriers (e.g., masks, impervious dressings) are worn or used by the patient to reduce the opportunity for transmission of pertinent microorganisms to other patients, personnel, and visitors and to reduce contamination of the environment; 2) personnel in the area to which the patient is to be taken are notified of the impending arrival of the patient and of the precautions to be used to reduce the risk of transmission of infectious microorganisms; and 3) patients are informed of ways by which they can assist in preventing the transmission of their infectious microorganisms to others.

Masks, Respiratory Protection, Eye Protection, Face Shields

Various types of masks, goggles, and face shields are worn alone or in combination to provide barrier protection. A mask that covers both the nose and the mouth, and goggles or a face shield are worn by hospital personnel during procedures and patient-care activities that are likely to generate splashes or sprays of blood, body fluids, secretions, or excretions to provide protection of the mucous membranes of the eyes, nose, and mouth from contact transmission of pathogens. The wearing of masks, eye protection, and face shields in specified circumstances to reduce the risk of exposures to bloodborne pathogens is mandated by the OSHA bloodborne pathogens final rule.(51) A surgical mask generally is worn by hospital personnel to provide protection against spread of infectious large-particle droplets that are transmitted by close contact and generally travel only short distances (up to 3 ft) from infected patients who are coughing or sneezing.

An area of major concern and controversy over the last several years has been the role and selection of respiratory protection equipment and the implications of a respiratory protection program for prevention of transmission of tuberculosis in hospitals. Traditionally, although the efficacy was not proven, a surgical mask was worn for isolation precautions in hospitals when patients were known or suspected to be infected with pathogens spread by the airborne route of transmission. In 1990, however, the CDC tuberculosis guidelines (18) stated that surgical masks may not be effective in preventing the inhalation of droplet nuclei and recommended the use of disposable particulate respirators, despite the fact that the efficacy of particulate respirators in protecting persons from the inhalation of *M tuberculosis* had not been demonstrated. By definition, particulate respirators included dust-mist (DM), dust-fume-mist (DFM), or high-efficiency particulate air (HEPA) filter respirators certified by the CDC National Institute for Occupational Safety and Health (NIOSH); because the generic term "particulate respirator" was used in the 1990 guidelines, the implication was that any of these respirators provided sufficient protection.(80)

In 1993, a draft revision of the CDC tuberculosis guidelines (22) outlined performance criteria for respirators and stated that some DM or DFM respirators might not meet these criteria. After review of public comments, the guidelines were finalized in October 1994,(23) with the draft respirator criteria unchanged. At that time, the only class of respirators that were known to consistently meet or exceed the performance criteria outlined in the 1994 tuberculosis guidelines and that were certified by NIOSH (as required by OSHA) were HEPA filter respirators. Subsequently, NIOSH revised the testing and certification requirements for all types of air-purifying respirators, including those used for tuberculosis control.(81) The new rule, effective in July 1995, provides a broader range of certified respirators that meet the performance criteria recommended by CDC in the 1994 tuberculosis guidelines. NIOSH has indicated that the N95 (N category at 95% efficiency) meets the CDC performance criteria for a tuberculosis respirator. The new respirators are likely to be available in late 1995. Additional information on the evolution of respirator recommendations, regulations to protect hospital personnel, and the role of various federal agencies in respiratory protection for hospital personnel has been published.(80)

Gowns and Protective Apparel

Various types of gowns and protective apparel are worn to provide barrier protection and to reduce opportunities for transmission of microorganisms in hospitals. Gowns are worn to prevent contamination of clothing and to protect the skin of personnel from blood and body fluid exposures. Gowns especially treated to make them impermeable to liquids, leg coverings, boots, or shoe covers provide greater protection to the skin when splashes or large quantities of infective material are present or anticipated. The wearing of gowns and protective apparel under specified circumstances to reduce the risk of exposures to bloodborne pathogens is mandated by the OSHA bloodborne pathogens final rule.(51)

Gowns are also worn by personnel during the care of patients infected with epidemiologically important microorganisms to reduce the opportunity for transmission of pathogens from patients or items in their environment to other patients or environments; when gowns are worn for this purpose, they are removed before leaving the patient's environment and hands are washed. Adequate data regarding the efficacy of gowns for this purpose, however, is not available.

Patient-Care Equipment and Articles

Many factors determine whether special handling and disposal of used patient-care equipment and articles are prudent or required, including the likelihood of contamination with infective material; the ability to cut, stick, or otherwise cause injury (needles, scalpels, and other sharp instruments [sharps]); the severity of the associated disease; and the environmental stability of the pathogens involved. (27,51,82-84) Some used articles are enclosed in containers or bags to prevent inadvertent exposures to patients, personnel, and visitors and to prevent contamination of the environment. Used sharps are placed in puncture-resistant containers; other articles are placed in a bag. One bag is adequate if the bag is sturdy and the article can be placed in the bag without contaminating the outside of the bag (85); otherwise, two bags are used.

The scientific rationale, indications, methods, products, and equipment for reprocessing patient-care equipment have been delineated in other publications.(68,84,86-91) Contaminated, reusable critical medical devices or patient-care equipment (i.e., equipment that enters normally sterile tissue or through which blood flows) or semicritical medical devices or patient-care equipment (i.e., equipment that touches mucous membranes) are sterilized or disinfected (reprocessed) after use to reduce the risk of transmission of microorganisms to other patients; the type of reprocessing is determined by the article and its intended use, the manufacturer's recommendations, hospital policy, and any applicable guidelines and regulations.

Noncritical equipment (i.e., equipment that touches intact skin) contaminated with blood, body fluids, secretions, or excretions is cleaned and disinfected after use, according to hospital policy. Contaminated disposable (single-use) patient-care equipment is handled and transported in a manner that reduces the risk of transmission of microorganisms and decreases environmental contamination in the hospital; the equipment is disposed of according to hospital policy and applicable regulations.

Linen and Laundry

Although soiled linen may be contaminated with pathogenic microorganisms, the risk of disease transmission is negligible if it is handled, transported, and laundered in a manner that avoids transfer of microorganisms to patients, personnel, and environments. Rather than rigid rules and regulations, hygienic and common sense storage and processing of clean and soiled linen are recommended.(27,83,92,93) The methods for handling, transporting, and laundering of soiled linen are determined by hospital policy and any applicable regulations.

Dishes, Glasses, Cups, and Eating Utensils

No special precautions are needed for dishes, glasses, cups, or eating utensils. Either disposable or reusable dishes and utensils can be used for patients on isolation precautions. The combination of hot water and detergents used in hospital dishwashers is sufficient to decontaminate dishes, glasses, cups, and eating utensils.

Routine and Terminal Cleaning

The room, or cubicle, and bedside equipment of patients on Transmission-Based Precautions are cleaned using the same procedures used for patients on Standard Precautions, unless the infecting microorganism(s) and the amount of environmental contamination indicates special cleaning. In addition to thorough cleaning, adequate disinfection of bedside equipment and environmental surfaces (e.g., bedrails, bedside tables, carts, commodes, doorknobs, faucet handles) is indicated for certain pathogens, especially enterococci, which can survive in the inanimate environment for prolonged periods of time.(94) Patients admitted to hospital rooms that previously were occupied by patients infected or colonized with such pathogens are at increased risk of infection from contaminated environmental surfaces and bedside equipment if they have not been cleaned and disinfected adequately. The methods, thoroughness, and frequency of cleaning and the products used are determined by hospital policy.

HICPAC ISOLATION PRECAUTIONS

There are two tiers of HICPAC isolation precautions. In the first, and most important, tier are those precautions designed for the care of all patients in hospitals, regardless of their diagnosis or presumed infection status. Implementation of these "Standard Precautions" is the primary strategy for successful nosocomial infection control. In the second tier are precautions designed only for the care of specified patients. These additional "Transmission-Based Precautions" are for patients known or suspected to be infected by epidemiologically important pathogens spread by airborne or droplet transmission or by contact with dry skin or contaminated surfaces.

Standard Precautions

Standard Precautions synthesize the major features of UP (Blood and Body Fluid Precautions) (27,28) (designed to reduce the risk of transmission of bloodborne pathogens) and BSI (29,30) (designed to reduce the risk of transmission of pathogens from moist body substances) and applies them to all patients receiving care in hospitals, regardless of their diagnosis or presumed infection status. Standard Precautions apply to 1) blood; 2) all body fluids, secretions, and excretions *except sweat*, regardless of whether or not they contain visible blood; 3) nonintact skin; and 4) mucous membranes. Standard Precautions are designed to reduce the risk of transmission of microorganisms from both recognized and unrecognized sources of infection in hospitals.

http://www.cdc.gov/ncidod/hip/ISOLAT/isopart2.htm

Transmission-Based Precautions

Transmission-Based Precautions are designed for patients documented or suspected to be infected with highly transmissible or epidemiologically important pathogens for which additional precautions beyond Standard Precautions are needed to interrupt transmission in hospitals. There are three types of Transmission-Based Precautions: Airborne Precautions, Droplet Precautions, and Contact Precautions. They may be combined for diseases that have multiple routes of transmission. When used either singularly or in combination, they are to be used in addition to Standard Precautions.

Airborne Precautions are designed to reduce the risk of airborne transmission of infectious agents. Airborne transmission occurs by dissemination of either airborne droplet nuclei (small-particle residue [5 μm or smaller in size] of evaporated droplets that may remain suspended in the air for long periods of time) or dust particles containing the infectious agent. Microorganisms carried in this manner can be dispersed widely by air currents and may become inhaled by or deposited on a susceptible host within the same room or over a longer distance from the source patient, depending on environmental factors; therefore, special air handling and ventilation are required to prevent airborne transmission. Airborne Precautions apply to patients known or suspected to be infected with epidemiologically important pathogens that can be transmitted by the airborne route.

Droplet Precautions are designed to reduce the risk of droplet transmission of infectious agents. Droplet transmission involves contact of the conjunctivae or the mucous membranes of the nose or mouth of a susceptible person with large-particle droplets (larger than 5 μm in size) containing microorganisms generated from a person who has a clinical disease or who is a carrier of the microorganism. Droplets are generated from the source person primarily during coughing, sneezing, or talking and during the performance of certain procedures such as suctioning and bronchoscopy. Transmission via large-particle droplets requires close contact between source and recipient persons, because droplets do not remain suspended in the air and generally travel only short distances, usually 3 ft or less, through the air. Because droplets do not remain suspended in the air, special air handling and ventilation are not required to prevent droplet transmission. Droplet Precautions apply to any patient known or suspected to be infected with epidemiologically important pathogens that can be transmitted by infectious droplets.

Contact Precautions are designed to reduce the risk of transmission of epidemiologically important microorganisms by direct or indirect contact. Direct-contact transmission involves skin-to-skin contact and physical transfer of microorganisms to a susceptible host from an infected or colonized person, such as occurs when personnel turn patients, bathe patients, or perform other patient-care activities that require physical contact. Direct-contact transmission also can occur between two patients (e.g., by hand contact), with one serving as the source of infectious microorganisms and the other as a susceptible host. Indirect-contact transmission involves contact of a susceptible host with a contaminated intermediate object, usually inanimate, in the patient's environment. Contact Precautions apply to specified patients known or suspected to be infected or colonized (presence of microorganism in or on patient but without clinical signs and symptoms of infection) with epidemiologically important microorganisms than can be transmitted by direct or indirect contact.

A synopsis of the types of precautions and the patients requiring the precautions is listed in Table 1.

EMPIRIC USE OF AIRBORNE, DROPLET, OR CONTACT PRECAUTIONS

In many instances, the risk of nosocomial transmission of infection may be highest before a definitive diagnosis can be made and before precautions based on that diagnosis can be implemented. The routine use of Standard Precautions for all patients should reduce greatly this risk for conditions other than those requiring Airborne, Droplet, or Contact Precautions. While it is not possible to prospectively identify all patients needing these enhanced precautions, certain clinical syndromes and conditions carry a sufficiently high risk to warrant the empiric addition of enhanced precautions while a more definitive diagnosis is pursued. A listing of such conditions and the recommended precautions beyond Standard Precautions is presented in Table 2.

The organisms listed under the column "Potential Pathogens" are not intended to represent the complete or even most likely diagnoses, but rather possible etiologic agents that require additional precautions beyond Standard Precautions until they can be ruled out. Infection control professionals are encouraged to modify or adapt this table according to local conditions. To ensure that appropriate empiric precautions are implemented always, hospitals must have systems in place to evaluate patients routinely, according to these criteria as part of their preadmission and admission care.

IMMUNOCOMPROMISED PATIENTS

Immunocompromised patients vary in their susceptibility to nosocomial infections, depending on the severity and duration of immunosuppression. They generally are at increased risk for bacterial, fungal, parasitic, and viral infections from both endogenous and exogenous sources. The use of Standard Precautions for all patients and Transmission-Based Precautions for specified patients, as recommended in this guideline, should reduce the acquisition by these patients of institutionally acquired bacteria from other patients and environments.

It is beyond the scope of this guideline to address the various measures that may be used for immunocompromised patients to delay or prevent acquisition of potential pathogens during temporary periods of neutropenia. Rather, the primary objective of this guideline is to prevent transmission of pathogens from infected or colonized patients in hospitals. Users of this guideline, however, are referred to the

http://www.cdc.gov/ncidod/hip/ISOLAT/isopart2.htm

"Guideline for Prevention of Nosocomial Pneumonia" (95,96) for the HICPAC recommendations for prevention of nosocomial aspergillosis and Legionnaires' disease in immunocompromised patients.

RECOMMENDATIONS

The recommendations presented below are categorized as follows:

Category IA. Strongly recommended for all hospitals and strongly supported by well-designed experimental or epidemiologic studies.

Category IB. Strongly recommended for all hospitals and reviewed as effective by experts in the field and a consensus of HICPAC based on strong rationale and suggestive evidence, even though definitive scientific studies have not been done.

Category II. Suggested for implementation in many hospitals. Recommendations may be supported by suggestive clinical or epidemiologic studies, a strong theoretical rationale, or definitive studies applicable to some, but not all, hospitals.

No recommendation; unresolved issue. Practices for which insufficient evidence or consensus regarding efficacy exists.

The recommendations are limited to the topic of isolation precautions. Therefore, they must be supplemented by hospital policies and procedures for other aspects of infection and environmental control, occupational health, administrative and legal issues, and other issues beyond the scope of this guideline.

I. Administrative Controls

A. Education

Develop a system to ensure that hospital patients, personnel, and visitors are educated about use of precautions and their responsibility for adherence to them. *Category IB*

B. Adherence to Precautions

Periodically evaluate adherence to precautions, and use findings to direct improvements. *Category IB*

II. Standard Precautions

Use Standard Precautions, or the equivalent, for the care of all patients. *Category IB*

A. Handwashing

(1) Wash hands after touching blood, body fluids, secretions, excretions, and contaminated items, whether or not gloves are worn. Wash hands immediately after gloves are removed, between patient contacts, and when otherwise indicated to avoid transfer of microorganisms to other patients or environments. It may be necessary to wash hands between tasks and procedures on the same patient to prevent cross-contamination of different body sites. *Category IB*

(2) Use a plain (nonantimicrobial) soap for routine handwashing. *Category IB*

(3) Use an antimicrobial agent or a waterless antiseptic agent for specific circumstances (e.g., control of outbreaks or hyperendemic infections), as defined by the infection control program. *Category IB* (See Contact Precautions for additional recommendations on using antimicrobial and antiseptic agents.)

B. Gloves

Wear gloves (clean, nonsterile gloves are adequate) when touching blood, body fluids, secretions, excretions, and contaminated items. Put on clean gloves just before touching mucous membranes and nonintact skin. Change gloves between tasks and procedures on the same patient after contact with material that may contain a high concentration of microorganisms. Remove gloves promptly after use, before touching noncontaminated items and environmental surfaces, and before going to another patient, and wash hands immediately to avoid transfer of microorganisms to other patients or environments. *Category IB*

C. Mask, Eye Protection, Face Shield

Wear a mask and eye protection or a face shield to protect mucous membranes of the eyes, nose, and mouth during procedures and patient-care activities that are likely to generate splashes or sprays of blood, body fluids, secretions, and excretions. *Category IB*

D. Gown

Wear a gown (a clean, nonsterile gown is adequate) to protect skin and to prevent soiling of clothing during procedures and patient-care activities that are likely to generate splashes or sprays of blood, body fluids, secretions, or excretions. Select a gown that is appropriate for the activity and amount of fluid likely to be encountered. Remove a soiled gown as promptly as possible, and wash hands to avoid transfer of microorganisms to other patients or environments. *Category IB*

E. Patient-Care Equipment

Handle used patient-care equipment soiled with blood, body fluids, secretions, and excretions in a manner that prevents skin and mucous membrane exposures, contamination of clothing, and transfer of microorganisms to other patients and environments. Ensure that reusable equipment is not used for the care of another patient until it has been cleaned and reprocessed appropriately. Ensure that single-use items are discarded properly. *Category IB*

F. Environmental Control

Ensure that the hospital has adequate procedures for the routine care, cleaning, and disinfection of environmental surfaces, beds, bedrails, bedside equipment, and other frequently touched surfaces, and ensure that these procedures are being followed. *Category IB*

G. Linen

Handle, transport, and process used linen soiled with blood, body fluids, secretions, and excretions in a manner that prevents skin and mucous membrane exposures and contamination of clothing, and that avoids transfer of microorganisms to other patients and environments. *Category IB*

H. Occupational Health and Bloodborne Pathogens

(1) Take care to prevent injuries when using needles, scalpels, and other sharp instruments or devices; when handling sharp instruments after procedures; when cleaning used instruments; and when disposing of used needles. Never recap used needles, or otherwise manipulate them using both hands, or use any other technique that involves directing the point of a needle toward any part of the body; rather, use either a one-handed "scoop" technique or a mechanical device designed for holding the needle sheath. Do not remove used needles from disposable syringes by hand, and do not bend, break, or otherwise manipulate used needles by hand. Place used disposable syringes and needles, scalpel blades, and other sharp items in appropriate puncture-resistant containers, which are located as close as practical to the area in which the items were used, and place reusable syringes and needles in a puncture-resistant container for transport to the reprocessing area. *Category IB*

(2) Use mouthpieces, resuscitation bags, or other ventilation devices as an alternative to mouth-to-mouth resuscitation methods in areas where the need for resuscitation is predictable. *Category IB*

I. Patient Placement

Place a patient who contaminates the environment or who does not (or cannot be expected to) assist in maintaining appropriate hygiene or environmental control in a private room. If a private room is not available, consult with infection control professionals regarding patient placement or other alternatives. *Category IB*

III. Airborne Precautions

In addition to Standard Precautions, use Airborne Precautions, or the equivalent, for patients known or suspected to be infected with microorganisms transmitted by airborne droplet nuclei (small-particle residue [5 μm or smaller in size] of evaporated droplets containing microorganisms that remain suspended in the air and that can be dispersed widely by air currents within a room or over a long distance). *Category IB*

A. Patient Placement

Place the patient in a private room that has 1) monitored negative air pressure in relation to the surrounding areas, 2) 6 to 12 air changes per hour, and 3) appropriate discharge of air outdoors or monitored high-efficiency filtration of room air before the air is circulated to other areas in the hospital.(23) Keep the room door closed and the patient in the room. When a private room is not available, place the patient in a room with a patient who has active infection with the same microorganism, unless otherwise recommended,(23) but with no other infection. When a private room is not available and cohorting is not desirable, consultation with infection control professionals is advised before patient placement. *Category IB*

B. Respiratory Protection

Wear respiratory protection (N95 respirator) when entering the room of a patient with known or suspected infectious pulmonary tuberculosis.(23,81) Susceptible persons should not enter the room of patients known or suspected to have measles (rubeola) or varicella (chickenpox) if other immune caregivers are available. If susceptible persons must enter the room of a patient known or suspected to have measles (rubeola) or varicella, they should wear respiratory protection (N95 respirator).(81) Persons immune to measles (rubeola) or varicella need not wear respiratory protection. *Category IB*

C. Patient Transport

Limit the movement and transport of the patient from the room to essential purposes only. If transport or movement is necessary, minimize patient dispersal of droplet nuclei by placing a surgical mask on the patient, if possible. *Category IB*

D. Additional Precautions for Preventing Transmission of Tuberculosis

Consult CDC "Guidelines for Preventing the Transmission of Tuberculosis in Health-Care Facilities"(23) for additional prevention strategies.

IV. Droplet Precautions

In addition to Standard Precautions, use Droplet Precautions, or the equivalent, for a patient known or suspected to be infected with microorganisms transmitted by droplets (large-particle droplets [larger than 5 μm in size] that can be generated by the patient during coughing, sneezing, talking, or the performance of procedures). *Category IB*

A. Patient Placement

Place the patient in a private room. When a private room is not available, place the patient in a room with a patient(s) who has active infection with the same microorganism but with no other infection (cohorting). When a private room is not available and cohorting is not achievable, maintain spatial separation of at least 3 ft between the infected patient and other patients and visitors. Special air handling and ventilation are not necessary, and the door may remain open. *Category IB*

B. Mask

In addition to wearing a mask as outlined under Standard Precautions, wear a mask when working within 3 ft of the patient. (Logistically, some hospitals may want to implement the wearing of a mask to enter the room.) *Category IB*

C. Patient Transport

Limit the movement and transport of the patient from the room to essential purposes only. If transport or movement is necessary, minimize patient dispersal of droplets by masking the patient, if possible. *Category IB*

V. Contact Precautions

In addition to Standard Precautions, use Contact Precautions, or the equivalent, for specified patients known or suspected to be infected or colonized with epidemiologically important microorganisms that can be transmitted by direct contact with the patient (hand or skin-to-skin contact that occurs when performing patient-care activities that require touching the patient's dry skin) or indirect contact (touching) with environmental surfaces or patient-care items in the patient's environment. *Category IB*

A. Patient Placement

Place the patient in a private room. When a private room is not available, place the patient in a room with a patient(s) who has active infection with the same microorganism but with no other infection (cohorting). When a private room is not available and cohorting is not achievable, consider the epidemiology of the microorganism and the patient population when determining patient placement. Consultation with infection control professionals is advised before patient placement. *Category IB*

B. Gloves and Handwashing

In addition to wearing gloves as outlined under Standard Precautions, wear gloves (clean, nonsterile gloves are adequate) when entering the room. During the course of providing care for a patient, change gloves after having contact with infective material that may contain high concentrations of microorganisms (fecal material and wound drainage). Remove gloves before leaving the patient's room and wash hands immediately with an antimicrobial agent or a waterless antiseptic agent.(72,94) After glove removal and handwashing, ensure that hands do not touch potentially contaminated environmental surfaces or items in the patient's room to avoid transfer of microorganisms to other patients or environments. *Category IB*

C. Gown

In addition to wearing a gown as outlined under Standard Precautions, wear a gown (a clean, nonsterile gown is adequate) when entering the room if you anticipate that your clothing will have substantial contact with the patient, environmental surfaces, or items in the patient's room, or if the patient is incontinent or has diarrhea, an ileostomy, a colostomy, or wound drainage not contained by a dressing. Remove the gown before leaving the patient's environment. After gown removal, ensure that clothing does not contact potentially contaminated environmental surfaces to avoid transfer of microorganisms to other patients or environments. *Category IB*

D. Patient Transport

Limit the movement and transport of the patient from the room to essential purposes only. If the patient is transported out of the room, ensure that precautions are maintained to minimize the risk of transmission of microorganisms to other patients and contamination of environmental surfaces or equipment. *Category IB*

E. Patient-Care Equipment

When possible, dedicate the use of noncritical patient-care equipment to a single patient (or cohort of patients infected or colonized with the pathogen requiring precautions) to avoid sharing between patients. If use of common equipment or items is unavoidable, then adequately clean and disinfect them before use for another patient. *Category IB*

F. Additional Precautions for Preventing the Spread of Vancomycin Resistance

Consult the HICPAC report on preventing the spread of vancomycin resistance for additional prevention strategies.(94)

Contents
Updated: February 18, 1997

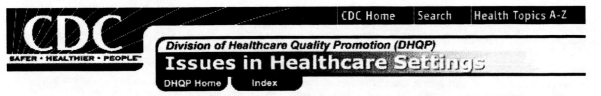

Table 2
Clinical Syndromes or Conditions Warranting Additional Empiric Precautions to Prevent Transmission of Epidemiologically Important Pathogens Pending Confirmation of Diagnosis*

Clinical Syndrome or Condition†	Potential Pathogens‡	Empiric Precautions
Diarrhea		
Acute diarrhea with a likely infectious cause in an incontinent or diapered patient	Enteric pathogens§	Contact
Diarrhea in an adult with a history of recent antibiotic use	*Clostridium difficile*	Contact
Meningitis	*Neisseria meningitidis*	Droplet
Rash or exanthems, generalized, etiology unknown		
Petechial/ecchymotic with fever	*Neisseria meningitidis*	Droplet
Vesicular	Varicella	Airborne and Contact
Maculopapular with coryza and fever	Rubeola (measles)	Airborne
Respiratory infections		
Cough/fever/upper lobe pulmonary infiltrate in an HIV-negative patient or a patient at low risk for HIV infection	*Mycobacterium tuberculosis*	Airborne
Cough/fever/pulmonary infiltrate in any lung location in a HIV-infected patient or a patient at high risk for HIV infection (23)	*Mycobacterium tuberculosis*	Airborne
Paroxysmal or severe persistent cough during periods of pertussis activity	*Bordetella pertussis*	Droplet
Respiratory infections, particularly bronchiolitis and croup, in infants and young children	Respiratory syncytial or parainfluenza virus	Contact
Risk of multidrug-resistant microorganisms		
History of infection or colonization with multidrug-resistant organisms‖	Resistant bacteria‖	Contact
Skin, wound, or urinary tract infection in a patient with a recent hospital or nursing home stay in a facility where multidrug-resistant organisms are prevalent	Resistant bacteria‖	Contact
Skin or Wound Infection		
Abscess or draining wound that cannot be covered	*Staphylococcus aureus*, group A streptococcus	Contact

* Infection control professionals are encouraged to modify or adapt this table according to local conditions. To ensure that appropriate empiric precautions are implemented always, hospitals must have systems in place to evaluate patients routinely according to these criteria as part of their preadmission and admission care.

† Patients with the syndromes or conditions listed below may present with atypical signs or symptoms (eg, pertussis in neonates and adults may not have paroxysmal or severe cough). The clinician's index of suspicion should be guided by the prevalence of specific conditions in the community, as well as clinical judgment.

‡ The organisms listed under the column "Potential Pathogens" are not intended to represent the complete, or even most likely, diagnoses, but rather possible etiologic agents that require additional precautions beyond Standard Precautions until they can be ruled out.

§ These pathogens include enterohemorrhagic *Escherichia coli* O157:H7, *Shigella*, hepatitis A, and rotavirus.

‖Resistant bacteria judged by the infection control program, based on current state, regional, or national recommendations, to be of special clinical or epidemiological significance.

Contents
Updated: February 18, 1997

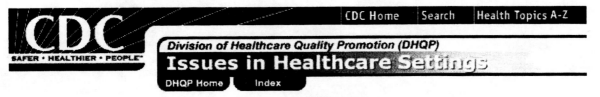

CDC Home | Search | Health Topics A-Z

Division of Healthcare Quality Promotion (DHQP)

Issues in Healthcare Settings

DHQP Home | Index

APPENDIX A

Type and Duration of Precautions Needed for Selected Infections and Conditions

Infection/Condition	Type*	Duration†
Abscess		
Draining, major *a*	C	DI
Draining, minor or limited *b*	S	
Acquired immunodeficiency syndrome *c*	S	
Actinomycosis	S	
Adenovirus infection, in infants and young children	D,C	DI
Amebiasis	S	
Anthrax		
Cutaneous	S	
Pulmonary	S	
Antibiotic-associated colitis (see *Clostridium difficile*)		
Arthropodborne viral encephalitides (eastern, western, Venezuelan equine encephalomyelitis; St Louis, California encephalitis)	S *d*	
Arthropodborne viral fevers (dengue, yellow fever, Colorado tick fever)	S *d*	
Ascariasis	S	
Aspergillosis	S	
Babesiosis	S	
Blastomycosis, North American, cutaneous or pulmonary	S	
Botulism	S	
Bronchiolitis (see respiratory infections in infants and young children)		
Brucellosis (undulant, Malta, Mediterranean fever)	S	
Campylobacter gastroenteritis (see gastroenteritis)		
Candidiasis, all forms including mucocutaneous	S	
Cat-scratch fever (benign inoculation lymphoreticulosis)	S	
Cellulitis, uncontrolled drainage	C	DI
Chancroid (soft chancre)	S	
Chickenpox (varicella; see F *e* for varicella exposure)	A,C	F *e*
Chlamydia trachomatis		
Conjunctivitis	S	
Genital	S	
Respiratory	S	
Cholera (see gastroenteritis)		
Closed-cavity infection		
Draining, limited or minor	S	
Not draining	S	
Clostridium		
C botulinum	S	
C difficile	C	DI

http://www.cdc.gov/ncidod/hip/ISOLAT/isoapp_a.htm

C perfringens		
Food poisoning	S	
Gas gangrene	S	
Coccidioidomycosis (valley fever)		
Draining lesions	S	
Pneumonia	S	
Colorado tick fever	S	
Congenital rubella	C	F *f*
Conjunctivitis		
Acute bacterial	S	
Chlamydia	S	
Gonococcal	S	
Acute viral (acute hemorrhagic)	C	DI
Coxsackievirus disease (see enteroviral infection)		
Creutzfeldt-Jakob disease	S *g*	
Croup (see respiratory infections in infants and young children)		
Cryptococcosis	S	
Cryptosporidiosis (see gastroenteritis)		
Cysticercosis	S	
Cytomegalovirus infection, neonatal or immunosuppressed	S	
Decubitus ulcer, infected		
Major *a*	C	DI
Minor or limited *b*	S	
Dengue	S *d*	
Diarrhea, acute-infective etiology suspected (see gastroenteritis)		
Diphtheria		
Cutaneous	C	CN *h*
Pharyngeal	D	CN *h*
Ebola viral hemorrhagic fever	C *i*	DI
Echinococcosis (hydatidosis)	S	
Echovirus (see enteroviral infection)		
Encephalitis or encephalomyelitis (see specific etiologic agents)		
Endometritis	S	
Enterobiasis (pinworm disease, oxyuriasis)	S	
Enterococcus species (see multidrug-resistant organisms if epidemiologically significant or vancomycin resistant)		
Enterocolitis, *Clostridium difficile*	C	DI
Enteroviral infections		
Adults	S	
Infants and young children	C	DI
Epiglottitis, due to *Haemophilus influenzae*	D	U(24 hrs)
Epstein-Barr virus infection, including infectious mononucleosis	S	
Erythema infectiosum (also see Parvovirus B19)	S	
Escherichia coli gastroenteritis (see gastroenteritis)		
Food poisoning		
Botulism	S	
Clostridium perfringens or welchii	S	
Staphylococcal	S	
Furunculosis-staphylococcal		
Infants and young children	C	DI
Gangrene (gas gangrene)	S	

Gastroenteritis

   Campylobacter species   S*j*

   Cholera   S*j*

   Clostridium difficile   C   DI

   Cryptosporidium species   S*j*

   Escherichia coli

     Enterohemorrhagic O157:H7   S*j*

       Diapered or incontinent   C   DI

     Other species   S*j*

   Giardia lamblia   S*j*

   Rotavirus   S*j*

     Diapered or incontinent   C   DI

   Salmonella species (including *S typhi*)   S*j*

   Shigella species   S*j*

     Diapered or incontinent   C   DI

   Vibrio parahaemolyticus   S*j*

   Viral (if not covered elsewhere)   S*j*

   Yersinia enterocolitica   S*j*

German measles (see rubella)

Giardiasis (see gastroenteritis)

Gonococcal ophthalmia neonatorum (gonorrheal ophthalmia,   S
  acute conjunctivitis of newborn)

Gonorrhea   S

Granuloma inguinale (donovanosis, granuloma venereum)   S

Guillain-Barré, syndrome   S

Hand, foot, and mouth disease (see enteroviral infection)

Hantavirus pulmonary syndrome   S

Helicobacter pylori   S

Hemorrhagic fevers (for example, Lassa and Ebola)   C *i*   DI

Hepatitis, viral

   Type A   S

     Diapered or incontinent patients   C   F *k*

   Type B-HBsAg positive   S

   Type C and other unspecified non-A, non-B   S

   Type E   S

Herpangina (see enteroviral infection)

Herpes simplex (*Herpesvirus hominis*)

   Encephalitis   S

   Neonatal *l* (see F *l* for neonatal exposure)   C   DI

   Mucocutaneous, disseminated or primary, severe   C   DI

   Mucocutaneous, recurrent (skin, oral, genital)   S

Herpes zoster (varicella-zoster)

   Localized in immunocompromised patient, or disseminated   A,C   DI *m*

   Localized in normal patient   S *m*

Histoplasmosis   S

HIV (see human immunodeficiency virus)   S

Hookworm disease (ancylostomiasis, uncinariasis)   S

Human immunodeficiency virus (HIV) infection *c*   S

Impetigo   C   U(24 hrs)

Infectious mononucleosis   S

Influenza	D [n]	DI
Kawasaki syndrome	S	
Lassa fever	C [i]	DI
Legionnaires' disease	S	
Leprosy	S	
Leptospirosis	S	
Lice (pediculosis)	C	U(24 hrs)
Listeriosis	S	
Lyme disease	S	
Lymphocytic choriomeningitis	S	
Lymphogranuloma venereum	S	
Malaria	S [d]	
Marburg virus disease	C [i]	DI
Measles (rubeola), all presentations	A	DI
Melioidosis, all forms	S	
Meningitis		
Aseptic (nonbacterial or viral meningitis; also see enteroviral infections)	S	
Bacterial, gram-negative enteric, in neonates	S	
Fungal	S	
Haemophilus influenzae, known or suspected	D	U(24 hrs)
Listeria monocytogenes	S	
Neisseria meningitidis (meningococcal) known or suspected	D	U(24 hrs)
Pneumococcal	S	
Tuberculosis [o]	S	
Other diagnosed bacterial	S	
Meningococcal pneumonia	D	U(24 hrs)
Meningococcemia (meningococcal sepsis)	D	U(24 hrs)
Molluscum contagiosum	S	
Mucormycosis	S	
Multidrug-resistant organisms, infection or colonization [p]		
Gastrointestinal	C	CN
Respiratory	C	CN
Pneumococcal	S	
Skin, wound, or burn	C	CN
Mumps (infectious parotitis)	D	F [q]
Mycobacteria, nontuberculosis (atypical)		
Pulmonary	S	
Wound	S	
Mycoplasma pneumonia	D	DI
Necrotizing enterocolitis	S	
Nocardiosis, draining lesions or other presentations	S	
Norwalk agent gastroenteritis (see viral gastroenteritis)		
Orf	S	
Parainfluenza virus infection, respiratory in infants and young children	C	DI
Parvovirus B19	D	F [r]
Pediculosis (lice)	C	U(24 hrs)
Pertussis (whooping cough)	D	F [s]
Pinworm infection	S	
Plague		
Bubonic	S	
Pneumonic	D	U(72 hrs)

Pleurodynia (see enteroviral infection)

Pneumonia

Adenovirus	D,C	DI
Bacterial not listed elsewhere (including gram-negative bacterial)	S	
Burkholderia cepacia in cystic fibrosis (CF) patients, including respiratory tract colonization	S *t*	
Chlamydia	S	
Fungal	S	
Haemophilus influenzae		
Adults	S	
Infants and children (any age)	D	U(24 hrs)
Legionella	S	
Meningococcal	D	U(24 hrs)
Multidrug-resistant bacterial (see multidrug-resistant organisms)		
Mycoplasma (primary atypical pneumonia)	D	DI
Pneumococcal	S	
Multidrug-resistant (see multidrug-resistant organisms)		
Pneumocystis carinii	S *u*	
Pseudomonas cepacia (see *Burkholderia cepacia*)	S *t*	
Staphylococcus aureus	S	
Streptococcus, group A		
Adults	S	
Infants and young children	D	U(24hrs)
Viral		
Adults	S	
Infants and young children (see respiratory infectious disease, acute)		
Poliomyelitis	S	
Psittacosis (ornithosis)	S	
Q fever	S	
Rabies	S	
Rat-bite fever (*Streptobacillus moniliformis* disease, *Spirillum minus* disease)	S	
Relapsing fever	S	
Resistant bacterial infection or colonization (see multidrug-resistant organisms)		
Respiratory infectious disease, acute (if not covered elsewhere)		
Adults	S	
Infants and young children *c*	C	DI
Respiratory syncytial virus infection, in infants and young children, and immunocompromised adults	C	DI
Reye's syndrome	S	
Rheumatic fever	S	
Rickettsial fevers, tickborne (Rocky Mountain spotted fever, tickborne typhus fever)	S	
Rickettsialpox (vesicular rickettsiosis)	S	
Ringworm (dermatophytosis, dermatomycosis, tinea)	S	
Ritter's disease (staphylococcal scalded skin syndrome)	S	
Rocky Mountain spotted fever	S	
Roseola infantum (exanthem subitum)	S	
Rotavirus infection (see gastroenteritis)		
Rubella (German measles; also see congenital rubella)	D	F *v*
Salmonellosis (see gastroenteritis)		
Scabies	C	U(24 hrs)
Scalded skin syndrome, staphylococcal (Ritter's disease)	S	
Schistosomiasis (bilharziasis)	S	

Shigellosis (see gastroenteritis)		
Sporotrichosis	S	
Spirillum minus disease (rat-bite fever)	S	
Staphylococcal disease (*S aureus*)		
Skin, wound, or burn		
Major *a*	C	DI
Minor or limited *b*	S	
Enterocolitis	S *j*	
Multidrug-resistant (see multidrug-resistant organisms)		
Pneumonia	S	
Scalded skin syndrome	S	
Toxic shock syndrome	S	
Streptobacillus moniliformis disease (rat-bite fever)	S	
Streptococcal disease (group A streptococcus)		
Skin, wound, or burn		
Major *a*	C	U(24 hrs)
Minor or limited *b*	S	
Endometritis (puerperal sepsis)	S	
Pharyngitis in infants and young children	D	U(24 hrs)
Pneumonia in infants and young children	D	U(24 hrs)
Scarlet fever in infants and young children	D	U(24 hrs)
Streptococcal disease (group B streptococcus), neonatal	S	
Streptococcal disease (not group A or B) unless covered elsewhere	S	
Multidrug-resistant (see multidrug-resistant organisms)		
Strongyloidiasis	S	
Syphilis		
Skin and mucous membrane, including congenital, primary, secondary	S	
Latent (tertiary) and seropositivity without lesions	S	
Tapeworm disease		
Hymenolepis nana	S	
Taenia solium (pork)	S	
Other	S	
Tetanus	S	
Tinea (fungus infection dermatophytosis, dermatomycosis, ringworm)	S	
Toxoplasmosis	S	
Toxic shock syndrome (staphylococcal disease)	S	
Trachoma, acute	S	
Trench mouth (Vincent's angina)	S	
Trichinosis	S	
Trichomoniasis	S	
Trichuriasis (whipworm disease)	S	
Tuberculosis		
Extrapulmonary, draining lesion (including scrofula)	S	
Extrapulmonary, meningitis *o*	S	
Pulmonary, confirmed or suspected or laryngeal disease	A	F *w*
Skin-test positive with no evidence of current pulmonary disease	S	
Tularemia		
Draining lesion	S	
Pulmonary	S	
Typhoid (*Salmonella typhi*) fever (see gastroenteritis)		
Typhus, endemic and epidemic	S	

http://www.cdc.gov/ncidod/hip/ISOLAT/isoapp_a.htm

Urinary tract infection (including pyelonephritis), with or without urinary catheter	S	
Varicella (chickenpox)	A,C	F *e*
Vibrio parahaemolyticus (see gastroenteritis)		
Vincent's angina (trench mouth)	S	
Viral diseases		
Respiratory (if not covered elsewhere)		
Adults	S	
Infants and young children (see respiratory infectious disease, acute)		
Whooping cough (pertussis)	D	F *s*
Wound infections		
Major *a*	C	DI
Minor or limited *b*	S	
Yersinia enterocolitica gastroenteritis (see gastroenteritis)		
Zoster (varicella-zoster)		
Localized in immunocompromised patient, disseminated	A,C	DI *m*
Localized in normal patient	S *m*	
Zygomycosis (phycomycosis, mucormycosis)	S	

Abbreviations:

* Type of Precautions: A, Airborne; C, Contact; D, Droplet; S, Standard; when A, C, and D are specified, also use S.

† Duration of precautions: CN, until off antibiotics and culture-negative; DI, duration of illness (with wound lesions, DI means until they stop draining); U, until time specified in hours (hrs) after initiation of effective therapy; F, see footnote.

a No dressing or dressing does not contain drainage adequately.

b Dressing covers and contains drainage adequately.

c Also see syndromes or conditions listed in Table 2.

d Install screens in windows and doors in endemic areas.

e Maintain precautions until all lesions are crusted. The average incubation period for varicella is 10 to 16 days, with a range of 10 to 21 days. After exposure, use varicella zoster immune globulin (VZIG) when appropriate, and discharge susceptible patients if possible. Place exposed susceptible patients on Airborne Precautions beginning 10 days after exposure and continuing until 21 days after last exposure (up to 28 days if VZIG has been given). Susceptible persons should not enter the room of patients on precautions if other immune caregivers are available.

f Place infant on precautions during any admission until 1 year of age, unless nasopharyngeal and urine cultures are negative for virus after age 3 months.

g Additional special precautions are necessary for handling and decontamination of blood, body fluids and tissues, and contaminated items from patients with confirmed or suspected disease. See latest College of American Pathologists (Northfield, Illinois) guidelines or other references.

h Until two cultures taken at least 24 hours apart are negative.

i Call state health department and CDC for specific advice about management of a suspected case. During the 1995 Ebola outbreak in Zaire, interim recommendations were published.(97) Pending a comprehensive review of the epidemiologic data from the outbreak and evaluation of the interim recommendations, the 1988 guidelines for management of patients with suspected viral hemorrhagic infections (16) will be reviewed and updated if indicated.

j Use Contact Precautions for diapered or incontinent children <6 years of age for duration of illness.

k Maintain precautions in infants and children <3 years of age for duration of hospitalization; in children 3 to 14 years of age, until 2 weeks after onset of symptoms; and in others, until 1 week after onset of symptoms.

l For infants delivered vaginally or by C-section and if mother has active infection and membranes have been ruptured for more than 4 to 6 hours.

m Persons susceptible to varicella are also at risk for developing varicella when exposed to patients with herpes zoster lesions; therefore, susceptibles should not enter the room if other immune caregivers are available.

n The "Guideline for Prevention of Nosocomial Pneumonia" (95,96) recommends surveillance, vaccination, antiviral agents, and use of private rooms with negative air pressure as much as feasible for patients for whom influenza is suspected or diagnosed. Many hospitals encounter logistic difficulties and physical plant limitations when admitting multiple patients with suspected influenza during community outbreaks. If sufficient private rooms are unavailable, consider cohorting patients or, at the very least, avoid room sharing with high-risk patients. See "Guideline for Prevention of Nosocomial Pneumonia" (95,96) for additional prevention and control strategies.

o Patient should be examined for evidence of current (active) pulmonary tuberculosis. If evidence exists, additional precautions are necessary (see tuberculosis).

p Resistant bacteria judged by the infection control program, based on current state, regional, or national recommendations, to be of special clinical and epidemiologic significance.

q For 9 days after onset of swelling.

http://www.cdc.gov/ncidod/hip/ISOLAT/isoapp_a.htm

^r Maintain precautions for duration of hospitalization when chronic disease occurs in an immunodeficient patient. For patients with transient aplastic crisis or red-cell crisis, maintain precautions for 7 days.

^s Maintain precautions until 5 days after patient is placed on effective therapy.

^t Avoid cohorting or placement in the same room with a CF patient who is not infected or colonized with *B cepacia*. Persons with CF who visit or provide care and are not infected or colonized with *B cepacia* may elect to wear a mask when within 3 ft of a colonized or infected patient.

^u Avoid placement in the same room with an immunocompromised patient.

^v Until 7 days after onset of rash.

^w Discontinue precautions *only* when TB patient is on effective therapy, is improving clinically, and has three consecutive negative sputum smears collected on different days, or TB is ruled out. Also see CDC "Guidelines for Preventing the Transmission of Tuberculosis in Health-Care Facilities."(23)

Contents

Updated: February 18, 1997

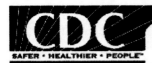

| CDC Home | Search | Health Topics A-Z |

Division of Healthcare Quality Promotion (DHQP)
Issues in Healthcare Settings

DHQP Home   Index

About DHQP

Antimicrobial Resistance

non-hospital settings

Bloodborne Pathogens

Child Care

Dialysis

Guidelines and Recommendations

-Infectious Diseases

Laboratory

Occupational Health

Outbreaks

Sterilization and Disinfection

Surveillance

Training

Antimicrobial Resistance
Multidrug-Resistant Organisms in Non-Hospital Healthcare Settings

What are "non-hospital healthcare settings"?

They refer to residential settings (e.g., long-term care and skilled nursing homes), home care, hemodialysis centers, and physicians' offices.

What are multidrug-resistant organisms?

They are bacteria and other microorganisms that have developed resistance to antimicrobial drugs. Common examples of these organisms include:

- **MRSA** - methicillin/oxacillin-resistant *Staphylococcus aureus*
- **VRE** - vancomycin-resistant enterococci
- **ESBLs** - extended-spectrum beta-lactamases (which are resistant to cephalosporins and monobactams)
- **PRSP** - penicillin-resistant *Streptococcus pneumoniae*

Which multidrug-resistant organisms are most commonly seen in non-hospital settings?

MRSA and VRE are the most commonly encountered multidrug-resistant organisms in patients residing in non-hospital healthcare facilities, such as nursing homes and other long-term care facilities. PRSP are more common in patients seeking care in outpatient settings such as physicians' offices and clinics, especially in pediatric settings. **back to top**

What is the difference between colonization and infection?

COLONIZATION means that the organism is present in or on the body but is not causing illness.

INFECTION means that the organism is present and is causing illness. **back to top**

What conditions increase the risk of acquiring these organisms?

There are several risk factors for both colonization and infection:

- severity of illness
- previous exposure to antimicrobial agents
- underlying diseases or conditions, particularly:
  - chronic renal disease
  - insulin-dependent diabetes mellitus
  - peripheral vascular disease
  - dermatitis or skin lesions
- invasive procedures, such as:
  - dialysis
  - presence of invasive devices
  - urinary catheterization
- repeated contact with the healthcare system

Page Index
- ▶ non-hospital settings
- ▶ multidrug-resistant organisms
- ▶ MDRO's in non-hospital settings
- ▶ colonization vs. infection
- ▶ risk of acquisition
- ▶ prevention and Control
- ▶ pre-admission screening
- ▶ outbreak management
- ▶ visitors/family
- ▶ family caregiver precautions
- ▶ additional reading

http://www.cdc.gov/ncidod/hip/Aresist/nonhosp.htm

- previous colonization of by a multidrug-resistant organism
- advanced age
  back to top

Should patients colonized or infected with these organisms be admitted to non-hospital healthcare facilities?

Non-hospital healthcare facilities can safely care for and manage these patients by following appropriate infection control practices. In addition, non-hospital healthcare facilities should be aware that persons with MRSA, VRE, and other infections may be protected by the Americans with Disabilities Act or other applicable state or local laws or regulations. **back to top**

What can be done to prevent or control transmission of these pathogens in my facility?

CDC's recommendations for preventing transmission of MRSA / VRE in hospitals consist of **standard precautions**, which **should be used for all patient care**. In addition, CDC recommends **contact precautions** when the facility (based on national or local regulations) deems the multidrug-resistant microorganism to be of special clinical and epidemiologic significance.

The components of contact precautions may be adapted for use in non-hospital healthcare facilities, especially if the patient has draining wounds or difficulty controlling body fluids.

In addition to standard and contact precautions, the following procedures also may be considered for non-hospital healthcare facilities:

- **Patient placement** - Place the patient in a private room, if possible. When a private room is not available, place the patient in a room with a patient who is colonized or infected with the same organism, but does not have any other infection (cohorting). Another option is to place an infected patient with a patient who does not have risk factors for infection.
- **Patient placement in dialysis facilities** - Dialyze the patient at a station with as few adjacent stations as possible (e.g., at the end or corner of the unit).
- **Group activities** - It is extremely important to maintain the patients' ability to socialize and have access to rehabilitation opportunities. Infected or colonized patients should be permitted to participate in group meals and activities if draining wounds are covered, bodily fluids are contained, and the patients observe good hygienic practices.

The following are recommended for prevention of VRE / MRSA in hospitals and may be adapted for use in non-hospital healthcare facilities:

- Obtain stool cultures or rectal swab cultures of roommates of patients newly found to be infected or colonized with VRE, and nasal swabs for MRSA.
- Adopt a policy for deciding when patients can be removed from isolation, e.g., VRE-negative results on at least three consecutive occasions, one or more weeks apart.
- Consult health departments regarding discharge requirements for patients with MRSA or VRE. **back to top**

Are there any recommendations for pre-admission screening in non-hospital settings?

CDC does not have recommendations for pre-admission screening.
However, the following options may be considered:

- Do NOT perform screening
- Screen high-risk patients on admission
  (Some evidence from a multicenter study suggests that screening before transfer leads to increased isolation and decreased transmission of VRE). **back to top**

How should clusters or outbreaks of infections be handled?

Consult with state or local health departments or an experienced infection control professional for reporting requirements and management of MRSA or VRE outbreaks.
back to top

If a patient in a facility is colonized or infected with MRSA or VRE, what do their visitors/family members need to know?

In general, healthy people are at low risk of getting infected with MRSA or VRE. Therefore, casual contact - such as kissing, hugging, and touching - is acceptable. Visitors should wash their hands before leaving an infected person's room. Also, disposable gloves should be worn if contact with body fluids is expected. (If excessive contact with body fluids is expected, gowns should also be worn.)
It is also acceptable for infants and children to have casual contact with these patients. **back to top**

What precautions should family caregivers take for infected persons in their homes?

Outside of healthcare settings, there is little risk of transmitting organisms to persons at risk of disease from MRSA / VRE, therefore, healthy people are at low risk of getting infected. In the home, the following precautions should be followed:

- Caregivers should wash their hands with soap and water after physical contact with the infected or colonized person and before leaving the home.
- Towels used for drying hands after contact should be used only once.
- Disposable gloves should be worn if contact with body fluids is expected and hands should be washed after removing the gloves.
- Linens should be changed and washed if they are soiled and on a routine basis.
- The patient's environment should be cleaned routinely and when soiled with body fluids.
- Notify doctors and other healthcare personnel who provide care for the patient that the patient is colonized/infected with a multidrug-resistant organism.
  back to top

ADDITIONAL READINGS

Antimicrobial resistance in long-term-care facilities. 1996 Leave CDC

back to top

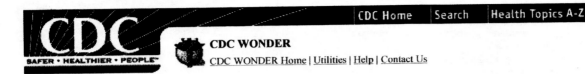

CDC WONDER

CDC WONDER Home | Utilities | Help | Contact Us

Warning:

This site is being maintained for historical purposes, but has had no new entries since October 1998. If you would like your search to include more recent articles, please visit the new prevention guidelines site,

CDC Recommends

at http://www.phppo.cdc.gov/CDCrecommends/AdvSearchV.asp.

Recommendations for Preventing the Spread of Vancomycin Resistance Recommendations of the Hospital Infection Control Practices Advisory Committee (HICPAC)

MMWR 44(RR12);1-13

Publication date: 09/22/1995

Table of Contents

Article

Summary

Since 1989, a rapid increase in the incidence of infection and colonization with vancomycin-resistant enterococci (VRE) has been reported by U.S. hospitals. This increase poses important problems, including a) the lack of available antimicrobial therapy for VRE infections, because most VRE are also resistant to drugs previously used to treat such infections (e.g., aminoglycosides and ampicillin), and b) the possibility that the vancomycin-resistant genes present in VRE can be transferred to other gram-positive microorganisms (e.g., Staphylococcus aureus). An increased risk for VRE infection and colonization has been associated with previous vancomycin and/or multiantimicrobial therapy, severe underlying disease or immunosuppression, and intraabdominal surgery. Because enterococci can be found in the normal gastrointestinal and female genital tracts, most enterococcal infections have been attributed to endogenous sources within the individual patient. However, recent reports of outbreaks and endemic infections caused by enterococci, including VRE, have indicated that patient-to-patient transmission of the microorganisms can occur either through direct contact or through indirect contact via a) the hands of personnel or b) contaminated patient-care equipment or environmental surfaces.

This report presents recommendations of the Hospital Infection Control Practices Advisory Committee for preventing and controlling the spread of vancomycin resistance, with a special focus on VRE. Preventing and controlling the spread of vancomycin resistance will require coordinated, concerted efforts from all involved hospital departments and can be achieved only if each of the following elements is addressed: a) prudent vancomycin use by clinicians, b) education of hospital staff regarding the problem of vancomycin resistance, c) early detection and prompt reporting of vancomycin resistance in enterococci and other gram-positive microorganisms by the hospital microbiology laboratory, and d) immediate implementation of appropriate infection-control measures to prevent person-to-person transmission of VRE.

INTRODUCTION

From 1989 through 1993, the percentage of nosocomial enterococcal infections reported to CDC's National Nosocomial Infections Surveillance (NNIS) system that were caused by vancomycin-resistant enterococci (VRE) increased from 0.3% to 7.9% (1). This overall increase primarily reflected the 34-fold increase in the percentage of VRE infections in patients in intensive-care units (ICUs) (i.e., from 0.4% to 13.6%), although a trend toward an increased percentage of VRE infections in non-ICU patients also was noted (1). The occurrence of VRE in NNIS hospitals was associated with larger hospital size (i.e., a hospital with greater than or equal to 200 beds) and university affiliation (1). Other hospitals also have reported increased endemic rates and clusters of VRE infection and colonization (2-8). The actual increase in the incidence of VRE in U.S. hospitals might be greater than reported because the fully automated methods used in many clinical laboratories cannot consistently detect vancomycin resistance, especially moderate vancomycin resistance (as manifested in the VanB phenotype) (9-11).

Vancomycin resistance in enterococci has coincided with the increasing incidence of high-level enterococcal resistance to penicillin and aminoglycosides, thus presenting a challenge for physicians who treat patients who have infections caused by these microorganisms (1,4). Treatment options are often limited to combining antimicrobials or experimental compounds that have unproven efficacy (12-14). The epidemiology of VRE has not been clarified; however, certain patient populations are at increased risk for VRE infection or colonization. These populations include critically ill patients or those with severe underlying disease or immunosuppression (e.g., patients in ICUs or in oncology or transplant wards); persons who have had an intraabdominal or cardio-thoracic surgical procedure or an indwelling urinary or central venous catheter; and persons who have had a prolonged hospital stay or received multiantimicrobial and/or vancomycin therapy (2-8). Because enterococci are part of the normal flora of the gastrointestinal and female genital tracts, most infections with these microorganisms have been attributed to the patient's endogenous flora (15). However, recent studies have indicated that VRE and other enterococci can be transmitted directly by patient-to-patient contact or indirectly by transient carriage on the hands of personnel (16) or by contaminated environmental surfaces and patient-care equipment (3,8,17).

The potential emergence of vancomycin resistance in clinical isolates of Staphylococcus aureus and Staphylococcus epidermidis also is a public health concern. The vanA gene, which is frequently plasmid-borne and confers high-level resistance to vancomycin, can be transferred in vitro from enterococci to a variety of gram-positive microorganisms (18,19), including S. aureus (20). Although vancomycin resistance in clinical strains of S. epidermidis or S. aureus has not been reported, vancomycin-resistant strains of Staphylococcus haemolyticus have been isolated (21,22).

In November 1993 and February 1994, the Subcommittee on the Prevention and Control of Antimicrobial-Resistant Microorganisms in Hospitals of CDC's Hospital Infection Control Practices Advisory Committee (HICPAC) responded to the increase in vancomycin resistance in enterococci by meeting with representatives from the American Hospital Association, the American Society for Microbiology, the Association for Professionals in Infection Control and Epidemiology, the Infectious Diseases Society of America, the Society for Healthcare Epidemiology of America, and the Surgical Infection Society. Meeting participants agreed with the need for prompt implementation of control measures; thus, recommendations to prevent the spread of VRE were developed. Public comments were solicited and incorporated into the draft recommendations. In November 1994, HICPAC ratified the following recommendations for preventing and controlling the spread of vancomycin resistance, with special focus on VRE. HICPAC recognizes that a) data are limited and additional research will be required to clarify the epidemiology of VRE and determine cost-effective control strategies, and b) many U.S. hospitals have concurrent problems with other antimicrobial-resistant organisms (e.g., methicillin-resistant S. aureus {MRSA} and beta-lactam and aminoglycoside-resistant gram-negative bacilli) that might have different epidemiologic features and require different control measures.

RECOMMENDATIONS

Each hospital -- through collaboration of its quality-improvement and infection-control programs; pharmacy and therapeutics committee; microbiology laboratory; clinical departments; and nursing, administrative, and housekeeping services -- should develop a comprehensive, institution-specific, strategic plan to detect, prevent, and control infection and colonization with VRE. The following elements should be addressed in the plan.

Prudent Vancomycin Use

Vancomycin use has been reported consistently as a risk factor for infection and colonization with VRE (2,4,7,8,17) and may increase the possibility of the emergence of vancomycin-resistant S. aureus (VRSA) and/or vancomycin-resistant S. epidermidis (VRSE). Therefore, all hospitals and other health-care delivery services, even those at which VRE have never been detected, should a) develop a comprehensive, antimicrobial-utilization plan to provide education for their medical staff (including medical students who rotate their training in different departments of the health-care facility), b) oversee surgical prophylaxis, and c) develop guidelines for the proper use of vancomycin (as applicable to the institution).

Guideline development should be part of the hospital's quality-improvement program and should involve participation from the hospital's pharmacy and therapeutics committee; hospital epidemiologist; and infection-control, infectious-disease, medical, and surgical staffs. The guidelines should include the following considerations:

- Situations in which the use of vancomycin is appropriate or acceptable:
  - For treatment of serious infections caused by beta-lactam- resistant gram-positive microorganisms. Vancomycin may be less rapidly bactericidal than are beta-lactam agents for beta-lactam- susceptible staphylococci (23,24).
  - For treatment of infections caused by gram-positive microorganisms in patients who have serious allergies to beta-lactam antimicrobials.
  - When antibiotic-associated colitis fails to respond to metronidazole therapy or is severe and potentially life-threatening.
  - Prophylaxis, as recommended by the American Heart Association, for endocarditis following certain procedures in patients at high risk for endocarditis (25).
  - Prophylaxis for major surgical procedures involving implantation of prosthetic materials or devices (e.g., cardiac and vascular procedures {26} and total hip replacement) at institutions that have a high rate of infections caused by MRSA or methicillin-resistant S. epidermidis. A single dose of vancomycin administered immediately before surgery is sufficient unless the procedure lasts greater than 6 hours, in which case the dose should be repeated. Prophylaxis should be discontinued after a maximum of two doses (27-30).
- Situations in which the use of vancomycin should be discouraged:
  - Routine surgical prophylaxis other than in a patient who has a life-threatening allergy to beta-lactam antibiotics (28).
  - Empiric antimicrobial therapy for a febrile neutropenic patient, unless initial evidence indicates that the patient has an infection caused by gram-positive microorganisms (e.g., at an inflamed exit site of Hickman catheter) and the prevalence of infections caused by MRSA in the hospital is substantial (31-37).
  - Treatment in response to a single blood culture positive for coagulase-negative staphylococcus, if other blood cultures taken during the same time frame are negative (i.e., if contamination of the blood culture is likely). Because contamination of blood cultures with skin flora (e.g., S. epidermidis) could result in inappropriate administration of vancomycin, phlebotomists and other personnel who obtain blood cultures should be trained to minimize microbial contamination of specimens (38-40).
  - Continued empiric use for presumed infections in patients whose cultures are negative for beta-lactam-resistant gram-positive microorganisms (41).
  - Systemic or local (e.g., antibiotic lock) prophylaxis for infection or colonization of indwelling central or peripheral intravascular catheters (42-48).
  - Selective decontamination of the digestive tract.
  - Eradication of MRSA colonization (49,50).
  - Primary treatment of antibiotic-associated colitis (51).
  - Routine prophylaxis for very low-birthweight infants (i.e., infants who weigh less than 1,500 g {3 lbs 4 oz}) (52).
  - Routine prophylaxis for patients on continuous ambulatory peritoneal dialysis or hemodialysis (48,53).
  - Treatment (chosen for dosing convenience) of infections caused by beta-lactam-sensitive gram-positive microorganisms in patients who have renal failure (54-57).
  - Use of vancomycin solution for topical application or irrigation.
- Enhancing compliance with recommendations:
  - Although several techniques may be useful, further study is required to determine the most effective methods for influencing the prescribing practices of physicians (58-61).
  - Key parameters of vancomycin use can be monitored through the hospital's quality assurance/improvement process or as part of the drug-utilization review of the pharmacy and therapeutics committee and the medical staff.

Education Programs

Continuing education programs for hospital staff (including attending and consulting physicians, medical residents, and students; pharmacy, nursing, and laboratory personnel; and other direct patient-care providers) should include information concerning the epidemiology of VRE and the potential impact of this pathogen on the cost and outcome of patient care. Because detection and containment of VRE require an aggressive approach and high performance standards for hospital personnel, special awareness and educational sessions might be indicated.

Role of the Microbiology Laboratory in the Detection, Reporting, and Control of VRE

The microbiology laboratory is the first line of defense against the spread of VRE in the hospital. The laboratory's ability to promptly and accurately identify enterococci and detect vancomycin resistance is essential for recognizing VRE colonization and infection and avoiding complex, costly containment efforts that are required when recognition of the problem is delayed. In addition, cooperation and communication between the laboratory and the infection-control program will facilitate control efforts.

Identification of Enterococci

Presumptively identify colonies on primary isolation plates as enterococci by using colonial morphology, a Gram stain, and a pyrrolidonyl arylamidase (PYR) test. Although identifying enterococci to the species level can help predict certain resistance patterns (e.g., Enterococcus faecium is more resistant to penicillin than is Enterococcus faecalis) and may help determine the epidemiologic relatedness of enterococcal isolates, such identification is not routinely necessary if antimicrobial susceptibility testing is performed. However, under special circumstances or as laboratory resources permit, biochemical tests can be used to differentiate between various enterococcal species. Although most commercially available identification systems adequately differentiate E. faecalis from other species of enterococci, additional tests for motility and pigment production are required to distinguish Enterococcus gallinarum (motile and nonpigmented) and Enterococcus casseliflavus (motile and pigmented) from E. faecium (nonmotile and nonpigmented).

Tests for Antimicrobial Susceptibility

Determine vancomycin resistance and high-level resistance to penicillin (or ampicillin) and aminoglycosides (62) for enterococci isolated from blood, sterile body sites (with the possible exception of urine), and other sites as clinically indicated. Laboratories routinely may test wound and urine isolates for resistance to vancomycin and penicillin or ampicillin if resources permit (see Screening Procedures for Detecting VRE in Hospitals Where VRE Have Not Been Detected).

- Laboratories that use disk diffusion should incubate plates for 24 hours and read zones of inhibition by using transmitted light (62,63).
- Minimum inhibitory concentrations can be determined by agar dilution, agar gradient dilution, broth macrodilution, or manual broth microdilution (62-64). These test systems should be incubated for 24 hours.
- The fully automated methods of testing enterococci for resistance to vancomycin currently are unreliable (9-11).

When VRE Are Isolated From a Clinical Specimen

Confirm vancomycin resistance by repeating antimicrobial susceptibility testing using any of the recommended methods (see Tests for Antimicrobial Susceptibility), particularly if VRE isolates are unusual in the hospital, OR streak 1 uL of standard inoculum (0.5 McFarland) from an isolated colony of enterococci onto brain heart infusion agar containing 6 ug/mL of vancomycin, incubate the inoculated plate for 24 hours at 35 C (95 F), and consider any growth indicative of vancomycin resistance (62,63,65). Immediately, while performing confirmatory susceptibility tests, notify the patient's primary caregiver, patient-care personnel, and infection-control personnel regarding the presumptive identification of VRE so that appropriate isolation precautions can be initiated promptly (see Preventing and Controlling VRE Transmission in All Hospitals). Follow this preliminary report with the (final) result of the confirmatory test. Additionally, highlight the report regarding the isolate to alert staff that isolation precautions are indicated.

Screening Procedures for Detecting VRE in Hospitals Where VRE Have Not Been Detected

In some hospital microbiology laboratories, antimicrobial susceptibility testing of enterococcal isolates from urine or nonsterile body sites (e.g., wounds) is not performed routinely; thus, identification of nosocomial VRE colonization and infection in hospitalized patients may be delayed. Therefore, in hospitals where VRE have not yet been detected, implementing special measures can promote earlier detection of VRE.

Antimicrobial susceptibility survey. Perform periodic susceptibility testing on an epidemiologic sample of enterococcal isolates recovered from all types of clinical specimens, especially from high-risk patients (e.g., those in an ICU or in an oncology or transplant ward). The optimal frequency of testing and number of isolates to be tested will vary among hospitals, depending on the patient population and number of cultures performed at the hospital. Hospitals that process large numbers of culture specimens need to test only a fraction (e.g., 10%) of enterococcal isolates every 1-2 months, whereas hospitals processing fewer specimens might need to test all enterococcal isolates during the survey period. The hospital epidemiologist can help design a suitable sampling strategy.

Culture survey of stools or rectal swabs. In tertiary medical centers and other hospitals that have many critically ill patients (e.g., ICU, oncology, and transplant patients) at high risk for VRE infection or colonization, periodic culture surveys of stools or rectal swabs of such patients can detect the presence of VRE. Because most patients colonized with VRE have intestinal colonization with this organism, fecal screening of patients is recommended even though VRE infections have not been identified clinically (2,4,16).

The frequency and intensity of surveillance should be based on the size of the population at risk and the specific hospital unit(s) involved. If VRE have been detected in other health-care facilities in a hospital's area and/or if a hospital's staff decides to determine whether VRE are present in the hospital despite the absence of recognized clinical cases, stool or rectal-swab culture surveys are useful. The cost of screening can be reduced by inoculating specimens onto selective media containing vancomycin (2,17,66) and restricting screening to those patients who have been in the hospital long enough to have a substantial risk for colonization (e.g., 5-7 days) or who have been admitted from a facility (e.g., a tertiary-care hospital or a chronic-care facility) where VRE have been identified.

After colonization with VRE has been detected, all the enterococcal isolates (including those from urine and wounds) from patients in the hospital should be screened routinely for vancomycin resistance, and efforts to contain the spread of VRE should be intensified (i.e., by strict adherence to handwashing and compliance with isolation precautions) (see Preventing and Controlling VRE Transmission in All Hospitals). Intensified fecal screening for VRE might facilitate earlier identification of colonized patients, leading to more efficient containment of the microorganism.

Preventing and Controlling Nosocomial Transmission of VRE

Eradicating VRE from hospitals is most likely to succeed when VRE infection or colonization is confined to a few patients on a single ward. After VRE have become endemic on a ward or have spread to multiple wards or to the community, eradication becomes difficult and costly. Aggressive infection-control measures and strict compliance by hospital personnel are required to limit nosocomial spread of VRE.

Control of VRE requires a collaborative, institution-wide, multidisciplinary effort. Therefore, the hospital's quality-assurance/improvement department should be involved at the outset to identify specific problems in hospital operations and patient-care systems and to design, implement, and evaluate appropriate changes in these systems.

Preventing and Controlling VRE Transmission in All Hospitals The following measures should be implemented by all hospitals, including those in which VRE have been isolated infrequently or not at all, to prevent and control transmission of VRE.

- Notify appropriate hospital staff promptly when VRE are detected (see When VRE Are Isolated From a Clinical Specimen).
- Inform clinical staff of the hospital's policies regarding VRE-infected or colonized patients. Because the slightest delay can lead to further spread of VRE and complicate control efforts, implement the required procedures as soon as VRE are detected. Clinical staff are essential to limiting the spread of VRE in patient-care areas; thus, continuing education regarding the appropriate response to the detection of VRE is critical (see Education Programs).
- Establish system(s) for monitoring appropriate process and outcome measures (e.g., cumulative incidence or incidence density of VRE colonization, rate of compliance with VRE isolation precautions and handwashing, interval between VRE identification in the laboratory and implementation of isolation precautions on the wards, and the percentage of previously colonized patients admitted to the ward who are identified promptly and placed on isolation precautions). Relay these data to the clinical, administrative, laboratory, and support staff to reinforce ongoing education and control efforts (67).
- Initiate the following isolation precautions to prevent patient-to-patient transmission of VRE:
  - Place VRE-infected or colonized patients in private rooms or in the same room as other patients who have VRE (8).
  - Wear gloves (clean, nonsterile gloves are adequate) when entering the room of a VRE-infected or colonized patient because VRE can extensively contaminate such an environment (3,8,16,17). When caring for a patient, a change of gloves might be necessary after contact with material that could contain high concentrations of VRE (e.g., stool).
  - Wear a gown (a clean, nonsterile gown is adequate) when entering the room of a VRE-infected or colonized patient a) if substantial contact with the patient or with environmental surfaces in the patient's room is anticipated, b) if the patient is incontinent, or c) if the patient has had an ileostomy or colostomy, has diarrhea, or has a wound drainage not contained by a dressing (8).
  - Remove gloves and gown before leaving the patient's room and immediately wash hands with an antiseptic soap or a waterless antiseptic agent (68-71). Hands can be contaminated via glove leaks (72-76) or during glove removal, and bland soap does not always completely remove VRE from the hands (77).
  - Ensure that after glove and gown removal and handwashing, clothing and hands do not contact environmental surfaces in the patient's room that are potentially contaminated with VRE (e.g., a door knob or curtain) (3,8).
- Dedicate the use of noncritical items (e.g., a stethoscope, sphygmomanometer, or rectal thermometer) to a single patient or cohort of patients infected or colonized with VRE (17). If such devices are to be used on other patients, adequately clean and disinfect these devices first (78).
- Obtain a stool culture or rectal swab from roommates of patients newly found to be infected or colonized with VRE to determine their colonization status, and apply isolation precautions as necessary. Perform additional screening of patients on the ward at the discretion of the infection-control staff.
- Adopt a policy for deciding when patients infected or colonized with VRE can be removed from isolation precautions. The optimal requirements remain unknown; however, because VRE colonization can persist indefinitely (4), stringent criteria might be appropriate, such as VRE-negative results on at least three consecutive occasions (greater than or equal to 1 week apart) for all cultures from multiple body sites (including stool or rectal swab, perineal area, axilla or umbilicus, and wound, Foley catheter, and/or colostomy sites, if present).
- Because patients with VRE can remain colonized for long periods after discharge from the hospital, establish a system for highlighting the records of infected or colonized patients so they can be promptly identified and placed on isolation precautions upon readmission to the hospital. This information should be computerized so that placement of colonized patients on isolation precautions will not be delayed because the patients' medical records are unavailable.
- Local and state health departments should be consulted when developing a plan regarding the discharge of VRE-infected or colonized patients to nursing homes, other hospitals, or home-health care. This plan should be part of a larger strategy for handling patients who have resolving infections and patients colonized with antimicrobial-resistant microorganisms.

Hospitals With Endemic VRE or Continued VRE Transmission

The following measures should be taken to prevent and control transmission of VRE in hospitals that have endemic VRE or continued VRE transmission despite implementation of measures described in the preceding section (see Preventing and Controlling VRE Transmission in All Hospitals).

- Focus control efforts initially on ICUs and other areas where the VRE transmission rate is highest (4). Such areas can serve as reservoirs for VRE, allowing VRE to spread to other wards when patients are well enough to be transferred.
- Where feasible, cohort the staff who provide regular, ongoing care to patients to minimize the movement/contact of health-care providers between VRE-positive and VRE-negative patients (4,8).
- Hospital staff who are carriers of enterococci have been implicated rarely in the transmission of this organism (8). However, in

conjunction with careful epidemiologic studies and upon the direction of the infection-control staff, examine personnel for chronic skin and nail problems and perform hand and rectal swab cultures of these workers. Remove from the care of VRE-negative patients those VRE-positive personnel linked epidemiologically to VRE transmission until their carrier state has been eradicated.

- Because the results of several enterococcal outbreak investigations suggest a potential role for the environment in the transmission of enterococci (3,8,16,17,79,80), institutions experiencing ongoing VRE transmission should verify that the hospital has adequate procedures for the routine care, cleaning, and disinfection of environmental surfaces (e.g., bed rails, bedside commodes, carts, charts, doorknobs, and faucet handles) and that these procedures are being followed by housekeeping personnel. To verify the efficacy of hospital policies and procedures, some hospitals might elect to perform focused environmental cultures before and after cleaning rooms that house patients who have VRE. All environmental culturing should be approved and supervised by the infection-control program in collaboration with the clinical laboratory (3,8,16,17,79,80).
- Consider sending representative VRE isolates to reference laboratories for strain typing by pulsed field gel electrophoresis or other suitable techniques to aid in defining reservoirs and patterns of transmission.

Detecting and Reporting VRSA and VRSE

The microbiology laboratory has the primary responsibility for detecting and reporting the occurrence of VRSA or VRSE in the hospital. All clinical isolates of S. aureus and S. epidermidis should be tested routinely, using standard methods, for susceptibility to vancomycin (62). If VRSA or VRSE is identified in a clinical specimen, confirm vancomycin resistance by repeating antimicrobial susceptibility testing using standard methods (62). Restreak the colony to ensure that the culture is pure. The most common causes of false-positive VRSA reports are susceptibility testing on mixed cultures and misidentifying VRE, Leuconostoc, S. haemolyticus, or Pediococcus as VRSA (81,82).

Immediately (i.e., while performing confirmatory testing) notify the hospital's infection-control personnel, the patient's primary caregiver, and patient-care personnel on the ward on which the patient is hospitalized so that the patient can be placed promptly on isolation precautions (depending on the site{s} of infection or colonization) adapted from previous CDC guidelines (83) and those recommended for VRE infection or colonization in this report (see Preventing and Controlling Nosocomial Transmission of VRE). Furthermore, immediately notify the state health department and CDC, and send the isolate through the state health department to CDC (telephone {404} 639-6413) for confirmation of vancomycin resistance.

References

References

1. CDC. Nosocomial enterococci resistant to vancomycin -- United States, 1989-1993. MMWR 1993;42:597-9.
2. Rubin LG, Tucci V, Cercenado E, Eliopoulos G, Isenberg HD. Vancomycin-resistant Enterococcus faecium in hospitalized children. Infect Control Hosp Epidemiol 1992;13:700-5.
3. Karanfil LV, Murphy M, Josephson A, et al. A cluster of vancomycin-resistant Enterococcus faecium in an intensive care unit. Infect Control Hosp Epidemiol 1992;13:195-200.
4. Handwerger S, Raucher B, Altarac D, et al. Nosocomial outbreak due to Enterococcus faecium highly resistant to vancomycin, penicillin, and gentamicin. Clin Infect Dis 1993;16:750-5.
5. Frieden TR, Munsiff SS, Low DE, et al. Emergence of vancomycin-resistant enterococci in New York City. Lancet 1993;342: 76-9.
6. Boyle JF, Soumakis SA, Rendo A, et al. Epidemiologic analysis and genotypic characterization of a nosocomial outbreak of vancomycin-resistant enterococci. J Clin Microbiol 1993;31: 1280-5.
7. Montecalvo MA, Horowitz H, Gedris C, et al. Outbreak of vancomycin-, ampicillin-, and aminoglycoside-resistant Enterococcus faecium bacteremia in an adult oncology unit. Antimicrob Agents Chemother 1994;38:1363-7.
8. Boyce JM, Opal SM, Chow JW, et al. Outbreak of multi-drug resistant Enterococcus faecium with transferable vanB class vancomycin resistance. J Clin Microbiol 1994;32:1148-53.
9. Tenover FC, Tokars J, Swenson J, Paul S, Spitalny K, Jarvis W. Ability of clinical laboratories to detect antimicrobial agent-resistant enterococci. J Clin Microbiol 1993;31:1695-9.
10. Sahm DF, Olsen L. In vitro detection of enterococcal vancomycin resistance. Antimicrob Agents Chemother 1990;34:1846-8.
11. Zabransky RJ, Dinuzzo AR, Huber MB, Woods GL. Detection of vancomycin resistance in enterococci by the Vitek AMS System. Diagn Microbiol Infect Dis 1994;20:113-6.
12. Moellering RC Jr. The Garrod lecture: the enterococcus -- a classic example of the impact of antimicrobial resistance on therapeutic options. J Antimicrob Chemother 1991;28:1-12.
13. Hayden MK, Koenig GI, Trenholme GM. Bactericidal activities of antibiotics against vancomycin-resistant Enterococcus faecium blood isolates and synergistic activities of combinations. Antimicrob Agents Chemother 1994;38:1225-9.
14. Mobarakai N, Landman D, Quale JM. In-vitro activity of trospectomycin, a new aminocyclitol antibiotic against multidrug-resistant Enterococcus faecium. J Antimicrob Chemother 1994;33:319-21.
15. Murray BE. The life and times of the enterococcus. Clin Microbiol Rev 1990;3:46-65.
16. Rhinehart E, Smith N, Wennersten C, et al. Rapid dissemination of beta-lactamase-producing aminoglycoside-resistant Enterococcus faecalis among patients and staff on an infant and toddler surgical ward. N Engl J Med 1990;323:1814-8.

SHEA Position Paper

Society for Healthcare Epidemiology of America and Infectious Diseases Society of America Joint Committee on the Prevention of Antimicrobial Resistance: Guidelines for the Prevention of Antimicrobial Resistance in Hospitals

David M. Shlaes, MD, PhD; Dale N. Gerding, MD; Joseph F. John, Jr, MD; William A. Craig, MD; Donald L. Bornstein, MD; Robert A. Duncan, MD; Mark R. Eckman, MD; William E. Farrer, MD; William H. Greene, MD; Victor Lorian, MD; Stuart Levy, MD; John E. McGowan, Jr, MD; Sindy M. Paul, MD; Joel Ruskin, MD; Fred C. Tenover, MD; Chatrchai Watanakunakorn, MD

ABSTRACT

Antimicrobial resistance results in increased morbidity, mortality, and costs of health care. Prevention of the emergence of resistance and the dissemination of resistant microorganisms will reduce these adverse effects and their attendant costs. Appropriate antimicrobial stewardship that includes optimal selection, dose, and duration of treatment, as well as control of antibiotic use, will prevent or slow the emergence of resistance among microorganisms. A comprehensively applied infection control program will interdict the dissemination of resistant strains (*Infect Control Hosp Epidemiol* 1997;18:275-291).

SUMMARY

Antimicrobial resistance results in increased morbidity, mortality, and costs of health care. Prevention of the emergence of resistance and the dissemination of resistant microorganisms will reduce these adverse effects and their attendant costs. Appropriate antimicrobial stewardship that includes optimal selection, dose, and duration of treatment, as well as control of antibiotic use, will prevent or slow the emergence of resistance among microorganisms. A comprehensively applied infection control program will interdict the dissemination of resistant strains. It therefore is recommended that hospitals, large and small, with and without perceived problems of bacterial resistance to antimicrobials, do the following:

- Establish a system for monitoring bacterial resistance and antibiotic usage;
- Establish practice guidelines and other institutional policies to control the use of antibiotics, and respond to data from the monitoring system;
- Adopt the recommendations of the Centers for Disease Control and Prevention's (CDC) "Guidelines for Isolation Precautions in Hospitals," as concerns the isolation of patients colonized or infected with resistant microorganisms;
- Utilize hospital committees to develop local policies and to evaluate and adopt, as appropriate, guidelines from state advisory boards and national

From Wyeth-Ayerst Research (Dr. Shlaes), Pearl River, New York; Veterans' Affairs Lakeside Medical Center (Dr. Gerding), Chicago, Illinois; UMDNJ-Robert Wood Johnson Medical School (Dr. John), New Brunswick, New Jersey; William S. Middleton Memorial Veterans' Hospital (Dr. Craig), Madison, Wisconsin; SUNY Health Science Center (Dr. Bornstein), Syracuse, New York; Lahey Clinic (Dr. Duncan), Burlington, Massachusetts; Duluth Clinic Limited (Dr. Eckman), Duluth, Minnesota; St Elizabeth Hospital (Dr. Farrer), Elizabeth, New Jersey; University Hospital (Dr. Greene), State University of New York, Stony Brook, New York; Bronx-Lebanon Hospital Center (Dr. Lorian), Bronx, New York; Tufts University School of Medicine (Dr. Levy), Boston, Massachusetts; Grady Memorial Hospital (Dr. McGowan), Atlanta, Georgia; New Jersey Department of Health (Dr. Paul), Trenton, New Jersey; Kaiser Permanente Medical Center (Dr. Ruskin), Los Angeles, California; Centers for Disease Control and Prevention (Dr. Tenover), Atlanta, Georgia; St. Elizabeth Hospital Medical Center (Dr. Watanakunakorn), Youngstown, Ohio.
Address reprint requests to David M. Shlaes, MD, Wyeth-Ayerst Research, 401 N Middletown Rd, Pearl River, NY 10965.
96-SR-183. Shlaes DM, Gerding DN, John JF Jr, Craig WA, Bornstein DL, Duncan RA, Eckman MR, Farrer WE, Greene WH, Lorian V, Levy S, McGowan JE Jr, Paul SM, Ruskin J, Tenover FC, Watanakunakorn C. Society for Healthcare Epidemiology of America and Infectious Diseases Society of America Joint Committee on the Prevention of Antimicrobial Resistance: guidelines for the prevention of antimicrobial resistance in hospitals. Infect Control Hosp Epidemiol 1997;18:275-291.

societies;

● Recognize that the financial well-being of the institution and the health of its patients are at stake and therefore that the hospital administration should be accountable for the implementation and enforcement of policies adopted by hospital committees;

● By measuring outcomes, evaluate the effectiveness of the policies that are put in place.

It is recommended that research to define the mechanism of transfer of bacteria and their resistance determinants among patient populations and to determine methods to prevent emergence and transfer of resistance, including control of antibiotic usage, be supported with increases in targeted research funding.

Antimicrobial resistance is costly in both human and financial terms. Infection with a resistant microorganism increases the cost of health care, length of hospital stay, and mortality compared to infections with organisms susceptible to common, inexpensive antimicrobials.[1,2] The Society for Healthcare Epidemi-ology of America (SHEA) and the Infectious Diseases Society of America (IDSA) have embarked on a joint project to make recommendations regarding the prevention and control of antimicrobial resistance. This task has assumed very broad boundaries and includes the prevention of emergence and control of dissemination of antibiotic-resistant pathogens in hospitals, in other institutions, in outpatient settings, and in both animal and human health.

There is convincing evidence that we share a single ecosystem globally in terms of resistance. The selection of resistance in one organism in one part of the world, even within an animal population, may have long-term, important implications for human health globally. Therefore, management of the problem of antimicrobial resistance within hospitals is a community responsibility, both within and outside of the hospital. The following recommendations are directed toward all hospitals, small to large, with and without currently perceived problems with antibiotic resistance. Good stewardship of antibiotic usage combined with strong infection control will be required. To achieve this, all levels of personnel within the hospital must be involved, from top administration down to individuals performing services and providing patient care. The recommendations promulgated in this set of guidelines reflect this approach.

This report, the first of a series that is emerging from this joint committee on antibiotics, is concerned with two major aspects of antibiotic resistance in hospitals: the selection of antibiotic-resistant organisms and the dissemination of resistance within the hospital setting. The basic genetics of bacteri-al resistance and the breadth of possibilities available to microorganisms to avoid the toxic effects of antibiotics are reviewed. Various methods of surveillance for resistance in the hospital are considered, and criteria that hospitals might use to identify resistant organisms of epidemiological importance are developed. The critical role of antibiotic use in the hospital in the selection of resistant bacteria is reviewed, and recommendations designed to avoid or retard the selection of resistant bacteria are provided. Specific isolation procedures for patients infected or, in some cases, colonized with resistant organisms that the hospital has chosen to attempt to control also are reviewed.

That infection control committees of hospitals have been struggling with these problems for many years is clear, and many feel frustrated with a real or perceived lack of administrative support. The relation between infection control and the hospital administration regarding these recommendations is examined. It is clear that, without the support of the administration, neither these recommendations nor those of local infection control committees will be of use in the struggle against antibiotic resistance. The guidelines seek to motivate administrators to invest in the infection control effort, given the convincing financial arguments favoring the control of antimicrobial resistance. We also provide an organizational framework for administrators so that they can appreciate their role as part of a team involved in providing the most efficient and highest-quality care for patients in their institutions.

One critical area requiring immediate attention is the existing database from which these and other guidelines are constructed. Clear recommendations have been made regarding further research that might provide the kind of data needed for rational decisions in the management of antimicrobial usage and infection control.

EMERGENCE OF ANTIMICROBIAL RESISTANCE IN HOSPITALS

Genetics of Resistance

Bacteria possess a remarkable number of genetic mechanisms for resistance to antimicrobials. They can undergo chromosomal mutations, express a latent chromosomal resistance gene, or acquire new genetic resistance material through direct exchange of DNA (by conjugation), through a bacteriophage (transduction), through extrachromosomal plasmid DNA (by conjugation), or by acquisition of DNA via transformation. The information encoded in this genetic material enables a bacterium to develop resistance through three major mechanisms: production of an enzyme

TABLE 1
EXAMPLES OF RESISTANCE MECHANISMS AND THEIR GENETIC BASES*

Antibiotic(s)	Mechanisms	Genetic Basis	Example Organisms

β-lactams
  Penicillins
  Cephalosporins
  Monobactams
  Carbapenems
	Altered penicillin-binding protein targets	Chromosomal	*Staphylococcus aureus*
			Streptococcus pneumoniae
			Staphylococcus epidermidis
			Haemophilus influenzae
			Neisseria gonorrhoeae
			Neisseria meningitidis
			Escherichia coli
			Pseudomonas aeruginosa

	Reduced permeability	Chromosomal	*P aeruginosa* *Enterobacter cloacae* *Serratia marcescens* *Klebsiella pneumoniae* *Klebsiella oxytoca*
	β-lactamase inactivation	Chromosomal and plasmid	*S aureus* *S epidermidis* Enterococci *P aeruginosa* *Enterobacteriaceae* *N gonorrhoeae* *N meningitidis*

Fluoroquinolones
  Ciprofloxacin
  Ofloxacin
  Norfloxacin
  Lomefloxacin
	Altered DNA gyrase target	Chromosomal	*S aureus*
			S epidermidis
			Enterobacteriaceae

	Efflux or reduced permeability	Chromosomal	*Enterobacteriaceae* *P aeruginosa*

Aminoglycosides
  Amikacin
  Gentamicin
  Tobramycin
	Modifying enzyme inactivation	Plasmid	Staphylococci
			Enterococci
			Streptococci
			Enterobacteriaceae

	Reduced permeability	Chromosomal	*Enterobacteriaceae* Pseudomonads *Bacteroides*
	Altered ribosomal target binding	Chromosomal	Streptococci

Macrolides and
  lincosamides
  Erythromycin
  Clindamycin
	Methylation of rRNA target	Chromosomal and plasmid	Streptococci
			S pneumoniae
			
			Enterococci
			Staphylococci

	Efflux	Plasmid	Staphylococci, streptococci

Tetracyclines
  Tetracycline
  Minocycline
  Doxycycline
	Efflux	Plasmid	Staphylococci
			Streptococci
			Enterococci
			Enterobacteriaceae
			Bacteroides
			Haemophilus

	Altered ribosomal target	Plasmid	*N gonorrhoeae* *Bacteroides* *Listeria* *Mycoplasma* *Ureaplasma*

(Continued on page 278)

TABLE 1 *(continued)*
EXAMPLES OF RESISTANCE MECHANISMS AND THEIR GENETIC BASES*

Antibiotic(s)	Mechanisms	Genetic Basis	Example Organisms
Glycopeptides Vancomycin Teicoplanin	Altered target	Chromosomal and plasmid	Enterococci Lactobacilli *Staphylococcus hemolyticus*
Folate inhibitors Trimethoprim-sulfamethoxazole	Altered targets	Chromosomal and plasmid	Staphylococci Streptococci *S pneumoniae* *Enterobacteriaceae* *Neisseria*
Rifampin	Altered DNA polymerase target	Chromosomal	Staphylococci Streptococci Enterococci *Enterobacteriaceae* *Mycobacterium tuberculosis* Pseudomonads
Chloramphenicol	Acetyltransferase inactivation	Chromosomal and plasmid	Staphylococci Streptococci *H influenzae* *S pneumoniae* *Enterobacteriaceae* *Neisseria*
	Efflux	Chromosomal and plasmid	*Enterobacteriaceae* Pseudomonads
Mupirocin	Altered target	Plasmid	Staphylococci

* Modified from Neu HC.[3]

that will inactivate or destroy the antibiotic; alteration of the antibiotic target site to evade action of the antibiotic; or prevention of antibiotic access to the target site. Examples of organisms that are known to possess resistance mechanisms of the various types are shown in Table 1, together with the genetic mechanism for the resistance.[3] It is not unusual for a single bacterial strain found in a hospital to possess several of these resistance mechanisms simultaneously.

Some resistance can be acquired by a single genetic mutation that can occur spontaneously, such as the DNA gyrase target alteration that results in fluoroquinolone resistance. Other resistance mechanisms are far more complex and consist of genes that encode production of highly specific enzymes that inactivate several antibiotics (eg, β-lactams or aminoglycosides). There is considerable speculation about the origin of these genes. Some genes can be found naturally occurring in other species of bacteria.[4] It is postulated that there is a substantial pool of antibiotic resistance genes (or related genes) in nature. This gene pool, to be of use to bacteria that are under selective antibiotic pressure, must be accessible, and the bacteria must possess the means to acquire the needed genetic information (gene pickup).

Transposons (so-called jumping genes) and plasmids provide two readily available means for gene transfer. One class of transposons, called integrons, consist of conserved DNA segments that flank a central region into which "cassettes" that encode antibiotic-resistance functions can be inserted. The 5' conserved segment encodes a site-specific recombinase or integrase, as well as one or more promoters that assure expression of the integrated resistance cassettes. Integron-type transposons provide a model for assembly of multiple antibiotic resistance genes from a variety of sources into R plasmids that have been found to display an ever-increasing array of resistance properties.[4,5]

Transposable elements and plasmids encode not only genetic information for inactivation of antimicrobials, they also may encode genes for the active efflux of antibiotics from the cell, the so-called sump pump mechanism of resistance. Efflux systems may be highly specific for single agents or may involve a variety of classes of antimicrobial agents. Many of the resistances previously thought to be due to permeability barriers subsequently have been found to be mediated by efflux pumps.[6,7]

Whereas some altered target-site resistance may be due to single mutations, as occur with fluoroquinolones and rifampin, target-site alterations for β-lactam resistance are more complex. Penicillins, cephalosporins, and other β-lactams act by inactivating a number of transpeptidases (or penicillin-binding proteins [PBPs]) essential for the cross-linking reactions of cell-wall synthesis.[8] Because there often are multiple PBP targets, resistance development is slow and often stepwise as each PBP is altered in its affinity for the β-lactam. Development of resistance may occur gradually with the slow accumulation of multiple amino acid substitutions through mutations; however, there also is evidence to support the acquisition of low-affinity PBP genes in *Neisseria gonorrhoeae* and *Neisseria meningitidis* from recombination with commensal *Neisseria* species. In the case of methicillin resistance in *Staphylococcus aureus*, a new PBP 2′ or *mecA* gene, which is part of a transposon, has been acquired by the *Staphylococcus*.

Clearly, bacteria have evolved a wide array of mechanisms to become resistant to antimicrobials and are adept at disseminating the resistance once it has been acquired. Analysis of organisms from the preantibiotic era suggests that evolution of multiresistant R plasmids has occurred over the past 50 years, a period that happens to coincide with the discovery and increasingly widespread use of antimicrobial agents. A causal association between these two temporally related phenomena is quite probable.

Virulence of Resistant Bacteria

Although it often has been stated that antibiotic-resistant bacteria tend to be less virulent than their susceptible parents,[9] this is not necessarily true, and even less virulent bacteria can be dangerous pathogens for some hospitalized patients. For example, bacteria that acquire mutations in genes responsible for vital functions, such as transport of small molecules, can be resistant to some antibiotics, such as aminoglycosides, and tend to be less virulent in animal models of infection.[10] However, some authors argue that such bacteria can be responsible for relapse of infection after treatment, because they are not treated effectively by the antibiotic nor are they cleared effectively by impaired host defenses.[11] Many resistant pathogens appear just as virulent as the susceptible parents in animal models and in patients, as is the case for methicillin-resistant *Staphylococcus aureus* (MRSA), for example.[12] Therefore, antimicrobial resistance per se may not render pathogenic bacteria easier to clear from infected sites. Further, there is evidence that they are transmitted from patient to patient in much the same way as susceptible bacteria, ie,

mainly through contact and occasionally through airborne droplets (see below).[13,14]

Surveillance for Resistant Bacterial Pathogens

A major role of the clinical microbiology laboratory is to provide antimicrobial susceptibility testing data on bacterial isolates to guide clinicians in their choice of anti-infective therapy. Susceptibility testing data can serve both as a guide to therapy and, in some instances, as an initial means of strain typing for investigations of potential outbreaks of infection. Other strain typing methods, such as pulsed-field gel electrophoresis, have better discriminatory ability. However, unusual antibiograms, especially multiply resistant patterns, can be helpful early in the course of an investigation for identifying outbreak-related isolates.

Microbiologists can aid in the prudent use of antimicrobial agents in their respective hospitals by testing and reporting drugs using the guidelines developed by the National Committee for Clinical Laboratory Standards (NCCLS; Executive Offices, 940 W Valley Rd, Ste 1400, Wayne, PA 19087) Subcommittee on Antimicrobial Susceptibility Testing in documents M2-A7, M7-A5, M11-A3, and M100-S6. Microbiologists should consult Tables 1 and 1A of NCCLS documents M2-A5 and M7-A3 for recommendations on which drugs to test against various classes of microorganisms. An example of such recommendations is given in Table 2 of this article. Prioritizing of susceptibility reports, in which extended-spectrum drugs such as imipenem are not reported unless resistance to other agents is documented, can contribute to prudent use. Microbiologists should work with infectious disease clinicians, pharmacists, hospital epidemiologists, infection control practitioners, and representatives of clinical departments to choose the drugs that will be tested and reported routinely. Sometimes choices will be limited by the instruments used in the microbiology laboratory for susceptibility testing, and this limitation should be part of discussions concerning the choice of drugs tested.

In conjunction with routine antimicrobial susceptibility testing for guiding antimicrobial chemotherapy, microbiologists also frequently are involved in programs for the surveillance of organisms with novel resistance patterns. There are two components to such surveillance. First, surveillance involves periodic review of minimum inhibitory concentrations (MIC) or zone diameter data for changes in resistance patterns. Changes indicating trends toward increasing resistance may be detected first by noting a decrease in the mean zone diameters around antibiotic disks using the Bauer-Kirby disk-diffusion method or by increases in the MICs of organisms, even though the

TABLE 2
GUIDELINES FOR TESTING BACTERIAL PATHOGENS FOR
ANTIMICROBIAL RESISTANCE*

Gram-Positive Organisms	Gram-Negative Organisms
Staphylococci	*Enterobacteriaceae*
Penicillin	Ampicillin
Oxacillin	Cefazolin or cephalothin
Vancomycin	Cefotetan or cefoxitin
Alternate agents as needed, including	Cefotaxime or ceftriaxone
Erythromycin	Gentamicin
Clindamycin	Amikacin
Trimethoprim-sulfamethoxazole	Ciprofloxacin
	Trimethoprim-sulfamethoxazole
	β-lactam–β-lactamase inhibitor combinations
Enterococci	*Pseudomonas* and *Acinetobacter*
Penicillin or ampicillin (β-lactamase test)	Ticarcillin or piperacillin
	Gentamicin
Vancomycin	Ceftazidime
High-level gentamicin and streptomycin (invasive isolates only)	Ampicillin/sulbactam
	Amikacin
	Imipenem
	Ciprofloxacin
	Trimethoprim-sulfamethoxazole
	Cefoperazone or aztreonam
Streptococcus pneumoniae	
Penicillin[†]	
Cefotaxime or ceftriaxone	
Vancomycin	
Alternate agents as needed, including	
Erythromycin	
Clindamycin	

* This guide is adapted from the National Committee for Clinical Laboratory Standards Document M100-S6 for initial susceptibility testing and reporting of antimicrobial agents for several bacterial pathogen groups. (Not all drugs should be reported routinely.)
[†] Laboratories may screen for penicillin resistance in pneumococci by using a 1-μg oxacillin disk. Organisms with zone diameters of ≥20 mm are considered susceptible to all β-lactam drugs. Isolates with zone diameters of ≤19 mm should be tested by a minimum inhibitory concentration method against both penicillin and cefotaxime or ceftriaxone, especially if the organism is causing invasive disease.

TABLE 3
MECHANISMS FOR THE APPEARANCE OR SPREAD OF
ANTIMICROBIAL RESISTANCE IN HOSPITAL ORGANISMS

Introduction of a resistant organism to a previously susceptible population
Acquisition of resistance by a susceptible strain
    Spontaneous mutation
    Genetic transfer
Expression of regulated resistance already present in the population
Selection of a resistant subpopulation
Dissemination or spread of resistant organisms

Modified from McGowan JE Jr.[15]

example, MICs of ceftazidime for *Klebsiella pneumoniae* may change from 0.1 μg/mL to 8 μg/mL, yet still would be classified as susceptible. Such changes potentially are important, and clinical microbiologists should alert clinicians, particularly infectious disease specialists and hospital epidemiologists, to such trends in their hospitals. Alternate methods of testing to confirm resistance mechanisms (eg, β-lactamase tests for *Haemophilus influenzae* and *N gonorrhoeae* or disk diffusion tests for extended-spectrum β-lactamases) also can be helpful for detecting borderline resistance.

The second component of surveillance is the reporting of novel resistance patterns to local, state, and national public health officials. Unusual resistance patterns, such as vancomycin-resistant *S aureus* or penicillin-resistant *N meningitidis*, would have major public health implications and should be acted on immediately. These should be reported to clinicians and hospital epidemiologists. Such unusual antibiotic-resistance patterns should be confirmed by the laboratory to rule out random laboratory errors. If the resistance profile is confirmed, laboratories should notify the state health department and the CDC. Clinical microbiologists and infectious disease clinicians need to keep abreast of other novel resistance patterns, particularly those that have the potential to spread rapidly.

Antimicrobial Use and Resistance

There are multiple mechanisms postulated by which antimicrobial resistance may appear and disseminate within hospital organisms (Table 3).[15] Three of the proposed mechanisms for resistance development are influenced by antimicrobial usage: acquisition of resistance, emergence of dormant resistance, and selection of resistant subpopulations. Often, the introduction of a resistant organism can be documented by contact tracing to an index case that was admitted to the hospital already infected or

categorical interpretations of the zone sizes or MIC results still may be within the susceptible range. For

colonized with the resistant organism. More frequently, however, the source of resistant organisms remains an enigma. Although the exact magnitude of the problem due to the spread of resistant organisms within the institution is unknown, it is clear that such spread can be minimized by early recognition and effective infection control practices. Regrettably, recognition of cross-infection often is slow, and containment and control measures often are inadequate or ineffective.

Several lines of evidence suggest that there is a causal association between antimicrobial usage in hospitals and antimicrobial resistance.[16] For some pathogens, selection of resistance during treatment or prophylaxis is thought to be a more important factor in the acquisition of infection by a resistant organism than is transmission from patient to patient.[17] Additional compelling observations are as follows:

1. Changes in antimicrobial usage are paralleled by changes in the prevalence of resistance.

2. Antimicrobial resistance is more prevalent in nosocomial bacterial strains than in those from community-acquired infections.

3. During outbreaks of nosocomial infection, patients infected with resistant strains are more likely than control patients to have received prior antimicrobials.

4. Areas within hospitals that have the highest rates of antimicrobial resistance also have the highest rates of antimicrobial use.

5. Increasing duration of patient exposure to antimicrobials increases the likelihood of colonization with resistant organisms.[16]

The above observations are derived from review of multiple published reports. However, questions remain unanswered because of the lack of uniformity of definitions of resistance, variation in susceptibility test methodologies, potential study selection biases, and failure to control for confounding variables, especially infection control measures.[18] These and other additional factors that may affect antimicrobial resistance are summarized in Table 4 and typify many of the characteristics of the changing hospital environment.

Recently, Stuart Levy, MD, proposed a provocative hypothesis: the intensity of antibiotic use in a population may be the most important factor in selection of resistance. Moreover, there may be a "threshold" for such selection[19] that may differ for an individual, as compared to a population, and from one population to another. This may explain why, in intensive-care units, where there is usually a small population undergoing intensive antibiotic therapy or prophylaxis, resistance tends to be more common, pathogens are more often multiply resistant, and spread within the population is more likely. The same concept might

TABLE 4
FACTORS THAT MAY INCREASE ANTIMICROBIAL RESISTANCE IN HOSPITALS

Greater severity of illness of hospitalized patients

More severely immunocompromised patients

Newer devices and procedures in use

Increased introduction of resistant organisms from the community

Ineffective infection control and isolation practices and compliance

Increased use of antimicrobial prophylaxis

Increased empiric polymicrobial antimicrobial therapy

High antimicrobial usage per geographic area per unit time

Modified from McGowan JE Jr.[18]

explain resistance problems in the poultry manufacturing industry and in other settings where antibiotic use is intensive within a small and confined population.

The growing emphasis on outpatient medical management has increased the severity of illness of those who are admitted to the hospital. Patients with advanced malignancies, organ transplantation, multiorgan failure, or human immunodeficiency virus infection are far more immunocompromised and constitute a larger portion of hospital patients than in the past. These patients often are colonized or infected with unusual opportunistic organisms that are far more resistant to antimicrobials—organisms such as *Pseudomonas, Stenotrophomonas, Acinetobacter, Enterobacter, Serratia,* coagulase-negative staphylococci, enterococci, *Candida,* phycomycetes, and *Aspergillus.*[20] These patients also are more likely to be treated with procedures (such as bone marrow transplantation) and devices (indwelling urinary and intravascular catheters) that increase the risk of infection by specific organisms. Increased treatment of patients in the community can lead to resistance in the community that is introduced to the hospital by patients on admission; methicillin-resistant staphylococci and ampicillin-resistant *Haemophilus* organisms are examples. Infection control and isolation practices vary from hospital to hospital. Their effective use can have considerable influence on reducing the persistence and spread of resistant organisms in the hospital. Changes in antimicrobial usage also may influence resistance. Policies such as systemic and gastrointestinal antimicrobial prophylaxis in intensive-care units[21] and empiric poly-antimicrobial treatment of febrile immunocompromised, as well as immunocompetent patients,[22,23] may add to the risk of antimicrobial resistance in hospital organisms. Taken together, the above factors have led to an increased percentage of hospitalized patients who

TABLE 5

ELEMENTS OF AN OPTIMAL ANTIMICROBIAL CONTROL
PROGRAM TO STUDY THE PREVENTION OR REDUCTION OF
ANTIMICROBIAL RESISTANCE

Precise definitions of antimicrobial resistance for
  antimicrobials and organisms

A system for monitoring the frequency of resistance (clinical
  and environmental)

A determination of which antimicrobial(s) to control

A method to achieve usage control

A determination of who will be responsible for maintaining
  control

A method to educate and enroll prescribers in the control
  process

A stable system of hospital infection control

A system to measure use of controlled and uncontrolled
  antimicrobials

A method to determine antimicrobial use per geographic area
  per unit time

Ability to distinguish community from nosocomial isolates

Ability to identify isolates by body site and hospital location

A method to assure that clinical care will not be harmed by
  control measures

Ability to identify known mechanisms of antimicrobial
  resistance

Ability to type organisms by phenotypic or genetic methods

receive antimicrobials and an increased number of antimicrobials per patient over the past 15 years.[24]

Notwithstanding the complexity of the problem and the need for better data-controlled studies, there nonetheless are sufficient reports of the association of antimicrobial usage in hospitals with emergence of antimicrobial resistance to implicate use as a causal factor in antimicrobial resistance.[15,16,18,20,25-28] Clearly, the degree to which such resistance occurs, and the organisms and drugs affected, is quite variable and not predictable for most drug-organism pairs. This is illustrated by the observation that the rate of ciprofloxacin resistance among MRSA is markedly higher than for methicillin-sensitive *S aureus* or gram-negative organisms.[28] In this case, the ciprofloxacin resistance mechanism has been determined, but it is not clear why these mutational changes apparently are more frequent in MRSA than in other organisms.[29-31] Thus, we need to examine carefully not only the relation of resistance to antimicrobial use for specific organism-drug pairs but also to determine the mechanism of that resistance as an indicator of possible causation.

Prevention of Emergence of Resistance

Prevention of the emergence of antimicrobial resistance and reduction of established resistance

are dual goals for which the methods are likely similar if not identical. Preventing the acquisition of resistance is assumed to be the easier task, although data regarding preventive strategies generally are lacking, whereas studies of actions taken once resistance has occurred are plentiful, if not consistent, regarding their efficacy. The elements of a good program for prevention of resistance generally include an active system of surveillance for resistance, an active and effective infection control program to minimize secondary spread of resistance, and an effective program of antimicrobial use stewardship. The latter element, sometimes referred to as "antibiotic control," most often is cited as a means to prevent and control resistance. Appropriate antimicrobial stewardship includes not only the limitation of use of inappropriate agents but also the appropriate selection, dosing, and duration of antimicrobial therapy to achieve optimal efficacy in managing infections.

The effectiveness of antimicrobial control as a means to prevent the emergence of resistance has been reviewed. The results of available studies are suggestive, but not conclusive.[32] However, because resistance among certain species such as enterococci has become so widespread that there are no longer any effective antimicrobial agents, the interest in antimicrobial control as a preventive measure has intensified. Past studies have been criticized for their selection biases, small size, limitation to single institutions, and failure to control for confounding variables.[32] Not only is the effect of antimicrobial control on microbial resistance not known, the most effective methods to achieve antimicrobial control also are not clear. The need for better data from larger and better controlled multicenter studies is apparent. In addition, the relation of antimicrobial resistance to the "defined drug density" (the amount of antimicrobial use per geographic unit per unit time) has been suggested as an evaluation measure that could be useful in relating resistance to use of antimicrobials.[19]

The elements suggested for inclusion in an effective antimicrobial control program to prevent or reduce antimicrobial resistance are shown in Table 5. Because of the complexity of multidrug resistance in many organisms, it can be predicted that not all control measures will succeed. For this reason, it is recommended that monitoring include many of the variables listed in Table 5 (such as mechanism of resistance, molecular typing of organisms, and complete resistance profiles), so that insights can be obtained regarding which control strategies are more likely to succeed than others. For example, multiply antimicrobial-resistant organisms may respond to control of one agent to which they are resistant, but they may not respond to control of other agents to which they also are resistant.

Initial control efforts are likely to be empiric, simply because the best strategies are not known yet. Uncontrolled resistance no longer can be tolerated. Managed-care networks are likely to demand control of resistance to improve patient-care quality and to reduce costs of healthcare. It is likely, given the trend toward greater outpatient care, that prevention and control of antimicrobial resistance will be as important in the outpatient arena as in the inpatient setting.

The ideal is to have all patients treated with the most effective, least toxic, and least costly antibiotic for the precise duration of time needed to cure or prevent an infection. This is the essence of good antimicrobial use stewardship. Four possible strategies to optimize use are shown in Table 6. The first of these involves the development of guidelines and treatment algorithms, designed to elucidate "pathways" of optimal use. Prescribers are educated to follow them and to seek expert guidance along the way from infectious disease specialists and pharmacists. To date, such programs have not been particularly effective, even with the addition of peer review.[32]

The second method of antimicrobial control, selective removal or control of use of specific agents or classes of agents, has been employed in numerous hospitals. Compliance with the restriction policy easily can be documented from pharmacy prescribing data, and favorable effects on the incidence and prevalence of specific resistant organisms have been documented.[32-40] More studies have been conducted on control of gentamicin resistance (mainly through the restriction of gentamicin and replacement with amikacin) than on any other antimicrobial.[33-38] Most have shown significant reductions in gentamicin resistance during restriction, but return of resistance with resumption of gentamicin use.[34-36] In some instances when this "replacement" strategy was employed, resistance to amikacin developed, and resistance problems became worse[41-43]; however, in most institutions, this did not occur.[33-38,44] Although such studies often were commercially sponsored to promote use of an alternative product, they still provide a model for future efforts to control antimicrobials in that the protocols employed for monitoring resistance and antimicrobial use in each institution were similar. In most instances, the mechanism of resistance to gentamicin was determined (usually plasmid-mediated transferable aminoglycoside inactivating enzymes), and the potential mechanism for amikacin resistance (a different aminoglycoside inactivating enzyme) was monitored.[34-36] Control measures were enforced rigidly and resulted in major usage changes, as had been described by others.[39] Organisms and

TABLE 6
PROPOSED METHODS TO CONTROL ANTIMICROBIAL USE TO PREVENT OR CONTROL ANTIMICROBIAL RESISTANCE

Optimal use of all antimicrobials

Selective removal, control, or restriction of antimicrobial agents or classes

Rotational or cyclic antimicrobial use

Use of combination antimicrobial therapy to prevent the emergence of resistance

plasmids were typed using molecular techniques, so that the presence of resistance genes in hospital organisms could be determined during and after antimicrobial changes.[34] Future studies should build on the wide experience of these studies in exploring the effect of control measures on resistance prevention and reduction. The pharmaceutical industry should be encouraged to explore ways in which they can provide support for studies that can lead to preservation of the effectiveness of their drugs in the clinical setting.

The third method suggested in Table 6 is rotational or cyclic antimicrobial use. Few data are available on its impact. The largest experience is reported for changes in aminoglycoside use.[45] Attempts to reintroduce or to cycle gentamicin following use of amikacin resulted in recurrence of gentamicin resistance in three institutions.[34,37,46] Gentamicin use in one of these institutions was reinstituted successfully, subsequently, at a time when the original resistance plasmid no longer was found in hospital organisms.[34] The potential of this strategy as a resistance prevention measure has not been explored adequately, but it is a distinctly testable hypothesis in intensive-care units. In addition to the caveats expressed previously regarding such attempts,[45] it also is important to note that the duration of the cycles and the preferred order in which agents are cycled is unknown. Testing this method will require a multicenter trial, because a large population will be needed to control for several confounding variables.

The last strategy suggested in Table 6, use of combination antimicrobial therapy to reduce emergence of resistance, is theoretically attractive and is the basis for current treatment of tuberculosis with multiple antimicrobials. It has not been adequately tested clinically to determine if overall institutional resistance can be reduced by the use of combination therapy for individual patients.[47] In one study of *Enterobacter*, no benefit in reducing emerging resistance was observed when combined third-generation cephalosporin and aminoglycoside therapy was used.[48] The risks include increased antimicrobial costs and the potential for increasing resistance by raising the number of antimicrobials and antimicrobial

TABLE 7
RECOMMENDATIONS FOR PREVENTION AND REDUCTION OF ANTIMICROBIAL RESISTANCE IN HOSPITALS

Recommendations	Strength of Recommendation*	Quality of Evidence†
It is recommended that hospitals have a system for monitoring antimicrobial resistance of both community and nosocomial isolates (by hospital location and patient site) on a monthly basis or at a frequency appropriate to the volume of isolates.	A	III
Monitoring use of antimicrobials by hospital location or prescribing service is recommended on a monthly basis or at a frequency appropriate to the prescription volume.	A	III
It is recommended that hospitals monitor the relationship between antimicrobial use and resistance, and assign responsibility through practice guidelines or other institutional policies.	A	II
It is recommended that hospitals apply Contact Precautions to specified patients known or suspected to be colonized or infected with epidemiologically important microorganisms that can be transmitted by direct or indirect contact.	A	III

* Categories for strength of recommendation: A, good evidence for support; B, moderate evidence for support; C, poor evidence to support.
† Categories reflecting the quality of evidence on which recommendations are based: I, evidence from at least one properly randomized controlled trial; II, evidence from at least one well-designed clinical trial without randomization, from cohort or case-controlled analytic studies (preferably from more than one center), from multiple time-series studies, or from dramatic results in uncontrolled experiments; III, evidence from opinions of respected authorities, based on clinical experience, descriptive studies, or reports from expert committees.

courses administered. The use of combination therapy is, however, already widespread for the treatment of seriously ill patients, so controlled trials to determine the effect on resistance prevention are reasonable.

In summary, antimicrobial resistance among some hospital organisms has increased to the point that no antimicrobials are available for treatment. This is a situation that cannot be tolerated. The need for preventive and corrective measures is urgent. There is an almost certain causal association between the use of antimicrobials and resistance to them. Alterations in antimicrobial usage have been shown to affect antimicrobial resistance rates, particularly for the aminoglycosides. Additional large-scale, well-controlled trials of regulation of antimicrobial use employing sophisticated epidemiological methods, molecular typing of organisms, and precise analysis of mechanisms of resistance are required to determine the best methods to prevent and control this emerging problem of antimicrobial resistance and to establish optimal antimicrobial use.

CONTROLLING THE DISSEMINATION OF RESISTANT BACTERIA IN HOSPITALS

The SHEA/IDSA Joint Committee on Antibiotics supports the CDC "Guideline for Isolation Precautions in Hospitals"[13] as it applies to preventing the selection and spread of resistant microorganisms. Our recommendations are summarized in Table 7. Clearly, isolation of individuals infected with organisms for which no effective parenteral therapy remains (80% of vancomycin-resistant enterococci) is recommended universally for all hospitals.[49] Beyond this clear recommendation, hospitals again will have to make choices. Will colonized patients be isolated, for example? In general, it is recommended[13] that hospitals choose which organisms are of special clinical and epidemiological importance to identify patients for isolation. That such policies be adopted and implemented is especially important for hospitals where such resistance is not yet perceived as problematic. How should hospitals carry out surveillance for resistant microorganisms to identify patients requiring isolation? These questions are discussed below.

The Colonized Patient

The recommendations from the CDC[13] are unclear on how to care for patients colonized with resistant organisms. The most conservative approach is to isolate patients colonized with those organisms the hospital has decided to control, because they may be an important reservoir for transmission to, and eventually infection of, other patients or even healthcare workers. On the other hand, colonized patients are difficult to identify, likely to have a smaller burden of organisms than infected patients, and therefore are less likely to be a source of transmission. Isolation, or even cohorting, of every patient colonized with a resistant, epidemiologically important microorganism may not be practical for some hospitals. When possible, patients colonized with such an organism, whether they have been recognized through a surveillance effort or by chance, should be handled in the same manner as patients clinically infected with those organisms. Readmission of patients colonized with resistant organisms represents a hidden reservoir that could be monitored and controlled.

Identification of Patients to Be Isolated Because of Colonization or Infection With Resistant Microorganisms

Definition of resistance. According to the CDC,[13] resistant bacteria are those judged by the infection control program, based on current state, regional, or national recommendations, to be of special clinical and epidemiological significance. In its most rigorous form, this should include a quantitative susceptibility testing system that is better able to detect resistance than a simple breakpoint testing system. Under such a system, any epidemiologically important isolate with an unusual and relevant (for the hospital) decrease in susceptibility to one or more antibiotics might prompt institution of isolation precautions for the colonized or infected patient. An example might be *Klebsiella pneumoniae* isolated from the sputum of a patient with pneumonia that has an MIC for cefotaxime or ceftriaxone of 2 μg/mL. Although this ordinarily might be called susceptible by the hospital laboratory and by currently accepted US laboratory guidelines, such as those furnished by the NCCLS, this MIC certainly is unusual for the species. Identifying such an isolate justifiably might call for isolation of the patient, especially because it is unlikely that treatment with cefotaxime or ceftriaxone would be successful.[50] A simple, user-friendly data entry and retrieval system called WHONET has been supported by the World Health Organization for use by hospitals that wish to survey quantitative susceptibility tests (MICs or zone sizes).[51] A recent feature of this system calls attention to unusual drug resistance as the results are being entered.

Hospitals should consider instituting isolation precautions for patients colonized or infected with multiply resistant microorganisms. This seems most important for hospitals where resistance is not yet perceived to be a problem, because it is in such hospitals that the emergence of resistance will have the greatest impact on quality and cost of patient care.[2] An example of this is MRSA (and perhaps even methicillin-resistant *Staphylococcus epidermidis*) currently resistant to all but one effective parenteral antibiotic. Increasingly, data indicate that spread of MRSA in hospitals where such strains are not endemic can be controlled by isolating infected and colonized patients.

CDC Isolation Precautions for Hospitals

All patients are cared for using Standard Precautions. Standard Precautions synthesize the major features of Universal (Blood and Body Fluid) Precautions (designed to reduce the risk of transmission of bloodborne pathogens) and Body Substance Isolation (designed to reduce the risk of transmission of pathogens from moist body substances)[52-54] and apply them to all patients receiving care in hospitals, regardless of their diagnosis or presumed infection or colonization status. Standard Precautions apply to blood,[1] all body fluids, secretions, and excretions, regardless of whether they contain visible blood, nonintact skin, and mucous membranes.[13] Standard Precautions are designed to reduce the risk of transmission of microorganisms from both recognized and unrecognized sources of infection in hospitals.

Transmission-Based Precautions. Transmission-Based Precautions are designed for patients documented or suspected to be infected or colonized with highly transmissible or epidemiologically important pathogens for which additional precautions beyond Standard Precautions are needed to interrupt transmission in hospitals. Of the three types of Transmission-Based Precautions discussed in the Hospital Infection Control Practices Advisory Committee (HICPAC) recommendations,[13] only Contact Precautions are thought to be relevant to the transmission of resistant bacteria other than *Mycobacterium tuberculosis*. SHEA supports the HICPAC recommendations for the prevention of transmission of resistant pathogens[13] (Table 7).

Contact Precautions. Contact Precautions are designed to reduce the transmission of epidemiologically important microorganisms by direct or indirect contact. Direct contact transmission involves skin-to-skin contact and physical transfer of microorganisms to a susceptible host from an infected or colonized person, such as occurs when personnel turn a patient, give a patient a bath, or perform other patient-care activities that require physical contact. Direct contact transmission also can occur between two patients (eg, by hand contact), with one serving as the source of infectious microorganisms and the other as the susceptible host. Indirect contact transmission involves contact of a susceptible host with a contaminated intermediate object, usually inanimate, in the patient's environment. *Clearly, the environment can be an important reservoir of resistant microorganisms.* Contact Precautions apply to specified patients known or suspected to be colonized or infected with epidemiologically important microorganisms that can be transmitted by direct or indirect contact.

IMPLEMENTATION OF POLICY TO CONTROL ANTIBIOTIC RESISTANCE
Overview

Despite a strategic vision among hospital epidemiologists and tactical tools within hospitals known to be effective in limiting antimicrobial use, the most difficult aspect of influencing the use of antimicrobial agents has been administrative implementation of guidelines and policies designed to change usage. Implementation, in this context, means the attainment of sustained performance of approved standards of good stewardship. Effective implementation remains a problem, because it is not clear what administrative level of approval and enforcement is needed to ensure sustained positive performance. It is likely that a hierarchy of decision-making groups working together will guarantee implementation of sound antibiotic stewardship guidelines best.[55]

It is important to be aware that control of microbial resistance is not implemented just through control of antimicrobial use, although this may be an essential component. There are very few studies on the relative effectiveness of strategies for implementation of antimicrobial control policies.[55] Most authorities suggest that the pharmacy and therapeutics (P&T) committee should be charged with developing formulary and antimicrobial controls through a variety of mechanisms. Such mechanisms often include approval of orders by the infectious disease service, use of antibiotic order forms, and use of a computerized database to correlate pharmacy and bacteriology results.[56] Ordinarily, the P&T committee submits its policies for executive board review and approval, although this measure is often a rubber stamp of the P&T recommendations. The involvement of hospital administration in this process varies.[57]

Approaches to Implementation

Historically, antibiotic control policies have been used to control costs.[56-58] A side benefit always has been assumed to be reduced selective pressure and thus less antimicrobial resistance. Reduction of antimicrobial resistance using cost-motivated controls has not been documented well.[59,60] Nevertheless, "bottom-up" systems that start with P&T committees within hospitals have been used with variable success in controlling antimicrobial use, as long as the control measures remain in effect or are accepted fully by prescribers.[61] Ultimately, regardless of the mechanisms for control, very few programs have been able to show changes among prescribers that are sustained over a substantial period of time.

Bottom-up approaches have advantages and disadvantages for implementation of changes. Some advantages include the ability to streamline control methods to local resistance problems, the backing of on-site infectious disease practitioners, and a democratic procedure involving clinicians, administrators, and other healthcare workers. Disadvantages include the inability to anticipate national and international resistance trends; the outside pressures brought by physicians, pharmaceutical buying groups, and pharmaceutical representatives; and the lack of consensus among clinicians and administrative personnel regarding the importance of a broad attack on antibiotic resistance and the roles they should play.

Modern electronic communications and computers are revolutionizing hospital practice. In some hospitals, all medication orders must be entered into computer terminals in the hospital or clinics. Such computerized order entry provides the opportunity for real-time physician-pharmacy interactions that otherwise would be impossible with a handwritten order. Although initial reports are encouraging, there is no consensus on the effect of computer-based drug utilization review on reducing antibiotic prescribing practices.[62,63] Regardless of the value of computer-based drug utilization, increasingly sophisticated interactions now possible with computerized ordering will have a profound effect on physician prescribing and education in the future.

Control of antimicrobial resistance requires the implementation of two processes: infection control practices to limit the spread of resistant microorganisms and hospital policies of good antimicrobial use stewardship, which may include antimicrobial usage controls. In outbreak situations, standard infection control measures usually have been shown to reduce the spread of resistant microorganisms.[64] The utility of infection control measures to reduce the *endemic* spread of resistant bacteria is much harder to demonstrate.[65] Nevertheless, all experts urge control measures in such situations.[65,66]

Multiple approaches have been employed to enforce hospital policies to limit or control antibiotic use (see Table 8). The primary motivation for antibiotic control has been to reduce the cost of certain agents[67]; only recently has the need for antibiotic control resulted from an escalation of antimicrobial resistance.[68,69] Previously, cost-benefit analyses could determine which antimicrobial to include or exclude from hospital formulary use. A more difficult determination using risk-benefit analysis—where risk, in part, includes the emergence of antimicrobial resistance—now has become necessary to decide if an agent should be deleted, restricted, or substituted. Proof of the efficacy of these approaches in establishing control of resistance is lacking. Recommendations for effective implementation of antibiotic control, therefore, remain empirical. Nevertheless, because effective implementation and enforcement of antibiotic control programs are the essential first steps to success, it seems prudent to build first a consensus of various interest groups.[61] Consensus of quality standards for antimicrobial prophylaxis in surgical procedures already has been developed. Implementation of these standards should prove effective in reducing the length of prophylaxis and the total volume of antimicrobial use.[70]

The British approach. The British Society for Antimicrobial Chemotherapy (BSAC) has conducted a large survey to assess national characteristics of control measures in British hospitals. They sampled microbiologists and pharmacists to determine the practice of control measures for their respective hospital[68]; 49% responded. Among respondent hospitals, 86% had a P&T committee, 79% had an antibiotic formulary, 62% had a policy for therapy, and 17% had an antibiotic committee. In 40%, compliance was monitored, and 88% believed their policies for antimicrobial prophylaxis and therapy were beneficial.

Policies included educational campaigns (52%), cost-control programs (50%), regulation of pharmaceutical promotions (48%), therapeutic substitutions (43%), automatic stop orders (26%), antibiotic utilization coordinators (11%), and antibiotic audit (11%). In a country that has had a national health service for years, how would antimicrobial gatekeepers feel about developing national policies for control? Interestingly, very few of the microbiologists (5.6%) and fewer pharmacists (0.7%) advocated a national policy. These attitudes are surprising, because a report with recommendations from the Working Party of the BSAC in 1982 probably resulted in the high prevalence of control measures.[68]

The minimum control measures that the BSAC now recommends are summarized as follows:

1. Updating of antibiotic formulary and policies with appropriate funding for staff and resources.

2. Widespread consultation before inception of antibiotic control programs and constructive feedback thereafter, thus ensuring "continuous consultation."

3. Representative committees to consider introduction of new antibiotics, with the authority to withhold these agents or to make these agents available.

4. Strict restriction of nonformulary agents.

5. Provisions for departments of microbiology (infectious diseases) and pharmacy to have adequate facilities, to ensure the success of educational programs, and to have adequate computer resources.

6. Appropriate personnel to monitor the adherence to policies and formularies.

7. Funded programs to assess and adopt auto-

TABLE 8
METHODS TO IMPLEMENT ANTIBIOTIC CONTROL OR RESTRICTION POLICIES

Written hospital guidelines
    National[49]
    Regional (state regulations)
    Local[68]
Educational efforts aimed at changing prescribing practices
  of physicians
    Face-to-face-presentations[72]
    Computer interactions[73]
    Pharmacy "Top 100" expenditures list
Restriction of hospital formulary through pharmacy and
  therapeutics committee
    Cyclic rotation of antimicrobials within a class[34]
    Antibiotic order forms[74,75]
    Antibiotic stop orders
      Therapeutic use
      Prophylactic use
    Restriction of use[77]
    Removal of specific agents[78]
    Review of medical record by pharmacists[79]
      Decentralized pharmacies
      PharmDs to interact with physicians[80]
    Usage feedback to physician[78]
    Computerized review
    Group purchasing practices
    Generic substitution[81]
Utilization review with guidelines for rational
  and appropriate usage
    Antibiotic utilization subcommittee
      Multidisciplinary teams[79]
Requirement of consultation with infectious diseases
  subspecialists for certain antimicrobial choices
    By telephone approval[78]
    By written audit[82,83]
Antimicrobial susceptibility reporting[84]
Reduction of pharmaceutical promotion[68]

matic stop orders, antibiotic prescription forms, and use of utilization coordinators.

8. Requirement of permission from administration for pharmaceutical promotions.

9. Susceptibility patterns should be published by microbiology laboratories.

10. Research into novel control measures should be encouraged with provision of adequate facilities, including computerized information systems.

Consensus-Building to Develop and Implement Antibiotic Control Policies

A new American approach. The British experience may not be applicable to hospitals in other countries. Thus, a recent document representing a new American approach, "Workshop to Prevent and Control the Emergence and Spread of Antibiotic-Resistant Microorganisms in Hospitals,"[65] has diverged from traditional approaches to implement control programs. In the document, the authors speak of a "striking lack of success in the prevention and control of antibiotic resistance despite career devotion by many health professionals to this objective." To quote further, "Despite guidelines promulgated by the CDC and professional societies, antibiotic-restriction policies, and the entreaties of their colleagues, physicians continue to prescribe antibiotics excessively and inappropriately. . . ." As the authors note, although many American hospitals have a strategic policy for prevention and control of antibiotic resistance, very few hospitals have made antibiotic resistance a strategic priority. Regardless of the reason for inaction by hospitals, we agree with the workshop participants that the time for complacency has long passed.

The workshop advanced two broad focus areas; each area involved strategic goals with steps, process measures, and countermeasures to ensure success. Listed here are those goals that involve implementation of an effective program of good antibiotic stewardship.

The following are strategies to optimize the prophylactic, empiric, and therapeutic use of antibiotics in the hospital, considering their impact on microbial environment, effectiveness, and cost:

Strategic goal 1: Optimize choice and duration of prophylactic antibiotic therapy.

Strategic goal 2: Optimize choice and duration of empiric antibiotic therapy.

Strategic goal 3: Improve antibiotic prescribing practices by educational and administrative means.

Strategic goal 4: Establish a system to monitor and provide feedback on the occurrence and impact of antibiotic resistance.

Strategic goal 5: Define and implement institutional or healthcare delivery-system guidelines for important types of antibiotic use.

The following are strategies for detecting, reporting, and preventing transmission of antibiotic-resistant microorganisms:

Strategic goal 1: Develop a system to recognize trends in antibiotic resistance and to report them promptly to hospital and physician leaders; medical, nursing, infection control, and pharmacy staffs; and others who need to know.

Strategic goal 2: Develop a system for rapid detection of resistant microorganisms in individual patients, with reporting to infection control staff for rapid response by caregivers.

Strategic goal 3: Increase adherence to policies and procedures, especially hand hygiene, barrier precautions, and environmental control measures.

Strategic goal 4: Incorporate detection, prevention, and control of antibiotic resistance into institutional strategic goals, and provide required resources.

Strategic goal 5: Develop a plan for identifying, transferring, discharging, and readmitting patients colonized with specified antimicrobial-resistant microorganisms.

A model using consensus for implementation. The potential for implementing many of the outlined steps, processes, and countermeasures exists at American hospitals. Leadership will be needed. This leadership should come from hospital epidemiologists, microbiologists, pharmacists, physicians, infection control practitioners, and others who participate in the hospital committees providing recommendations. Hospital epidemiologists and others will need to present substantiating information to hospital administration on the morbidity, mortality, expense, and increased length of stay associated with antibiotic resistance. Hospital management will need to become invested in, and accountable for, the control of antibiotic resistance in hospitals, because certain processes and countermeasures are painful and expensive.

With the resistance crisis upon us, incremental change is likely to be ineffective, and a mass mobilization is needed to curb the existing level of resistance. The current system of antibiotic use has resulted in the problem we face. Counteracting forces constantly will come into play, eg, the use of vancomycin for highly penicillin-resistant *Streptococcus pneumoniae* will increase the selective pressure for the emergence of vancomycin-resistant enterococci. The expanding population of neutropenic patients will increase the need for extended-spectrum cephalosporins and thus the likelihood of emergence of extended-spectrum β-lactamases. Companies that develop new antimicrobials for use against resistant organisms may oppose efforts to restrict their use.

Hospitals, led by their committees with the support of hospital management, should develop policies based on their local resistance characteristics, antibiotic usage patterns, input from a state department of health advisory board or other similar body, and input from national organizations (Figure). Hospital-specific formal guidelines then would be delivered from these committees to the hospital administration for implementation. Staff compliance in individual facilities should be compared to quality improvement standards, and these outcomes should be the basis for continuous quality improvement.

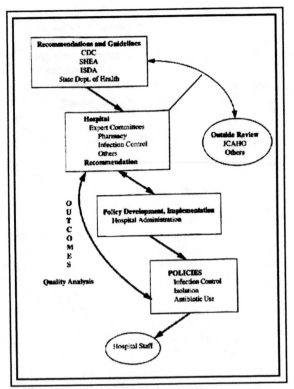

FIGURE. Flow of information, recommendations, and policies for the development of hospital policies to prevent the emergence and dissemination of resistance. Expert committees of the hospital, taking into account the recommendations and guidelines of outside agencies, develop hospital-specific recommendations and guidelines that are forwarded to the hospital administration. The responsibility of the administration is to develop or approve policies and to implement them within the hospital. These then are communicated to the hospital staff. Implementation is monitored by outcomes analysis and quality analysis. These data are analyzed by the expert hospital committees for further action and are communicated to outside agencies such as the Centers for Disease Control and Prevention, the Society for Healthcare Epidemiology of America, and the Infectious Diseases Society of America, as well as to oversight agencies such as the Joint Commission on Accreditation of Healthcare Organizations (JCAHO). Outside review by JCAHO and other agencies is aimed specifically at the implementation of recommendations, guidelines, and proposed policies, the primary responsibility of hospital administration.

SHEA proposes that data provided by hospitals be utilized by state and national organizations, such as state health departments, the CDC, SHEA, and IDSA, to feed back information important to the hospital for evaluating its own antimicrobial-resistance policy. A state-supervised system of surveillance, like the one recently described in New Jersey, also would provide trends in emergence and spread of antibiotic-resistant organisms.[71] The Joint Commission on the Accreditation of Healthcare Organizations, or a similar review organization skilled in oversight functions, should take into account the priority hospitals give to antimicrobial resistance; policies, procedures, and

TABLE 9
RECOMMENDATIONS FOR FUTURE STUDIES TO EXAMINE MEANS TO PREVENT AND REDUCE THE DEVELOPMENT AND DISSEMINATION OF ANTIMICROBIAL RESISTANCE

The development and testing of protocols for measuring the effect of a variety of antimicrobial usage controls is recommended for use in multiple hospitals to determine the most effective ways to prevent and reduce antimicrobial resistance in specific species to specific antimicrobials.

Pharmaceutical industry and governmental support for such studies is recommended and encouraged.

It is recommended that educational methods, including those that are interactive and computer-based, be developed to improve the appropriateness of antimicrobial prescribing.

It is recommended that protocols to evaluate antimicrobial resistance include the ability to relate resistance rates to the "defined drug density" (the amount of antimicrobial used per geographic area per unit time).

The transfer of resistance determinants in situ in a patient population is very poorly understood. First, the genetics of resistance transfer, the construction of composite transposons, and the actual mechanism of dissemination of these elements in situ, especially intergeneric transfer within the gram-positive bacteria, all should be studied further.

Methods for interdicting transfer of resistance requires further study, especially in the behavioral area. Novel approaches to this area are needed.

The efficacy of various levels of infection control precautions should be documented by controlled trials.

Controlled studies of behavior modification, including novel approaches, to permit the efficient application of recommended guidelines within hospitals are recommended.

The efficacy of quality improvement approaches to control of resistance should be studied.

measurements hospitals put into place; and evidence of ongoing review of data to judge the effectiveness of the plan.

These recommendations are a beginning of a national program to control antimicrobial resistance in hospitals. Similar standards can be applied to long-term–care facilities, private offices, and ambulatory-care clinics. Methods of implementation that are shown in cooperative studies to be useless in controlling resistance will be rescinded at the state level and abridged in subsequent CDC guidelines. The process thus allows for continuous quality improvement in implementing guidelines and policies to control antimicrobial use and resistance.

THE FUTURE

Recognizing that our recommendations frequently are based on inadequate data, we call for funding for additional studies that will allow us to preserve better our antimicrobial arsenal in the future. Toward this goal, we echo the recommendations of the American Society for Microbiology Task Force on Antimicrobial Resistance. We support, in addition, the recommendations of previous National Institutes of Health workshops regarding new research directions in antimicrobial resistance. Our specific recommendations in this regard are summarized in Table 9.

REFERENCES

1. Shlaes DM, Levy S, Archer G. Antimicrobial resistance: new directions. *ASM News* 1991;57:455-463.
2. Phelps CE. Bug/drug resistance. *Med Care* 1988;27:194-203.
3. Neu HC. The crisis in antibiotic resistance. *Science* 1992;257:1064-1073.
4. Davies J. Inactivation of antibiotics and the dissemination of resistance genes. *Science* 1994;264:375-382.
5. Stokes HW, Hall RM. A novel family of potentially mobile DNA elements encoding site-specific gene integration functions: integrons. *Mol Microbiol* 1989;3:1669-1683.
6. Nikaido H. Prevention of drug access to bacterial targets: permeability barriers and active efflux. *Science* 1994;264:382-388.
7. Levy SB. Active efflux mechanisms of antibiotic resistance. *Antimicrob Agents Chemother* 1992;36:695-703.
8. Spratt BG. Resistance to antibiotics mediated by target alterations. *Science* 1994;264:388-393.
9. Musher DM, Baughn RE, Templeton GB, Minuth JN. Emergence of variant forms of *Staphylococcus aureus* after exposure to gentamicin and infectivity of the variants in experimental animals. *J Infect Dis* 1977;136:360-369.
10. Musher DM, Baughn RE, Merrell GL. Selection of small-colony variants of *Enterobacteriaceae* by in vitro exposure to aminoglycosides: pathogenicity for experimental animals. *J Infect Dis* 1979;140:209-214.
11. Balwitt JM, van Langevelde P, Vann JM, Proctor RA. Gentamicin-resistant menadione and hemin auxotrophic *Staphylococcus aureus* persist within cultured epithelial cells. *J Infect Dis* 1994;170:1033-1037.
12. Muder RR, Brennen C, Wagener MW, et al. Methicillin-resistant staphylococcal colonization and infection in a long term care facility. *Ann Intern Med* 1991;114:107-112.
13. Garner JS, Hospital Infection Control Practices Advisory Committee, Centers for Disease Control and Prevention. Guideline for isolation precautions in hospitals. *Infect Control Hosp Epidemiol* 1996;17:53-80.
14. Wingard E, Shlaes JH, Mortimer EA, Shlaes DM. Colonization and cross-colonization of nursing home patients with trimethoprim-resistant gram-negative bacilli. *Clin Infect Dis* 1993;16:75-81.
15. McGowan JE Jr. Antibiotic resistance in hospital bacteria: current patterns, modes for appearance or spread, and economic impact. *Rev Med Microbiol* 1991;2:161-169.
16. McGowan JE Jr. Antimicrobial resistance in hospital organisms and its relation to antibiotic use. *Rev Infect Dis* 1983;5:1033-1048.
17. Olson B, Weinstein RA, Nathan C, Gaston MA, Kabins SA. Epidemiology of endemic *Pseudomonas aeruginosa*: why infection control efforts have failed. *J Infect Dis* 1987;150:808-816.
18. McGowan JE Jr. Is antimicrobial resistance in hospital microorganisms related to antibiotic use? *Bull NY Acad Med* 1987;63:253-268.
19. Levy SB. Balancing the drug-resistance equation. *Trends Microbiol* 1994;2:341-342.
20. Courcol RJ, Pinkas M, Martin GR. A seven-year survey of antibiotic susceptibility and its relationship with usage. *J Antimicrob Chemother* 1989;23:441-451.
21. Duncan RA, Steger KA, Craven DE. Selective decontamination of the digestive tract: risks outweigh benefits for intensive care

unit patients. *Semin Respir Infect* 1993;8:308-324.
22. Hughes WT, Armstrong D, Bodey GP, et al. Guidelines for the use of antimicrobial agents in neutropenic patients with unexplained fever. *J Infect Dis* 1990;161:381-396.
23. Kim JH, Gallis HA. Observations on spiraling empiricism: its causes, allure, and perils with particular reference to antibiotic therapy. *Am J Med* 1989;87:201-206.
24. Pallares R, Dick R, Wenzel RP, Adams JR, Nettleman MD. Trends in antimicrobial utilization at a tertiary teaching hospital during a 15-year period (1978-1992). *Infect Control Hosp Epidemiol* 1993;14:376-382.
25. Conus P, Francioli P. Relationship between ceftriaxone use and resistance of *Enterobacter* species. *J Clin Pharm Ther* 1992;17:303-305.
26. Moller JK. Antimicrobial usage and microbial resistance in a university hospital during a seven-year period. *J Antimicrob Chemother* 1989;24:983-992.
27. Ballow CH, Schentag JJ. Trends in antibiotic utilization and bacterial resistance report of the national nosocomial resistance surveillance group. *Diagn Microbiol Infect Dis* 1992;15:375-425.
28. Coronado VG, Edwards JR, Culver DH, Gaynes RP. Ciprofloxacin resistance among nosocomial *Pseudomonas aeruginosa* and *Staphylococcus aureus* in the United States. *Infect Control Hosp Epidemiol* 1995;16:71-75.
29. Goswitz JJ, Willard KE, Fasching CE, Peterson LR. Detection of *gyrA* gene mutations associated with ciprofloxacin resistance in methicillin-resistant *Staphylococcus aureus*: analysis by polymerase chain reaction and automated direct DNA sequencing. *Antimicrob Agents Chemother* 1992;36:1166-1169.
30. Ferrero L, Cameron B, Manse B, et al. Cloning and primary structure of *Staphylococcus aureus* DNA topoisomerase, IV: a primary target of fluoroquinolones. *Mol Microbiol* 1994;13:641-653.
31. Ferrero L, Cameron B, Crouzet J. Analysis of *gyrA* and *grlA* mutations in stepwise-selected ciprofloxacin-resistant mutants of *Staphylococcus aureus*. *Antimicrob Agents Chemother* 1995;39:1554-1558.
32. McGowan JE Jr. Do intensive hospital antibiotic control programs prevent the spread of antibiotic resistance? *Infect Control Hosp Epidemiol* 1994;15:478-483.
33. Betts RF, Valenti WM, Chapman SW, et al. Five-year surveillance of aminoglycoside usage in a university hospital. *Ann Intern Med* 1984;100:219-222.
34. Gerding DN, Larson TA, Hughes RA, et al. Aminoglycoside resistance and aminoglycoside usage: ten years of experience in one hospital. *Antimicrob Agents Chemother* 1991;35:1284-1290.
35. Berk SL, Alvarez S, Ortega G, et al. Clinical and microbiological consequences of amikacin use during a 42-month period. *Arch Intern Med* 1986;146:538-541.
36. Young EJ, Sewell CM, Koza MA, Clarridge JE. Antibiotic resistance patterns during aminoglycoside restriction. *Am J Med Sci* 1985;290:223-227.
37. King JW, White MC, Todd JR, Conrad SA. Alterations in the microbial flora and in the incidence of bacteremia at a university hospital after adoption of amikacin as the sole formulary aminoglycoside. *Clin Infect Dis* 1992;14:908-915.
38. van Landuyt HW, Boelaert J, Glibert B, Gordts B, Verbruggen AM. Surveillance of aminoglycoside resistance: European data. *Am J Med* 1986;80(suppl 6B):76-81.
39. Bamberger DM, Dahl SL. Impact of voluntary vs enforced compliance of third-generation cephalosporin use in a teaching hospital. *Arch Intern Med* 1992;152:554-557.
40. Pear SM, Williamson TH, Bettin KM, Gerding DN, Galgiani JN. Decrease in nosocomial *Clostridium difficile*-associated diarrhea by restricting clindamycin use. *Ann Intern Med* 1994;120:272-277.
41. Hammond JMJ, Potgieter PD, Forder AA, Plumb H. Influence of amikacin as the primary aminoglycoside on bacterial isolates in the intensive care unit. *Crit Care Med* 1990;18:607-610.
42. Friedland IR, Funk E, Khoosal M, Klugman KP. Increased resistance to amikacin in a neonatal unit following intensive amikacin usage. *Antimicrob Agents Chemother* 1992;36:

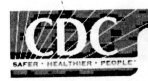

Campaign to
Prevent Antimicrobial Resistance in Healthcare Settings

Fact Sheet
12 Steps to Prevent Antimicrobial Resistance Among Dialysis Patients

Campaign Home

by patient type

by tool type

Overview

Why a Campaign?

Goals & Methods

Partnerships

Get Involved!

Web Resources

Contact Us

Prevent Infection

Step 1. Vaccinate Staff and Patients
‣ Get influenza vaccine
‣ Give influenza and pneumococcal vaccine to patients in addition to routine vaccines (e.g. hepatitis B)

Step 2. Get the Catheters out
Hemodialysis
‣ Use catheters only when essential
‣ Maximize use of fistulas/grafts
‣ Remove catheters when they are no longer essential
Peritoneal Dialysis
‣ Remove/replace infected catheters

Step 3. Optimize Access Care
‣ Follow established KDOQI and CDC Guidelines for access care
‣ Use proper insertion and catheter-care protocols
‣ Remove access device when infected
‣ Use the correct catheter

Diagnose and Treat Infection Effectively

141

Step 4. Target the Pathogen
▸ Obtain appropriate cultures
▸ Target empiric therapy to likely pathogens
▸ Target definitive therapy to known pathogens
▸ Optimize timing, regimen, dose, route, and duration

Step 5. Access the Experts
▸ Consult the appropriate expert for complicated infections

Use Antimicrobials Wisely

Step 6. Use local data
▸ Know your local antibiogram
▸ Get previous microbiology results when patients transfer to your facility

Step 7. Know when to say "no" to vanco
▸ Follow CDC guidelines for vancomycin use
▸ Consider 1st generation cephalosporins instead of vancomycin

Step 8. Treat infection, not contamination or colonization
▸ Use proper antisepsis for drawing blood cultures
▸ Get one peripheral vein blood culture, if possible
▸ Avoid culturing vascular catheter tips
▸ Treat bacteremia, not the catheter tip

Step 9. Stop Antimicrobial Treatment
▸ When infection is treated
▸ When infection is not diagnosed

Prevent transmission

Step 10: Follow Infection Control Precautions
▸Use standard infection control precautions for dialysis centers
▸Consult local infection control experts

Step 11: Practice Hand Hygiene
▸Wash your hands or use an alcohol-based handrub
▸Set an example

Step 12: Partner With Your Patients
▸Educate on access care and infection control measures
▸Re-educate regularly

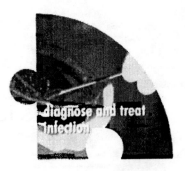

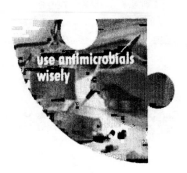

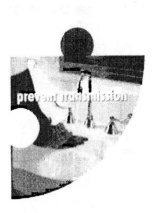

DHQP Home | DHQP Index

NCID Home | **CDC Home** | **CDC Search** | **CDC Health Topics A-Z**

SUPPLEMENT

APIC GUIDELINES FOR INFECTION CONTROL PRACTICE

The publication of this supplement was made possible by an educational grant from Johnson & Johnson Medical, Inc.

The Association for Professionals in Infection Control and Epidemiology, Inc. (APIC) Board of Directors and Guidelines Committee are pleased to present the "APIC Guideline for Selection and Use of Disinfectants."

William A. Rutala, PhD, MPH, CIC, was selected to revise the previously published "APIC Guideline for Selection and Use of Disinfectants" because of his recognized expertise in infection control and extensive research with disinfectants. Initial drafts were reviewed by the APIC Guidelines Committee, key individuals, and professional organizations before the publication of the draft document in the August 1995 issue of AJIC, soliciting further comments. All written comments were reviewed by the APIC Guidelines Committee and revisions were made. The Guideline was finalized by the Committee in February 1996 and approved by the APIC Board of Directors in March 1996.

The APIC Board of Directors and the APIC Guidelines Committee express our sincere gratitude to the author and to all who provided their assistance in the guideline development and review process.

APIC guideline for selection and use of disinfectants*

William A. Rutala, PhD, MPH, CIC
1994, 1995, and 1996 APIC Guidelines Committee
Association for Professionals in Infection Control and Epidemiology, Inc.

From the Statewide Infection Control Program, Division of Infectious Diseases, University of North Carolina School of Medicine, and Hospital Epidemiology, Occupational Health, and Safety Program, University of North Carolina Hospitals, Chapel Hill, N.C.

Reprint requests: APIC National Office, 1016 16th St. N.W., 6th Floor, Washington, DC 20036; phone (202) 296-2742. Volume discount available.

*The 1996 version supercedes the 1990 guideline.

AJIC Am J Infect Control 1996;24:313-42.

The need for appropriate disinfection and sterilization has been emphasized by numerous articles documenting infection after improper reprocessing of patient care items. Because it is unnecessary to sterilize all patient care items, hospital policies must identify whether disinfection or sterilization is indicated on the basis of each item's intended use. In 1982 the Centers for Disease Control and Prevention (CDC) prepared a "Guideline for Hospital Environmental Control," which provided specific directions for the selection and use of disinfectants.[1] A revised version of

313

this guideline, entitled "Guideline for Handwashing and Hospital Environmental Control, 1985," was published in November 1985.[2] This latter guideline did not recommend chemical germicides that were formulated for use on medical equipment or environmental surfaces in health care facilities. Rather, the revised CDC guideline focused on strategies for disinfection and sterilization of medical (equipment used in the health care setting.

The purpose of this revised Association for Professionals in Infection Control and Epidemiology, Inc. (APIC) Guideline, which is an updated version of previous publications,[3-6] is to assist health care professi~onals in their decisions involving the judicious selection and proper use of specific disinfectants. In the preparation of this guideline, articles in the scientific literature were used to augment the manufacturers' label claims because these claims were not consistently verifiables[7] Disinfectant failures noted at variance to label claims may be caused by deficiencies in testing methods[7] or by improperly conducted tests8 In addition, in-use testing has not been incorporated into all Environmental Protection Agency (EPA) methods (e.g., Association of Official Analytical Chemists [AOAC] tuberculocidal activity test), and fa:ilures have been demonstrated when some disinfectants are subjected to conditions, such as dilution, age, and presence of organic matter, that challenge their antimicrobial activity.[9] It should also be recognized that EPA registration claims are based on microbicidal efficacy data submitted by manufacturers. The EPA does not independently test disinfectants before their registration, but in 1990 the EPA resumed postregistration testing of chemical sterilants to ensure that they satisfy their registered label claims.

DEFINITIONS

For the purpose of this guideline, the following definitions will be used:

Sterilization is the complete elimination or destruction of all forms of microbial life. It is accomplished by either physical or chemical processes. Steam under pressure, dry heat, low temperature sterilization processes (ethylene oxide [ETO] gas, plasma sterilization) and liquid chemicals are the principal sterilizing agents used. The term *sterilization is* intended to convey an absolute meaning, not a relative one.

Disinfection describes a process that eliminates

BACTERIALSPORES
Bacillus subtilis
⇓
MYCOBACTERIA
Mycobacterium tuberculosis
⇓
NONLIPID OR SMALLVIRUSES
poliovirus
4
FUNGI
Trichophyton spp.

VEGETATIVE BACTERIA
Pseudomonas aeruginosa
Staphylococcus aureus
⇓
LIPID OR MEDIUM-SIZED VIRUSES
herpes simplex virus
hepatitis B virus
human immunodeficiency virus

Fig. 1. Descending order of resistance to germicidal chemicals. This hierarchy considers broad classifications of microbial categories. It is considered a rough guide to general susceptibility of microorganisms to disinfectants. Adapted from Favero MS, Bond WV. Chemical disinfection of medical and surgical materials. In: Block SS, ed. Disinfection, sterilization and preservation. 4th ed. Philadelphia: Lea & Febiger, 1991:621.

many or all pathogenic microorganisms, with the exception of bacterial spores, from inanimate objects. In health care settings, this is generally accomplished by the use of liquid chemicals or wet pasteurization. The efficacy of disinfection is affected by a number of factors, each of which may nullify or limit the efficacy of the process. Some of the factors that have been shown to affect disinfection efficacy are the previous cleaning of the object, the organic load on the object, the type (Fig. 1) and level of microbial contamination, the concentration of and exposure time to the germicide, the physical configuration of the object (e.g., crevices, hinges, lumens), and the temperature and pH of the disinfection process. More extensive consideration of these and other factors that affect both disinfection and sterilization may be found in several references.3, [6, 10-13] Chemical disinfectants can be classified by several schemes. This guideline uses the terminology used by the CDC's "Guideline for Handwashing and Hospital

Table 1. Classification of devices, processes, and germicidal products

Device classification	Devices (examples)	Spaulding process classification	EPA product classification
Critical (enters sterile tissue or vascular system)	Implants, scalpels, needles, other surgical instruments, etc.	*Sterilization*—sporicidal chemical; prolonged contact	Sterilant/disinfectant
Semicritical (touches mucous membranes [except dental])	Flexible endoscopes, laryngoscopes, endotracheal tubes, and other similar instruments	*High-level disinfection*—sporicidal chemical; short contact	Sterilant/disinfectant
	Thermometers, hydrotherapy tanks	*Intermediate-level disinfection*	Hospital disinfectant with label claim for tuberculocidal activity
Noncritical (touches intact skin)	Stethoscopes, tabletops, bedpans, etc.	*Low-level disinfection*	Hospital disinfectant without label claim for tuberculocidal activity

Modified from Favero MS, Bond WW. Chemical disinfection of medical and surgical materials. In: Block SS, ed. Disinfection, sterilization and preservation. 4th ed. Philadelphia: Lea & Febiger 1991:627.

ronmental Control, 1985,"[2] in which the levels of disinfection are defined as *sterilization, high-level disinfection, intermediate-level disinfection*, and *low-level disinfection*. These terms were also used in the CDC's "Guidelines for the Prevention of Transmission of Human Immunodeficiency Virus and Hepatitis B Virus to Health-Care and Public-Safety Workers."[14]

High-level disinfection can be expected to destroy all microorganisms, with the exception of high numbers of bacterial spores. *Intermediate-level disinfection* inactivates *Mycobacterium tuberculosis*, vegetative bacteria, most viruses, and most fungi, but it does not necessarily kill bacterial spores. *Low-level disinfection* can kill most bacteria, some viruses, and some fungi, but it cannot be relied on to kill resistant microorganisms such as tubercle bacilli or bacterial spores.

Cleaning is the removal of all foreign material (e.g., soil, organic material) from objects. It is normally accomplished with water, mechanical action, and detergents or enzymatic products. Failure to remove foreign matter (e.g., lubricants, soils) from an object before a disinfection or sterilization process is likely to render the process ineffective.[15-18] Meticulous physical cleaning must precede disinfection and sterilization procedures. Studies have shown that manual and mechanical cleaning of endoscopes achieves approximately a 4 log reduction of contaminating organisms.[15] Thus cleaning alone is very effective in reducing the number of microorganisms present on contaminated equipment. A *germicide* is an agent that destroys microorganisms, particularly pathogenic organisms ("germs"). Other agents designated by

words with the suffix *-cide* (e.g., virucide, fungicide, bactericide, sporicide, tuberculocide) destroy the microorganisms identified by the prefix. For example, a *bactericide* is an agent that kills bacteria.[1, 10, 11, 19] Chemicals used for the purpose of destroying all forms of microbial life, including fungal and bacterial spores, are called *chemical sterilants*. These same chemical sterilants may also be part of the high-level disinfection process when used for shorter exposure periods. A *disinfectant* is a germicide that inactivates virtually all recognized pathogenic microorganisms but not necessarily all microbial forms (e.g., bacterial endospores) on inanimate objects. As of June 1993, the Food and Drug Administration (FDA) has primary responsibility for the premarket review of safety and efficacy requirements for liquid chemical germicides that are sterilants intended for use on critical and semicritical devices. The EPA has primary responsibility for premarket review of general-purpose disinfectants used on noncritical items.[20] An *antiseptic* is a chemical germicide formulated for use on skin or tissue and should not be used to decontaminate inanimate objects. The selection and use of antiseptics are extensively discussed in another publication.[21] Antiseptics are registered and regulated by the FDA.

A RATIONAL APPROACH TO DISINFECTION AND STERILIZATION

In 1968 a rational approach to disinfection and sterilization of patient care items or equipment was devised by E. H. Spaulding.[11] This classification scheme is so clear and logical that it has been retained, refined, and successfully used by infection control professionals (ICPs) and others when planning methods for disinfection or sterilization.[1-4, 10] Spaulding[11] believed that the nature of disinfection could be understood more readily if instruments and items for patient care were divided into three categories according to degree of risk of infection involved in the use of the items. The three categories of items he described were as follows: *critical, semicritical,* and *noncritical.* Table 1 correlates the three device classifications (critical, semicritical, and noncritical) with Spaulding's process classification and the EPA's product classifications.

Critical Items

Items assigned to the *critical* category present a high risk of infection if contaminated with any microorganism, including bacterial spores. It is critical that objects entering sterile tissue or the vascular system be kept sterile. This category includes surgical instruments, cardiac and urinary catheters, implants, and needles. Most of the items in this category should be purchased as sterile or should be sterilized by steam under pressure if possible. If heat labile, the object may be treated with ETO or other low temperature sterilization processes. Table 2 lists several germicides categorized as chemical sterilants. These include 2% glutaraldehyde-based formulations, 6% stabilized hydrogen peroxide, and peracetic acid. Chemical sterilants can be relied on to produce sterility only if adequate cleaning precedes treatment and if proper guidelines with regard to organic load, contact time, temperature, and pH are met.

Semicritical Items

Semicritical items are those objects that come in contact with mucous membranes or skin that is not intact. These items must be free of all microorganisms, with the exception of high numbers of bacterial spores. Intact mucous membranes are generally resistant to infection by common bacterial spores but are susceptible to other organisms, such as tubercle bacilli and viruses. Respiratory therapy and anesthesia equipment, endoscopes, and cervical diaphragm fitting rings are included in this category. Semicritical items generally require high-level disinfection with wet pasteurization or chemical disinfectant. Glutaraldehyde, stabilized hydrogen peroxide, chlorine, and peracetic acid are dependable high-level disinfectants, provided the factors influencing germicidal

procedures are considered (Table 2). Heat sterilization is the preferred method of between-patient processing of heat-stable medical instruments because it provides the widest margin of safety, even though high-level disinfection with a liquid chemical disinfectant would provide a patient-safe device. When selecting a disinfectant for use with certain patient care items, the chemical compatibility after extended use with the items must also be considered. For example, although chlorine is considered a high-level disinfectant, it is generally not used for disinfecting semicritical items because of its corrosive effects.

It is recommended that semicritical items be rinsed with sterile water after disinfection to prevent contamination with organisms that may be present in tap water, such as nontuberculous mycobacteria and *Legionella.*[2, 5, 22-26] In circumstances under which a sterile water rinse is not feasible, a tap water rinse should be followed by an alcohol rinse and forced-air drying.[22, 24, 27, 28] Introduction of forced-air drying significantly reduces bacterial contamination of stored endoscopes, presumably by removing the wet environment favorable for bacterial growth.[18, 27]

Some semicritical items (e.g., hydrotherapy tanks used for patients whose skin is not intact, thermometers) may require only intermediate-level disinfection. Intermediate-level disinfectants (e.g., chlorine, phenolics, iodophor) inactivate *M. tuberculosis,* vegetative bacteria, most viruses, and most fungi but do not necessarily kill bacterial spores.

Noncritical Items

Noncritical items come in contact with intact skin but not with mucous membranes. Intact skin acts as an effective barrier to most microorganisms, and sterility is not critical. Examples of noncritical items include bedpans, blood pressure cuffs, crutches, bed rails, linens, some food utensils, bedside tables, and patient furniture. Most noncritical reusable items may be disinfected where they are used and do not need to be transported to a central processing area. There is generally little risk of transmitting infectious agents to patients by means of noncritical items[29]; however, these items could potentially contribute to secondary transmission by contaminating hands of health care workers or by contact with medical equipment that subsequently comes in contact with patients.[10, 30] The low-level disinfectants listed in Table 2 may be used for noncritical items.

Table 2. Methods of sterilization and disinfection

Object	Sterilization		Disinfection		
	Critical items (will enter tissue or vascular system or blood will flow through them)		High-level (semicritical items [except dental[a]] will come in contact with mucous membrane or nonintact skin)	Intermediate-level (some semicritical items[b] and noncritical items)	Low-level (noncritical items; will come in contact with intact skin)
	Procedure	Exposure time (hr.)	Procedure (exposure time ≥ 20 min.)[c, d]	Procedure (exposure time ≤ 10 min.)	Procedure (exposure time ≤ 10 min.)
Smooth hard surface[b]	A	MR	C	G[e]	H
	B	MR	D	H	I
	C	MR	E	J	J
	D	6	F[f]	K	K
	E	MR	G		L
Rubber tubing and catheters[d]	A	MR	C		
	B	MR	D		
	C	MR	E		
	D	6	F[f]		
	E	MR			
Polyethylene tubing and catheters[d, g]	A	MR	C		
	B	MR	D		
	C	MR	E		
	D	6	F[f]		
	E	MR			
Lensed instruments	B	MR	C		
	C	MR	D		
	D	6	E		
	E	MR			
Thermometers (oral and rectal)[h]				H[h]	
Hinged instruments	A	MR	C		
	B	MR	D		
	C	MR	E		
	D	6			
	E	MR			

Adapted from Simmons BP. Guideline for hospital environmental control. Am J Infect Control 1983;11:97-115.

A, Heat sterilization, including steam or hot air (see manufacturer's recommendations).

B, Ethylene oxide gas (see manufacturer's recommendations).

C, Glutaraldehyde-based formulations (2%). (Caution should be exercised with all glutaraldehyde formulations when further in-use dilution is anticipated.).

D, Stabilized hydrogen peroxide 6% (will corrode copper, zinc, and brass).

E, Peracetic acid, concentration variable but ≤1% is sporicidal.

F, Wet pasteurization at 70° C for 30 minutes after detergent cleaning.

G, Sodium hypochlorite (5.2% household bleach) 1:50 dilution (1000 ppm free chlorine).

H, Ethyl or isopropyl alcohol (70% to 90%).

I, Sodium hypochlorite (5.2% household bleach) 1:500 dilution (100 ppm free chlorine).

J, Phenolic germicidal detergent solution (follow product label for use-dilution).

K, Iodophor germicidal detergent solution (follow product label for use-dilution).

L, Quaternary ammonium germicidal detergent solution (follow product label for use-dilution).

MR, Manufacturer's recommendations.

[a]Semicritical dental items (e.g. handpieces, amalgam condensers) should be heat sterilized; refer to text for details.

[b]See text for discussion of hydrotherapy.

[c]The longer the exposure to a disinfectant, the more likely it is that all microorganisms will be eliminated. Ten minutes' exposure is not adequate to disinfect many objects, especially those that are difficult to clean because they have narrow channels or other areas that can harbor organic material and bacteria. Twenty minutes' exposure is the minimum time needed to reliably kill *M. tuberculosis* and nontuberculous mycobacteria with glutaraldehyde.

[d]Tubing must be completely filled for chemical disinfection; care must be taken to avoid entrapment of air bubbles during immersion.

[e]Used in laboratory where cultures or concentrated preparations or microorganisms have spilled. This solution may destroy some surfaces.

[f]Pasteurization (washer disinfector) of respiratory therapy and anesthesia equipment is a recognized alternative to high-level disinfection. Some data challenge the efficacy of some pasteurization units (J Hosp Infect 1983;4:119-208).

[g]Thermostability should be investigated when appropriate.

[h]Do not mix rectal and oral thermometers at any stage of handling or processing.

CHANGES SINCE 1981

As a guide to the appropriate selection and use of disinfectants, a table was prepared by the CDC in 1981 and is presented here in modified form (Table 2). This current table contains several changes from the original CDC guideline[1] and one change from the 1990 APIC Guideline.[5] First, formaldehyde-alcohol has been deleted as a chemical sterilant and high-level disinfectant because, with the exception of dialysis equipment, it no longer has a role in disinfection strategies. It is corrosive, irritating, toxic, and not commonly used.[31, 32] Second, the chemical sterilant demand-release chlorine dioxide[33-35] is deleted from the table because it is no longer commercially available, and peracetic acid[36, 37] has been added to the table. Third, 3% phenolic and iodophors have been deleted as high-level disinfectants because of their unproven efficacy against bacterial endospores, *M. tuberculosis*, and some fungi.[34] Fourth, isopropyl and ethyl alcohols have been excluded as high-level disinfectants because of their inability to inactivate bacterial spores and because of the inability of isopropyl alcohol to inactivate hydrophilic viruses.[38] Fifth, a 1:16 dilution of 2.0% glutaraldehyde–7.05% phenol–1.2% sodium phenate (which contains 0.13% glutaraldehyde, 0.44% phenol, and 0.075% sodium phenate when diluted) has been deleted as a high-level disinfectant because of numerous scientific publications that demonstrate a lack of bactericidal activity in the presence of organic matter; a lack of fungicidal, tuberculocidal, and sporicidal activity; and reduced virucidal activity.[34, 39-47] This product and another diluted glutaraldehyde were removed from the marketplace by the EPA, FDA, and Federal Trade Commission in 1991. Sixth, the exposure time required to achieve high-level disinfection has been changed from a period of 10 to 30 minutes to a period of 20 minutes or more.[15, 39, 41, 42, 48-51]

PROBLEMS WITH DISINFECTION AND STERILIZATION OF HEALTH CARE EQUIPMENT

Concerns with Spaulding scheme

One problem associated with the Spaulding scheme is that of oversimplification. For example, the system does not consider problems with processing complicated medical equipment, which is often heat labile, or problems of inactivating certain microorganisms. In some situations, it is therefore still difficult to choose a level of disinfection after considering the categories of risk to patients. This is especially true for a few medical devices (e.g., arthroscopes, laparoscopes) in the critical category because there is a controversy regarding whether we should sterilize or high-level disinfect these patient care items.[22,52] Sterilization would not be a problem if these items could be steam sterilized, but most of these items are heat labile, and sterilization is achieved by using ETO, which may be too time-consuming for routine use between patients. Whereas new technology is making it easier to sterilize these items, evidence that sterilization of these items improves patient care by reducing the infection risk is lacking.[53-55] Presumably these reasons account for the fact that many procedures done with arthroscopes and laparoscopes are performed with equipment that has been processed by high-level disinfection, not sterilization.[22, 53] Ideally, biopsy forceps or other cutting instruments that break the mucosal barrier and laparoscopes, arthroscopes, and other scopes that enter normally sterile tissue should be subjected to a sterilization process before each use.[23]

This is also true for equipment in the semicritical category such as flexible endoscopes, which may be heat labile and with which there may be difficulty in exposing organisms to a sterilization process. For example, is the endoscope used for upper gastrointestinal tract examination still a semicritical item when it is used with sterile biopsy forceps or when it is used in a patient who is bleeding heavily from esophageal varices? Provided that high-level disinfection is achieved and all microorganisms with the exception of a high number of bacterial spores have been removed from the endoscope, then the endoscope should not represent an infection risk and should remain in the semicritical category.[56]

Several other problems are associated with the disinfection of patient care items.[6] The optimal contact times and disinfection schemes are not known for all equipment. For this reason, disinfectant strategies for several semicritical items (e.g., endoscopes, applanation tonometers, cryosurgical instruments, diaphragm fitting rings) are highly variable and are discussed further in this guideline. Although additional studies are needed to determine whether simplified disinfecting procedures are efficacious in a clinical setting, it is prudent to follow the CDC and the APIC guidelines until studies have defined effective alternative processes.[2, 5, 57, 58]

Endoscopes

High-level disinfection can be expected to destroy all microorganisms, with the exception of high numbers of bacterial spores. An immersion time of ≥20 minutes in 2% glutaraldehyde is required to adequately disinfect semicritical items such as endoscopes between patient procedures, particularly in view of the disputed tuberculocidal efficacy of glutaraldehyde-based disinfectants.[15, 39, 41, 42, 48-51] Flexible endoscopic instruments are particularly difficult to disinfect and easy to damage because of their intricate design and delicate materials. It must be highlighted that meticulous cleaning must precede any sterilization or disinfection procedures or outbreaks of infection may occur.

Examining reports of nosocomial infections related only to endoscopes, one finds that 281 infections were transmitted by gastrointestinal endoscopy and 96 were transmitted by bronchoscopy. The clinical spectrum of these infections ranged from asymptomatic colonization to death. *Salmonella* species and *Pseudomonas aeruginosa* were repeatedly identified as causative agents of infections transmitted by gastrointestinal endoscopy, and *M. tuberculosis*, atypical mycobacteria, and *P. aeruginosa* were the most common causes of infections transmitted by bronchoscopy. Major reasons for transmission were inadequate cleaning, improper selection of a disinfecting agent, or failure to follow recommended cleaning and disinfection procedures.[59] One multistate investigation found that 23.9% of the bacterial cultures from the internal channels of 71 gastrointestinal endoscopes grew 100,000 colonies or more of bacteria after completion of all disinfection or sterilization procedures and before use in the next patient.[60] Automatic endoscope reprocessing machines have also been linked to outbreaks of infection[61] or colonization.[62] Outbreaks involving endoscopic accessories,[63, 64] such as suction valves and biopsy forceps, support a recommendation that if such an item cannot be cleaned of all foreign matter, it should be steam sterilized, when heat stable.[65]

Clearly, there is a need for further development and redesign of automated endoscope reprocessing machines[66] and endoscopes[67] so they do not represent a potential source of infectious agents. A redesigned endoscope was introduced that includes a reusable endoscope without channels and a sterile sheath set comprising a single disposable unit: a sheath; air, water, and suction channels; a distal window; and a cover for the endoscope control body. All contaminated surfaces, including the channels, are then discarded, thereby eliminating any concern for cross-transmission of infectious agents from the previous patients. Fur-

ther clinical trials and microbiologic evaluations are needed to document the comparability, cost-effectiveness, safety, and reduced infection risk of this system.

Recommendations for the cleaning and disinfection of endoscopic equipment have been published and should be followed.[23, 24, 68, 69] In general, endoscope disinfection involves six steps, which are as follows: (1) clean—mechanically clean external surfaces, ports, and internal channels with water and a detergent or enzymatic detergent; (2) rinse and drain channels; (3) disinfect—immerse endoscope in high-level disinfectant and perfuse disinfectant into the suction/biopsy channel and air and water channels and expose for at least 20 minutes; (4) rinse—the endoscope and channels should be rinsed with sterile water; if this is not feasible use tap water followed with an alcohol rinse; (5) dry—the insertion tube and inner channels should be dried by means of forced air after disinfection and before storage; and (6) store— the endoscope should be stored in a way that prevents recontamination.

FDA labeling requirements

As mentioned, the FDA now regulates the efficacy claims for chemical sterilants. All chemical sterilants (e.g., glutaraldehyde-based solutions) that are used for sterilization or high-level disinfection and come in contact with medical devices require premarket clearance from the FDA (called 510[K] -named after that section of the Food, Drug and Cosmetic Act describing the process). In April 1994 a chemical sterilant manufacturer received the first 510(K) clearance for its glutaraldehyde-based solutions from the FDA. The time and temperature specified for one formulation of 2.4% alkaline glutaraldehyde with a high-level disinfection claim (100% kill of *M. tuberculosis*) was 45 minutes at 25° C (77° F). One would expect similar competitive 2% alkaline glutaraldehyde products to have comparable label claims. Additionally, the FDA requires that the manufacturers provide additional use instructions to the health care worker.

The data required by the FDA are quite rigorous, requiring the quantitative tuberculocidal test and 100% kill of *M. tuberculosis* for high-level disinfectant claims. Because the quantitative test does not allow for cleaning, is conducted in the presence of 2% horse serum (a protein load), and uses an extremely high number of organisms (100,000 to 1,000,000), it is necessary to have an extended immersion time (e.g., 45 minutes) and elevated temperature (25° C) to inactivate 100% of the mycobacteria. Several investigators, however, have shown that cleaning alone of endoscopic equipment is extremely effective in eliminating microbial contaminants. These studies have shown a mean 4 log (99.99%) reduction in microbial contaminants with cleaning alone.[70-73] Cleaning is a very effective adjuvant because it removes pathogenic microorganisms on inanimate objects and also removes organic matter that may interfere with the microbicidal activity of the germicide. Because neither the manufacturers nor the FDA has control over the cleaning techniques, a specific label statement cannot be made with respect to the potential decrease in immersion time. In the absence of cleaning and the presence of proteinaceous materials with high microbial loads, immersion in a 2.4% alkaline glutaraldehyde for 45 minutes at 25° C may be necessary for 100% tuberculocidal kill. This statement should not be interpreted to mean that prolonged immersion is an adequate substitute for proper cleaning before high-level disinfection or sterilization.

When proper cleaning is used, multiple studies demonstrate that *M. tuberculosis* is effectively destroyed by a 20-minute immersion time[15, 39, 41, 42, 48-51] in glutaraldehyde and other chemical sterilants at 20° C. The "APIC Guideline for Infection Prevention and Control in Flexible Endoscopy" recommendation of 20 minutes or longer at 20° C for high-level disinfection presumes precleaning with an enzymatic detergent[74] or detergent that removes debris and significantly reduces microbial contaminants.

Laparoscopes and arthroscopes

Although high-level disinfection appears to be the minimum standard for processing laparoscopes and arthroscopes between patients,[22, 52, 53, 75] there continues to be debate regarding this practice.[55, 76] Proponents of high-level disinfection refer to membership surveys[53] or institutional experiences[54] involving more than 117,000 and 10,000 laparoscopic procedures, respectively, that cite a low risk of infection (< 0.3%) when high-level disinfection is used for gynecologic laparoscopic equipment. Only one infection in the membership survey series was believed to be related to spores. In addition, studies conducted by Corson et al.[77, 78] demonstrated growth of common skin microorganisms (e.g., *Staphylococcus epidermidis*, diphtheroids) from the umbilical area even after skin preparation with povidone-iodine and ethyl alcohol. Similar organisms were recovered in some cases from the pelvic serosal surfaces and from the laparoscopic telescopes, suggesting

that the microorganisms were probably carried from the skin into the peritoneal cavity. Proponents of sterilization focus on the possibility of transmitting infection by spore-forming organisms. Researchers have proposed several reasons why sterility was not necessary for all laparoscopic equipment; these include the following: limited number of organisms (usually < 10) introduced into the peritoneal cavity, minimal damage to inner abdominal structures with little devitalized tissue, tolerance of the peritoneal cavity to small numbers of spore-forming bacteria, simplicity of cleaning and disinfection of equipment, relative nature of surgical sterility, and lack of epidemiologic evidence that high-level disinfection increases the infection risk.[54]

As with laparoscopes and other equipment that enters sterile body sites, arthroscopes ideally should be sterilized before use. In the United States, however, they commonly undergo high-level disinfection.[22, 53] Presumably this is because the incidence of infection is low and the few infections that occur are probably unrelated to the use of high-level disinfection rather than sterilization. In a retrospective study of 12,505 arthroscopic procedures, Johnson and associates[55] found an infection rate of 0.04% (five infections) when arthroscopes were soaked in 2% glutaraldehyde for 15 to 20 minutes. Interestingly, four infections were caused by *Staphylococcus aureus*, and the other was an anaerobic streptococcal infection. Because these organisms are very susceptible to 2% glutaraldehyde, the source of these infections was probably the patient's skin. Although only limited data are available, there is no evidence to demonstrate that high-level disinfection of arthroscopes poses an infection risk to the patient. Although the debate regarding high-level disinfection versus sterilization of laparoscopes and arthroscopes will go unsettled until there are well-designed, randomized clinical trials, the CDC and APIC guidelines are appropriate.[2, 5] That is, laparoscopes, arthroscopes, and other scopes that enter normally sterile tissue should be subjected to a sterilization procedure before each use; if this is not feasible, they should receive at least high-level disinfection. If high-level disinfection is used, a sterile water rinse is required to prevent contamination with tap water organisms. After rinsing, the scopes must be dried according to a method that does not recontaminate the item.

Tonometers, diaphragm fitting rings, cryosurgical instruments

Disinfection strategies for other semicritical items (e.g., applanation tonometers, cryosurgical instruments, and diaphragm fitting rings) are highly variable. For example, one study revealed that no uniform technique was in use for disinfection of applanation tonometers, with disinfectant contact times varying from less than 15 seconds to 20 minutes.[22] Concern regarding transmission of viruses (e.g., herpes simplex virus [HSV], adenovirus 8, HIV) by tonometer tips has prompted CDC disinfection recommendations.[57] These recommendations are that the instrument be wiped clean and disinfected for 5 to 10 minutes with either 3% hydrogen peroxide, 500 parts per million (ppm) chlorine, 70% ethyl alcohol, or 70% isopropyl alcohol. After disinfection, the device should be thoroughly rinsed in tap water and dried before use. Although these disinfectants and exposure times should kill microorganisms of relevance in ophthalmology, each of these disinfectants has not been tested against all relevant pathogens.[79] The American Academy of Ophthalmology also has developed specific guidelines for preventing infection in ophthalmology practice, but they only consider certain infectious agents (e.g., HIV, herpes, adenovirus).[80] Because a short and simple cleaning procedure is desirable in the clinical setting, swabbing the tonometer tip with a 70% isopropyl alcohol wipe is sometimes practiced.[79] Preliminary reports suggest that wiping the tonometer tip with an alcohol swab and then allowing the alcohol to evaporate may be an effective means of eliminating HSV-1, HIV-1, and adenovirus 8.[79, 81, 82] Because these studies involved only a few replicates and were conducted in a controlled laboratory setting, further studies are needed before this technique can be recommended. In addition, two studies have found that disinfection of pneumotonometer tips between uses with a 70% isopropyl alcohol wipe contributed to outbreaks of epidemic keratoconjunctivitis caused by adenovirus type 8.[83, 84] Therefore it is recommended that the tonometer be immersed in the germicides listed here for at least 5 minutes.

No studies have evaluated disinfection techniques for other items that contact mucous membranes, such as diaphragm fitting rings, cryosurgical probes, or vaginal probes used in sonographic scanning. Lettau et al.[58] of the CDC supported a diaphragm fitting ring manufacturer's recommendation, which involved a soap-and-water wash followed by a 15-minute, 70% alcohol immersion. This disinfection method should be adequate to inactivate HIV-1, hepatitis B virus (HBV), and HSV, even though alcohols are not classified as high-level disinfectants because their activity against picornaviruses is somewhat limited.[38] There are no data on the inactivation of

human papillomavirus by alcohol or other disinfectants because in vitro replication of complete virions has not been achieved. Thus, although isopropyl alcohol for 15 minutes should kill microorganisms of relevance in gynecology, there are no clinical studies that provide direct support for this procedure. Cryosurgical probes should be high-level disinfected. A condom may be used to cover the vaginal probe used in sonographic scanning. A new condom should be used to cover the probe with each new patient; because condoms may fail, however, high-level disinfection of the probe is necessary after each use.

Dental Instruments

Scientific articles and increased publicity about the potential for transmitting infectious agents in dentistry have focused attention on dental instruments as possible agents for disease transmission.[85, 86] The American Dental Association recommends that surgical and other instruments that normally penetrate soft tissue or bone (e.g., forceps, scalpels, bone chisels, scalers, and surgical burs) are classified as critical and must be sterilized or discarded after each use. Instruments that are not intended to penetrate oral soft tissues or bone (e.g., amalgam condensers, air/water syringes) but may come in contact with oral tissues are classified as semicritical and should also be sterilized after each use.[87] This is consistent with the recommendations from the CDC and the FDA.[88, 89] Handpieces that cannot be heat sterilized should be retrofitted to attain heat tolerance. Handpieces that cannot be retrofitted and thus cannot be heat sterilized should not be used.[89] Chemical disinfection is not recommended for critical or semicritical dental instruments that can be heat sterilized. Methods of sterilization that may be used for critical and semicritical dental instruments and materials that are heat stable include the following: steam under pressure (autoclave), heat/chemical vapor, and dry heat, following manufacturers' recommendations. ETO may not be an effective means of sterilization because it may be difficult to ensure that the internal portions of the handpieces are adequately cleaned and dried before ETO processing. Consideration must be given to the effect that a sterilization process may have on instruments and materials.

Uncovered operatory surfaces (e.g., countertops, chair switches, light handles) should be disinfected between patients. This can be accomplished by use of a disinfectant that is registered with the EPA as a "hospital disinfectant." There are several categories of such products.[87, 90, 91] If

Table 3. Inactivation of HBV and HIV by disinfectants

Disinfectant	Concentration inactivating 10^6 HBV in ST, 10 min., 20° C*	Concentration inactivating 10^5 HIV in ST, ≤10 min., 25° C†
Ethyl alcohol	ND	50%
Glutaraldehyde	2%	ND
Glutaraldehyde-phenate	0.13% glutaraldehyde—0.44% phenol	ND
Hydrogen peroxide	ND	0.3%
Iodophor	80 ppm	ND
Isopropyl alcohol	70%	35%
Paraformaldehyde	ND	0.5%
Phenolic	ND	0.5%
Sodium hypochlorite	500 ppm	50 ppm

ST, Suspension test; *ND*, no data.
*Data from Bond et al.[92]
†Data from Martin et al.[95] Also see Sattar and Springthorpe[99] for data concerning activity of other disinfectants against HIV.

waterproof surface covers are used to prevent contamination of surfaces and are carefully removed and replaced between patients, the protected surfaces do not need to be disinfected between patients but must be disinfected at the end of the day.

Disinfection of devices contaminated with HBV, HIV, or *M. tuberculosis*

Should we sterilize or high-level disinfect semicritical medical devices contaminated by blood from patients infected with HIV or HBV or by respiratory secretions from a patient with pulmonary tuberculosis? The CDC recommendation for high-level disinfection is appropriate because experiments have demonstrated the effectiveness of high-level disinfectants to inactivate these and other pathogens that may contaminate semicritical devices (Table 3).* Nonetheless, some hospitals modify their disinfection procedures when the endoscopes have been used with a patient known or suspected to be infected with HIV, HBV, or *M. tuberculosis*.[22, 104] This practice is inconsistent with the concept of universal precautions, which presumes that all patients are potentially infected with blood-borne pathogens.[97] Several studies have highlighted the inability to distinguish HIV- or HBV-infected patients from noninfected patients on clinical grounds.[105-107] It is also likely that in many patients mycobacterial infection is not immediately clinically apparent. It should be noted that in most cases hospitals gas-sterilized endoscopic instruments because they believed that this practice reduced the risk of infection.[22, 104] ETO is not routinely used for endoscope sterilization because of the lengthy processing

*References 33, 39, 48, 70-72, and 92-103.

time. Endoscopes and other semicritical devices should be managed the same way regardless of whether the patient is infected with *M. tuberculosis*, HIV, or HBV.

Inactivation of *Clostridium difficile*

Some investigators have also recommended the use of dilute solutions of hypochlorite for routine environmental disinfection of rooms of patients with *C. difficile*–associated diarrhea or colitis.[108] This practice would appear unnecessary because studies have shown that patients without symptoms constitute an important reservoir within the hospital and that person-to-person transmission is the principal means of transmission between patients. Handwashing, barrier precautions, and meticulous environmental cleaning may therefore be equally effective in preventing the spread of *C. difficile*.[109]

Contaminated endoscopes such as colonoscopes can serve as vehicles of transmission. For this reason, investigators have studied commonly used disinfectants and exposure times to assess whether current practices may be placing patients at risk. Data demonstrate that 2% glutaraldehyde reliably kills *C. difficile* spores with short exposure times (≤20 minutes).[46, 110, 111]

Inactivation of Creutzfeldt-Jakob disease (CJD) agent

The only infectious agent that requires unique decontamination recommendations is the prion CJD.[112] CJD is a degenerative neurologic disorder with an incidence rate of one new case in 1 million people per year.[113] Infectivity is tissue dependent with the brain, spinal cord, and eye suspected to have the highest infectivity.[114] It has been transmitted iatrogenically by means of implanted brain electrodes that were disinfected with ethanol and formaldehyde after use on a patient known to have CJD. Iatrogenic transmission has been observed in recipients of contaminated human growth hormone, gonadotropin, and corneal, pericardial and dura mater grafts.[113, 115] The need for special recommendations is due to an extremely resistant subpopulation of prions[116] and the protection afforded this tissue-associated virus. Although discrepancies exist between different studies, they all agree that these prions resist normal inactivation methods. Steam sterilization for at least 30 minutes at a temperature of 132° C (121° C ineffective) in a gravity displacement sterilizer has been recommended as the preferred method for the treatment of contaminated material. When a prevacuum sterilizer is used, 18 minutes at 134° to 138° C has been found to be effective. Immersion in 1 N sodium hydroxide (which is caustic) for 1 hour at room temperature followed by steam sterilization at 121° C for 30 minutes is an alternative procedure for critical and semicritical items.[117-122] Because noncritical patient care items or surfaces (e.g., autopsy tables, floors) have not been involved in disease transmission,[29] these surfaces may be disinfected with either bleach (undiluted, or up to 1:10 dilution) or 1 N sodium hydroxide at room temperature for 15 minutes or less.[117] A formalin–formic acid procedure is required for inactivating virus infectivity in tissue samples from patients with CJD.[123]

OSHA blood-borne pathogen standard

In December 1991, the Occupational Safety and Health Administration (OSHA) promulgated a standard entitled "Occupational Exposure to Bloodborne Pathogens; Final Rule" to eliminate or minimize occupational exposure to blood-borne pathogens.[124] One component of this requirement is that all equipment, environmental surfaces, and working surfaces should be cleaned and decontaminated with an appropriate disinfectant after contact with blood or other potentially infectious materials. Although the OSHA standard does not specify the type of disinfectant or procedure, the OSHA compliance document[125] suggests that a germicide must be tuberculocidal to kill HBV. The document thus suggests that a tuberculocidal agent should be used to clean blood spills on noncritical surfaces. This recommendation is inconsistent with data that demonstrate that non-tuberculocidal quaternary ammonium compounds inactivate HBV.[103] Nonetheless, to follow the OSHA compliance document a tuberculocidal

disinfectant (e.g., phenolic, chlorine) would be needed to clean a blood spill. This has caused concern among housekeeping managers, who try to find disinfectant detergents claiming to be tuberculocidal on the assumption that such products would be effective in eliminating transmission of HBV. This directive can be questioned on a practical level for three reasons. First, nontuberculocidal disinfectants such as quaternary ammonium compounds inactivate HBV.[103] Second, noncritical surfaces are rarely involved in disease transmission.[29] Third, the exposure times that manufacturers use to achieve their label claims are not used in health care settings to disinfect noncritical surfaces. For example, to make a label claim against HIV, HBV, or *M. tuberculosis*, a manufacturer must demonstrate inactivation of these organisms when exposed to a disinfectant for 10 minutes. This exposure cannot be practically achieved in a health care setting without immersion. Alternatively, a hospital could use the scientific literature and use any EPA-registered hospital disinfectant (e.g., phenolic, chlorine, quaternary ammonium compounds) for cleaning blood spills on noncritical surfaces. However, this practice could result in an OSHA citation for noncompliance with the rule.

Toxicologic and environmental concerns

Health hazards associated with the use of germicides in health care vary from mucous membrane irritation to death, with the latter involving accidental ingestion by mentally disturbed patients.[126] Although variations exist in the degree of toxicity, as discussed in this document and elsewhere,[4, 127, 128] all disinfectants should be used for the intended purpose only.

Some water and sewer jurisdictions have excluded the disposal of certain chemical germicides (e.g., glutaraldehyde, formaldehyde, phenol) by means of the sewer system. These rules are intended to minimize environmental harm. If hospitals exceed the maximum allowable concentration for a given chemical (e.g., ≤5.0 mg/L), they have three options. First, they can switch to alternative products. For example, they can change from glutaraldehyde to hydrogen peroxide for high-level disinfection or from phenolics to quaternary ammonium compounds for low-level disinfection. Second, the hospitals can collect the disinfectant and dispose of it as a hazardous chemical. Third, they can use a commercially available small-scale treatment system that may neutralize chemicals such as formaldehyde.

153

AJIC
August 1996

European authors have suggested that disinfection by heat rather than chemicals should be used for instruments and ventilation therapy equipment. For example, flushing and washer disinfectors are automated and closed equipment used to clean and disinfect objects from bedpans and washbowls to surgical instruments and anesthesia tubes. Items such as bedpans and urinals can be cleaned and disinfected in flushing disinfectors with a short cycle of a few minutes. They clean by flushing with warm water, possibly with a detergent, and then disinfect by flushing the items with hot water at approximately 90° C, or with steam. Because this machine empties, cleans, and disinfects, manual cleaning is eliminated, fewer disposable items are needed, and less chemical germicides are used. They are available and used in many European countries. Surgical instruments and anesthesia equipment that are more difficult to clean are run in washer-disinfectors with the use of a detergent by use of a longer cycle of 20 to 30 minutes. These machines also disinfect by hot water at approximately 90° C.[129] The stated disadvantages for chemical disinfection include the following: the toxic side effects for the patient caused by chemical residues on the instrument or object; occupational exposure to toxic chemicals; and the danger of recontamination by rinsing the instrument with microbially contaminated tap water.[130]

Transmissible resistance to germicides

Antibiotic resistance among bacteria has been of growing concern in recent years. Of special concern is the increased incidence of infections caused by methicillin-resistant *S. aureus*, vancomycin-resistant *Enterococcus*, multiple-drug-resistant *M. tuberculosis*, and multiple-drug-resistant gram-negative bacilli.

Chromosomal-mediated antibiotic resistance may confer resistance to broad classes of antibiotics (e.g., methicillin-resistant *S. aureus* [MRSA] exhibits resistance to all penicillins and cephalosporins). Many studies have demonstrated that plasmid-mediated resistance may also include multiple drugs. For these reasons, concern has been raised that antibiotic-resistant bacteria might also exhibit cross-resistance to antiseptics and disinfectants.

Several investigators have studied disinfectant resistance in MRSA and methicillin-susceptible *S. aureus* (MSSA). Brumfitt et al.[131] found MRSA more resistant than MSSA strains to chlorhexidine, propamidine, and the quaternary ammonium compound—centrimide. Al-Masaudi et al.[132] reported MRSA and MSSA strains to be equally susceptible to phenols and chlorhexidine but found that MRSA strains were slightly more resistant to quaternary ammonium compounds. Townsend et al.[133-135] demonstrated that a *S. aureus* plasmid carrying gentamicin resistance also encoded resistance to propamidine and quaternary ammonium compounds. Studies have established the involvement of a plasmid locus, *qacA*, in providing protection against quaternary ammonium compounds. Tennant et al.[136, 137] propose that staphylococci evade destruction because the protein specified by the *qacA* determinant is a cytoplasmic membrane–associated protein involved in an efflux system that actively reduces intracellular accumulation in intracellular targets of toxicants such as quaternary ammonium compounds. It has been shown that the presence of the RP1 plasmid in *Escherichia coli* or *P. aeruginosa* does not increase resistance to phenols or quaternary ammonium compounds.[138] Plasmid-mediated resistance to formaldehyde has been demonstrated in *Serratia marcescens*[139] and to hexachlorophene in *P. aeruginosa*.[140]

The literature provides ample evidence of plasmid-mediated resistance to antiseptics and disinfectants. However, these observations have no clinical relevance because even for the more resistant strains the concentrations of disinfectants used in practice are much higher than the observed minimum inhibitory concentrations (MICs). For example, phenolics are used as surface disinfectants at concentrations of approximately 400 ppm and quaternary ammonium compounds at concentrations of approximately 500 ppm. Resistant bacterial strains described in the literature have exhibited MICs less than 15 ppm (µg/ml) for phenolics and quaternary ammonium compounds.[131, 132]

In fact, Rutala et al.[141] found antibiotic-resistant hospital strains of common nosocomial pathogens (i.e., *P. aeruginosa*, *Klebsiella pneumoniae*, *E. coli*, *S. aureus*, *S. epidermidis*, and Enterococcus) to be equally susceptible to disinfectants as antibiotic-sensitive strains by use of the Use-Dilution Method. Other investigators have also been unable to demonstrate a relationship between antibiotic resistance and germicide resistance when the disinfectants are used at the manufacturers' recommended use-dilution. Anderson et al.[142] found similar time-kill curves for vancomycin-resistant and vancomycin-susceptible enterococci by use of a quaternary ammonium compound. Best[143] reported similar inactivation of *M. tuberculosis* and multiple-drug–resistant *M. tuberculosis* (MDR-TB) with 70% ethyl alcohol, 2% glutaraldehyde, 5000 ppm chlorine, and povidone-iodine. Thus vancomycin-resistant enterococcus (VRE), MRSA, and MDR-TB are as sensitive to commonly used hospital disinfectants as drug-sensitive strains at use concentrations.

For these reasons, the CDC does not recommend any special strategies or germicides with higher potencies for cleaning noncritical surfaces in rooms of patients who are infected with multi-antibiotic-resistant organisms such as vancomycin-resistant enterococci. Any EPA-registered germicidal detergent is appropriate for this purpose.[144]

Is there a "double standard" for patient care and processing patient equipment?

Are health care facilities' practices for disinfection consistent in intent and application? For example, semicritical equipment (e.g., endoscopes) should be high-level disinfected between patients; however, some institutions choose to sterilize semicritical equipment when used on certain infectious patients. This may lead to a "double standard" of patient care and is inconsistent with the principle of universal precautions[97] when equipment used on patients with known specific infectious diseases (e.g., tuberculosis, HIV infection) is sterilized, but the same equipment is only high-level–disinfected for other patients. Under these circumstances, sterilization should not be performed in the belief that it is providing a greater margin of safety. In contrast, it is not a double standard of patient care to sterilize endoscopes in one hospital area (e.g., operating room) and high-level disinfect in another area (e.g., gastroenterology clinic) because the outcome is equivalent from an infectious disease transmission perspective.

DISINFECTION

A great number of disinfectants are used in the health care setting, including alcohol, chlorine and chlorine compounds, formaldehyde, glutaraldehyde, hydrogen peroxide, iodophors, phenolics, and quaternary ammonium compounds. These disinfectants are not interchangeable, and the following overview of the performance characteristics of each is intended to provide the user with information to select an appropriate disinfectant and to use it in the safest and most efficient way. It should be recognized that excessive costs may be attributed to the use of incorrect concentrations and inappropriate germicides. In addition, some disinfectants are formulated in combinations (e.g., hydrogen peroxide and peracetic acid) that may alter their antimicrobial activity. Each formulation of active and inert ingredients is considered a unique product and must undergo the EPA registration approval process, the FDA premarket clearance process, or both. Finally, occupational skin diseases among cleaning personnel have been associated with the use of several disinfectants, such as formaldehyde, glutaraldehyde, chlorine, phenol, and others, and precautions (e.g., gloves, proper ventilation, etc.) should be used to minimize exposure.[145, 146]

Alcohol

In the sphere of hospital disinfection, *alcohol* refers to two water-soluble chemical compounds whose germicidal characteristics are generally underrated; these are *ethyl alcohol* and *isopropyl alcohol*.[147] These alcohols are rapidly bactericidal, rather than bacteriostatic, against vegetative forms of bacteria[148, 149]; they are also tuberculocidal,[147, 150] fungicidal,[34, 151, 152] and virucidal[33, 38, 92-96, 153] but do not destroy bacterial spores. Isopropyl alcohol (20%) has also been shown to be effective in killing the cysts of *Acanthamoeba culbertsoni*.[154] Their cidal activity drops sharply when diluted below 50% concentration, and the optimum bactericidal concentration is in the range of 60% to 90% by volume.[148] The most feasible explanation for the antimicrobial action is denaturation of proteins.

Alcohols are not recommended for sterilizing medical and surgical materials, principally because of their lack of sporicidal action and their inability to penetrate protein-rich materials. Fatal postoperative wound infections with *Clostridium* have occurred when alcohols were used to sterilize surgical instruments contaminated with bacterial spores.[155] Ethyl and isopropyl alcohols are therefore not high-level disinfectants because of their inability to inactivate bacterial spores and because of isopropyl alcohol's inability to kill hydrophilic viruses (e.g., echovirus, coxsackievirus).[38] Alcohols have been used effectively to disinfect oral and rectal thermometers[156, 157] and fiberoptic endoscopes.[158, 159] Alcohol wipes have been used for years to disinfect small surfaces, such as rubber stoppers of multiple-dose medication vials. Furthermore, alcohol is occasionally used to disinfect external surfaces of equipment (e.g., stethoscopes, ventilators, manual ventilation

Table 4. Preparation and stability of chlorine solutions

	Desired chlorine concentration			
	5000 ppm	1000 ppm	500 ppm	100 ppm
Dilution of bleach (5.25% NaOCl) prepared fresh for use within 24 hr	1:10*	1:50	1:100	1:500
Dilution of bleach (5.25% NaOCl) prepared fresh and used for 1-30 days	1:5†	1:25	1:50	1:250

*To achieve a 1:10 dilution, add one part bleach to nine parts water.
†To achieve a 1:5 dilution, add one part bleach to four parts water.

bags[160]), cardiopulmonary resuscitation manikins,[161] or medication preparation areas. Two recent studies demonstrated the effectiveness of 70% isopropyl alcohol to disinfect reusable transducer heads in a controlled environment.[162, 163] In contrast, Beck-Sague and Jarvis[164] described three outbreaks that occurred when alcohol was used to disinfect transducer heads in an intensive care unit setting. The disadvantages of using alcohols on equipment are that they damage the shellac mounting of lensed instruments, tend to cause rubber and certain plastic tubing to swell and harden after prolonged and repeated use, discolor rubber and plastic tiles,[147] and damage tonometer tips (through deterioration of the glue) after the equivalent of 1 working year of routine use.[165] Lingel and Coffey[166] also found that tonometer biprisms soaked in alcohol for 4 days acquired rough front surfaces that could potentially cause corneal damage. This roughening appeared to be caused by a weakening of the cementing substances used to fabricate the biprisms. Corneal opacification has been reported when tonometer tips were swabbed with alcohol immediately before intraocular pressure measurements were taken.[167] Alcohols are flammable and consequently must be stored in a cool, well-ventilated area. They also evaporate rapidly, which makes extended contact times difficult to achieve unless the items are immersed.

Chlorine and chlorine compounds

Hypochlorites, the most widely used of the *chlorine* disinfectants, are available in liquid (e.g., sodium hypochlorite) and solid (e.g., calcium hypochlorite, sodium dichloroisocyanurate) forms. They have a broad spectrum of antimicrobial activity and are inexpensive and fast acting. Use of hypochlorites in hospitals is limited by their corrosiveness, inactivation by organic matter, and relative instability. The microbicidal activity of chlorine is largely attributable to undissociated hy-

pochlorous acid (HOCl). The dissociation of hypochlorous acid to the less microbicidal form (hypochlorite ion, OCl^-) is dependent on pH. As the pH increases, more hypochlorite ion is formed, and microbicidal activity decreases.[168, 169] A potential hazard is the production of the carcinogen bis-chloromethyl ether when hypochlorite solutions come into contact with formaldehyde[170] and production of the animal carcinogen trihalomethane when hyperchlorinated.[168] A mixture of sodium hypochlorite with acid will also produce a rapid evolution of toxic chlorine gas.

An alternative compound that releases chlorine and is used in the hospital setting is chloramine-T. The advantage of this compound over hypochlorites is that it retains chlorine longer and therefore exerts a more prolonged bactericidal effect. Sodium dichloroisocyanurate tablets are also stable, and the microbicidal activity of solutions prepared from these tablets may be greater than that of sodium hypochlorite solutions containing the same total available chlorine.[171-174]

The exact mechanism by which free chlorine destroys microorganisms has not been elucidated. The postulated mechanism of chlorine disinfection is the inhibition of some key enzymatic reactions within the cell, protein denaturation, and inactivation of nucleic acids.[168]

Low concentrations of free chlorine have biocidal effects on mycoplasma (25 ppm)[175] and vegetative bacteria (<1 ppm) within seconds in the absence of organic matter.[168] Higher concentrations (1000 ppm) of chlorine are required to kill *M. tuberculosis* according to the AOAC tuberculocidal test.[39] Because household bleach contains 5.25% sodium hypochlorite, or 52,500 ppm available chlorine, a 1:1000 dilution of household bleach provides about 50 ppm available chlorine, and a 1:50 dilution of household bleach provides about 1000 ppm (Table 4). A concentration of 100 ppm will kill 99.9% of *Bacillus subtilis* spores within 5 minutes[176] and will destroy fungal agents in less than 1 hour.[168] Klein and DeForest[38] reported that 25 different viruses were inactivated in 10 minutes with 200 ppm available chlorine.

Some data are available for chlorine dioxide to substantiate manufacturers' bactericidal, fungicidal, tuberculocidal, sporicidal, and virucidal label claims.[33-35, 39] In 1986, a chlorine dioxide product was voluntarily removed from the market when its use was found to cause dialyzer membrane leaks, which allowed bacteria to migrate from the dialysis fluid side of the dialyzer to the blood side in cellulose-based membranes.[177]

Inorganic chlorine solution is used for disinfecting tonometer heads and for spot disinfection of countertops and floors. A 1:10[10, 178, 179] or 1:100 dilution of 5.25% sodium hypochlorite (household bleach) or an EPA-registered hospital disinfectant[5] can be used for decontamination of blood spills. Either of these methods will minimize the risk of employee exposure to blood. Because hypochlorites and other germicides are substantially inactivated in the presence of blood,[180] the surface should be cleaned before an EPA-registered disinfectant or a 1:10 solution of household bleach is applied (see discussion of OSHA bloodborne pathogen standard). At least 500 ppm available chlorine for 10 minutes is recommended for decontamination of cardiopulmonary resuscitation training manikins.[181] Full-strength bleach has been recommended for the disinfection of needles and syringes in needle-exchange programs for the prevention of blood-borne pathogen spread among intravenous drug–using population. The difference in the recommended concentrations of bleach reflects the difficulty of cleaning the interior of needles and syringes and the use of needles and syringes for parenteral injection.[182] Clinicians should not alter their use of chlorine on surfaces on the basis of testing methods that do not simulate actual disinfection practices.[183]

Chlorine has long been favored as the preferred disinfectant for water treatment. Hyperchlorination of a *Legionella*-contaminated hospital water system resulted in a dramatic decrease (30% to 1.5%) in the isolation of *Legionella pneumophila* from water outlets and a cessation of nosocomial legionnaires' disease in the affected unit.[184] Chloramine T[185] and hypochlorites[186] have been evaluated in disinfecting hydrotherapy equipment.

Hypochlorite solutions in tap water at pH 8.0 or greater are stable for a period of 1 month when stored at room temperature (23° C) in closed, opaque plastic containers.[168, 187] During 1 month at room temperature, the free available chlorine levels of solutions in opened and closed polyethylene containers are reduced maximally to 40% to 50% of the original concentration. On the basis of these data, one investigator recommended that if a user wished to have a solution containing 500 ppm of available chlorine at day 30, a solution initially containing 1000 ppm of chlorine should be prepared (Table 4). After 30 days there was no decomposition of the sodium hypochlorite solution when it was stored in a closed brown bottle.[187]

Formaldehyde

Formaldehyde is used as a disinfectant and a sterilant in both its liquid and its gaseous states. The liquid form will be considered briefly in this section, and a review of formaldehyde as a gas sterilant may be found elsewhere.[188] Formaldehyde is sold and used principally as a water-based solution called *formalin*, which is 37% formaldehyde by weight. The aqueous solution is a bactericide, tuberculocide, fungicide, virucide, and sporicide.[38, 189-191] OSHA indicated that formaldehyde should be handled in the workplace as a potential carcinogen, and it set an employee exposure standard for formaldehyde that limits an 8-hour time-weighted average exposure to a concentration of 0.75 ppm.[31, 32] For this reason, employees should have limited direct contact with formaldehyde. These considerations limit the role of formaldehyde in sterilization and disinfection processes.

Formaldehyde inactivates microorganisms by alkylating the amino and sulfhydryl groups of proteins and the ring nitrogen atoms of purine bases.[10] Although formaldehyde-alcohol is a chemical sterilant and formaldehyde is a high-level disinfectant, formaldehyde's hospital uses are limited by its irritating fumes and the pungent odor that is apparent at very low levels (< 1 ppm). For these reasons and others, including carcinogenicity, this germicide is excluded from Table 2. When it is used, direct employee exposure is generally limited; however, significant exposures to formaldehyde have been documented for employees of renal transplant units[192, 193] and students in a gross anatomy laboratory.[194] Formaldehyde is used in the health care setting for preparing viral vaccines (e.g., poliovirus, influenza), as an embalming agent, and for preserving anatomic specimens. In the past it was used, especially as a mixture of formaldehyde and ethanol, for sterilizing

AJIC
August 1996

surgical instruments. A survey conducted in 1992 found that formaldehyde was the disinfectant used for reprocessing hemodialyzers by 40% of the hemodialysis centers in the United States, a 54% decrease from 1983.[195] If formaldehyde is used at room temperature, the CDC recommends a concentration of 4% with a minimum exposure time of 24 hours to disinfect disposable hemodialyzers that are reused on the same patient.[196] Aqueous formaldehyde solutions (1% to 2%) have been used to disinfect the internal fluid pathways.[197] To minimize a potential health hazard to patients undergoing dialysis, the dialysis equipment must be thoroughly rinsed and tested for residual formaldehyde before use. Other disinfectants that are available for dialysis systems are chlorine-based disinfectants, glutaraldehyde-based disinfectants, peracetic acid, and peracetic acid with hydrogen peroxide.[196] Some dialysis systems use hot water disinfection for the control of microbial contamination.[196]

Paraformaldehyde

Paraformaldehyde, a solid polymer of formaldehyde, may be vaporized by heat for the gaseous decontamination of laminar-flow biologic safety cabinets when maintenance work or filter changes require access to the sealed portion of the cabinet.

Glutaraldehyde

Glutaraldehyde is a saturated dialdehyde that has gained wide acceptance as a high-level disinfectant and chemical sterilant. Aqueous solutions of glutaraldehyde are acidic and generally in this state are not sporicidal. Only when the solution is "activated" (made alkaline) by alkalizing agents to a pH of 7.5 to 8.5 does the solution become sporicidal. Once activated, these solutions have a shelf life of 14 to 28 days because of the polymerization of the glutaraldehyde molecules at alkaline pH levels. This polymerization blocks the active sites (aldehyde groups) of the glutaraldehyde molecules, which are responsible for its biocidal activity.

Novel glutaraldehyde formulations (e.g., glutaraldehyde-phenate, potentiated acid glutaraldehyde, stabilized alkaline glutaraldehyde) have been produced that have overcome the problem of rapid loss of stability (e.g., use life 28 to 30 days) while generally maintaining excellent microbicidal activity.[34, 198-202] It should be realized, however, that antimicrobial activity is dependent not only on age but also on use conditions, such as dilution and organic stress. Manufacturers' literature for these preparations suggest that the neutral or alkaline glutaraldehydes possess microbicidal and anticorrosion properties superior to those of acid glutaraldehydes. A few published reports substantiate these claims.[203-205] The use of glutaraldehyde-based solutions in hospitals is widespread because of their advantages, which include the following: excellent biocidal properties; activity in the presence of organic matter (20% bovine serum); noncorrosive action on endoscopic equipment, thermometers, and rubber or plastic equipment; and noncoagulation of proteinaceous material.

The biocidal activity of glutaraldehyde is a consequence of its alkylation of sulfhydryl, hydroxyl, carboxyl, and amino groups of microorganisms, which alters RNA, DNA, and protein synthesis.[206]

The in vitro inactivation of microorganisms by glutaraldehydes has been extensively investigated and reviewed.[206] Several investigators showed that 2% aqueous solutions of glutaraldehyde, buffered to a pH of 7.5 to 8.5 with sodium bicarbonate, were effective in killing vegetative bacteria in less than 2 minutes; *M. tuberculosis*, fungi, and viruses in less than 10 minutes; and spores of *Bacillus* and *Clostridium* species in 3 hours.[206-208] Spores of *C. difficile* are more rapidly killed (e.g., 20 minutes) by 2% glutaraldehyde.[46, 110, 111] Concern has been raised about the mycobactericidal prowess of glutaraldehydes because a single investigator using the quantitative suspension test reported that 2% glutaraldehyde inactivated only 2 to 3 logs *M. tuberculosis* in 20 minutes at 20° C.[48] However, all other investigators[15, 39, 41, 42, 49-51] using various test methods, including a quantitative suspension test, have found much greater levels of *M. tuberculosis* inactivation by use of 2% glutaraldehyde. For example, several investigators have demonstrated that glutaraldehyde solutions inactivate 2.4 to >5.0 logs *M. tuberculosis* in 10 minutes (including multidrug-resistant *M. tuberculosis*) and 4.0 to 6.4 logs *M. tuberculosis* at 20 minutes.[15, 39, 41, 42, 49-51] One study reports the isolation of glutaraldehyde-resistant mycobacteria in endoscope washers; however, the clinical significance of this observation is unclear at present.[209] Rubbo et al.[189] showed that 2% alkaline glutaraldehyde has slower action against *M. tuberculosis* than alcohols, formaldehydes, iodine, and phenol. Collins[51] demonstrated that suspensions of *Mycobacterium avium*, *Mycobacterium intracellulare*, and *Mycobacterium gordonae* were more resistant to disinfection by a 2% alkaline glutaraldehyde (estimated time to sterility 60 minutes) than were virulent *M. tuberculosis* organisms (estimated time to sterility 25 minutes). Collins[51] also showed that the rate of kill was directly proportional to the temperature and the sterility of a standardized suspension of *M. tuberculosis* could not be achieved within 10 minutes. On the basis of these data, 20 minutes at room temperature with a 2% glutaraldehyde is the minimum exposure time needed to reliably kill organisms such as *M. tuberculosis* that are resistant to disinfectants. Glutaraldehyde preparations that are diluted to less than 2% glutaraldehyde should be used as chemical sterilants only after independent verification of their label claims.

There are two publications that evaluate the ability of 2% glutaraldehyde to kill oocytes of *Cryptosporidium* in 30 minutes or 60 minutes.[210, 211] One study found 2% glutaraldehyde to be effective against *Cryptosporidium pavum* at 60 minutes,[210] but another study questioned the ability of glutaraldehyde to kill *Cryptosporidium* in 30 minutes.[211]

Glutaraldehyde is used most commonly as a high-level disinfectant for medical equipment such as endoscopes,[22] respiratory therapy equipment,[212] dialyzers,[213] transducers, anesthesia equipment, spirometry tubing,[214] and hemodialysis proportioning and dialysate delivery systems.[215] Glutaraldehyde is noncorrosive to metal and does not damage lensed instruments, rubber, or plastics. Glutaraldehyde should not be used for cleaning noncritical surfaces; it is too toxic and expensive for this application. Dilution of glutaraldehyde commonly occurs during use. One study showed a glutaraldehyde concentration decline from 2.4% to 1.5% after 10 days in manual and automatic baths used for endoscopes.[216] Others have shown the glutaraldehyde level to fall below 1%, to as low as 0.27%, on day 4 of reuse.[217] These data emphasize the need to ensure that semicritical equipment is disinfected with a minimum effective concentration (MEC) of glutaraldehyde. Most studies suggest that 1.0% glutaraldehyde is the minimum effective concentration when used as a high-level disinfectant,[41, 204, 205] although one investigator using atypical mycobacteria showed that the MEC should be 1.5%.[216] Test strips are available for determining whether an effective concentration of active ingredients (e.g., glutaraldehyde) is present despite repeated use and dilution. The glutaraldehyde test kits have been preliminarily evaluated for accuracy and range,[218, 219] and most test strips are constructed to indicate a concentration above 1.5%. The frequency of testing should be based on how frequently the solutions are used (e.g., if used daily, test daily), but the strip should not be used to extend the use life beyond the expiration date. The solution should be considered unsafe when a dilution of 1% glutaraldehyde or lower is measured.

Proctitis believed to be caused by glutaraldehyde exposure from residual endoscope solution contaminating the air-water channel has been reported and is preventable by thorough endoscope rinsing.[220] Similarly, keratopathy was reported to be caused by ophthalmic instruments that were inadequately rinsed after soaking in 2% glutaraldehyde.[221]

Health care workers can become exposed to elevated levels of glutaraldehyde vapor when equipment is processed in poorly ventilated rooms, when spills occur, or when there are open immersion baths. In these situations, the level of glutaraldehyde in the air could reach its ceiling limit of 0.2 ppm. Engineering and work practice controls that may be used to combat these problems include the following: improved ventilation (7 to 15 air exchanges per hour); use of ducted exhaust hoods or ductless fume hoods with absorbents for glutaraldehyde vapor[222]; tight-fitting lids on immersion baths; and personal protective equipment (e.g., gloves [nitrile rubber, butyl rubber, polyethelyne], goggles) to minimize skin or mucous membrane contact. Some workers have been fitted with a half-face respirator with organic vapor filters[223] or offered a type "C" supplied air respirator with a full facepiece operated in a positive-pressure mode.[224] Even though enforcement of the ceiling limit was suspended on March 23, 1993, by a United States Court of Appeals,[225] it is prudent to limit employee exposure to 0.2 ppm because at this level glutaraldehyde is irritating to the eyes, throat, and nose.[226-228] The American Conference of Governmental Industrial Hygienists issued a "Notice of Intended Changes" in which it was proposed that the ceiling threshold limit value for glutaraldehyde be reduced from 0.2 ppm to 0.05 ppm.[222] Epistaxis, allergic contact dermatitis, asthma, and rhinitis have also been reported in health care workers exposed to glutaraldehyde.[223, 229, 230] Some automated machines for endoscope disinfection reduce employee exposure to glutaraldehyde.[73] Dosimeters are available for measuring glutaraldehyde levels in the workplace.

Hydrogen peroxide

The literature contains limited accounts of the properties, germicidal effectiveness, and potential uses for stabilized *hydrogen peroxide* in the hospital setting. Reports ascribing good germicidal activity to hydrogen peroxide have been published and attest to its bactericidal,[231] virucidal,[232] tuberculocidal,[39] sporicidal,[233] and fungicidal properties.[234] Synergistic sporicidal effects were observed when spores were exposed to a combination of hydrogen peroxide (5.9% to 23.6%) and peracetic acid.[235]

Hydrogen peroxide works by the production of destructive hydroxyl free radicals. These can attack membrane lipids, DNA, and other essential cell components.[234]

Commercially available 3% hydrogen peroxide is a stable and effective disinfectant when used on inanimate surfaces. It has been used in concentrations from 3% to 6% for the disinfection of soft contact lenses (3% for 2 to 3 hours),[234, 236, 237] tonometer biprisms,[166] and ventilators.[238] Corneal damage from a hydrogen peroxide–disinfected tonometer tip that was not properly rinsed has been reported.[239] Hydrogen peroxide has also been instilled into urinary drainage bags in an attempt to eliminate the bag as a source of bladder bacteriuria and environmental contamination.[240, 241] Although the instillation of hydrogen peroxide into the bag reduced microbial contamination of the bag, this procedure did not reduce the incidence of catheter-associated bacteriuria.[241]

Concentrations of hydrogen peroxide from 6% to 25% have promise as chemical sterilants. In one recent study, 6% hydrogen peroxide was significantly more effective in the high-level disinfection of the flexible endoscopes than was the 2% glutaraldehyde solution.[73] Hydrogen peroxide has not been widely used for endoscope disinfection, however, because there continues to be concerns that its oxidizing properties may be harmful to some components of the endoscope.[73] The use of hydrogen peroxide for high-level disinfection of semicritical items warrants further study. Chemical irritation resembling pseudomembranous colitis, caused by either 3% hydrogen peroxide or a 2% glutaraldehyde, has been infrequently reported.[242] An epidemic of pseudomembrane-like enteritis and colitis in seven patients in a gastrointestinal endoscopy unit was also associated with use of 3% hydrogen peroxide.[243]

Iodophors

Iodine solutions or tinctures have long been used by health professionals, primarily as antiseptics on skin or tissue. Iodophors, on the other hand, have enjoyed use both as antiseptics and disinfectants. An *iodophor* is a combination of iodine and a solubilizing agent or carrier; the resulting complex provides a sustained-release reservoir of iodine and releases small amounts of free iodine in aqueous solution. The best known and most widely used iodophor is povidone-iodine, a compound of polyvinylpyrrolidone with iodine. This product and other iodophors retain the germicidal efficacy of iodine but, unlike iodine, are generally nonstaining and are relatively free of toxicity and irritancy.[244]

Several reports that documented intrinsic microbial contamination of povidone-iodine and poloxamer-iodine[245-247] caused a reappraisal of concepts concerning the chemistry and use of iodophors.[248] It seems that "free" iodine (I_2) is the principal contributor to the bactericidal activity of iodophors, and dilutions of iodophors demonstrate more rapid bactericidal action than a full-strength povidone-iodine solution. The reason that has been suggested for the observation that dilution can increase bactericidal activity is that the dilution of povidone-iodine results in weakening of the iodine linkage to the carrier polymer, with an accompanying increase of free iodine in solution.[246] Iodophor therefore must be used per the manufacturer's recomendations to achieve maximum antimicrobial activity.

Iodine is able to penetrate the cell walls of microorganisms quickly. It is believed that iodine's lethal effects result from a disruption of protein and nucleic acid structure and synthesis.

Published reports on the in vitro antimicrobial efficacy of iodophors demonstrate that iodophors are bactericidal, virucidal, and mycobactericidal but may require prolonged contact times to kill certain fungi and bacterial spores.* Manufacturers' data demonstrate that commercial iodophors are not sporicidal but are tuberculocidal, fungicidal, virucidal, and bactericidal at recommended use dilutions.

In addition to their use as an antiseptic, iodophors have been used for the disinfection of blood culture bottles and medical equipment such as hydrotherapy tanks, thermometers, and endoscopes. Antiseptic iodophors are not suitable for use as hard-surface disinfectants because of concentration differences. Iodophors formulated as antiseptics contain significantly less free iodine than do those formulated as disinfectants.[10]

*References 11, 34, 38, 39, and 249-252.

Peracetic acid

Peracetic acid, or peroxyacetic acid, in low concentrations (0.001% to 0.2%) is characterized by a very rapid action against all microorganisms, including bacterial spores. A special advantage of peracetic acid is that its decomposition products (i.e., acetic acid, water, oxygen, hydrogen peroxide) are not harmful, and it leaves no residue. It remains effective in the presence of organic matter and is sporicidal even at low temperatures. Peracetic acid can corrode copper, brass, bronze, plain steel, and galvanized iron, but these effects can be reduced by additives and pH modification. Peracetic acid is considered unstable, particularly when diluted. For example, a 1% solution loses half its strength through hydrolysis in 6 days, whereas 40% peracetic acid loses 1% to 2% of its activity per month.[253, 254]

Little is known about the mechanism of action of peracetic acid, but it is believed to function in the same manner as other oxidizing agents. It denatures proteins, disrupts the cell wall permeability, and oxidizes sulfhydryl and sulfur bonds in proteins, enzymes, and other metabolites.[253]

The combination of peracetic acid and hydrogen peroxide has been used for disinfecting hemodialyzers.[255] The percentage of centers using a peracetic acid–hydrogen peroxide–based disinfectant for reprocessing dialyzers increased from 5% in 1983 to 52% in 1992.[195] A study showed that patients treated in dialysis units that disinfected dialyzers with a peracetic acid, hydrogen peroxide, acetic acid mixture or with glutaraldehyde had a higher mortality rate than did patients treated in units that used formalin or in units that did not reuse dialyzers. Although the cause of this elevated mortality risk is currently not known, some believe that the germicide is not the causative element, but rather the germicide may be a surrogate indicator of other problems.[256] An automated machine using peracetic acid to chemically process medical, surgical, and dental instruments (e.g., endoscopes, arthroscopes) is used in the United States.[257, 258] Manufacturer's data demonstrated that this system inactivates *Bacillus subtilis* and *Clostridium sporogenes* when the solution is heated to 50° C with an exposure time of 12 minutes or less.[259] Three recent studies have demonstrated that a peracetic acid processor is rapidly sporicidal and bactericidal, and these data suggest the automatic endoscope processor is suitable for processing medical devices such as flexible and rigid scopes.[260-262]

A new product that contains 0.35% peracetic acid has been formulated as a possible alternative to glutaraldehyde and preliminary studies have shown that it has excellent sporicidal and mycobactericical activity.[263, 264]

Phenolics

Phenol (carbolic acid) has occupied a prominent place in the field of hospital disinfection since its initial use as a germicide by Lister in his pioneering work on antiseptic surgery. In the past 30 years, however, work has concentrated on the numerous phenol derivatives (or *phenolics*) and their antimicrobial properties. Phenol derivatives originate when a functional group (e.g., alkyl, phenyl, benzyl, halogen) replaces one of the hydrogen atoms on the aromatic ring. Two of the phenol derivatives that are commonly found as constituents of hospital disinfectants are *ortho*-phenylphenol and *ortho*-benzyl-*para*-chlorophenol. The antimicrobial properties of these compounds and many other phenol derivatives are much improved from the parent chemical. Phenolics are assimilated by porous materials, and the residual disinfectant may cause tissue irritation. In 1970 Kahn[265] reported that skin depigmentation is caused by phenolic germicidal detergents containing *para*-tertiary-butylphenol and *para*-tertiary-amylphenol.

At higher concentrations, phenol acts as a gross protoplasmic poison, penetrating and disrupting the cell wall and precipitating the cell proteins. Low concentrations of phenol and higher–molecular weight phenol derivatives cause bacterial death by the inactivation of essential enzyme systems and leakage of essential metabolites from the cell wall.[266]

Published reports on the antimicrobial efficacy of commonly used phenolic detergents show that phenolics are bactericidal, fungicidal, viricidal, and tuberculocidal.* Data show that three phenolic detergents are bactericidal and tuberculocidal,[268] and another phenol (containing 50% cresol) has little or no virucidal effect against coxsackie B4, echovirus 11, and poliovirus 1.[270] Similarly, Klein and DeForest[38] made the observation that 12% *ortho*-phenylphenol fails to inactivate any of the three hydrophilic viruses after a 10-minute exposure time, although 5% phenol is lethal for these viruses. A 0.5% dilution of a phenolic (2.8% *ortho*-phenylphenol and 2.7% *ortho*-benzyl-*para*-chlorophenol) has been shown to inactivate HIV,[95] and a 2% solution of a phenolic (15% *ortho*-phenylphenol and 6.3% *para*-tertiary-amylphenol) inactivated all but one of 11 fungi tested.[34] Manufacturers' data from tests with the standardized AOAC methods demonstrate that

*References 4, 11, 34, 39, 95, 99, 266-270.

commercial phenolic detergents are not sporicidal but are tuberculocidal, fungicidal, virucidal, and bactericidal at their recommended use dilutions. Generally, these efficacy claims against microorganisms have not been verified by independent laboratories or the EPA. Attempts to substantiate the bactericidal label claims of phenolic detergents with use of the AOAC method have failed.[7,271] These same studies, however, have shown extreme variability of test results among laboratories testing identical products.

This class of compounds is used for decontamination of the hospital environment, including laboratory surfaces, and for noncritical medical and surgical items. Phenolics are not recommended for semicritical items because of the lack of published efficacy data for many of the available formulations and because the residual disinfectant on porous materials may cause tissue irritation even when thoroughly rinsed.

The use of phenolics in nurseries has been justifiably questioned because of the occurrence of hyperbilirubinemia in infants placed in nurseries that use phenolic detergents.[272] In addition, Doan et al.[273] demonstrated microbilirubin level increases in phenolic-exposed infants compared with nonexposed infants when the phenolic was prepared according to the manufacturer's recommended dilution. If phenolics are used to clean nursery floors, they must be diluted according to the recommendation on the product label. Based on these observations, phenolics should not be used to clean infant bassinets and incubators during the stay of an infant. If phenolics are used to terminally clean infant bassinets and incubators, the surfaces should be rinsed thoroughly with water and dried before the infant bassinets and incubators are reused.

Quaternary ammonium compounds

The *quaternary ammonium compounds* have enjoyed wide use as disinfectants and until recently as antiseptics. Benzalkonium chloride ([N]-alkyl [C14 50%, C12 40%, C16 10%] dimethyl benzyl ammonium chloride) was the first commercially available quaternary ammonium compound. This first-generation quaternary ammonium compound, which was introduced in 1935, received acclaim for its microbicidal activity and good detergent action. Common environmental factors, however, such as hard water, soap, anionic residues, and proteinaceous soils, were subsequently found to reduce benzalkonium chloride's effectiveness.

The elimination of such solutions as antiseptics on skin and tissue was recommended by the CDC[1] because of several outbreaks of infections associated with in-use contamination.[274-281] There have also been a few reports of nosocomial infections associated with contaminated quaternary ammonium compounds used to disinfect patient care supplies or equipment such as cystoscopes or cardiac catheters.[279, 282, 283] The quaternary ammonium compounds are good cleaning agents, but materials such as cotton and gauze pads make them less microbicidal because these materials absorb the active ingredients. As with several other germicides (e.g., phenolics, iodophors), gram-negative bacteria have been found to grow in the compounds.[284]

Chemically, the quaternary ammonia compounds are organically substituted ammonium compounds in which the nitrogen atom has a valence of five, four of the substituent radicals (R1 through R4) are alkyl or heterocyclic radicals of a given size or chain length, and the fifth substituent radical (X-) is a halide, sulfate, or similar radical.[285]

Each compound exhibits its own antimicrobial characteristics, so there has been a search for one compound with outstanding antimicrobial properties. The first significant improvement in quaternary ammonium compound technology, referred to as the second-generation quaternary ammonium compound or dual quaternary ammonium compound, was introduced in 1955. The dual quaternary ammonium compound is a combination of ethyl benzyl chloride quaternary ammonium compounds and a modified alkyl chain–distribution dimethyl benzyl ammonium chloride quaternary ammonium compound. Performance in the presence of hard water was purportedly improved.

The third-generation quaternary ammonium compounds, which are referred to as dialkyl or twin-chain quaternary ammonium compounds (such as dodecyl dimethyl ammonium chloride), were introduced in 1965. These quaternary ammonium compounds remained active in hard water and were tolerant of anionic residues.

The bactericidal action of quaternary ammonium compounds has been attributed to inactivation of energy-producing enzymes, denaturation of essential cell proteins, and disruption of the cell membrane. Evidence offered in support of these and other possibilities is provided by Sykes[285] and Petrocci.[286]

Results from manufacturers' data sheets and

from published scientific literature indicate that the quaternary ammonium compounds sold as hospital disinfectants are fungicidal, bactericidal, and virucidal against lipophilic viruses; they are not sporicidal and generally are not tuberculocidal or virucidal against hydrophilic viruses.* Attempts to reproduce the manufacturers' bactericidal and tuberculocidal claims with a limited number of quaternary ammonium compounds by means of the AOAC tests have failed.[7, 39, 271] These same studies, however, showed extreme variability of test results among laboratories testing identical products.

The quaternary ammonium compounds are commonly used in ordinary environmental sanitation of noncritical surfaces such as floors, furniture, and walls.

EMERGING TECHNOLOGIES FOR DISINFECTION AND STERILIZATION

Several other disinfectants and sterilants and sterilization processes are being investigated and may be incorporated into our armamentarium of disinfection and sterilization in the future. The paucity of published studies on disinfectants makes the microbicidal activity of new products difficult to assess. For example, one new high-level disinfectant (*ortho*-phthalaldehyde) requires further evaluation[288] before it can be considered for use on endoscopes.

Reprocessing of heat-labile medical equipment is a major problem in hospitals. ETO has been the sterilant of choice for sterilizing heat-labile medical equipment. Despite ETO's excellent properties, it is toxic, mutagenic, and a suspected carcinogen. Until recently ETO sterilizers combined ETO with a chlorofluorocarbon (CFC) stabilizing agent, most commonly in a ratio of 12% ETO mixed with 88% CFC (referred to as 12/88 ETO). For several reasons health care organizations are exploring the use of new low temperature sterilization technologies.[289] First, CFCs were to be phased out in December 1995 under provisions of the Clean Air Act.[290] CFCs were classified as a class I substance under the Clean Air Act because of scientific evidence linking them to destruction of the earth's ozone layer. Second, some states (e.g., California, New York, Michigan) require the use of ETO abatement technology to reduce the amount of ETO being released into ambient air by 90% to 99.9%. Third, OSHA regulates the acceptable vapor levels of ETO (i.e., 1 ppm averaged over 8

hours) because of concerns that ETO exposure represents an occupational hazard. These constraints have led to the recent development of alternative technologies for low temperature sterilization in the health care setting.

Alternative technologies to ETO with CFC include the following: 100% ETO; ETO with a different stabilizing gas such as carbon dioxide or hydrochlorofluorocarbons; vaporized hydrogen peroxide; gas plasmas; ozone; and chlorine dioxide. These new technologies should be compared against the characteristics of an ideal low-temperature ($< 60°$ C) sterilant.[289] Although it is apparent that all technologies will have limitations,[291] understanding the limitations imposed by restrictive device designs (e.g., long, narrow lumens) is critical for proper application of new sterilization technology.[292] For example, the development of increasingly small and complex endoscopes presents a difficult challenge for current sterilization processes. This occurs because microorganisms must be in direct contact with the sterilant for inactivation to occur. There are peer-reviewed scientific data demonstrating concerns about the efficacy of several of the low-temperature sterilization processes (i.e., gas plasma, vaporized hydrogen peroxide, ETO), particularly when the test organisms are challenged in the presence of serum and salt and a narrow lumen vehicle.[292, 294]

RECOMMENDATIONS

A. Cleaning, disinfecting, and sterilizing patient care equipment: All objects to be high-level disinfected or sterilized should first be thoroughly cleaned to remove all organic matter (e.g., blood, tissue) and other residue.
B. Indications for sterilization and high-level disinfection (recommendations B.1. and B.4. per 1985 CDC guideline[2] and recommendation B.5 per 1993 CDC guideline).[88]
  1. Critical medical devices or pieces of patient care equipment that enter normally sterile tissue or the vascular system or through which blood flows should be sterilized before each use.
  2. Endoscope accessories: Biopsy forceps or other cutting instruments that break the mucosal barrier should be sterilized. Other endoscope accessories (e.g., suction valves) should be sterilized after each patient use; if this is not feasible, they should receive at least high-level disinfection. Please refer to the "APIC Guideline for Infection Preven-

*References 11, 34, 37, 39, 42, 44, 99, 286, 287.

AJIC
August 1996

tion and Control in Flexible Endoscopy" for additional recommendations.[23]

3. Laparoscopes, arthroscopes, and other scopes that enter normally sterile tissue should be subjected to a sterilization procedure before each use; if this is not feasible, they should receive at least high-level disinfection. Disinfection should be followed by a rinse with sterile water.

4. Equipment that touches mucous membranes (e.g., endoscopes, endotracheal tubes, anesthesia breathing circuits, and respiratory therapy equipment) should receive high-level disinfection.

5. Dental instruments that penetrate soft tissue or bone (e.g., forceps, scalpels, bone chisels, scalers, and burs) are classified as critical and should be sterilized or discarded after each use. Dental instruments that are not intended to penetrate oral soft tissue or bone (e.g., amalgam condensers, air-water syringes) but may come into contact with oral tissues are classified as semicritical and should be sterilized after each use. If the semicritical instrument could be damaged by the sterilization process, the instrument should be high-level disinfected. Noncritical surfaces, such as uncovered operatory surfaces (e.g., countertops, chair switches), should be disinfected between patients with an intermediate-level or low-level disinfectant.

C. Chemical methods for sterilization (Table 2): When sterilization is indicated and other sterilization methods (e.g., steam or ETO) cannot be used, any one of three liquid chemical sterilants (see Table 2) may be used. The manufacturer's instructions for use will specify the recommended exposure time.

D. Selection and use of high-level disinfectants for semicritical patient care items.

1. Solutions containing glutaraldehyde, hydrogen peroxide, chlorine, and peracetic acid can achieve high-level disinfection if objects are properly cleaned before disinfection. See Table 2 for recommended concentrations. The disinfectant or chemical sterilant selected should have no or minimal deleterious effects on the object (e.g., chlorine may corrode metals; see Table 2).

2. The exact time for disinfecting semicritical items is somewhat elusive at present because of conflicting label claims and lack of agreement in published literature, especially regarding the mycobactericidal activity of glutaraldehydes. The longer the exposure of an item to a disinfectant, the more likely it is that all contaminating microorganisms will be inactivated. Unfortunately, with extended exposure to a disinfectant it is also more likely that delicate and intricate instruments such as endoscopes may be damaged. Medical equipment such as endoscopes, which are difficult to clean and disinfect because of narrow channels or other areas that can harbor organisms (e.g., crevices, joints), should be exposed to a high-level disinfectant for at least 20 minutes at room temperature after cleaning.

E. Selection and use of low-level disinfectants for noncritical patient care items.

1. Solutions for use on noncritical patient care equipment and recommended concentrations are listed in Table 2.

2. The contact time is 10 minutes or less.

3. Phenolics should not be used to clean infant bassinets and incubators during the stay of an infant. If phenolics are used to terminally clean infant bassinets and incubators, the surfaces should be rinsed thoroughly with water and dried before the infant bassinets and incubators are reused.

F. Processing patient care equipment contaminated with HIV or HBV.

1. Standard sterilization and disinfection procedures for patient care equipment (as recommended in this guideline) are adequate to sterilize or disinfect instruments or devices contaminated with blood or other body fluids from persons infected with blood-borne pathogens, including HIV. No changes in procedures for cleaning, disinfecting, or sterilizing need to be made.

2. Noncritical environmental surfaces contaminated with blood or bloody body fluids should be cleaned before an EPA-registered disinfectant/detergent is applied for disinfection. Persons cleaning spills should wear disposable gloves and other personal protective equipment as indicated.

G. Processing CJD-contaminated patient care equipment

1. The only infectious agent that requires unique decontamination recommendations is the CJD prion. The need for such recommendations is due to an extremely resistant subpopulation of prions and the protection afforded this tissue-associated agent.

2. Critical and semicritical CJD-contaminated care equipment should preferably be steam sterilized for at least 30 minutes at a temperature of 132° C (121° C is not effective) in a gravity displacement sterilizer. A prevacuum sterilizer used for 18 minutes at 134° C to 138° C has also been found to be effective. Immersion in 1 N sodium hydroxide (which is caustic) for 1 hour at room temperature followed by steam sterilization at 121° C for 30 minutes is an alternative procedure for critical and semicritical items. Because noncritical patient care items or surfaces (e.g., autopsy tables, floors) have not been involved in disease transmission, these surfaces may be disinfected with either bleach (undiluted, or up to 1:10 dilution) or 1 N sodium hydroxide at room temperature for 15 minutes or less. A formalin–formic acid procedure is required for inactivating virus infectivity in tissue samples from patients with CJD.

H. Method of processing reusable transducers: After transducers are cleaned, they may be sterilized with ETO or disinfected with a high-level disinfectant. Alternatively, transducer heads may be disinfected with 70% isopropyl alcohol. However, the disinfection procedure must be adhered to rigorously, and this is best accomplished in a controlled setting. The transducers should be stored in a manner to prevent recontamination before use.

I. The selection and use of disinfectants in the health care field is dynamic, and products may become available that were not in existence when this guideline was written. As newer disinfectants become available, persons or committees responsible for selecting disinfectants should be guided by information in the scientific literature.

I gratefully acknowledge Ms. Eva P. Clontz for her invaluable assistance in preparing this manuscript.

References

1. Simmons BP. Guideline for hospital environmental control. AJIC Am J Infect Control 1983;11:97-115.
2. Garner JS, Favero MS. Guideline for handwashing and hospital environmental control, 1985. AJIC Am J Infect Control 1986;14:110-26.
3. Rutala WA. Disinfection, sterilization and waste disposal. In: Wenzel RP, ed. Prevention and control of nosocomial infections. Baltimore: Williams and Wilkins, 1987:257-82.
4. Rutala WA. Disinfection, sterilization and waste disposal. In: Wenzel RP, ed. Prevention and control of nosocomial infections. 2nd ed. Baltimore: Williams and Wilkins, 1993:460-95.
5. Rutala WA. APIC guideline for selection and use of disinfectants. AJIC Am J Infect Control 1990;18:99-117.
6. Rutala WA. Selection and use of disinfectants in health care. In: Mayhall CG, ed. Hospital epidemiology and infection control. Baltimore: Williams and Wilkins, 1995: 913-36.
7. Rutala WA, Cole EC. Ineffectiveness of hospital disinfectants against bacteria: a collaborative study. Infect Control 1987;8:501-6.
8. Myers T. Failing the test: germicides or use-dilution methodology? ASM News 1988;54:19-21.
9. Robison RA, Bodily HL, Robinson DF, Christensen RP. A suspension method to determine reuse life of chemical disinfectants during clinical use. Appl Environ Microbiol 1988;54:158-64.
10. Favero MS, Bond WW. Chemical disinfection of medical and surgical materials. In: Block SS, ed. Disinfection, sterilization and preservation. 4th ed. Philadelphia: Lea & Febiger, 1991:617-41.
11. Spaulding EH. Chemical disinfection of medical and surgical materials. In: Lawrence CA, Block SS, eds. Disinfection, sterilization and preservation. Philadelphia: Lea & Febiger, 1968:517-31.
12. Bean HS. Types and characteristics of disinfectants. J Appl Bacteriol 1967;30:6-16.
13. Russell AD. Factors influencing the efficacy of antimicrobial agents. In: Russell AD, Hugo WB, Ayliffe GAJ, eds. Principles and practice of disinfection, preservation and sterilisation. Oxford: Blackwell Scientific Publications, 1992:89-113.
14. Centers for Disease Control. Guidelines for the prevention of transmission of human immunodeficiency virus and hepatitis B virus to health-care and public-safety workers. MMWR 1989;38(S-6):1-37.
15. Rutala WA, Weber DJ. FDA labeling requirements for disinfection of endoscopes: a counterpoint. Infect Control Hosp Epidemiol 1995;16:231-5.
16. Lewis DL, Arens M. Resistance of microorganisms to disinfection in dental and medical devices. Nature Medicine 1995;1:1-3.
17. Parker HH IV, Johnson RD. Effectiveness of ethylene oxide for sterilization of dental handpieces. J Dent 1995;23:113-5.
18. Muscarella LF. Sterilizing dental equipment. Nature Medicine 1995;1:1223-4.
19. Block SS. Definition of terms. In: Block SS, ed. Disinfection, sterilization and preservation. 4th ed. Philadelphia: Lea & Febiger, 1991:18-25.
20. Food and Drug Administration, Public Health Service, Environmental Protection Agency. Memorandum of understanding between the Food and Drug Administration, Public Health Service, and the Environmental Protection Agency. Washington, DC: FDA, PHS, EPA, June 4 1993.
21. Larson EL. APIC guideline for handwashing and hand antisepsis in health care settings. AJIC Am J Infect Control 1995;23:251-69.
22. Rutala WA, Clontz EP, Weber DJ, Hoffmann KK. Disinfection practices for endoscopes and other semicritical items. Infect Control Hosp Epidemiol 1991;12:282-8.
23. Martin MA, Reichelderfer M. APIC guideline for infection prevention and control in flexible endoscopy. AJIC Am J Infect Control 1994;22:19-38.

APIC State-of-the-Art Report: The role of infection control during construction in health care facilities

Judene Mueller Bartley, MS, MPH, CIC
The 1997, 1998, and 1999 APIC Guidelines Committees

The Association for Professionals in Infection Control and Epidemiology, Inc (APIC), is a multidisciplinary organization of more than 12,000 health care professionals who practice infection control and epidemiology within a variety of health care settings.

This report reviews issues the infection control professional should consider related to construction and renovation projects in health care facilities. Preventing transmission of infectious agents to vulnerable patient populations, health care workers, and visitors remains an important component of infection control programs. Environmental dispersal of microorganisms during construction, resulting in nosocomial infections, has been described previously, and select examples are provided in Table I as a reminder that there is a solid, scientific basis for these concerns. Environmental airborne contaminants and infectious agents are closely related to water and moisture-related conditions and figure prominently in construction activity. Weems et al have established construction activity as an independent variable for infectious risks in such circumstances. Construction-related outbreak literature will not be revisited in detail; however, pertinent citations will identify resources as appropriate. (AJIC Am J Infect Control 2000;28:156-69)

Section I outlines the broad semiregulatory foundation for direct infection control participation in strategic planning for construction. Section II describes initial steps of planning through policy development, and suggests initial, basic elements for inclusion. Section III examines the infection control implications of the *process in detail and is structured on the typical stages* of construction. Section IV addresses common questions related to remediation after environmental emergencies or special structural design issues that remain somewhat controversial or unresolved. Recommendations are provided from a variety of reasonable and practical sources not always available as published controlled studies. Section V identifies a number of future research areas that remain important challenges. Terms and abbreviations used frequently throughout the text are highlighted in Table II.

I. CURRENT BASIS OF STRATEGIC PLANNING AND THE ROLE OF INFECTION CONTROL

AIA Guidelines

The current authority for construction design for federal and state health care providers is the 1996–1997 edition of the *Guidelines for Design and Construction of Hospitals and Health Care Facilities.* The American Institute of Architects (AIA) Academy of Architecture for Health publishes this consensus document with concurrence from the US Department of Health and Human Services. Many states adopt the Guidelines in their entirety as minimum standards for design and construction.[19] Prior editions of the Guidelines required construction and renovation assessments during project planning related to specific risks. The new AIA Guidelines strongly support infection control input at the initial stages of planning and design by requiring a new element termed an Infection Control Risk Assessment (ICRA) for broad and long-range involvement of infection control/epidemiology leadership.[19]

The AIA Guidelines state that "Design and planning for such [renovation and new construction] projects shall require consultation from infection control and safety personnel. Early involvement in the conceptual phase helps ascertain the risk for susceptible patient and disruption of essential patient services." Each subsequent section requires an ICRA (eg, numbers and type of isolation rooms) and is predicated upon an "infection control risk assessment" by the infection control committee or a multidisciplinary group designated for that purpose. An ICRA provides for strategic, proactive design to mitigate environmental sources of microbes and for prevention of infection through architectural design (eg, handwashing facilities, separation of patients with communicable diseases), as well as specific needs of the population served by the facility.

Reprint requests: APIC, 1275 K Street NW, Suite 1000, Washington, DC 20005-4006.

doi:10.1067/mic.2000.106055

156

Table 1. Selected events of nosocomial infection associated with the dispersal of microorganisms during construction

Year, author	Organism	Population	Epidemiologic factors
Airborne			
1976 Aisner et al[1]	*Aspergillus* spp	Acute leukemia	Fireproofing insulation
1982 Lentino et al[2]	*Aspergillus* spp	BMT; renal	Road construction; window air conditioners
1985 Krasinski et al[3]	*Rhizopus; Aspergillus*	Neonatal	False ceiling
1987 Streifel et al[4]	*Penicillium* spp	BMT	Rotted wood cabinet
1987 Weems et al[5]	*Rhizopus; Mucor* sp;	Hematologic BMT	Construction activity
1990 Fox et al[6]	*Penicillium* sp; *Cladosporium* sp	OR	Ventilation duct fiberglass insulation
1991 Arnow et al[7]	*Aspergillus* sp	Cancer-melanoma	Tiles; humidified cell incubators; air filters
1993 Flynn et al[8]	*Aspergillus terreus*	ICU	ICU renovation; elevators
1994 Gerson et al[9]	*Aspergillus* sp	General	Carpeting
1995 Alvarez et al[10]	*Scedosporium prolificans (inflatum)*	Neutropenic hematology	Construction, presumed environmental
1996 Pittet et al[11]	*Aspergillus* sp	COPD	Air filter replacement
Waterborne			
1976 Haley et al[12]	*Legionella* spp	Immunosuppressed	Soil; water
1980 Dondero et al[13]	*Legionella* spp	Adults, employees	Cooling towers
1980 Crane et al[14]	*Pseudomonas paucimobilis*	ICU	Potable water used to fill flush water bottles
1985 Claesson et al[15]	Group A *Streptococcus*	Maternity	Shower head
1993 Sniadeck et al[16]	*Mycobacterium xenopi*	Endoscopy-pseudo	Potable water; scopes
1997 Dearborn et al[17]	*Stachybotrys atra*	Infants	Water-damaged homes
1997 Fridkin et al[18]	*Acremonium kiliense*	Ambulatory surgery	Vent system humidifier

BMT, Bone marrow transplant; *OR*, operating room; *ICU*, intensive care unit; *COPD*, chronic obstructive pulmonary disease.

To carry out an ICRA in the design phase, AIA identifies a multidisciplinary planning group that should involve, at minimum, the health systems' infection control/epidemiology department, the infection control committee (or committee charged with development and review of the infection control policy), and administrators representing special program needs. The planning group's charge is to consider communicable disease prevalence in the community while recognizing the importance of disease variation and distribution across geographic regions and to weigh the availability of public support agencies, as well as to consider the needs of health systems that manage patients with communicable disease, patients who are severely immunosuppressed, or both.

Implementation

The role of infection control is multifaceted and will be required throughout and after completion of the construction project. Infection control staff members provide important leadership and a communication link with program administrators, architects, and engineers. Completion of an ICRA is only the first step; input also is needed in early stages of project design as well as during later blueprint reviews. For example, early coordination with facility management during construction phase identifies necessary support structures required to prevent and control airborne contamination, thus avoiding costly rework or redesign. Newer design challenges include "retrofitting" older buildings into offices and clinics to meet needs for patient examination and instrument cleaning rooms, laboratories, and storage. In the absence of clear-cut rules or regulations, infection control staff members serve to bridge gaps with health agencies and facility administration regarding infection control guidelines and essential design features needed for safe practice. The ICRA sets the scene for involving infection control and supports continuing implementation of infection control principles.[20-33]

II. CONSTRUCTION AND RENOVATION POLICY

A comprehensive construction and renovation policy (CRP) operationalizes the facility's ICRA, ensures management's understanding of the ICRA, and specifies essential participants. A well-designed policy will ensure timely notification of the infection control professional and designated committee(s) for early program planning efforts. In addition, the CRP calls for infection control to evaluate the project from conception through completion and supports a systematic approach for project management. The policy should be submitted for approval by the facility's board of trustees and reviewed/approved periodically.

Elements

Numerous publications have identified a common set of elements to address the planning, designing, and

Table 2. Terms and abbreviations

Term or abbreviation	Description
AIA Guidelines	American Institute of Architects: 1996–1997 Guidelines for Design and Construction of Hospitals and Healthcare Facilities
AII	Airborne infection isolation room (old isolation room)
ANSI	American National Standards Institute
ASHRAE	American Society of Heating, Refrigerating, and Air Conditioning Engineers Inc
BMT	Bone marrow transplant
CFU/m³	Colony forming units per cubic meter (of air)
CRP	Construction and renovation policy
HEPA–filter	High efficiency particulate air filters (99% of .3 micron size particles)
High efficiency	Filtration at 95% efficiency
HVAC	Heating ventilation air conditioning (air handler or air handling unit)
ICRA	Infection control risk assessment
LDRP	Labor/delivery/recovery/postpartum
PE	Protected environment (old protective isolation room)
PPE	Personal protective equipment
SSI	Surgical site infection
UVGI	Ultraviolet germicidal irradiation
VAP	Ventilator-associated pneumonia

monitoring processes. These topics are grouped and itemized below, though many options for development and effective implementation of each have been described in the literature.[20-34]

- Authority and responsibility for establishing internal and subcontractor coordination of (1) construction preparation and demolition; (2) intraconstruction operations and maintenance; (3) project completion and postconstruction cleanup; and (4) monitoring
- Authority and communication lines to determine if or how patient unit closure will occur
- Planning for air handling and water systems/plumbing as appropriate
- Expectations for contractor accountability in the event of breaches in infection control practices and related written agreements
- Patient area risk assessment; criteria for emergency work interruptions (stop and start processes)
- Education: for whom and by whom
- Occupational health expectations for subcontractors before start, as needed
- Traffic patterns for patients, health care workers, and visitors
- Transport and approval for disposal of waste materials
- Emergency preparedness plans for major utility failures with infection control implications, including location and responsibilities.

Process

The CRP must ensure continuous input from infection control into the structural design process to identify appropriate and timely infection control practices. The CRP should require:

- routine submission of scheduled project lists from facility management to infection control, enabling infection control to be proactively aware of projects and to anticipate infection control needs.
- submission of an "infection control (IC) permit" or "project approval signature block" before the beginning of projects, beyond required project lists.[31] Formats may range from simple checklists to questionnaires designed to assist staff members in assessing risks and identifying prevention strategies.
- submission of an IC permit designed to assess the complexity of the project as a matrix of risk groups (patients and environment).

The score determines needed interventions based on:
- construction activity—project complexity in terms of dust generation and duration of activity.
- patients—assessment of the population at risk and location in terms of invasive procedures.

The matrix grid format immediately leads to identifying:
- number and types of necessary controls and IC interventions.
- signatures of all parties, thus providing accountability for the mutually agreed upon plan.[31]

III. INFECTION CONTROL IMPLICATIONS FOR CONSTRUCTION AND RENOVATION

Planning—design and preconstruction

IC participation is critical in the initial planning and approval meetings during the design phase. Issues frequently addressed include budget, space constraints including storage and equipment cleaning areas, air-handling units, handwashing facilities, appropriate finishes, specific products with infectious implications, and applicable regulations. Infection control professionals (ICPs) should be prepared to support their position and recommendations with published citations whenever feasible, especially when a recommendation is not budget neutral.[20,21,26,33-35] ICPs frequently work with consultants during the planning phase, including architectural and construction companies in a "partnering" process. Consulting an environmental expert might also be necessary if the size and complexity of construction provides considerable risk to highly susceptible patients because of location, prolonged time of construction, work conducted over continuous shifts, and likelihood of air handlers sustaining frequent interruptions. These variables increase risks to patients and personnel and may require monitoring. If appropriate, budgets for environmental consultants and anticipated testing or environmental monitoring needs to be considered at the earliest stage of planning.

Design and structure. IC should ensure that major design components are addressed as appropriate and justified by relevant guidelines, standards, codes, and regulations.[19,24,36-48] Guidance for many elements is described in the resources already referenced; asterisked items below are requirements for new construction addressed in the 1996-1997 AIA Guidelines.[19] Major design components that need to be addressed include:

- Design to support IC practice.*
- Design, number, and type of isolation rooms (ie, airborne infection isolation [AII] or protective environment [PE]).* (AIA Guidelines outline the design characteristics for AII, including no requirement for anterooms, nor support for "reversible" ventilation [ie, rooms "switched" from negative to positive air pressure]; the AIA appendix provides suggestions for PE design.[19-21] These designs are deliberately consistent with Centers for Disease Control and Prevention guidelines regarding tuberculosis and pneumonia.[38,39])
- Heating, ventilation, and air conditioning systems (HVAC), including recommended ventilation and filtration charts.*
- Mechanical systems involving water supply and plumbing.*
- Number, type, and placement of handwashing fixtures,* clinical sinks,* dispensers for handwashing soap,* paper towels, and lotion.
- Sharps disposal unit placement.
- Accommodation for personal protection equipment.*
- Surfaces: ceiling tiles, walls, counters, floor covering, and furnishings.*
- Utility rooms: soiled, clean, instrument processing, holding, workrooms.*

- Storage of movable and modular equipment.

Preparation for demolition and construction. The project teams provide ongoing planning and monitoring during area preparation and throughout the demolition, construction, cleanup, preparation for return to service, and final project review.[19,21,26,34,42,43] Before construction begins, the focus of preparations should be on isolation of the construction/renovation area. Some sources categorize projects in terms of minor or major risk based on the level of needed barriers; checklists are developed accordingly.[26,28-34,49-51]

Type and extent of construction. Project complexity varies with time, numbers of workers, whether contractors work continuous shifts, scope and degree of activity (high or low dust generation), and proximity to patients with varying degrees of risk for infection. Internal renovations may require as much consideration as external construction. Patient areas or units that cannot be closed or that are adjacent to a major renovation require special planning, (eg, operating room additions adjacent to an active surgical suite). These situations may justify environmental monitoring beyond visual inspection to detect increased airborne contamination and to plan interventions.[5,21,25,28-30,39,51-54]

External excavation is ideally conducted during off-hours so that air handlers can be shut down and sealed; the goal is to protect the intake as much as possible. Small projects require similar planning and vary by degree, but preparation still requires early communication with facility management. Specific educational needs (eg, Occupational Safety and Health Administration [OSHA]) regulations and health issues for patients and workers need to be addressed. A summary of common issues is provided below within 3 major categories of tasks; items will vary by facility, but the final customized list should be appended to the CRP.[5,21,22,26,33,43,49,51]

Dust and debris control.

- Medical waste containers (sharps or other medical regulated waste): These should be removed by the facility before start of the project.
- Barrier systems: The area should be isolated, as the project requires. Small, short duration projects generating minimal dust may use fire-rated plastic sheeting, but should be sealed at full ceiling height with at least 2-foot overlapping flaps for access to entry. Any project that produces moderate to high levels of dust requires rigid, dust-proof, and fire-rated barrier walls (eg, drywall) with caulked seams for a tight seal. Large, dusty projects need an entry vestibule for clothing changes and tool storage. The entry area should have gasketed doorframes; tight seals should be maintained at the full perimeter of walls and wall penetrations. An inter-

im plastic dust barrier may be required to protect the area while the rigid impervious barrier is being constructed. Cleaning is required at completion of the barrier construction; plans should also describe a terminal barrier removal process that minimizes dust dispersal.[33,34,43]

- Traffic control: Designated entry and exit procedures must be defined. Egress paths should be free of debris; designated elevators should be used during scheduled times; and only authorized personnel should be allowed to enter the construction zone. Signage should direct pedestrian traffic away from the construction area and materials.[5,21,26,34]

- Demolition: Debris should be removed in carts with tightly fitted covers, using designated traffic routes. Efforts should be made to minimize use of elevators with transport during the lowest period of activity. Debris should be removed daily and at times specified by agreements. If chutes are used to direct debris outside, HEPA-filtered negative air machines should be used, and the chute opening should be sealed when not in use. Filters should be bagged and sealed before being transported out of the construction area.[5,21,22,33]

- Exterior windows: Windows should be sealed to minimize infiltration from excavation debris.

- Visual monitoring: Compliance with barrier maintenance includes education of staff for simple clues (eg, accumulation of visible dust evidenced by footprints, opened doors/windows evidenced by presence of insects and flies, wet ceiling tiles, etc).[21,26,55]

Ventilation and environmental control.

- Air system flow: It should be determined whether the construction area uses fresh/outside or recirculated air; filters should be added or return vents covered as needed with filter material or plastic. Air must flow from clean to dirty areas.[19,20,21,33,34,43]

- Negative air pressure: The air within the construction area must be negative with respect to surrounding areas and with no disruption of air systems of adjacent areas. Constant negative pressure within the zone should be monitored with an alarmed device, which must be maintained and monitored by construction personnel. Exhaust from construction air should be directed outside with no recirculation if possible. If the exhaust must tie into a recirculated air system, a pre-filter and high efficiency filter (95%) should be used before exhaust to prevent contamination of the ducts. Fans should be turned off before opening ductwork and necessary interruptions (eg, fire drills) should be planned for to minimize risk.[20-22,33,34,43,51]

- Adjacent areas: The status of sealed penetrations and intact ceilings should be verified.

- Air exchange rates and pressure relationships: It should be verified that the facility can:
  - maintain proper rates in critical areas near construction activity.
  - ensure air is not being recirculated without filtration from the construction area elsewhere.
  - provide accountability for and frequency of testing air pressure throughout the project.[20-22,26,33]

- Vibration or disturbances: Drilling and other sources of vibration have potential to dislodge dust collected above suspended or false ceilings; vibrations loosen corrosion within water pipes as well. Plans should require vacuuming of affected areas and flushing debris from water systems before reoccupancy.[5,21,50,55,56]

- Specification of temperature and humidity ranges: Determine limits as appropriate.[20-22,35]

- Monitoring must consider risks of malfunction or complete loss of utilities. Both visual cues and particulate air monitoring may be used. The type and frequency of monitoring, evaluation of results, and follow-up action by designated parties are essential to planning.[20,21,26,33,57]

Contamination of patient rooms, supplies, equipment, and related areas.

- Worksite garb: Contractor personnel clothing should be free of loose soil and debris before leaving the construction area. If protective apparel is not worn, a HEPA-filtered vacuum should be used to remove dust from clothing before leaving the barricade. Personal protective equipment (eg, face shields, gloves, respirators) are worn as appropriate. Contractors entering invasive procedure areas should be provided with disposable jump suits and head and shoe coverings. Protective clothing should be removed before exiting the work area. Tools and equipment should be damp wiped before entry and exit from the work areas.[20-22,26,33]

- Barriers around construction should be monitored to maintain protection of in-use patient care areas as described. Patient doors adjacent to construction area should be kept closed, with appropriate traffic control.[20-22,26]

- Storage should be designated for construction materials.[22,33,43]

- Contractor cleaning: The construction zone should be maintained in a clean manner by contractors and swept or HEPA-vacuumed daily or more frequently as needed to minimize dust. Adjacent areas should be damp mopped daily or more frequently as needed. Walk-off mats may minimize tracking of heavy dirt and dust from construction areas.[21,26,33,43]

- Facility cleaning: Contracts should clearly specify responsibilities and expectations for routine and terminal cleaning before opening the newly renovated or construction zone.[21,22,25,51]

Intraconstruction and the role of IC. Once renovation or construction has begun, the ICP should be available to provide maintenance and operational input. Frequency of input or meetings will depend on the scope of the project. Specific concerns need to be customized in each project and include IC practices, education, and monitoring. The ICP is vital in educating and supporting "users/owners" to manage their area under construction (eg, educating staff members on how to monitor their own performance as much as possible). In more complex projects, the ICP may assist directly or make provisions for items already outlined. A number of areas involving specific ICP involvement are discussed below.

Environmental rounds. An efficient method to integrate key IC and life safety issues is the use of rounds, using simple checklists based on the items addressed above. ICPs can advise or participate in rounds, which should be scheduled as often as necessary and include a variety of observable "indicators" such as barriers (doors, signage), air handling (windows closed), project area (debris, cleaning), traffic control, and dress code. It may be necessary on occasion to schedule rounds after normal hours or on weekends if that is when construction or renovation is scheduled.[20-22,26,33,34,43,49,51]

Outcome or process measures. Projects may be approached as performance improvement initiatives using outcome measures (eg, surgical site infection rates) or process measures (measuring compliance) using visual observations, airborne particulate monitors, satisfaction surveys, etc.[51-54]

Impact on special areas. Patients requiring AII need close monitoring to ensure negative pressure relationships are maintained, particularly when there is potential for disruption of pressure relationships.[20,21,58-61] Intake areas such as emergency departments need planning to triage potentially infectious patients.[19,45,62] If highly susceptible patients cannot be relocated, indicators should be identified to trigger planned intervention.[5,21,25,26-29,33,52-54] Immunosuppressed populations in bone marrow transplantation units or protected environments, intensive care units, etc, require special planning. The goal is to minimize patient exposure to major construction activity; therefore, nonemergency admissions should be avoided during periods of major excavation. If delaying admissions is not an option, patients should be located in areas as remote as possible from construction activity.[20,21,26]

Patient location and transport. Health care providers should plan patient care activities to minimize exposure to construction sites.[20-21] At least one study found that critically ill, ventilator-dependent patients transported from the ICU for diagnostic or therapeutic procedures was an independent risk factor for development of ventilator-associated pneumonia.[63] To decrease exposure for patients during construction activities the following should be considered:

- Provide treatment in the patient's room.
- Transport via an alternate route.
- Schedule transport or procedures during periods with minimal construction activity.
- Minimize waiting and procedure times near construction zones.
- Mask patient or provide other barriers (eg, covering open wounds) based on patient's clinical status.

Interruption of utility services. Utility services may be interrupted during any type of construction. Infectious agents may contaminate air-handling units, medical vacuum, and water systems after planned or unplanned power disruptions. IC provides input into emergency preparedness to reduce the potential risks of contamination.[20-22,42,57] Response plans should include assessment of the population at risk and cleanup should focus on steps to prevent, detect, and reduce risk from infectious hazards. For example, as power is reestablished after an interruption, dampers and fans of air handling units resume operation. Dust and particulate matter released during this process may transmit allergenic or infectious agents such as *Aspergillus* sp to patients and staff.[3,5,20-22,26,33,50,64] Therefore, IC policies for areas in which invasive procedures are performed should require sufficient time to clear the air of potential contaminants before resuming the room(s) use. Ventilation time should be based on the number of air changes per hour required by the area. The National Institute for Occupational Safety and Health (NIOSH) chart for removal efficiency of airborne contaminants may provide guidance, but its use should be tempered by its assumptions.[39] In the event of major contamination of patient care areas, plans should specify responsibilities for these decisions as well as for intensified cleaning, environmental surveillance of airborne infectious agents, and restriction of water use until testing or flushing determines safe usage.

Worker risk assessment and education. Health risk evaluations for potential exposures depend on the type of construction planned. Facility staff overseeing or working with outside contractors should assist in determining potential environmental risks for facility workers or contractors. Policies should include provisions for training and by whom (facility or contractor). Training must be appropriate to the task (eg, staff entering air systems for preventive maintenance [changing filters] should be alerted to the potential for airborne dust containing spores of microorganisms and arrange to first turn off fans and don a mask). Staff members working in sanitary or septic sewage systems, drainage pipes, etc, should be alerted to the risks of moisture and fungal contamination.[20-22,57,65-67] Agreements should be developed appropriate to the project regarding provisions for pertinent health protection, vaccinations, tuberculosis assessment/PPD skin testing, or related education before workers begin construction. Requirements will vary with degree of environmental risk and proximity to patient population.

Documentation of health/training issues. As agreements are completed, they should provide evidence that workers have received appropriate health protection as noted above and should include the following information:

- Facility exposure control plan(s) for IC, hazardous chemicals, and life safety.
- How to seek help and report exposures (eg, first aid location and initial steps to report exposures).
- Use of particulate respirators or other PPE.
- Risk prevention for unexpected safety issues, such as noxious fumes, asbestos, etc.[22,66,67]

The facility should be satisfied that provisions have been made for effective IC education designed to address facility-specific needs related to potential infectious risk exposures as described above.[45-48]

Postconstruction and cleanup

Project checklists. Check-off lists of expected practices identified at the beginning of the project should be reviewed for items agreed upon before the area is returned to full service or patient occupancy. A useful tool during review is the contractor's "punchlist" that will ensure missed details have been addressed (eg, installations of soap dispensers or designated types of handwashing/sink controls).[33,34]

Postconstruction agreements. Cleanup agreements (eg, cleaning, air balancing, filter changes, flushing of water systems, etc) and other utility service checks/ cleaning must be established in the early planning phase as discussed in Section II. These include at minimum[33,34]:

- Contractor cleaning to include area clearance, cleaning, and decontamination/wipedown.
- Cleaning after removal of partitions around construction area, minimizing dust production.
- Facility-based routine/terminal cleaning before returning area to service.
- Provision of time frames for facility review (eg, 2 weeks) after completion of the project to ensure all issues were addressed properly.[33,34]
- Systematic review of outcomes in the facility's designated review process, whether by contract or committee structure. Items may range from sealed

cabling/electrical penetrations and ceiling tile replacements to the completed punchlist.
- Cleaning and replacement of filters and other equipment if affected by major or minor disruptions or conditions that could have contaminated the air or water supply.[4,23,33,68,69]

Steps before occupancy: Checklists specific to the project should be developed for a walk-through just before occupancy. Core IC issues for inclusion are listed below as applicable. The designated team should do the following:

- Check that sinks are properly located and functioning.
- Verify that sinks in critical patient care areas have properly functioning fixtures.
- Check for the presence/absence of aerators in these fixtures according to facility policy.
- Test whether soap and towel dispensers are filled and functioning.
- Check whether surfaces in procedure/service areas are appropriate for use (eg, smooth, nonporous, water-resistant).
- Verify that air balancing has been completed according to specifications.
- Test whether air flows into negative pressure rooms or out of positive pressure rooms.

Monitoring activities during construction[20,23]

There are currently no recommendations for routine environmental culturing during construction. Enhanced targeted patient surveillance (eg, respiratory illnesses consistent with aspergillosis or legionellosis) near construction areas should be part of the ICRA. Other control measures previously discussed need to be continuously monitored.

However, when an outbreak associated with construction is suspected or identified, water or air sampling may be indicated. It is vitally important to establish a hypothesis with clear and measurable goals. Culturing or sampling procedures should be defined before initiation (eg, asbestos, fungal, or particulates). Sampling procedures relative to the suspected agent(s) and sources should be used. The investigator must be cognizant of the many pitfalls associated with the interpretation of environmental data. Therefore, as part of the investigation planning, it is important to establish parameters for interpreting collected data.*

IV. ENVIRONMENTAL EMERGENCIES AND REMEDIATION

Environmental emergencies may occur during construction disruptions; when they occur, timely IC con-

*References 5, 6, 23, 25, 27–29, 38, 41, 45, 51–53, 56, 59, 70-75

sultation is critical. Practical applications of IC principles, generalized from experience in related industries, are offered here within stated limitations. In addition, other structural design issues which lack support if AIA Guidelines or scientific studies will be addressed.

Contamination of ventilation in surgical suites or other invasive areas

Sealing and air intakes. If nearby drilling or excavation occur during surgical activity, it is critical to check for tight room sealing to reduce the potential for air and water leakage. Because operating rooms usually have separate air handlers, the air intakes should be located to determine need for additional protection or sealing during periods of highest construction activity.[20–22,35,51,52]

Operating room ventilation and tuberculosis. AIA guidelines recommend bronchoscopy procedures be performed in treatment rooms meeting AII room ventilation requirements or in a space that exhausts directly to the outside. Optimum methods for managing patients with active tuberculosis requiring urgent surgical intervention have not yet been determined. However, the number of operating room air changes provides increased dilution of potential contaminants. NIOSH ventilation charts are included in the Centers for Disease Control and Prevention 1994 Guidelines and may assist in calculating percentages of particles removed by time and ventilation rates; this offers some guidance for the time needed to air a room, but the underlying assumptions need study as noted earlier.[39] Modifying the pressure relationships of the room to neutral or negative risks overall pressure imbalances, has not been studied for effectiveness, and is not recommended by the AIA.[19]

Air handlers, ducts, and filters. If air handlers are replaced, old ducts must be replaced or cleaned, and the issue should be treated as fundamental to the projected budget. Contaminated ducts have been implicated in outbreaks (eg, the operating room outbreak caused by *Penicillium* reported by Fox et al.[6] The American Society of Heating, Refrigerating, and Air Conditioning Engineers Inc is including language in HVAC system surface standards to prevent future duct lining problems.[40] Experiences vary, but it is important to clean ducts filled with debris observed during inspections, especially on the return air ducts. Hermann and Streifel recommend semiannual inspections of air-handling units for filter integrity.[75] However, definitive evidence specifying frequency of preventive cleaning is lacking.

Water contamination

Water contamination risks and prevention strategies are addressed in multiple sources.[20–23,57,65,76-77] IC should focus on maintaining a dynamic water flow that meets local standards. Water pressure "shock" may send a surge of debris when pressure loss is restored after a rupture.[78] Massive amounts of loosened scale may be released when domestic valves are returned to service after being off during construction or disruptions. If decontamination is necessary, systematic flushing of the water system assists in removing debris shaken loose by drilling or disruptions.

- *Legionella* sp: If testing is warranted because of high-risk populations and suspicion of *Legionella* sp exposure in the facility, major intervention methods should include chlorinating, hot water flushing, or copper-silver ionization treatment.[69,79-82] The last appears to have advantages over prior methods because of penetration of biofilms and reduced pipe corrosion; concerns for heavy metal (silver ions) accumulation remain and warrant additional study.[73,83]

- Fungus: Water seepage and damage are difficult to manage in an occupied building.[69] Reports of moisture/water sources leading to airborne spread of infectious agent(s) have been cited.[17,18,84] Several suggestions for detection and treatment are offered.[4,33,68] Prevention of fungal growth takes on increased importance after any type of flooding or utility failure related to water. Brace and Streifel have both published useful case studies and similar information is available from on-line sources.[33,34] Suggested cleanup protocols after water exposure are summarized here, but the basic approach is one of identifying moisture, followed by cleaning and thorough drying of surfaces.

General remediation procedure after water contamination. A systematized approach to prevent fungal growth in buildings caused by floods, roof leaks, sewage backup, steam leaks, and groundwater infiltration includes the following steps, modified according to the extent of damage sustained[33,34]:

- Inventory of water-damaged areas of the building, materials, and furnishings, paying particular attention to carpeting under cabinets and furnishings.

- Use of moisture meters (electronic wet test meter) to identify extent of water damage to drywall.

- Environmental sampling to monitor stages of cleanup and remediation.

- Removal of materials within 24-48 hours of water damage.

- Decontamination by spraying with chlorine-based mist or diluted bleach, followed by drying.

- Ventilation balancing to reduce supply air volume to effect a negative air pressure area, sealing off area with tape, and checking airflow with a smoke stick. Mobile HEPA machines may assist in providing the needed negative air balance in areas being remediated.

- Wall areas to be treated are identified and opened (eg, strip off vinyl covering) for drying.
- Decontamination of opened wall area is accomplished with 1:9 dilution of copper-8-quinolinolate compound, using a pressurized spray pump.[33,52]
- Remove surface soil with a detergent (eg, diluted tri-sodium phosphate), followed by use of a liquid disinfectant (eg, diluted bleach).
- Ceilings are vacuumed with a HEPA filtered vacuum cleaner. Walls and ceiling are closed and covered with standard wall finishing materials when the area is completely dry. Brace reported filling the spaces with aerosol foam; Streifel did not.[33,34]

Surfaces: design or disruption/damage issues

Design. Ideally, surfaces are designed to include cleanability; problems can be avoided if surfaces near plumbing fixtures are smooth, nonporous, and water-resistant.[19,85] Operating and delivery rooms, isolation and sterile processing areas also need smooth finishes, free of fissures or open joints and crevices that retain or permit passage of dirt particles. After disruptions, care should be taken to note penetrations (ducts, pipes), with attention to proper replacement, including tight seals.[19-23]

Flooding accidents. Cleaning and decontamination are required for major leaks occurring from the outside, such as broken pipes containing potable water or sprinkler water systems with added chemicals (ethylene glycol). Specific suggestions are itemized below for ceilings, walls, floors, and carpeting.

Ceiling tiles/porous materials. Water leaks or floods that wet acoustical ceiling tiles or fireproofing and filter materials may produce reservoirs of fungal spores.[1,32,34,52]

- If major water damage has occurred and porous tiles were not removed within 24-48 hours, tiles should be discarded/replaced.
- If tiles are nonporous, or if moisture is a result of small steam leaks, tiles can be cleaned with dilute bleach and air dried before replacement.[33]

Walls. When replacement options exist, the ICP should consider that smooth paint surfaces are easier for cleaning.[19,85] (The potential for antimicrobial effects present in copper paints has been published.[86] However, concerns for unknown efficacy and potential long-term toxicity have yet to be characterized and validated before efficacy can be established.[87]) Vinyl wall coverings risk moisture problems from condensation and have potential for fungal growth on the substrate. Wall cleaning under different conditions is based on the protocol described earlier:

- Water damage addressed in less than 24 hours: Vinyl-covered drywall laths/plaster/plasterboard should be stripped and examined. Portions of drywall may need to be removed to determine the extent of damage with a moisture meter. In some cases, especially if minor water damage was sustained, only minimal cleaning may be required.
- Water damage not addressed within 24–48 hours: If major flooding has occurred and material has not been removed within 24–28 hours, there is increasing probability that damage has already led to microbial growth, and more extensive effort may be required.
- Removal should be done under controlled conditions (area sealed off and removal done under negative air pressure).
- Water-soaked areas should be removed approximately 12 in above water mark and discarded, while allowing opened areas to dry.
- Hard surfaces are cleaned with diluted bleach solution without rinsing.
- Area may be sprayed from top to bottom with a dilution of copper-8-quinolinolate compound.[33,34,52]
- Wall is sealed and finished with standard materials after installing new 12 in wall piece.[33,34]

Floors. Desirable features include surfaces easily cleaned and wear-resistant according to usage. For example, if the floor is subject to frequent wet-cleaning methods, it should not be physically affected by germicidal disinfectants. Floor surfaces subject to traffic when wet (eg, kitchens) should have nonslip surfaces and be resistant to food acids (to avoid discoloration), and the perimeters should be tightly sealed.[20,21,85] After water disruptions, the perimeter should be closely examined for signs of long-standing moisture and possible fungus contamination.

Carpeting. Esthetic considerations related to stains and odor control support recommendations to avoid carpeting in areas of frequent spillage or heavy contamination; however, carpets have not generally been associated with nosocomial infection.[88-90] Carpets require regular vacuuming, shampooing, or extraction depending on use, material, and degree of soiling; cleaning should follow manufacturers' directions for proper cleaning materials, dilution (due to potential for discoloration), and frequency of cleaning techniques.[55,88] Contamination of carpeting after saturation with water or during demolition has been reported as a reservoir for nosocomial fungal infection.[9,91]

- Major damage from flooding: Carpeting and padding exposed to sewage should be discarded and the area disinfected with diluted bleach. If it is wet from steam or water leaks for greater than 24-48 hours, it is potentially already contaminated with fungi and may need to be discarded. If it is wet from steam or potable water leaks, but for *less than 24–48 hours*, protocols require cleaning and disinfection principles similar to those described earlier:

- Remove furniture, extract with water, shampoo with diluted surfactant/detergent.
- Soak with diluted bleach solution (1:10); rinse and extract with clean water to remove bleach; commercial steam cleaning is an alternative to bleach.
- Dry within 12–24 hours of treatment using floor or exhaust fans to aid in drying.[33]

Furnishings, fixtures, and equipment

Furniture. Modular furniture not easily moved should be installed on raised platforms or suspended in some manner to achieve a minimum 6-in to 12-in clearance from the floor to pull out for cleaning or to clean underneath. Attention must be paid to storage units with electrical or computer connections.[85]

Upholstered furniture should be treated the same as carpeting (including disposal) in the event of major soaking and contamination as a result of floods, leaks, or sewage. If it is affected by only steam moisture, it can be dried. Hardwood with intact laminate can be cleaned and disinfected with dilute bleach. If laminated furniture that has exposed particle board beneath the surface or other furniture composed of pressed wood or chip board becomes soaked, it should be discarded.[33]

Handwashing facilities/sinks. This section merits consideration primarily for design and cleaning issues; but plumbing disruptions or lack of preventive maintenance pose risks of contamination as well.

- Number and design: AIA Guidelines for new construction recommend the minimum number of handwashing facilities for patient rooms as one in the toilet room; they recommend handwashing facilities in the patient room only when the toilet room serves more than 2 beds.[19] Having a sink in a patient/resident room and in the toilet room (whether private or shared) supports essential IC practices. Whereas there is support for the ideal, IC plays a critical role in recommending proper placement of handwash facilities, and in both rooms.[85] In addition, IC support for a sink standard of minimum dimensions may prevent installation of small "cup" sinks that challenge proper handwashing.[85] AIA guidelines describe permissible types of controls for handwashing facilities in various areas.[19,21]
- Placement: Improper placement can add to the environmental reservoir of contaminants. Sinks need to be convenient and accessible, but nearby surfaces should also be nonporous to resist fungal growth.[33,85] One source recommends a minimum

distance of 15 ft from all inpatient beds/bassinets and 25 ft from outpatient chairs, stretcher, and treatment areas to ensure access.[85] Handwashing facilities should also be situated to avoid splashing (suggesting at least 36 in from patients or clean supplies), or equipped with a splash guard to avoid splash contamination.[85]

- Cabinets: Areas beneath sinks should not be considered storage areas due to proximity to sanitary sewer connections and risk of leaks or water damage. Clean or sterile patient items should be not be placed beneath sanitary sewer pipe connections or stored with soiled items; cleaning materials are the only items acceptable to be stored under sinks, from a regulatory aspect.[85] Facilities may develop design standards excluding storage space beneath sinks, thus preventing misuse and need for cleaning. As noted earlier, cabinet construction materials need to be nonporous to resist fungal growth.
- Aerators: Aerated sink faucets located near patients, particularly in intensive care units, may be a risk because of their ability to enhance growth of waterborne microorganisms. The faucet aerator has been identified as a reservoir and possible source of infection within the hospital. Rutala notes that the most convincing evidence for the role of faucet aerators is provided by Fierer et al (1967). In this study, premature infants became infected with *Pseudomonas aeruginosa* from delivery room resuscitation equipment contaminated by a faucet aerator.[87] Rutala concludes that the degree of importance of aerators as reservoirs for nosocomial pathogens remains unknown. Because *Legionella* sp grow well in the sediment formed in aerators, Freije recommends aerator removal.[50] Proper sink design and dimensions can reduce splashing and risks of general contamination, while eliminating concerns for aerators completely.

Flush sinks/hoppers. Clinical sinks are frequently located in soiled utility rooms for disposal of body fluids and liquids but warrant similar considerations for moisture and contamination.[92] Splash guards are valuable but inclusion may depend on sink usage and design. If staff members are not routinely required to use face protectors, a splash guard should be required.

Whirlpool or spa-like (Jacuzzi) bathing facilities. Various types of bathing facilities are now available for mothers in birthing rooms; recommendations for cleaning have been compared with hydrotherapy tanks and equipment cleaning procedures.[93] However, plumbing for Jacuzzi tubs or similar spa-like tubs have longer piping with higher siphons, resulting in risks for trapped contaminated water after apparent draining;

AJIC
April 2000

the trapped water may be flushed into the tub with its next use. Communication with state regulators, cleaning and disinfecting the tub and jets with specific spa-cleaning products, and proper draining and flushing sequences are essential when considering installation.[92-95]

Eyewash stations. OSHA directs proper use and placement of eyewash stations with distance determined by the pH of the involved chemicals. Source water in stationary eyewash stations may stand unused in the incoming pipes at room temperature for long periods, providing a reservoir for potential pathogens.[87] After a report of Acanthamoeba in eyewash stations, OSHA issued a bulletin recommending cleaning and disinfection methods.[96] The schedule follows the American National Standards Institute Z358-1981 recommendations for flushing the system 3 minutes each week.[44]

Placement of sharps containers. Location of disposal containers should consider ease of visibility to avoid overfilling and should be within easy horizontal reach of the user. Systems should have secure locking and enable easy replacement. When containers are fixed to a wall, the vertical height should allow the worker to view the opening or access the container. NIOSH recommendations suggest ergonomic considerations for installation heights or creative approaches for specialty areas.[97] Sufficient temporary storage space for filled containers must be in design planning.[47,92]

V. RESEARCH NEEDS

The role of IC continues to expand and interacts closely with safety and occupational health functions. Studies from indoor air quality research have an increasing impact on current practice. Industrial experiences continue to be evaluated for health care facility application. Some items identified throughout the text but not yet resolved are summarized below and offered for consideration:

- Surgical suite contamination: Many issues remain unanswered and require further study including the effectiveness of laminar air flow, ultraviolet germicidal irradiation, and the approach to managing *Mycobacterium tuberculosis* or other airborne pathogens in the operating room. Designs of future operating rooms to control all sources of environmental contamination are being studied in current IAQ building research.[98]
- Surgical suite air handling systems: Certification and recertification requirements for operating room air handling systems remain unresolved. Frequency of testing HEPA filters, systems, and air pressure balancing for operating rooms has not been determined or recommended.

- Ambulatory care sites: There is a need to identify optimal engineering controls for current ambulatory care surgery settings to improve outcomes; there is also need for further delineation of the role of mobile HEPA units, UVGI, etc, in clinics and non-traditional care settings, especially for highly susceptible, ambulatory patients.
- Fans: Concerns have been raised regarding use of fans in patient care areas. No studies or regulations have directly addressed this issue in terms of infection risk(s).
- Aerators: The degree of risk associated with aerator installation has not yet been determined and may be resolved by examining other methods of water purification or sink design.
- Plumbing and preventive maintenance systems: Better methods to reduce or eliminate *Legionella* sp. contamination in potable water systems continue to be sought. In the setting of continued low-level contamination, determination of the dose-response relationship from potable water exposures resulting in disease remains elusive. This remains key to preventive water system treatments, as well for clearer indications for environmental surveillance cultures.
- Role and methods of air monitoring: A number of major issues need clarification including (1) determination of electronic versus other sampling methodologies, and (2) need for standards and guidelines for sampling designs according to circumstances and related methodologies (eg, total particulate versus bioparticulates). The development of standards for certain patient care areas needs correlation to disease outcomes.
- Efficacy of remediation protocols: Controlled studies on the efficacy and safety of current or newer antifungal treatments after severe water damage are needed. Clearer determinations regarding the safety of damaged drywall left in place, versus its removal, needs further elaboration. Other studies are needed to determine the efficacy and safety of other types of materials for remediation.
- Ventilation and pressure relationships: Whereas the need for negative air pressure is clear, new studies are needed to determine the ideal room pressure differential related to actual infectious agent transmission and risk for developing actual disease. This is an area beginning to be addressed.[99]

In conclusion, the role of IC/epidemiology in construction and renovation remains a challenging and exciting one and is the ultimate demonstration of its multidisciplinary nature. Interaction and integration of efforts with other disciplines enables disease prevention for patients and health care workers to remain the focus and driving force during construction/renovation processes.

References

1. Aisner J, Schimpff SC, Bennett JE, Young MV, Wirnik PH. *Aspergillus* infections in cancer patients: association with fireproofing materials in a new hospital. JAMA 1976;235:411–12.

2. Lentino JR, Rosenkranz MA, Michaels JA, Kurup VP, Rose HD, Rytel MW. Nosocomial aspergillosis: a retrospective review of airborne disease secondary to road construction and contaminated air conditioners. Am J Epidemiol 1982;116:430–7.

3. Krasinski K, Holzman RS, Hanna B, Greco MA, Graff M, Bhogal M. Nosocomial fungal infection during hospital renovation. Infect Control Hosp Epidemiol 1985;6:278–82.

4. Streifel AJ, Stevens PP, Rhame FS. In-hospital source of airborne *Penicillium* species spores. J Clin Microbiol 1987;25:1–4.

5. Weems JJ Jr, Davis BJ, Tablan OC, Kaufman L, Martone WJ. Construction activity: an independent risk factor for invasive aspergillosis and zygomycosis in patients with hematologic malignancy. Infect Control 1987;8:71–5.

6. Fox BC, Chamberlin L, Kulich P, Rae EJ, Webster LR. Heavy contamination of operating room air by *Penicillium* species: identification of the source and attempts at decontamination. AJIC Am J Infect Control 1990;18:300–6.

7. Arnow PM, Sadigh MC, Weil D, Chudy R. Endemic and epidemic aspergillosis associated with in-hospital replication of *Aspergillus* organisms. J Infect Dis 1991 Nov;164:998–1002.

8. Flynn PM, Williams BG, Hethrington SV, Williams BF, Giannini MA, Pearson TA. *Aspergillus terreus* during hospital renovation [letter]. Infect Control Hosp Epidemiol 1993;14:363–5.

9. Gerson SL, Parker P, Jacobs MR, Creger R, Lazarus HM. Aspergillosis due to carpet contamination [letter]. Infect Control Hosp Epidemiol 1994;15:221–3.

10. Alvarez M, Lopez Ponga B, Raon C, Garcia Gala J, Porto MC, Gonzales M, et al. Nosocomial outbreak caused by *Scedosporium prolificans (inflatum)*: four fatal cases in leukemic patients. J Clin Microbiol 1995;33;3290–5.

11. Pittet D, Huguenin T, Dharan S, Sztajzel-Boissard J, Ducel G, Thorens JB, et al. Unusual case of lethal pulmonary aspergillosis in patients with chronic obstructive pulmonary disease. Am J Respir Crit Care Med 1996;154(2 Pt1):541–4.

12. Haley CE, Cohen ML, Halter J, Meyer RD. Nosocomial legionnaires' disease: a continuing common-source epidemic at Wadsworth Medical Center [abstract]. Ann Intern Med 1979;90:583–6.

13. Dondero TJ Jr, Rendtorff RC, Mallison GF, Weeks RM, Levy JS, Wong EW, et al. An outbreak of legionnaires' disease associated with a contaminated air-conditioning cooling tower. N Engl J Med;302:365–70.

14. Crane LC, Tagle LC, Palutke WA. Outbreak of *Pseudomonas paucimobilis* in an intensive care facility. JAMA 1981;246:985–7.

15. Claesson BEB, Claesson UL-E. An outbreak of endometritis in a maternity unit caused by spread of group A streptococci from a showerhead. J Hosp Infect 1995;6:304–11.

16. Sniadeck DH, Ostroff SM, Karlix MA, Smithwick RW, Schwartz B, Sprauer MA, et al. Nosocomial pseudo-outbreak of *Mycobacterium xenopi* due to contaminated potable water supply: lessons in prevention. Infect Control Hosp Epidemiol 1993;14:637–41.

17. Dearborn DG, Infeld MD, Smith PG, Brooks LJ, Carroll-Pankhurst DC, Kosik R, et al. Update: pulmonary hemorrhage/hemosiderosis among infants. MMWR Morb Mortal Wkly Rep 1997;46(2)33–5.

18. Fridkin SK, Kremer FB, Bland LA, Padhye A, McNeil MM, Jarvis WR. *Acremonium kiliense* endophthalmitis that occurred after

cataract extraction in an ambulatory surgical center and as traced to an environmental reservoir. Clin Infect Dis 1996;22:222–7.

19. American Institute of Architects Academy of Architecture for Health. 1996–1997 guidelines for design and construction of hospitals and healthcare facilities. Washington (DC): The American Institute for Architects Press; 1996.

20. Bartley J. Air (HVAC/Laminar Flow). In: Olmsted R, editor. APIC: infection control and applied epidemiology: principles and practice. 1996. St Louis (MO): Mosby; 1996. p. 103:1–9.

21. Bartley J. Construction. In: Olmsted R, editor. APIC: infection control and applied epidemiology: principles and practice. 1996. St Louis (MO): Mosby; 1996. p. 104:1–6.

22. Streifel AJ. Maintenance and engineering; biomedical engineering. In: Olmsted R, editor. APIC: infection control and applied epidemiology: principles and practice. 1996. St Louis (MO): Mosby; 1996. p. 111:1–7.

23. Bartley J. Water. In: Olmsted R, editor. APIC: infection control and applied epidemiology: principles and practice. 1996. St Louis (MO): Mosby; 1996. p. 118:1–4.

24. McDonald L. Regulatory/accrediting/guideline setting agencies. In: Olmsted R, editor. APIC: infection control and applied epidemiology: principles and practice. 1996. St Louis (MO): Mosby; 1996. p. 121:1–4.

25. Haberstich N. Prevention of infection during major construction and renovation in the surgery department of a large hospital. AJIC Am J Infect Control 1987;15:36A–38A.

26. Carter CD, Barr BA. Infection control issues in construction and renovation. Infect Control Hosp Epidemiol 1997;18:587–96.

27. Turner G, Sumner R, Ornelas L, Martin M. Controlling construction dust in the hospital environment; a quality improvement project [abstract]. AJIC Am J Infect Control 1995;23:115.

28. Brown S, Detzler L, Myers J, Swift S. The impact of environmental controls and air quality monitoring on surgical site infection rates during operating room construction [abstract]. AJIC Am J Infect Control 1996;24:140.

29. Gartner K, Blank M, Volosky R. Keeping the air clean—lessons from a construction project [abstract]. AJIC Am J Infect Control 1996;24:111.

30. Kennedy V, Barnard B, Hackett B. Use of a risk matrix to determine level of barrier protection during construction activities [abstract]. AJIC Am J Infect Control 1996;24:111.

31. Kennedy V, Barnard B, Hackett B. Use of a risk matrix to determine level of barrier protection during construction activities. Hosp Infect Control 1997;2:27–8.

32. Harvey MA, Critical care-unit bedside design and furnishing: impact on nosocomial infections. Infect Control Hosp Epidemiol 1998;19:597–601.

33. University of Minnesota Extension Service, University of Minnesota Building Research Consortium, IAQ Project, Department Env. Health and Safety. Health Care Construction and IAQ, Minneapolis (MN): Sept 15–16, 1997. Components available from: URL: *http://www.dehs.umn.edu/*.

34. Brace SE. Infection control during construction: planning is key. Healthcare Facilities Management Series (#094300). Chicago (IL): ASHE of American Hospital Association; 1993.

35. Bartley J. Environmental control: operating room air quality. Today's OR Nurse 1993;15:11–7.

36. American Society of Heating, Refrigerating and Air Conditioning Engineers. Systems and equipment handbook. Air cleaners for particulate contaminants. Atlanta (GA): ASHRAE Inc; 1996. p. 24.9–24.11.

37. Health Care Finance Administration. Medicare and Medicaid programs; hospital conditions of participation 1986. Baltimore (MD): Department of Health and Human Services; 1986.

38. Tablan OC, Anderson LJ, Arden NH, Butler BR, McNeil MM, the

Back to: Contents Page

Bacterial Pneumonia

Part I. Issues On Prevention Of Nosocomial Pneumonia, 1994

I. Etiologic Agents

The reported distribution of etiologic agents causing nosocomial pneumonia varies between hospitals because of differences in patient populations and diagnostic methods employed.(2-10) In general, however, bacteria have been the most frequently isolated pathogens.(2-6,9,11-13) Schaberg et al reported that in 1986-1989, aerobic bacteria comprised at least 73%, and fungi 4%, of isolates from sputum and tracheal aspirates from pneumonia patients at the University of Michigan Hospitals and hospitals participating in the National Nosocomial Infection Surveillance System (NNIS); very few anaerobic bacteria and no viruses were reported, probably because anaerobic and viral cultures were not performed routinely in the reporting hospitals (Table 1).(3) Similarly, cultures of bronchoscopic specimens from mechanically ventilated patients with pneumonia have rarely yielded anaerobes.(5-7,9,11,14,15) Only the report by Bartlett, which was based mainly on cultures of transtracheal aspirates from patients not receiving mechanically assisted ventilation, showed a predominance of anaerobes.

Nosocomial bacterial pneumonias are frequently polymicrobial,(4,7,9,11,12,15-19) and gram-negative bacilli are the usual predominant organisms (Table 1).(2-6,9,11-13) However, *Staphylococcus aureus* (especially methicillin-resistant *S. aureus*)(5,7,10,15,20,21) and other gram-positive cocci, including *Streptococcus pneumoniae*,(5,7) have recently emerged as significant isolates.(14) In addition, *Haemophilus influenza* has been isolated from mechanically ventilated patients with pneumonia that occurs within 48-96 hours after intubation.(3-5,12,15,22) In NNIS hospitals, *Pseudomonas aeruginosa, Enterobacter* sp., *Klebsiella pneumoniae, Escherichia coli, Serratia marcescens*, and *Proteus* spp. comprised 50% of the isolates from cultures of respiratory tract specimens from patients for whom nosocomial pneumonia was diagnosed by using clinical criteria; *S. aureus* accounted for 16%, and *H. influenzae*, for 6% (Table 1).(3) Fagon and co-workers reported that gram-negative bacilli were present in 75% of quantitative cultures of protected-specimen brushings (PSB) from patients who had received mechanically assisted ventilation and acquired nosocomial pneumonia; 40% of the cultures were polymicrobial.(5) In the report by Torres et al, 20% of pathogens recovered from cultures of PSB, blood, pleural fluid, or percutaneous lung aspirate were gram-negative bacilli in pure culture, and 17% were polymicrobial; however, 54% of specimens did not yield any microorganism, probably because of receipt of antibiotics by patients.(6)

II. Diagnosis

Nosocomial bacterial pneumonia has been difficult to diagnose.(7,8,16,23-32) Frequently, the criteria for diagnosis have been fever, cough, and development of purulent sputum, in combination with radiologic evidence of a new or progressive pulmonary infiltrate, a suggestive Gram's stain, and cultures of sputum, tracheal aspirate, pleural fluid, or blood.(3,4,23,25,33-36) Although clinical criteria together with cultures of sputum or tracheal specimens may be sensitive for bacterial pathogens, they are highly nonspecific, especially in patients with mechanically assisted ventilation;(8,9,12-15,18,24-26,39,31,37-42) on the other hand, cultures of blood or pleural fluid have very low sensitivity.(8,18,19,43)

Because of these problems, a group of investigators recently formulated consensus recommendations for standardization of methods to diagnose pneumonia in clinical research studies of ventilator-associated pneumonia.(44-46) These methods involve bronchoscopic techniques, e.g., quantitative culture of PSB,(5,7-9,13,15,27,31,38,41,47,48) bronchoalveolar lavage (BAL),(7,12,41,447,49-54) and protected BAL (pBAL).(14) The reported sensitivities and specificities of these methods have ranged between 70% to 100% and 60% to 100%, respectively, depending on the tests or diagnostic criteria they were compared with. Because these techniques are invasive, they may cause complications such as hypoxemia, bleeding, or arrhythmia.(8,13,42,44,52,55,56) In addition, the sensitivity of the PSB procedure may decrease for patients receiving antibiotic therapy.(9,13,27) Nonbronchoscopic (NB) procedures, e.g., NB-pBAL(12,27,57,58) or NB-PSB,(13) which utilize blind catheterization of the distal airways, and quantitative culture of endotracheal aspirate,(59,60) have been developed recently. Of these, endotracheal aspirate culture appears to be the most practical. The use of these bronchoscopic and nonbronchoscopic diagnostic tests can be a major step in better defining the epidemiology of nosocomial pneumonia, especially in patients with mechanically assisted ventilation; however, further studies are needed to determine each test's applicability in daily clinical practice.

III. Epidemiology

NNIS reports that pneumonias (diagnosed on the basis of the CDC surveillance definition of nosocomial pneumonia) account for

http://www.cdc.gov/ncidod/hip/pneumonia/1_bactpn.htm

approximately 15% of all hospital-associated infections and are the second most common nosocomial infections after those of the urinary tract.(2,61) In 1984, the overall incidence of lower respiratory tract infection was 6 per 1,000 discharged patients.(2) The incidence per 1,000 discharged patients ranged from 4.2 in nonteaching to 7.7 in university-affiliated hospitals, probably reflecting institutional differences in the level of patients' risk for acquiring nosocomial pneumonia.

Nosocomial bacterial pneumonia often has been identified as a postoperative infection.(62,63) In the Study of the Efficacy of Nosocomial Infection Control in the 1970s, 75% of reported cases of nosocomial bacterial pneumonia occurred in patients who had had a surgical operation; the risk was 38 times greater for thoracoabdominal procedures than for those involving other body sites.(63) More recent epidemiologic studies, including NNIS studies, have identified other subsets of patients at high risk of developing nosocomial bacterial pneumonia: patients with endotracheal intubation and/or mechanically assisted ventilation, depressed level of consciousness (particularly those with closed-head injury), prior episode of a large-volume aspiration, or underlying chronic lung disease, and patients >70 years of age. Other risk factors include 24-hour ventilator-circuit changes, fall-winter season, stress-bleeding prophylaxis with cimetidine with or without antacid, administration of antimicrobials, presence of a nasogastric tube, severe trauma, and recent bronchoscopy.(6,34,35,64-74)

Recently, NNIS stratified the incidence density of nosocomial pneumonia by patients' use of mechanical ventilator and type of intensive care unit (ICU). From 1986 to 1990, the median rate of ventilator-associated pneumonia per 1,000 ventilator-days ranged from 4.7 in pediatric ICUs to 34.4 in burn ICUs.(66) In contrast, the median rate of nonventilator-associated pneumonia per 1000 ICU-days ranged from 0 in pediatric and respiratory ICUs to 3.2 in trauma ICUs.

Nosocomial pneumonia has been associated with high fatality rates. Crude mortality rates of 20%-50% and attributable mortality rates of 30%-33% have been reported; in one study, pneumonia comprised 60% of all deaths due to nosocomial infections.(17,35,74-80) Patients receiving mechanically assisted ventilation have higher mortality rates than do patients not receiving ventilation support; however, other factors, such as a patient's underlying disease(s) and organ failure, are stronger predictors of death in patients with pneumonia.(34,74)

Analyses of pneumonia-associated morbidity have shown that pneumonia could prolong hospitalization by 4-9 days.(79-83) A conservative estimate of the direct cost of excess hospital stay due to pneumonia is $1.2 billion a year for the nation.(83) Because of its reported frequency, associated high fatality rate, and attendant costs, nosocomial pneumonia is a major infection control problem.

IV. Pathogenesis

Bacteria may invade the lower respiratory tract by aspiration of oropharyngeal organisms, inhalation of aerosols containing bacteria, or, less frequently, by hematogenous spread from a distant body site. In addition, bacterial translocation from the gastrointestinal tract has been recently hypothesized as a mechanism for infection. Of these routes, aspiration is believed to be the most important for both nosocomial and community-acquired pneumonia.

In radioisotope-tracer studies, 45% of healthy adults were found to aspirate during sleep.(84) Persons with abnormal swallowing, such as those who have depressed consciousness, respiratory tract instrumentation and/or mechanically assisted ventilation, or gastrointestinal tract instrumentation or diseases, or who have just undergone surgery, are particularly likely to aspirate.(6,34,35,63,85-87)

The high incidence of gram-negative bacillary pneumonia in hospitalized patients appears to be the result of factors that promote colonization of the pharynx by gram-negative bacilli and the subsequent entry of these organisms into the lower respiratory tract.(33,88-91) Whereas aerobic gram-negative bacilli are recovered infrequently or are found in small numbers in pharyngeal cultures of healthy persons, (88,92) colonization dramatically increases in patients with coma, hypotension, acidosis, azotemia, alcoholism, diabetes mellitus, leukocytosis, leukopenia, pulmonary disease, or nasogastric or endotracheal tubes in place, and in patients given antimicrobial agents. (33,91,93,94)

Oropharyngeal or tracheobronchial colonization by gram-negative bacilli begins with the adherence of the microorganisms to the host's epithelial cells.(90,95-97) Adherence may be affected by multiple factors related to the bacteria (presence of pili, cilia, capsule, or production of elastase or mucinase), host cell (surface proteins and polysaccharides), and environment (pH and presence of mucin in respiratory secretions).(89,90,95,98-107) The exact interactions among these factors have not been fully elucidated, but studies indicate that certain substances, such as fibronectin, can inhibit the adherence of gram-negative bacilli to host cells.(98,100,108) Conversely, certain conditions, such as malnutrition, severe illness, or post-operative state, can increase adherence of gram-negative bacteria. (89,98,102,107,109)

Besides the oropharynx, the stomach has been postulated to be an important reservoir of organisms that cause nosocomial pneumonia. (34,110-114) The stomach's role may vary depending on the patient's underlying conditions and on prophylactic or therapeutic interventions.(22,111,115-118) In healthy persons, few bacteria entering the stomach survive in the presence of hydrochloric acid at pH<2. (119,120) However, when gastric pH increases from the normal levels to ≥4, microorganisms are able to multiply to high concentrations in the stomach.(117,119,121-123) This can occur in patients with advanced age,(121) achlorhydria,(119) ileus, or upper gastrointestinal disease, and in patients receiving enteral feeding, antacids, or histamine-2 H-2 antagonists.(111,117,118,123-125) The contribution of other factors, such as duodeno-gastric reflux and the presence of bile, to gastric colonization in patients with impaired intestinal motility has been suggested and needs further investigation.(116)

http://www.cdc.gov/ncidod/hip/pneumonia/1_bactpn.htm

Bacteria can also gain entry into the lower respiratory tract of hospitalized patients through inhalation of aerosols generated primarily by contaminated respiratory-therapy or anesthesia-breathing equipment.(126-129) Outbreaks related to the use of respiratory-therapy equipment have been associated with contaminated nebulizers, which are humidification devices that produce large amounts of aerosol droplets <4μm via ultrasound, spinning disk, or the Venturi mechanism.(126,129,130) When the fluid in the reservoir of a nebulizer becomes contaminated with bacteria, the aerosol produced may contain high concentrations of bacteria that can be deposited deep in the patient's lower respiratory tract.(126,130,131) Because endotracheal and tracheal tubes provide direct access to the lower respiratory tract, contaminated aerosol inhalation is particularly hazardous for intubated patients. In contrast to nebulizers, bubble-through or wick humidifiers mainly increase the water-vapor (or molecular-water) content of inspired gases. Although heated bubble-through humidifiers generate aerosol droplets, they do so in quantities that may not be clinically significant;(127,132) wick humidifiers do not generate aerosols.

Rarely, bacterial pneumonia can result from hematogenous spread of infection to the lung from another infection site, e.g., pneumonia resulting from purulent phlebitis or right-sided endocarditis. Another mechanism, translocation of bacteria via the passage of viable bacteria from the lumen of the gastrointestinal tract through epithelial mucosa to the mesenteric lymph nodes and to the lung, has been shown in animal models.(133) Translocation is postulated to occur in patients with immunosuppression, cancer, or burns;(133) however data are lacking regarding this mechanism in humans.(134)

V. Risk Factors and Control Measures

Several large studies have examined potential risk factors for nosocomial bacterial pneumonia (Table 2).(6,34,35,135,136) Although specific risk factors may differ between study populations, they can be grouped into the following general categories: 1) host factors such as extremes of age and severe underlying conditions, including immunosuppression; 2) factors, such as administration of antimicrobials, admission to the ICU, underlying chronic lung disease, or coma, that enhance colonization of the oropharynx and/or stomach by microorganisms; 3) conditions favoring aspiration or reflux, including endotracheal intubation, insertion of nasogastric tube, or supine position; 4) conditions requiring prolonged use of mechanical ventilatory support with potential exposure to contaminated respiratory equipment and/or contact with contaminated or colonized hands of healthcare workers; and 5) factors that impede adequate pulmonary toilet, such as surgical procedures involving the head, neck, thorax, or upper abdomen, and immobilization due to trauma or illness.(6,33-35,62,73,74,135)

A. Oropharyngeal, Tracheal, and Gastric Colonization

The association between colonization of the oropharynx(88,137), trachea(138), or stomach(110,111,117,123) and predisposition to gram-negative bacillary pneumonia prompted attempts to prevent infection either by prophylactic local application of antimicrobial agent(s) (139,140) or by utilizing the phenomenon of local bacterial interference.(141,142) Although early work suggested that the former method, use of aerosolized antimicrobials, could eradicate common gram-negative pathogens from the upper respiratory tract,(138) superinfection occurred in some patients receiving this therapy.(139-141,143,144) The latter method, bacterial interference (with alpha-hemolytic streptococci), has been successfully used by some investigators to prevent oropharyngeal colonization by aerobic gram-negative bacilli. (141) However, the efficacy of this method for use in general has not been evaluated.

The administration of antacids and H-2 blockers for prevention of stress bleeding in critically ill, postoperative, and/or mechanically ventilated patients has been associated with gastric bacterial overgrowth in many studies.(34,112,113,118,122,123,145-147) Sucralfate, a cytoprotective agent that has little effect on gastric pH and may have bactericidal properties of its own, has been suggested as a potential substitute for antacids and H-2 blockers.(148-150) The results of clinical trials comparing the risk of pneumonia in patients receiving sucralfate to that in patients given antacids and/or H-2 blockers have been variable.(112,118,147,148,151-153) In most randomized trials, ICU patients receiving mechanically assisted ventilation and antacids with or without H-2 blockers had increased gastric pH, high bacterial counts in the gastric fluid, and increased risk of pneumonia compared with patients given sucralfate.(112,118,147,148,151) In one report with a large number of study patients, the incidence of early-onset pneumonia (occurring < or = 4 days after intubation) did not differ between patient groups, but late-onset pneumonia occurred in 5% of 76 patients who received sucralfate, 16% of 69 given antacids, and 21% of 68 who received an H-2 blocker.(147) On the other hand, a meta-analysis of data from eight earlier studies (154) and a later study comparing sucralfate with ranitidine(153) did not show a strong association between nosocomial pneumonia and drugs that raise gastric pH. Further comparative studies are underway in which bronchoscopy with PSB or BAL is utilized for the diagnosis of pneumonia.

Selective decontamination of the digestive tract (SDD) is another strategy designed to prevent bacterial colonization and lower respiratory tract infection in mechanically ventilated patients.(155-179) SDD is aimed at preventing oropharyngeal and gastric colonization with aerobic gram-negative bacilli and *Candida* spp., without altering the anaerobic flora (Table 3). A variety of SDD regimens use a combination of locally administered nonabsorbable antibiotic agents such as polymyxin and an aminoglycoside (tobramycin, gentamicin, or, rarely, neomycin), or a quinolone (norfloxacin or ciprofloxacin), coupled with either amphotericin B or nystatin. The local antimicrobial preparation is applied as a paste to the oropharynx and given orally or via the nasogastric tube four times a day. In addition, in many studies, a systemic (intravenous) antimicrobial such as cefotaxime or trimethoprim is administered to the patient.

While most clinical trials,(155-158,160-167,169,170,175-177) including two meta-analyses,(171,178) of SDD have demonstrated a decrease in the rates of nosocomial respiratory infections, these trials have been difficult to assess because they have differed in study design and population, and many have had short follow-up periods (Table 3). In most of these studies, the diagnosis of pneumonia was based on clinical criteria; bronchoscopy with BAL or PSB was used in only a few studies.(159,162,173,175-177,179)

Two recently published large double-blind, placebo-controlled trials demonstrated no benefit from SDD.(173,174) In one, a large French multicenter study by Gastinne et al, a significant decrease in incidence of gram-negative bacillary pneumonia was not accompanied by a decrease in pneumonia from all causes.(173) In the other study, by Hammond et al, no differences were noted between patients randomized to SDD or to placebo; however, both patient groups received intravenous cefotaxime.(174)

Although an earlier meta-analysis suggested a trend toward decreased mortality in patients given SDD,(171) a more recent and more extensive analysis highlights the equivocal effect of SDD on patient mortality, as well as the high cost of using SDD to prevent pneumonia or death (i.e., in order to prevent one case of nosocomial pneumonia, or one death due to nosocomial pneumonia, 6 [range: 5-9] or 23 [range: 13-39] patients, respectively, would have to be given SDD).(178) Furthermore, there are concerns over the development of antimicrobial resistance and superinfection with gram-positive bacteria and other antibiotic-resistant nosocomial pathogens. (156,158,159,161,175,180) Thus, currently available data do not justify the routine use of SDD for prevention of nosocomial pneumonia in ICU patients. SDD may be ultimately useful for specific subsets of ICU patients, such as those with trauma or severe immunosuppression, e.g., bone-marrow transplant recipients.

A new approach advocated to prevent oropharyngeal colonization in patients receiving enteral nutrition is to reduce bacterial colonization of the stomach by acidifying the enteral feed.(181) Although the absence of bacteria from the stomach has been confirmed in patients given acidified enteral feeding, the effect on the incidence of nosocomial pneumonia has not been evaluated.(181)

B. Aspiration of Oropharyngeal and Gastric Flora

Clinically significant aspiration usually occurs in patients who have one or more of the following conditions: a depressed level of consciousness, dysphagia due to neurologic or esophageal disorders, an endotracheal (naso- or oro-tracheal), tracheostomy, or enteral (naso- or oro-gastric) tube in place, and receipt of enteral feeding.(35,84,85,182-186) Placement of an enteral tube may increase nasopharyngeal colonization, cause reflux of gastric contents, or allow bacterial migration via the tube from the stomach to the upper airway.(183,186-188) When enteral feedings are administered, gross contamination of the enteral solution during preparation(189-191) and elevated gastric pH(70,192,193), may lead to gastric colonization with gram-negative bacilli. In addition, gastric reflux and aspiration may occur because of increased intragastric volume and pressure.(70,117,183)

Prevention of pneumonia in such patients may be difficult, but methods that make regurgitation less likely (for example, placing the patient in a semirecumbent position by elevating the head of the bed and withholding enteral feeding when the residual volume in the stomach is large or if bowel sounds are not heard upon auscultation of the abdomen) may be beneficial.(185,194-197) On the other hand, administering enteral nutrition intermittently in small boluses rather than continuously,(70,193) using flexible, small-bore enteral tubes, (186,198) or placing the enteral tube below the stomach (e.g., in the jejunum)(199,200) have yielded equivocal results.

C. Mechanically Assisted Ventilation and Endotracheal Intubation

Patients receiving continuous, mechanically assisted ventilation have 6-21 times the risk of developing nosocomial pneumonia compared with patients not receiving ventilatory support.(34,63,65,75) Data from the study by Fagon and co-workers indicate that the risk of developing ventilator-associated pneumonia increases by 1% per day.(5) This increased risk is partly due to carriage of oropharyngeal organisms upon passage of the endotracheal tube into the trachea during intubation, as well as to depressed host defenses secondary to the patient's severe underlying illness.(6,34,35,201) In addition, bacteria can aggregate on the surface of the tube over time and form a glycocalyx (biofilm) that protects the bacteria from the action of antimicrobial agents or host defenses.(202) Some investigators believe that these bacterial aggregates may become dislodged by ventilation flow, tube manipulation, or suctioning and subsequently embolize into the lower respiratory tract and cause focal pneumonia.(203,204) Removing tracheal secretions by gentle suctioning and using aseptic technique to reduce cross-contamination to patients from contaminated respiratory therapy equipment or contaminated or colonized hands of personnel have been utilized traditionally to help prevent pneumonia in patients receiving mechanically assisted ventilation.

The risk of pneumonia is also increased by the direct access of bacteria to the lower respiratory tract, often because of leakage around the endotracheal tube cuff,(86,205) which allows pooled secretions above the cuff to enter the trachea.(206) In one recent study, the occurrence of nosocomial pneumonia was delayed and decreased in intubated patients whose endotracheal tubes had a separate dorsal lumen that allowed drainage (by suctioning) of secretions in the space above the endotracheal tube cuff and below the glottis.(206) However, further studies are needed to determine the cost-benefit ratio of using this device.

D. Cross-Colonization Via Hands of Personnel

Pathogens causing nosocomial pneumonia, such as gram-negative bacilli and *Staphylococcus aureus*, are ubiquitous in the hospital, especially in intensive or critical care areas.(207,208) Transmission of these microorganisms to patients frequently occurs via healthcare workers' hands that become contaminated or transiently colonized with the microorganisms.(209-215) Procedures such as tracheal suctioning and manipulation of ventilator circuit or endotracheal tubes increase the opportunity for cross-contamination.(215,216) The risk of cross-contamination can be reduced by using aseptic technique and sterile or disinfected equipment when appropriate(65) and eliminating pathogens from the hands of personnel.(65,215,217-219)

In theory, adequate handwashing is an effective way of removing transient bacteria from the hands,(218,219) but personnel compliance with handwashing has been generally poor.(220-223) For this reason, the routine use of gloves has been advocated to help prevent cross-contamination.(224,225) Routine gloving (in addition to gowning) was associated with a decrease in the incidence of nosocomial respiratory syncytial virus (RSV)(226) and other ICU infections.(228) However, nosocomial pathogens can colonize gloves(228) and outbreaks have been traced to healthcare workers who did not change gloves after contact with one patient and before providing care to another.(229,230) In addition, gloved hands may get contaminated via leaks in the gloves.(231)

E. Contamination of Devices Used on the Respiratory Tract

Devices used on the respiratory tract for respiratory therapy (e.g., nebulizer), diagnostic examination (e.g., bronchoscope or spirometer), or administration of anesthesia are potential reservoirs or vehicles for infectious microorganisms.(65,232-236) Routes of transmission may be from device to patient,(127,129,234-244) from one patient to another,(245,246) or from one body site to the lower respiratory tract of the same patient via hand or device.(233,246-248) Contaminated reservoirs of aerosol-producing devices, e.g., nebulizers, can allow the growth of hydrophilic bacteria that may be subsequently aerosolized during device use.(126,129,130,242) Gram-negative bacilli such as *Pseudomonas* spp., *Xanthomonas* spp., *Flavobacterium* spp., *Legionella* spp., and nontuberculous mycobacteria can multiply to substantial concentrations in nebulizer fluid(241,249-251) and increase the device-user's risk of acquiring pneumonia.(127-130,241,242,252,253)

Proper cleaning and sterilization or disinfection of reusable equipment are important components of a program to reduce infections associated with respiratory therapy and anesthesia equipment.(234,235,237-240,242,254-259) Many devices or parts of devices used on the respiratory tract have been categorized as semicritical in the Spaulding classification system for appropriate sterilization or disinfection of medical devices because they come into direct or indirect contact with mucous membranes but do not ordinarily penetrate body surfaces (See Appendix A), and the associated infection risk following the use of these devices in patients is less than that associated with devices that penetrate normally sterile tissues.(260) Thus, if it is not possible or cost-effective to sterilize these devices by steam autoclave or ethylene oxide,(261) they can be subjected to high-level disinfection by pasteurization at 75ş for 30 min,(262-265) or by using liquid chemical disinfectants approved by the Environmental Protection Agency (EPA) as sterilants/disinfectants and cleared for marketing for use on medical instruments by the Food and Drug Administration.(225,266-268)

When rinsing is needed (to remove residual liquid chemical sterilant/disinfectant) after a respiratory device has been chemically disinfected, sterile water has been preferred because tap or locally prepared distilled water may harbor microorganisms that can cause pneumonia.(249,250,269-272) In some hospitals, a tap-water rinse followed by air-drying with or without an alcohol rinse (to hasten drying) is used.(273) In theory, if complete drying is achieved following a tap-water rinse, the risk of nosocomial pneumonia associated with the use of the device is probably low. Drying has been shown to lower the level of microbial contamination of gastrointestinal endoscopes and washed hands.(274-276) However, many semicritical items used on the respiratory tract (e.g., corrugated tubing, jet or ultrasonic nebulizers, bronchoscopes) are difficult to dry and the degree of dryness of a device is difficult to assess.(265) Data are lacking regarding the safety of routinely using tap water for rinsing (followed by drying) reusable semicritical respiratory devices after their disinfection or between their uses on the same patient.(242,258,273,277)

1. *Mechanical Ventilators, Breathing Circuits, Humidifiers, Heat-Moisture Exchangers and In-Line Nebulizers*

a. *Mechanical ventilators.* The internal machinery of mechanical ventilators used for respiratory therapy is not considered an important source of bacterial contamination of inhaled gas.(278) Thus, routine sterilization or high-level disinfection of the internal machinery is considered unnecessary. Using high-efficiency bacterial filters at various positions in the ventilator breathing circuit had been advocated previously.(279,280) Filters interposed between the machinery and the main breathing circuit can eliminate contaminants from the driving gas and prevent retrograde contamination of the machine by the patient but may also alter the functional specifications of the breathing device by impeding high gas flows.(279-281) Placement of a filter or condensate trap at the expiratory-phase tubing of the mechanical-ventilator circuit may help prevent cross-contamination of the ventilated patient's immediate environment,(247,282) but the importance of such filters in preventing nosocomial pneumonia needs further evaluation.

b. *Breathing circuits, humidifiers, and heat-moisture exchangers* . Most U.S. hospitals currently use ventilators with either bubble-through or wick humidifiers that produce either insignificant(132,283) or no aerosols, respectively, for humidification. Thus, they do not seem to pose an important risk for pneumonia in patients. In addition, bubble-through humidifiers are usually heated to temperatures that reduce or eliminate bacterial pathogens.(283,284) Sterile water, however, is still generally used to fill these humidifiers(285) because tap or distilled water may harbor microorganisms, such as *Legionella* spp., that are more heat-resistant than other bacteria.(252,271)

The potential risk for pneumonia in patients using mechanical ventilators with heated bubble-through humidifiers stems primarily from the condensate that forms in the inspiratory-phase tubing of the ventilator circuit as a result of the difference in the temperatures of the inspiratory-phase gas and ambient air; condensate formation increases if the tubing is unheated.(286) The tubing and condensate can rapidly become contaminated, usually with bacteria that originate from the patient's oropharynx.(286) In the study by Craven et al, 33% of inspiratory circuits were colonized with bacteria from patients' oropharynx within 2 hours and 80% within 24 hours of use.(286) Spillage of the contaminated condensate into the patient's tracheobronchial tree, as can occur during procedures in which the tubing may be moved (e.g., suctioning, adjusting the ventilator setting, or feeding or caring for the patient), may increase the risk of pneumonia in the patient. Thus, in many hospitals, healthcare workers are trained to prevent such spillage and to drain the fluid periodically. Microorganisms contaminating ventilator-circuit condensate can be transmitted to other patients via hands of the healthcare worker handling the fluid, especially if the healthcare worker fails to wash his or her hands after handling the condensate.

http://www.cdc.gov/ncidod/hip/pneumonia/1_bactpn.htm

The role of ventilator-tubing changes in preventing pneumonia in patients using mechanical ventilators with bubble-through humidifiers has been investigated. Initial studies of in-use contamination of mechanical ventilator circuits with humidifiers have shown that neither the rate of bacterial contamination of inspiratory-phase gas nor the incidence of pneumonia was significantly increased when tubing was changed every 24 hours rather than every 8 or 16 hours.(287) Craven et al later showed that changing the ventilator circuit every 48 hours rather than 24 hours did not result in an increase in contamination of the inspiratory-phase gas or tubing of the ventilator circuits.(288) In addition, the incidence of nosocomial pneumonia was not significantly higher when circuits were changed every 48 hours than when changes were done every 24 hours.(288) More recent reports suggest that the risk of pneumonia may not increase when the interval for circuit change is prolonged beyond 48 hours. Dreyfuss and others showed that the risk of pneumonia (8 [29%] of 28) was not significantly higher when the circuits were never changed for the duration of use by the patient, than (11 [31%] of 35) when the circuits were changed every 48 hours.(289)

These findings indicate that the recommended daily change in ventilator circuits may be extended to $\geq$48 hours. This change in recommendation is expected to result in large savings in device use and personnel time for U.S. hospitals.(285,288) The maximum time, however, that a circuit can be safely left unchanged on a patient has yet to be determined.

Condensate formation in the inspiratory-phase tubing of a ventilator breathing circuit can be decreased by elevating the temperature of the inspiratory-phase gas with a heated wire in the inspiratory-phase tubing. However, in one report, three cases of endotracheal- or tracheostomy-tube blockage by dried-up patient secretions were attributed to the decrease in the relative humidity of inspired gas that results from the elevation of the gas temperature.(290) Until further data are available about the frequency of the occurrence of such cases, users of heated ventilator tubing should be aware of the advantages and potential complications of using heated tubing.

Condensate formation can be eliminated by using a heat-moisture exchanger (HME) or a hygroscopic condenser humidifier ("artificial nose").(291-296) An HME recycles heat and moisture exhaled by the patient, and eliminates the need for a humidifier. In the absence of a humidifier, no condensate forms in the inspiratory-phase tubing of the ventilator circuit. Thus, bacterial colonization of the tubing is prevented, and the need to routinely change the tubing periodically is obviated.(216) Some models of HMEs are equipped with bacterial filters, but the advantage of these filters remains unknown. HMEs can increase the dead space and resistance to breathing, may leak around the endotracheal tube, and may result in drying of sputum and blockage of the tracheo-bronchial tree.(297) Although recently developed HMEs with humidifiers increase airway humidity without increasing colonization with bacteria,(293,298) more studies are needed to determine whether the incidence of pneumonia is decreased.(299-302)

c. *Small-Volume ("In-Line") Medication Nebulizers* . Small-volume medication nebulizers that are inserted in the inspiratory circuit of mechanical ventilators can produce bacterial aerosols.(242) If they become contaminated by condensate in the inspiratory tubing of the breathing circuit, they can increase the patient's risk of pneumonia because the nebulizer aerosol is directed through the endotracheal tube and bypasses many of the normal host defenses against infection.(286)

2. *Large-Volume Nebulizers*. Nebulizers with large-volume (>500 cc) reservoirs, including those used in intermittent positive-pressure breathing (IPPB) machines and ultrasonic or spinning-disk room-air "humidifiers," pose the greatest risk of pneumonia to patients, probably because of the total amount of aerosol they generate.(237-241,252,303) These reservoirs can become contaminated by hands of personnel, unsterile humidification fluid, or inadequate sterilization or disinfection between uses.(126) Once introduced into the reservoir, various bacteria, including *Legionella* spp., can multiply to sufficiently large numbers within 24 hours to pose a risk of infection in patients who receive inhalation therapy.(128,129,241,253,303) Sterilization or high-level disinfection of these reservoirs can eliminate vegetative bacteria from their reservoirs and make them safe for patient use.(260) Unlike nebulizers attached to IPPB machines, however, room-air "humidifiers" have a high cost-benefit ratio: evidence of clinical benefits from their use in hospitals is lacking, and the potential cost of daily sterilization or disinfection of, and use of sterile water to fill, such devices is substantial.

3. *Hand-Held Small-Volume Medication Nebulizers*. Small-volume medication nebulizers for administration of bronchodilators, including those that are hand-held, can produce bacterial aerosols. Hand-held nebulizers have been associated with nosocomial pneumonia, including Legionnaires' disease, resulting from contamination with medications from multidose vials(304) or *Legionella*-contaminated tap water used for rinsing and filling the reservoir.(258)

4. *Suction Catheters, Resuscitation Bags, Oxygen Analyzers, and Ventilator Spirometers*. Tracheal suction catheters can introduce microorganisms into a patient's lower respiratory tract. Currently, there are two types of suction-catheter systems used in U.S. hospitals, the open single-use catheter system and the closed multi-use catheter system. Studies comparing the two systems have involved small numbers of patients; results suggest that the risk of catheter contamination or pneumonia is not different between patients on whom the single-use suction method is used and those on whom the closed multi-use catheter system is used.(305-307) While advantages of cost and decreased environmental contamination have been attributed to the use of the closed-suction system,(308,309) larger studies are needed to weigh the advantages and disadvantages of one system over the other.(310)

Reusable resuscitation bags are particularly difficult to clean and dry between uses; microorganisms in secretions or fluid left in the bag may be aerosolized and/or sprayed into the lower respiratory tract of the patient on whom the bag is used; in addition, contaminating microorganisms may be transmitted from one patient to another via hands of staff members.(311-313) Oxygen analyzers and ventilator spirometers have been associated with outbreaks of gram-negative respiratory tract colonization and pneumonia resulting from patient-to-patient transmission of organisms via hands of personnel.(233,245) These devices require sterilization or high-level disinfection between uses on different patients. Education of physicians, respiratory therapists, and nursing staff regarding the associated risks and appropriate care of these devices is essential.

5. *Anesthesia Equipment.* The contributory role of anesthesia equipment in outbreaks of nosocomial pneumonia was reported before hospitals implemented routine after-use cleaning and disinfection/sterilization of reusable anesthesia-equipment components that may become contaminated with pathogens during use. (314,315)

a. *Anesthesia machine.* The internal components of anesthesia machines, which include the gas sources and outlets, gas valves, pressure regulators, flowmeters, and vaporizers, are not considered an important source of bacterial contamination of inhaled gases.(316) Thus, routine sterilization or high-level disinfection of the internal machinery is considered unnecessary.

b. *Breathing system or patient circuit.* The breathing system or patient circuit, through which inhaled and/or exhaled gases flow to and from a patient (and may include the tracheal tube or face mask, inspiratory and expiratory tubing, y-piece, CO_2 absorber and its chamber, the anesthesia ventilator bellows and tubing, humidifier, adjustable pressure-limiting valve, and other devices and accessories), can become contaminated with microorganisms that may originate from the patient's oropharynx or trachea. Recommendations for in-use care, maintenance, and reprocessing (i.e., cleaning and disinfection or sterilization) of the components of the breathing system have been published.(317,318) In general, reusable components of the breathing system that directly touch the patient's mucous membranes (e.g., face mask or tracheal tube) or become readily contaminated with the patient's respiratory secretions (e.g., y-piece, inspiratory and expiratory tubing and attached sensors) are cleaned and subjected to high-level disinfection or sterilization between patients. The other parts of the breathing system (e.g., carbon dioxide absorber and its chamber), for which an appropriate and cost-effective schedule of reprocessing has not been firmly determined,(319) are changed, cleaned, and sterilized or subjected to high-level disinfection periodically, according to published guidelines(317,318) and/or their manufacturers' instructions.

Using high-efficiency bacterial filters at various positions in the patient circuit, e.g., at the y-piece or on the inspiratory and expiratory sides of the patient circuit, has been advocated(317,320,321) and shown to decrease contamination of the circuit.(321-323) However, the use of bacterial filters to prevent nosocomial pulmonary infections has not been shown effective and needs further study.(324-326)

6. *Pulmonary Function Testing Apparatus.*

a. *Internal parts of pulmonary function testing apparatus* . In general, the internal parts of pulmonary function testing apparatus are not considered an important source of bacterial contamination of inhaled gas.(327) However, because of concern about possible carry-over of bacterial aerosols from an infectious patient-user of the apparatus to the next patient,(246,328) placement of bacterial filters (that remove exhaled bacteria) between the patient and the testing equipment has been recently advocated.(246,329) More studies are needed to evaluate the need for and efficacy of these filters in preventing nosocomial pneumonia.(330)

b. *Tubing, rebreathing valves, and mouthpieces.* Tubing, connectors, rebreathing valves, and mouthpieces may become contaminated with patient secretions during use of the pulmonary function testing apparatus. Thus, they are cleaned and subjected to high-level disinfection or sterilization between uses on different patients.

F. Thoracoabdominal Surgical Procedures

Certain patients are at high risk of developing postoperative pulmonary complications, including pneumonia. These persons include those who are more than 70 years of age, are obese, or have chronic obstructive pulmonary disease.(331-334) Abnormal pulmonary function tests (especially decreased maximum expiration flow rate), a history of smoking, the presence of tracheostomy or prolonged intubation, or protein depletion that can cause respiratory-muscle weakness are also risk factors.(62,68,136) Patients who undergo surgery of the head, neck, thorax, or abdomen may suffer from impairment of normal swallowing and respiratory clearance mechanisms as a result of instrumentation of the respiratory tract, anesthesia, or increased use of narcotics and sedatives;(332,335,336) patients who undergo upper abdominal surgery usually suffer from diaphragmatic dysfunction that results in decreased functional residual capacity of the lungs, closure of airways, and atelectasis.(337, 338) Interventions aimed at reducing the postoperative patient's risk of pneumonia have been developed. These include deep breathing exercises, chest physiotherapy, use of incentive spirometry, IPPB, and continuous positive airway pressure (CPAP) by face mask.(339-349) Studies evaluating the relative efficacy of these modalities have shown variable results, and have been difficult to compare because of differences in outcome variables assessed, patient populations studied, and study design.(339,341,342,348-350) Nevertheless, many studies have found deep breathing exercises, use of incentive spirometry, and IPPB as advantageous maneuvers, especially in patients with preoperative pulmonary dysfunction.(342,343,345,346,348-350) In addition, control of pain that interferes with cough and deep breathing during the immediate postoperative period has been shown to decrease the incidence of pulmonary complications after surgery; several methods of controlling pain have been used; these include intramuscular or intravenous (including patient-controlled) administration, or regional (e.g., epidural) analgesia.(351-358)

G. Other Prophylactic Measures

1. *Vaccination of Patients.* Although pneumococci are not a major cause of nosocomial pneumonia, they have been identified as etiologic agents of serious nosocomial pulmonary infection and bacteremia.(359-361) The following factors render patients at high risk of complications from pneumococcal infections: => 65 years of age, chronic cardiovascular or pulmonary disease, diabetes mellitus, alcoholism, cirrhosis, cerebrospinal fluid leaks, immunosuppression, functional or anatomic asplenia, or HIV infection. Pneumococcal

http://www.cdc.gov/ncidod/hip/pneumonia/1_bactpn.htm

vaccine is effective in preventing pneumococcal disease.(362,363) Because two-thirds or more of patients with serious pneumococcal disease have been hospitalized at least once within 5 years before their pneumococcal illness, offering pneumococcal vaccine in hospitals, e.g., at the time of patient discharge, should contribute substantially to preventing the disease.(362,364)

2. *Prophylaxis with Systemic Antimicrobial Agents.* Systemic antimicrobial administration has been a prevalent practice in the prevention of nosocomial infections,(365) including pneumonia,(366) especially in patients who are weaned off mechanical ventilators, postoperative, and/or critically ill.(367) However, the efficacy of such practice is questionable and the potential for superinfection, which may result from any antimicrobial therapy, is a problem.(74,91,366-371)

3. *Use of "Kinetic Beds" or Continuous Lateral Rotational Therapy (CLRT) for the Immobilized State.* Use of kinetic beds or CLRT is a maneuver for prevention of pulmonary and other complications from prolonged immobilization or bed rest, such as in patients with acute stroke, critical illness, head injury or traction, blunt chest trauma, and/or mechanically assisted ventilation.(372-377) This involves the use of a bed that turns continuously and slowly (from < or = 40 for CRLT to > or = 40 for kinetic therapy) along its longitudinal axis. Among the hypothesized benefits are improved drainage of secretions within the lungs and lower airways, increased tidal volume, and reduction of venous thrombosis with resultant pulmonary embolization.(378-381) However, the efficacy in preventing pneumonia needs further evaluation because studies have yielded variable results.(372-376) In addition, the studies either involved small numbers of patients,(373) lacked adequate randomization,(372) had no clear definition of pneumonia,(372) did not distinguish between community-acquired and nosocomial pneumonia,(373,377) or did not adjust for possible confounding factors such as mechanical ventilation, endotracheal intubation, nasogastric intubation, and enteral feeding.(372)

Continue to: Recommendations for Prevention and Control of Bacterial Pneumonia

Back to: Contents Page

DHQP Home | DHQP Index
CDC Home | CDC Search | CDC Health Topics A-Z

This page last reviewed March 26, 1996

Centers for Disease Control and Prevention
National Center for Infectious Diseases
Division of Healthcare Quality Promotion

http://www.cdc.gov/ncidod/hip/pneumonia/1_bactpn.htm

186

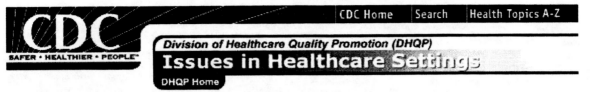

Back to: **Contents Page**

Legionnaires' Disease

Part I. Issues on Prevention of Nosocmial Pneumonia, 1994

Legionnaires' disease is a multisystem illness, with pneumonia, caused by *Legionella* spp. In contrast, Pontiac fever is a self-limited influenza-like illness, without pneumonia, that is associated with *Legionella* spp.(382)

I. Epidemiology

Since identification of the etiologic agent, numerous outbreaks of nosocomial Legionnaires' disease have been reported and have provided the opportunity to study the epidemiology of epidemic legionellosis. In contrast, the epidemiology of sporadic (i.e., nonoutbreak-related) nosocomial Legionnaires' disease has not been well elucidated. However, data suggest that when one case is recognized, the presence of additional cases should be suspected. Of 196 cases of nosocomial Legionnaires' disease reported in England and Wales during 1980 to 1992, 69% occurred during 22 nosocomial outbreaks (defined as two or more cases occurring at an institution during a 6-month period). (383) Nine per cent of cases occurred >6 months before or after a hospital outbreak. Another 13% were in hospitals where other sporadic cases (but no outbreaks) were identified. Only 9% occurred at institutions where no outbreaks or additional sporadic cases were identified.

The overall proportion of nosocomial pneumonias due to *Legionella* spp. in the North America has not been determined, although individual hospitals have reported ranges of 0%-14%.(384-386) Because diagnostic tests for *Legionella* spp. infection are not routinely performed on all patients with hospital-acquired pneumonia in most U.S. hospitals, these ranges probably underestimate the incidence of Legionnaires' disease.

Legionella spp. are commonly found in a variety of natural and man-made aquatic environments(387,388) and may enter hospital water systems in low or undetectable numbers.(389,390) Cooling towers, evaporative condensers, heated potable-water-distribution systems within hospitals, and locally produced distilled water can provide a suitable environment for legionellae to multiply. Factors known to enhance colonization and amplification of legionellae in man-made water environments include temperatures of 25-42ṣC,(392-396) stagnation,(397) scale and sediment,(393) and the presence of certain free-living aquatic amoebae that are capable of supporting intracellular growth of legionellae.(398,399)

A person's risk of acquiring legionellosis following exposure to contaminated water depends on a number of factors, including the type and intensity of exposure and the exposed person's health status.(400-402) Persons with severe immunosuppression or chronic underlying illnesses, such as hematologic malignancy or end-stage renal disease, are at markedly increased risk for legionellosis.(402-405) Persons in the later stages of acquired immunodeficiency syndrome are also probably at increased risk of legionellosis, but data are limited because of infrequent testing of patients.(402) Persons with diabetes mellitus, chronic lung disease, or non-hematologic malignancy, those who smoke cigarettes, and the elderly are at moderately increased risk.(382) Nosocomial Legionnaires' disease has also been reported among patients at children's hospitals.(406,407)

Underlying disease and advanced age are not only risk factors for acquiring Legionnaires' disease but also for dying from the illness. In a multivariate analysis of 3,524 cases reported to CDC from 1980 through 1989, immunosuppression, advanced age, end-stage renal disease, cancer, and nosocomial acquisition of disease were each independently associated with a fatal outcome.(402) The mortality rate among 803 persons with nosocomially acquired cases was 40% compared with 20% among 2,721 persons with community-acquired cases,(402) probably reflecting increased severity of underlying disease in hospitalized patients.

II. Diagnosis

The clinical spectrum of disease due to *Legionella* spp. is broad and ranges from asymptomatic infection to rapidly progressive pneumonia. Legionnaires' disease cannot be distinguished clinically or radiographically from pneumonia caused by other agents,(408,409) and evidence of infection with other respiratory pathogens does not rule out the possibility of concomitant *Legionella* spp. infection.(410-412)

The diagnosis of legionellosis may be confirmed by any one of the following: culture isolation of *Legionella* from respiratory secretions or tissues, or microscopic visualization of the bacterium in respiratory secretions or tissue by immunofluorescent microscopy; and, for legionellosis due to L. *pneumophila serogroup 1, detection of L. pneumophila serogroup-1 antigens in urine by radioimmunoassay, or*

http://www.cdc.gov/ncidod/hip/pneumonia/1_legion.htm

observation of a four-fold rise in L. pneumophila serogroup-1 antibody titer to >= 1:128 in paired acute and convalescent serum specimens by use of an indirect immunofluorescent antibody test (IFA).(413,419) A single elevated antibody titer does not confirm a case of Legionnaires' disease because IFA titers >= 1:256 are found in 1-16% of healthy adults.(411,414-417)

Because the above tests complement each other, performing each test when Legionnaires' disease is suspected increases the probability of confirming the diagnosis.(418) However, because none of the laboratory tests is 100% sensitive, the diagnosis of legionellosis is not ruled out even if one or more of the tests are negative.(418,419) Of the available tests, the most specific is culture isolation of Legionella spp. from any respiratory tract specimen.(420,421)

III. Modes of Transmission

Inhalation of aerosols of water contaminated with Legionella spp. is believed to be the primary mechanism of entry of these organisms into a patient's respiratory tract.(382) In several hospital outbreaks, patients were considered to be infected through exposure to contaminated aerosols generated by cooling towers, showers, faucets, respiratory therapy equipment, and room-air humidifiers.(11,241,258,422-428) In other studies, aspiration of contaminated potable water or pharyngeal colonizers has been proposed as the mode of transmission to certain patients.(426,429-431) Person-to-person transmission, however, has not been observed.

IV. Definition of Nosocomial Legionnaires' Disease

*The incubation period for Legionnaires' disease is generally 2-10 days;(432) thus, for epidemiologic purposes, in this document and in the accompanying recommendations by the HICPAC, laboratory-confirmed legionellosis that occurs in a patient who has spent > or = 10 days continuously in the hospital prior to onset of illness is considered **definite** nosocomial Legionnaires' disease, and laboratory-confirmed infection that occurs 2-9 days after hospitalization is **possible** nosocomial infection.*

V. Prevention and Control Measures

A. Prevention of Legionnaires' Disease in Hospitals with No Identified Cases (Primary Prevention)

Prevention strategies in healthcare facilities with no cases of nosocomial legionellosis have varied by institution, depending on the immunologic status of the patients, the design and construction of the facility, resources available for implementation of prevention strategies, and state and local regulations.

There are at least two schools of thought regarding the most appropriate and cost-effective approach to prevent nosocomial legionellosis, especially in hospitals where no cases or only sporadic cases of the illness are detected. However, a study comparing the cost-benefit ratios of these strategies has not been done.

The first approach is based on periodic, routine culturing of water samples from the hospital's potable water system, for Legionella spp. (433,434) When ≥30% of the samples obtained are culture-positive for Legionella spp., the hospital's potable water system is decontaminated(434) and diagnostic laboratory tests for legionellosis are made available to clinicians in the hospital's microbiology department so that active surveillance for cases can be instituted.(434,435) This approach is based on the premise that no cases of nosocomial legionellosis can occur in the absence of Legionella spp. from the potable water system, and, conversely, once Legionella spp. are cultured from the water, cases of nosocomial legionellosis may occur.(429,436) Proponents of this strategy indicate that when physicians are informed that the potable water system of the hospital is culture-positive for Legionella spp., they are more inclined to conduct the necessary tests for legionellosis.(435) A potential advantage of this approach is the lower cost of culturing a limited number of water samples, if the testing is done infrequently, compared with the cost of routine laboratory diagnostic testing for legionellosis in all patients with nosocomial pneumonia in hospitals that have had no cases of nosocomial legionellosis.

The main argument against this approach is that in the absence of cases, the relationship between the results of water cultures and the risk of legionellosis remains undefined. The bacterium has been frequently present in hospital water systems,(437) often without being associated with known cases of disease.(271,385,438,439) In a study of 84 hospitals in Quebec, 68% were found to be colonized with Legionella spp., and 26% were colonized at >30% of sites sampled; however, cases of Legionnaires' disease were rarely reported from these hospitals.(271) Similarly, at one hospital where active surveillance for legionellosis and environmental culturing for Legionella spp. were done, no cases of legionellosis occurred in a urology ward during a 3.5-month period when 70% of water samples from the ward were culture-positive for L. pneumophila serogroup 1.(385) Interpretation of the results of routine culturing of water may be confounded by variable culture results among sites sampled within a single water system and by fluctuations in the concentration of Legionella spp. in the same site.(440,441) In addition, the risk of illness following exposure to a given source may be influenced by a number of factors other than the presence or concentration of organisms; these include the degree to which contaminated water is aerosolized into respirable droplets, the proximity of the infectious aerosol to potential host, the susceptibility of the host, and the virulence properties of the contaminating strain.(442-444) Thus, data are insufficient to assign a level of risk of disease even on the basis of the number of colony-forming units detected in samples from the hospital environment. By routinely culturing water samples, many hospitals will have to be committed to water-decontamination programs to eradicate Legionella spp. Because of this problem, routine monitoring of water from the hospital's potable water system and from aerosol-producing devices is not widely recommended.(445)

http://www.cdc.gov/ncidod/hip/pneumonia/1_legion.htm

The second approach to prevent and control nosocomial legionellosis is by a) maintaining a high index of suspicion for legionellosis and appropriately using diagnostic tests for legionellosis in patients with nosocomial pneumonia who are at high risk of developing the disease and dying from the infection,(385,446) b) initiating an investigation for a hospital source of Legionella spp. upon identification of one case of definite or two cases of possible nosocomial Legionnaires' disease, and c) routinely maintaining cooling towers and using only sterile water for filling and terminal rinsing of nebulization devices.

Measures aimed at creating an environment that is not conducive to survival or multiplication of Legionella spp. have been advocated and utilized in hospitals where cases of nosocomial legionellosis have been identified; these include routine maintenance of potable water at > or = 50§C or <20§C at the tap or chlorination of heated water to achieve 1-2 mg/L free residual chlorine at the tap, especially in areas where immunosuppressed and other high-risk patients are located.(385,429,440,447-450) However, the cost-benefit ratio of such measures in hospitals with no identified cases of legionellosis needs further study.

B. Prevention of Legionnaires' Disease in Hospitals with Identified Cases (Secondary Prevention)

The indications for a full-scale environmental investigation to search for and subsequently decontaminate identified sources of Legionella spp. in hospital environments remain to be elucidated, and probably vary from hospital to hospital. In institutions where as few as 1-3 nosocomial cases are identified over a period of up to several months, intensified surveillance for Legionnaires' disease has frequently detected numerous additional cases.(404,423,426,448) This suggests the need for a low threshold for initiating an investigation following the identification of nosocomial, laboratory-confirmed cases of legionellosis. However, when developing a strategy to respond to such an identification, infection-control personnel should consider the level of risk of nosocomial acquisition of, and mortality from, Legionella spp. infection at their particular hospital.

An epidemiologic investigation of the source of Legionella spp. involves several important steps, including retrospective review of microbiologic and medical records; active surveillance to identify all recent or ongoing cases of legionellosis; identification of potential risk factors (including environmental exposures for infection, such as showering or use of respiratory-therapy equipment) by line listing of cases, analysis by time, place, and person, and comparison with appropriate controls; collection of water samples from environmental sources implicated by the epidemiologic investigation and from other potential sources of aerosolized water; and subtype-matching between legionellae isolated from patients and environmental samples.(428,452-454) The latter step can be crucial in supporting epidemiologic evidence of a link between human illness and a specific source.(455)

In hospitals where the heated-water system has been identified as the source of the organism, the system has been decontaminated by pulse (one-time) thermal disinfection or superheating (i.e., flushing for at least 5 minutes each distal outlet of the hot-water system with water at 65§C) and hyperchlorination (flushing all outlets of the hot-water system with water containing >= 10 mg/L free residual chlorine). (150,546-458) Following either of these procedures, most hospitals maintain heated water at >= 50§C or <20§C at the tap or chlorinate heated water to achieve 1-2 mg/L free residual chlorine at the tap.(385,429,440,447-450) Additional measures, such as physical cleaning or replacement of hot-water storage tanks, water-heaters, faucets, and showerheads, may be required because scale and sediment that provide organisms protection from the biocidal effects of heat and chlorine, may accumulate in them.(393,450) Alternative methods for control and eradication of legionellae in water systems, such as treatment of water with ozone, ultraviolet light, or heavy metal ions, have limited the growth of legionellae under laboratory and/or operating conditions.(391,459-463) However, further data are needed regarding the efficacy of these methods before they can be considered standard. In hospitals where the cooling towers are contaminated, measures for decontamination have been previously published.(464)

For highly immunocompromised patients, other preventive measures have been used. At one hospital, immunosuppressed patients were restricted from taking showers, and, for these patients, only sterile water was used for drinking or flushing nasogastric tubes.(430) In another hospital, a combined approach, consisting of continuous heating, particulate filtration, ultraviolet treatment, and monthly pulse hyperchlorination of the water supply of the bone-marrow transplant unit, was used to decrease the incidence of Legionnaires' disease. (459)

In view of the high cost of an environmental investigation and of instituting control measures to eradicate Legionella spp. from sources in the hospital(465,466) and the differential risk, based on host factors, for acquiring nosocomial legionellosis and of having severe and fatal infection with the microorganism, the decision to search for and the choice of procedures to eradicate hospital environmental sources of Legionella spp. should take into account the type of patient population served by the hospital.

Continue to: <u>Recommendations for Prevention and Control of Legionnaires' Disease</u>

Back to: <u>Contents Page</u>

Back to: **Contents Page**

Aspergillosis

Part I. Issues on Prevention of Nosocmial Pneumonia, 1994

I. Epidemiology

Aspergillus spp. are ubiquitous fungi, commonly occurring in soil, water, and decaying vegetation. *Aspergillus* spp. have been cultured from unfiltered air, ventilation systems, contaminated dust dislodged during hospital renovation and construction, horizontal surfaces, food, and ornamental plants.(467)

A. fumigatus and *A. flavus* are the most frequently isolated *Aspergillus* spp. in patients with proven aspergillosis.(468) Nosocomial aspergillosis has been recognized increasingly as a cause of severe illness and mortality in highly immunocompromised patients, e.g., patients undergoing chemotherapy and/or organ transplantation, including bone-marrow transplantation for hematologic and other malignant neoplasms.(469-473)

The most important nosocomial infection due to *Aspergillus* spp. is pneumonia.(474,495) Hospital outbreaks of pulmonary aspergillosis have occurred mainly in granulocytopenic patients, especially in bone-marrow transplant units.(474-480) Although invasive aspergillosis has been reported in recipients of solid-organ transplants (e.g., heart or kidney),(481-485) the incidence of *Aspergillus* spp. infections in these patients has been lower than in recipients of bone-marrow transplants, probably because granulocytopenia is less severe in solid-organ transplant recipients and the use of corticosteroids has decreased with the introduction of cyclosporine.(483,486) In solid-organ transplant recipients, the efficacy of infection control measures, such as provision of protected environments and prophylaxis with antifungal agents, in preventing aspergillosis has not been well evaluated.(483,484,486,489) In one study of heart-transplant recipients, protective isolation of patients alone failed to prevent fungal infections.(490)

The reported attributable mortality from invasive pulmonary aspergillosis has varied, depending on the patient population studied. Rates have been as high as 95% in recipients of allogeneic bone-marrow transplants and patients with aplastic anemia, compared with rates of 13-80% in leukemic patients.(491-493)

II. Pathogenesis

In contrast to most bacterial pneumonias, the primary route of acquiring *Aspergillus* spp. infection is by inhalation of the fungal spores. In severely immunocompromised patients, primary *Aspergillus* spp. pneumonia results from local lung tissue invasion.(468,494,495) Subsequently, the fungus may disseminate via the bloodstream to involve multiple other deep organs.(468,495,496) A role for nasopharyngeal colonization with *Aspergillus* spp., as an intermediate step before invasive pulmonary disease, has been proposed, but remains to be elucidated.(488,497,498) On the other hand, colonization of the lower respiratory tract by *Aspergillus* spp., especially in patients with preexisting lung disease such as chronic obstructive lung disease, cystic fibrosis, or inactive tuberculosis, has predisposed patients to invasive pulmonary and/or disseminated infection.(468,495,499)

III. Diagnosis

Diagnosing pneumonia due to *Aspergillus* spp. is often difficult without performing invasive procedures. Bronchoalveolar lavage has been a useful screening test,(500-502) but lung biopsy is still considered the most reliable technique.(503) Histopathologic demonstration of tissue invasion by fungal hyphae has been required in addition to isolation of *Aspergillus* spp. from respiratory tract secretions because the latter, by itself, may indicate colonization.(504) However, when *Aspergillus* spp. is grown from the sputum of a febrile, granulocytopenic patient with a new pulmonary infiltrate, it is highly likely that the patient has pulmonary aspergillosis.(497,505) Routine blood cultures are remarkably insensitive for detecting *Aspergillus* spp.,(506) and systemic antibody responses in immunocompromised patients are likely to be unreliable indicators of infection.(507-509) Antigen-based serologic assays are now being developed in an attempt to allow for the rapid and specific diagnosis of *Aspergillus* spp. infections; however, their clinical usefulness is presently undefined.(510,511)

IV. Risk Factors and Control Measures

The major risk factor for invasive aspergillosis is severe and prolonged granulocytopenia, both disease- and therapy-induced.(512) Since bone-marrow transplant recipients experience the most severe degree of granulocytopenia, they probably constitute the population at highest risk of developing invasive aspergillosis.(492,513) The tendency of bone-marrow transplant recipients to develop severe granulocytopenia (<1,000 polymorphonuclears/uL) is associated with the type of graft they receive. While both autologous and allogeneic bone-marrow transplant recipients are severely granulocytopenic for up to 4 weeks after the transplant procedure, allogeneic-transplant recipients may, in addition, develop acute or chronic graft-versus-host disease. The latter may occur up to several months after the procedure, and the disease and/or its therapy (often with high doses of corticosteroids, cyclosporine, and other immunosuppressive agents) may result in severe granulocytopenia. Consequently, in developing strategies to prevent invasive *Aspergillus* spp. infection in bone-marrow-transplant patients, infection control personnel should consider exposures of the patient to the fungus not only during the patient's immediate posttransplantation period, but also other exposures (eg, at home or in an ambulatory-care setting) subsequent to the immediate posttransplant period, when the patient (especially allogeneic-transplant recipients) may again manifest severe granulocytopenia. To help address this problem, various studies are now in progress to evaluate newer methods of enhancing host resistance to invasive fungal (and other) infections, and of eliminating or suppressing respiratory fungal colonization of the upper respiratory tract. These methods include, respectively, the use of granulocyte-colony-stimulating factors and intranasal application of amphotericin B, or oral or systemic antifungal drug prophylaxis.(467,514-517) For solid-organ transplant recipients, risk factors for invasive aspergillosis have not been as extensively studied. In one study of liver-transplant recipients, risk factors for invasive infection with *Aspergillus* spp. identified by univariate analysis included preoperative and postoperative receipt of steroids and antimicrobial agents, and prolonged duration of transplant surgery.(518)

The presence of aspergilli in the hospital environment is the major extrinsic risk factor for the occurrence of opportunistic invasive *Aspergillus* spp. infection.(487,519) Environmental disturbances due to construction and/or renovation activities in and around hospitals markedly raise the airborne *Aspergillus* spp. spore counts in such hospitals and have been associated with nosocomial aspergillosis. (476,478,479,520-523) In addition, aspergillosis in high-risk immunosuppressed patients has been associated with other hospital environmental reservoirs, including bird droppings in air ducts supplying high-risk patient areas,(524) and contaminated fireproofing material or damp wood.(478,525)

A single case of nosocomial *Aspergillus* spp. pneumonia is often difficult to link to a specific environmental exposure. However, additional cases may remain undetected without an active search that includes an intensive retrospective review of microbiologic, histopathologic, and postmortem records; notification of clinicians caring for high-risk patients; and establishment of a system for prospective surveillance for additional cases. When additional cases are detected, the likelihood is increased that a hospital environmental source of *Aspergillus* spp. can be identified.(476,478,520-525) Previous investigations have shown the importance of construction activities and/or fungal "contamination" of hospital air-handling systems as major sources for outbreaks.(474,476,478,520-524) New molecular typing techniques, namely karyotyping(526) and DNA endonuclease profiling (now available for *A. fumigatus*),(527) may significantly aid in identifying the source of an outbreak.

Outbreaks of invasive aspergillosis reinforce the importance of maintaining an environment as free of *Aspergillus* spp. spores as possible for patients with severe granulocytopenia. To achieve this goal, specialized services in many large hospitals, in particular bone-marrow transplant services, have installed "protected environments" for the care of their high-risk, severely granulocytopenic patients, and increased their vigilance during hospital construction and routine maintenance of hospital air-filtration and ventilation systems, to prevent exposing high-risk patients to bursts of fungal spores.(476,478,520-524,528-533)

While the exact configuration and specifications of the protected environments may vary between hospitals, these patient-care areas are built to minimize fungal spore counts in air by maintaining a) high-efficiency filtration of incoming air by using central or point-of-use HEPA filters that are 99.97% efficient in filtering 0.3 μ-sized particles, b) directed room airflow-- from intake on one side of the room, across the patient, and out through the exhaust on the opposite side of the room, c) positive room-air pressure relative to the corridor, d) well-sealed rooms, and e) high rates of room-air changes (range: 15 to >400 per hour) although air-change rates at the higher levels may pose problems of patient comfort.(474,529-531,533-535) The oldest and most studied protected environment is a room with laminar airflow, consisting of a bank of HEPA filters along an entire wall through which air is pumped by blowers into the room at a uniform velocity (90 ± 20 feet/minute), forcing the air to move in a laminar, or at least unidirectional, pattern.(536) The air usually exits at the opposite end of the room, and ultra-high air-change rates (100-400 per hour) are achieved.(474,528) The net effects are essentially sterile air in the room, minimal air turbulence, minimal opportunity for microorganism build-up, and a consistently clean environment.(474)

The efficacy of a laminar-airflow system in decreasing or eliminating the risk of nosocomial aspergillosis in high-risk patients has been demonstrated.(474,529,534,535) However, such a system is costly to install and maintain. Less expensive alternative systems with lower air-change rates (10-15 per hour) have been utilized in some centers.(530,531,537) However, studies comparing the efficacy of these alternative systems with laminar-airflow rooms in eliminating *Aspergillus* spp. spores and preventing nosocomial aspergillosis are limited. One institution employing cross-flow ventilation, point-of-use high-efficiency filters, and 15 air changes per hour reported that cases of nosocomial aspergillosis in patients housed in these rooms have occurred, albeit at a low rate (3.4%).(531,537) The infections, however, were due to *A. flavus*-- a species that was never cultured from the room air, suggesting that the patients were probably exposed to fungal spores when they were allowed outside their rooms.(531)

Copper-8-quinolinolate has been used on environmental surfaces contaminated with *Aspergillus* spp. to control a reported outbreak,(538) and incorporated in fireproofing material of a newly constructed hospital(531) to help decrease the environmental spore burden, but its general applicability is yet to be established.

Continue to: **Recommendations for Prevention and Control of Nosocomial Pulmonary Aspergillosis**

http://www.cdc.gov/ncidod/hip/pneumonia/1_asper.htm

Back to: Contents Page

RSV Infection

Part I. Issues on Prevention of Nosocmial Pneumonia, 1994

I. Epidemiology

RSV infection is most common during infancy and early childhood, but may also occur in adults.(563,566,575,576) Infection usually causes mild or moderately severe upper respiratory illness. However, life-threatening pneumonia or bronchiolitis has been reported in children with chronic cardiac and pulmonary disease, immunocompromised patients, and the elderly.(548,550,565,566,577,578)

Recent surveillance of 10 U.S. hospital laboratories performing cultures for RSV suggests that community outbreaks occur yearly between December and March, last from 3-5 months, and are associated with increased hospitalization and deaths among infants and young children.(579) During community outbreaks of RSV, children admitted to the hospital with respiratory symptoms often serve as reservoirs for RSV.(554,556)

II. Diagnosis

The clinical characteristics of RSV infection, especially in neonates, are often indistinguishable from those of other viral respiratory tract infections.(566,567) Culture of RSV from respiratory secretions remains the "gold standard" for diagnosis. Although rapid antigen-detection kits utilizing direct immunofluorescence or enzyme-linked immunosorbent assay are available and can provide results within hours, the benefit of using these tests to identify infected patients depends on the sensitivity and specificity of the test. The reported sensitivity and specificity of RSV enzyme immunoassays vary between 80% and 95%, and may even be lower in actual practice.(580-583) In general, once laboratory-confirmed cases of RSV infection are identified in a hospital, a presumptive diagnosis of RSV infection in subsequent cases with manifestations suggestive of RSV infection may be acceptable for infection control purposes.

III. Modes of Transmission

RSV is present in large numbers in the respiratory secretions of symptomatic persons infected with the virus and can be transmitted directly via large droplets during close contact with such persons, or indirectly via RSV-contaminated hands or fomites.(554,584,585) The portal of entry is usually the conjunctiva or the nasal mucosa.(586) Inoculation by RSV-contaminated hands is the usual way of depositing the virus onto the eyes or nose.(554,584-586) Hands can become contaminated through handling of infected persons' respiratory secretions or contaminated fomites.(584,585)

In nosocomial RSV outbreaks in which the viral isolates were typed, more than one strain of RSV has often been identified,(555,564,587) suggesting multiple sources of the virus. Potential sources include patients, hospital staff, and visitors. Because infected infants shed large amounts of virus in their respiratory secretions and easily contaminate their immediate surroundings, they are a major reservoir for RSV. (588) Hospital staff may become infected after exposure in the community(589) or in the hospital, and in turn, infect patients, other health-care workers, or hospital visitors.(567,590)

IV. Control Measures

Various combinations of control measures ranging from the simple to the complex have been effective, to some degree or other, in preventing and controlling nosocomial RSV infection.(226,590-597) Successful programs have had two elements in common: implementation of contact-isolation precautions, and compliance with these precautions by healthcare personnel. In theory, strict handwashing should prevent most nosocomial RSV infections. However, health-care workers' handwashing practices have always been poor.(221-222) Thus, other preventive measures are usually relied upon to prevent RSV infection.

The basic precautions that have been associated with decreased incidence of nosocomial RSV infections are gloving and gowning.(226) Gloving has helped decrease transmission probably because gloves remind patient-care personnel to comply with handwashing and other precautions, and deter persons from touching their eyes or noses. The benefits from gloving, however, are offset if gloves are not changed

http://www.cdc.gov/ncidod/hip/pneumonia/1_rsv.htm

between patients or after contact with contaminated fomites, and if hands are not adequately washed after glove removal.(229) Gowning, in combination with gloving, during contact with RSV-infected infants or their immediate environment has been used successfully to prevent infection.(226) In addition, the use of eye-nose goggles rather than masks has protected healthcare workers from infection; however, eye-nose goggles are not widely available and are inconvenient to wear.(594,598)

Additional measures may be indicated to control ongoing nosocomial transmission of RSV or to prevent transmission to patients at high risk for serious complications of infections, such as those with compromised cardiac, pulmonary, or immune systems. The following additional control measures have been used in various combinations: (1) use of private rooms for infected patients OR cohorting of infected patients, with or without pre-admission screening by rapid laboratory diagnostic tests; (2) cohorting of personnel; (3) exclusion of healthcare workers who have symptoms of upper respiratory tract infection from the care of uninfected patients at high risk of severe or fatal RSV infection, e.g., infants; (4) limiting visitors; and (5) postponing admission of patients at high risk of complications from RSV infection.(224,591,593,595,597) Although the exact role of each of these measures has not been fully elucidated, their use for control of outbreaks seems prudent.

Continue to: <u>Recommendations for Prevention and Control of RSV Infection</u>

Back to: <u>Contents Page</u>

<u>DHQP Home</u> | <u>DHQP Index</u>
<u>CDC Home</u> | <u>CDC Search</u> | <u>CDC Health Topics A-Z</u>

This page last reviewed March 26, 1996

<u>Centers for Disease Control and Prevention</u>
National Center for Infectious Diseases
Division of Healthcare Quality Promotion

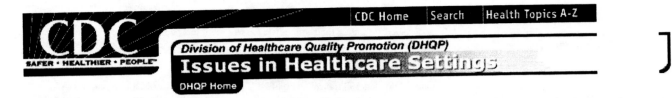

Influenza

PART I. Issues on Prevention of Nosocmial Pneumonia, 1994

I. Epidemiology

Pneumonia in patients with influenza may be due to the influenza virus itself, secondary bacterial infection, or a combination of both.(599-601) Influenza-associated pneumonia can occur in any person, but is more common in the very young or old and in persons in any age group with immunosuppression or certain chronic medical conditions such as severe underlying heart or lung disease.(576,602-604)

Influenza typically occurs annually in the winter between December and April; peak activity in a community usually lasts from 6 to 8 weeks during this period.(605,606) During influenza epidemics in the community, nosocomial outbreaks can occur and are often characterized by abrupt onset and rapid transmission.(607,609) Most reported institutional outbreaks of influenza have occurred in nursing homes; however, hospital outbreaks have been reported on pediatric and chronic-care wards, as well as on medical and neonatal intensive care units.(557,610-613)

Influenza is believed to be spread from person to person by direct deposition of virus-laden large droplets onto the mucosal surfaces of the upper respiratory tract of an individual during close contact with an infected person, as well as by droplet nuclei or small-particle aerosols.(614-617) The extent to which transmission may occur by virus-contaminated hands or fomites is unknown; however, it is not the primary mode of spread.(618)

The most important reservoirs of influenza virus are infected persons, and the period of greatest communicability is during the first 3 days of illness; however, the virus can be shed before onset of symptoms, and up to 7 or more days after illness onset.(451,557,605)

II. Diagnosis

Influenza is clinically indistinguishable from other febrile respiratory illnesses, but during outbreaks with laboratory-confirmed cases, a presumptive diagnosis of the infection can be made in cases with similar manifestations.(619) In the past, diagnosis of influenza was made by virus isolation from nasopharyngeal secretions or by serologic conversion, but recently developed rapid diagnostic tests that are similar to culture in sensitivity and specificity allow early diagnosis and treatment of cases and provide a basis for prompt initiation of antiviral prophylaxis as part of outbreak control.(620-625)

III. Prevention and Control of Influenza

Vaccination of persons at high risk for complications of influenza is currently the most effective measure for reducing the impact of influenza, and should be done before the influenza season each year. High-risk persons include those > or = 65 years of age; those in long-term-care units; those with chronic disorders of the pulmonary or cardiovascular systems, those with diabetes mellitus, renal dysfunction, hemoglobinopathies, or immunosuppression; and children 6 months-18 years of age who are receiving long-term aspirin therapy. Patients with musculo-skeletal disorders that impede adequate respiration may also be at high risk of developing complications of influenza. When high vaccination rates are achieved in closed or semi-closed settings, the risk of outbreaks is reduced because of induction of herd immunity.(629,630)

When an institutional outbreak is caused by influenza type A, antiviral agents may be used both for treatment of ill persons and as prophylaxis for others.(642) Two related antiviral agents, amantadine hydrochloride and rimantadine hydrochloride, are effective against influenza type A, but not influenza type B, virus.(544,632-634) These agents can be used to prevent influenza type A (1) as short-term prophylaxis after late vaccination of high-risk persons; (2) as prophylaxis for persons for whom vaccination is contraindicated; (3) as prophylaxis for immunocompromised persons who may not produce protective levels of antibody in response to vaccination; (4) as prophylaxis for unvaccinated healthcare workers who provide care to high-risk patients, either for the duration of influenza activity in the community or until immunity develops after vaccination; and (5) when vaccine strains do not closely match the epidemic virus strain.(642)

Amantadine has been available in the United States for many years; rimantadine has been approved for use since 1993. Both drugs protect

http://www.cdc.gov/ncidod/hip/pneumonia/1_flu.htm

against all naturally-occurring strains of type A influenza virus; thus, antigenic changes in the virus that may reduce vaccine efficacy do not alter the effectiveness of amantadine or rimantadine. Both drugs are 70-90% effective in preventing illness if taken before exposure to influenza A virus.(632,635) In addition, they can reduce the severity and duration of illness due to influenza type A when administered within 24-48 hours after onset of symptoms.(636,637) These drugs can limit nosocomial spread of influenza type A if they are administered to all or most patients when influenza type A illnesses begin in a facility.(610,638,639)

Compared to rimantadine, amantadine has been associated with a higher incidence of adverse central nervous system (CNS) reactions such as mild and transitory nervousness, insomnia, impaired concentration, mood changes, and light-headedness. These symptoms have been reported in 5%-10% of healthy young adults receiving 200 mg of amantadine per day.(544,632) In the elderly, CNS side effects may be more severe; in addition, dizziness and ataxia are more common in this age group.(640,641) Dose reductions of both amantadine and rimantadine are recommended for certain patient groups, such as persons > or = 65 years of age and/or those who have renal insufficiency. The drug package insert for amantadine or rimantadine contains important information regarding administration of either drug. Guidelines for the use of these drugs and considerations for the selection of amantadine or rimantadine have been developed by the Advisory Committee for Immunization Practices.(642)

Emergence of amantadine- and rimantadine-resistant strains of influenza A virus has been observed in persons who have received these drugs for treatment of the infection.(643,644) Because of the potential risk of transmission of resistant viral strains to contacts of persons receiving amantadine or rimantadine for treatment,(644,645) to the extent possible, infected persons taking either drug should avoid contact with others during treatment and for 2 days after discontinuing treatment.(645,646) This is particularly important if the contacts are uninfected high-risk persons.(645,647)

Vaccination of high-risk patients and of hospital personnel before the influenza season is the primary focus of efforts to prevent and control nosocomial influenza.(628,631,648) The decision to use amantadine or rimantadine as an adjunct to vaccination in the prevention and control of nosocomial influenza is based in part on results of virologic and epidemiologic surveillance in the hospital and the community. When outbreaks of influenza type A occur in a hospital, and antiviral prophylaxis of high-risk persons and/or treatment of cases is undertaken, administration of amantadine or rimantadine is begun as early in the outbreak as possible to reduce transmission. (610,631,642,647)

Measures other than vaccination and chemoprophylaxis have been recommended for control of nosocomial influenza outbreaks. Because influenza can be transmitted during contact with an infected person, contact-isolation precautions, placing a patient symptomatic with influenza in a private room, cohorting og patients with nfluenza-like illness, and masking upon entering a room with person with suspected or proven influenza have been recommended.(224) Handwashing, gloving, and gowing by health-care workers during the patient's symptomatic period have also been recommended, but the exact role of these measures in preventing influenza transmission remains to be elucidated.(224,609,649) Although influenza can be transmitted via the airborne route, the efficacy of placing infected persons in room with negative pressure in relation to their immediate environment has not been assessed. In addition, this measure may be impractical during institutional outbreaks that occur in the midst of a community epidemic of influenza because many newly admitted patients and healthcare workers may be infected with the virus; thus, the hospital would face the lofistical problem of accommodating all ill persons in rooms with special ventilation. Although controlled studies are not available to measure their effectiveness, the following additional measures have been recommended for consideration, particularly dring severe outbreaks: (1) curtailment or elimination of elective admissions, both medical and surgical; (2) restriction of cardiobascular and pulmonary sugery; (3) restriction of hospital visitors, especially those the acute respitaroty illnesses; and (4) work restriction for healthcare workers with acute respiratory illness.(649)

Continue to: Recommendations for Prevention and Control of Influenza
Back to: Contents Page

DHQP Home | DHQP Index
CDC Home | CDC Search | CDC Health Topics A-Z

This page last reviewed March 26, 1996

Centers for Disease Control and Prevention
National Center for Infectious Diseases
Division of Healthcare Quality Promotion

http://www.cdc.gov/ncidod/hip/pneumonia/1_flu.htm

195

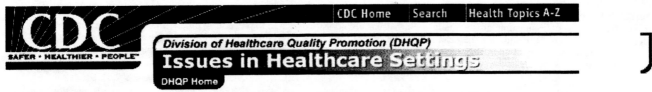

Back to: Contents Page

Bacterial Pneumonia

Recommendations for Prevention of Nosocomial Bacterial Pneumonia

I. STAFF EDUCATION AND INFECTION SURVEILLANCE

A. Staff Education

Educate healthcare workers regarding nosocomial bacterial pneumonias and infection control procedures to prevent their occurrence.(655-661) *CATEGORY IA*

B. Surveillance

1. Conduct surveillance for bacterial pneumonia in ICU patients at high risk for nosocomial bacterial pneumonia (eg, patients with mechanically assisted ventilation, selected postoperative patients) to determine trends and identify potential problems.(6,34,35,62,662-664) Include data regarding the causative microorganisms and their antimicrobial susceptibility patterns.(2,3) Express data as rates (eg, number of infected patients or infections per 100 ICU days or per 1,000 ventilator-days) to facilitate intra-hospital comparisons and determining trends.(66,665-667) *CATEGORY IA*

2. Do not **routinely** perform surveillance cultures of patients or of equipment or devices used for respiratory therapy, pulmonary-function testing, or delivery of inhalation anesthesia.(65,668,669)*CATEGORY IA*

II. INTERRUPTION OF TRANSMISSION OF MICROORGANISMS

A. Sterilization or disinfection, and Maintenance of Equipment and Devices

1. General Measures

a. Thoroughly clean all equipment and devices to be sterilized or disinfected.(266,267,670) *CATEGORY IA*

b. Sterilize or use high-level disinfection for semicritical equipment or devices, i.e., items that come into direct or indirect contact with mucous membranes of the lower respiratory tract (See examples, Appendix A). High-level disinfection can be achieved either by wet heat pasteurization at 76şC for 30 minutes or by using liquid chemical disinfectants approved as sterilants/disinfectants by the Environmental Protection Agency and cleared for marketing for use on medical instruments by the Office of Device Evaluation, Center for Devices and Radiologic Health, Food and Drug Administration.(260,262,264,267,671) Follow disinfection with appropriate rinsing, drying, and packaging, taking care not to contaminate the items in the process. *CATEGORY IB*

c. (1) Use sterile (not distilled, nonsterile) water for rinsing reusable semicritical equipment and devices used on the respiratory tract after they have been chemically disinfected.(241,249,250,258,269) *CATEGORY IB*

(2) *No Recommendation* for using tap water (as an alternative to sterile water) to rinse reusable semicritical equipment and devices used on the respiratory tract, after they have been subjected to high-level disinfection, whether or not rinsing is followed by drying with or without the use of alcohol.(241,249,250,258,269,273,277) *UNRESOLVED ISSUE*

d. Do not reprocess an equipment or device that is manufactured for single use only, unless data show that reprocessing the equipment or device poses no threat to the patient, is cost-effective, and does not change the structural integrity or function of the equipment or device. (672,673) *CATEGORY IB*

2. Mechanical Ventilators, Breathing Circuits, Humidifiers and Heat-Moisture Exchangers

http://www.cdc.gov/ncidod/hip/pneumonia/2_bactpn.htm

a. Mechanical Ventilators

Do not routinely sterilize or disinfect the internal machinery of mechanical ventilators.(126,128,674) *CATEGORY IA*

b. Ventilator Circuits with Humidifiers

(1) Do not routinely change more frequently than every 48 hours the breathing circuit, including tubing and exhalation valve, and the attached bubbling or wick humidifier of a ventilator that is in use on an individual patient.(34,283,288) *CATEGORY IA*

(2) *No Recommendation* for the maximum length of time after which the breathing circuit and the attached bubbling or wick humidifier of a ventilator in use on a patient should be changed.(289) *UNRESOLVED ISSUE*

(3) Sterilize reusable breathing circuits and bubbling or wick humidifiers, or subject them to high-level disinfection between their uses on different patients.(259,260,262,264,267) *CATEGORY IB*

(4) Periodically drain and discard any condensate that collects in the tubing of a mechanical ventilator, taking precautions not to allow condensate to drain toward the patient. Wash hands after performing the procedure or handling the fluid. (215,282,286) *CATEGORY IB*

(5) *No Recommendation* for placing a filter or trap at the distal end of the expiratory-phase tubing of the breathing circuit to collect condensate.(247,282) *UNRESOLVED ISSUE*

(6) Do not place bacterial filters between the humidifier reservoir and the inspiratory-phase tubing of the breathing circuit of a mechanical ventilator. *CATEGORY IB*

(7) Humidifier fluids

a) Use sterile water to fill bubbling humidifiers.(132,241,249,250,286) *CATEGORY II*

b) Use sterile, distilled, or tap water to fill wick humidifiers.(249,250,286) *CATEGORY II*

c) *No Recommendation* for preferential use of a closed, continuous-feed humidification system. *UNRESOLVED ISSUE*

c. Ventilator Breathing Circuits with Hygroscopic Condenser-Humidifiers or Heat-Moisture Exchangers

(1) *No Recommendation* for preferential use of hygroscopic condenser-humidifier or heat-moisture exchanger rather than a heated humidifier to prevent nosocomial pneumonia.(298-302) *UNRESOLVED ISSUE*

(2) Change the hygroscopic condenser-humidifier or heat-moisture exchanger according to manufacturer's recommendation and/or when evidence of gross contamination or mechanical dysfunction of the device is present.(298) *CATEGORY IB*

(3) Do not routinely change the breathing circuit attached to a hygroscopic condenser-humidifier or heat-moisture exchanger while it is in use on a patient.(298,301) *CATEGORY IB*

3. Wall humidifiers

a. Follow manufacturers' instructions for use and maintenance of wall oxygen humidifiers unless data show that the modification in their use or maintenance poses no threat to the patient and is cost-effective.(675-679) *CATEGORY IB*

b. Between patients, change the tubing, including any nasal prongs or mask, used to deliver oxygen from a wall outlet. *CATEGORY IB*

4. Small-Volume Medication Nebulizers: "In-line" and Hand-held Nebulizers

a. (1) Between treatments on the same patient, disinfect, rinse with sterile water, or air-dry small-volume medication nebulizers.(242-258) *CATEGORY IB*

2) *No Recommendation* for using tap water as an alternative to sterile water to rinse reusable small-volume medication nebulizers between treatments on the same patient.(242,258,273) *UNRESOLVED ISSUE*

b. Between patients, replace nebulizers with those that have undergone sterilization or high-level disinfection.(126,128,129,269,680) *CATEGORY IB*

c. Use only sterile fluids for nebulization, and dispense these fluids aseptically.(238,241,249,250,258,269,304) *CATEGORY IA*

d. If multidose medication vials are used, handle, dispense, and store them according to manufacturers' instructions.(238,304,680-682) *CATEGORY IB*

5. Large-volume Nebulizers and Mist Tents

a. Do not use large-volume room-air humidifiers that create aerosols (eg, by venturi principle, ultrasound, or spinning disk) and thus are really nebulizers, unless they can be sterilized or subjected to high-level disinfection at least daily and filled only with sterile water.(239-241,252,303,683) *CATEGORY IA*

b. Sterilize large-volume nebulizers that are used for inhalation therapy, eg, for tracheostomized patients, or subject them to high-level disinfection between patients and after every 24 hours of use on the same patient.(126,128,129) *CATEGORY IB*

c. (1) Use mist-tent nebulizers and reservoirs that have undergone sterilization or high-level disinfection and replace them between patients. (684) *CATEGORY IB*

(2) *No Recommendation* regarding the frequency of changing mist-tent nebulizers and reservoirs while in use on one patient. *UNRESOLVED ISSUE*

6. Other Devices Used in Association with Respiratory Therapy

a. Between patients, sterilize or subject to high-level disinfection portable respirometers, oxygen sensors, and other respiratory devices used on multiple patients.(233,245) *CATEGORY IB*

b. (1) Between patients, sterilize or subject to high-level disinfection reusable hand-powered resuscitation bags (for example, Ambu bags). (255,311-313) *CATEGORY IA*

(2) *No Recommendation* regarding the frequency of changing hydrophobic filters placed on the connection port of resuscitation bags. *UNRESOLVED ISSUE*

7. Anesthesia Machines and Breathing Systems or Patient Circuits

a. Do not routinely sterilize or disinfect the internal machinery of anesthesia equipment.(316) *CATEGORY IA*

b. Clean and then sterilize or subject to high-level liquid chemical disinfection or pasteurization reusable components of the breathing system or patient circuit (eg, tracheal tube or face mask; inspiratory and expiratory breathing tubing; y-piece; reservoir bag; humidifier and tubing) between uses on different patients, by following the device manufacturer's instructions for their reprocessing.(260,264,267,317,685) *CATEGORY IB*

c. *No Recommendation* for the frequency of routinely cleaning and disinfecting unidirectional valves and carbon dioxide absorber chambers.(317-319) *UNRESOLVED ISSUE*

d. Follow published guidelines and/or manufacturers' instructions regarding in-use maintenance, cleaning, and disinfection or sterilization of other components or attachments of the breathing system or patient circuit of anesthesia equipment.(317,318) *CATEGORY IB*

e. Periodically drain and discard any condensate that collects in the tubing of a breathing circuit, taking precautions not to allow condensate to drain toward the patient. After performing the procedure or handling the fluid, wash hands with soap and water or with a waterless handwashing preparation.(218,219,686,687) *CATEGORY IB*

f. *No Recommendation* for placing a bacterial filter in the breathing system or patient circuit of anesthesia equipment.(1,317,318,321-326,688) *UNRESOLVED ISSUE*

8. Pulmonary-Function Testing Equipment

a. Do not routinely sterilize or disinfect the internal machinery of pulmonary-function testing machines between uses on different patients.

(327,328) *CATEGORY II*

b. Sterilize or subject to high-level liquid chemical disinfection or pasteurization reusable mouthpieces and tubing or connectors between uses on different patients, OR follow device manufacturer's instructions for their reprocessing.(260,261,263-267) *CATEGORY IB*

B. Interruption of Person-to-Person Transmission of Bacteria

1. Handwashing

Wash hands after contact with mucous membranes, respiratory secretions, or objects contaminated with respiratory secretions, whether or not gloves are worn. Wash hands before and after contact with a patient who has an endotracheal or tracheostomy tube in place, and before and after contact with any respiratory device that is used on the patient, whether or not gloves are worn.(210,212,218,219,231,689,690) *CATEGORY IA*

2. Barrier Precautions

a. Wear gloves for handling respiratory secretions or objects contaminated with respiratory secretions of any patient.(226,227) *CATEGORY IA*

b. Change gloves and wash hands between patients; after handling respiratory secretions or objects contaminated with secretions from one patient and before contact with another patient, object, or environmental surface; and between contacts with a contaminated body site and respiratory tract of, or respiratory device on, the same patient.(226,228-230) *CATEGORY IA*

c. Wear a gown when soiling with respiratory secretions from a patient is anticipated, and change the gown after such contact and before providing care to another patient.(226) *CATEGORY IB*

3. Care of Patients with Tracheostomy

a. Perform tracheostomy under sterile conditions. *CATEGORY IB*

b. When changing a tracheostomy tube, use aseptic technique and replace the tube with one that has undergone sterilization or high-level disinfection. *CATEGORY IB*

4. Suctioning of Respiratory Tract Secretions

a. *No Recommendation* for wearing sterile rather than clean gloves when suctioning a patient's respiratory secretions. *UNRESOLVED ISSUE*

b. If the open suction system is employed, use a sterile single-use catheter. *CATEGORY II*

c. Use only sterile fluid to remove secretions from the suction catheter if the catheter is to be used for re-entry into the patient's lower respiratory tract.(691) *CATEGORY IB*

d. *No Recommendation* for preferential use of the multi-use closed-system suction catheter or the single-use open-system catheter for prevention of pneumonia.(305-308,310) *UNRESOLVED ISSUE*

e. Change suction collection tubing (up to the canister) between patients. *CATEGORY IB*

f. Change suction collection canisters between uses on different patients except when used in short-term care units. *CATEGORY IB*

III. MODIFYING HOST RISK FOR INFECTION

A. Precautions for Prevention of Endogenous Pneumonia

Discontinue enteral-tube feeding and remove devices such as endotracheal, tracheostomy, and/or enteral (i.e., oro- or naso-gastric, or jejunal) tubes from patients as soon as the clinical indications for these are resolved.(6,34,35,85-87,117,183,185,186,202,692) *CATEGORY IB*

http://www.cdc.gov/ncidod/hip/pneumonia/2_bactpn.htm

1. Prevention of Aspiration Associated with Enteral Feeding

a. If there is no contraindication to the maneuver, elevate at an angle of 30-45° the head of the bed of a patient at high risk of aspiration pneumonia, eg, a person receiving mechanically assisted ventilation and/or has an enteral tube in place.(74,185) *CATEGORY IB*

b. Routinely verify appropriate placement of the feeding tube.(693-695) *CATEGORY IB*

c. Routinely assess the patient's intestinal motility (eg, by auscultating for bowel sounds and measuring residual gastric volume or abdominal girth) and adjust the rate and volume of enteral feeding to avoid regurgitation.(692) *CATEGORY IB*

d. *No Recommendation* for the preferential use of small-bore tubes for enteral feeding.(694) *UNRESOLVED ISSUE*

e. *No Recommendation* for administering enteral feeding continuously or intermittently.(70,193,198) *UNRESOLVED ISSUE*

f. *No Recommendation* for preferentially placing the feeding tubes, eg, jejunal tubes, distal to the pylorus.(199,200) *UNRESOLVED ISSUE*

2. Prevention of Aspiration Associated with Endotracheal Intubation

a. *No Recommendation* for using orotracheal rather than nasotracheal tube to prevent nosocomial pneumonia.(699) *UNRESOLVED ISSUE*

b. *No Recommendation* for routinely using an endotracheal tube with a dorsal lumen above the endotracheal cuff to allow drainage (by suctioning) of tracheal secretions that accumulate in the patient's subglottic area.(206) *UNRESOLVED ISSUE*

c. Before deflating the cuff of an endotracheal tube in preparation for tube removal, or before moving the tube, ensure that secretions are cleared from above the tube cuff. *CATEGORY IB*

3. Prevention of Gastric Colonization

a. If stress-bleeding prophylaxis is needed for a patient with mechanically assisted ventilation, use an agent that does not raise the patient's gastric pH.(22,34,112,118,122,147-154) *Category II*

b. *No Recommendation* for selective decontamination of a critically ill, mechanically ventilated, or ICU patient's digestive tract with oral and/or intravenous antimicrobials to prevent gram-negative bacillary (or *Candida* spp.) pneumonia.(155-180) *UNRESOLVED ISSUE*

c. *No Recommendation* for routine acidification of gastric feedings to prevent nosocomial pneumonia.(181) *UNRESOLVED ISSUE*

B. Prevention of Postoperative Pneumonia

1. Instruct preoperative patients, especially those at high risk of developing pneumonia, regarding frequent coughing, taking deep breaths, and ambulating as soon as medically indicated in the postoperative period.(346,348) High-risk patients include those who will receive anesthesia, especially those who will have an abdominal, thoracic, head, or neck operation, or who have substantial pulmonary dysfunction, such as patients with chronic obstructive lung disease, a musculoskeletal abnormality of the chest, or abnormal pulmonary function tests. (331-334,337,338) *CATEGORY IB*

2. Encourage postoperative patients to cough frequently, take deep breaths, move about the bed, and ambulate unless it is medically contraindicated.(345,346,348) *CATEGORY IB*

3. Control pain that interferes with coughing and deep breathing during the immediate postoperative period by using systemic analgesia, (352,701) including patient-controlled analgesia,(353-355) with as little cough-suppressant effect as possible; appropriate support for abdominal wounds, such as tightly placing a pillow across the abdomen; or regional (eg, epidural) analgesia.(356-358) *CATEGORY IB*

4. Use an incentive spirometer or intermittent positive pressure breathing on patients at high risk of developing postoperative pneumonia. (See III-B-1 above for definition of high-risk patients.)(339,342,343,346,348,349) *CATEGORY II*

C. Other Prophylactic Procedures for Pneumonia

1. Vaccination of Patients

Vaccinate patients at high risk for complications of pneumococcal infections with pneumococcal polysaccharide vaccine. High-risk patients include persons > or = 65 years old; adults with chronic cardiovascular or pulmonary disease, diabetes mellitus, alcoholism, cirrhosis, or cerebrospinal fluid leaks; and children and adults with immunosuppression, functional or anatomic asplenia, or HIV infection.(362-364) *CATEGORY IA*

2. Antimicrobial Prophylaxis

Do not routinely administer systemic antimicrobial agents to prevent nosocomial pneumonia.(74,91,201,366-370,702) *CATEGORY IA*

3. Use of Rotating "Kinetic" Beds or Continuous Lateral Rotational Therapy

No Recommendation for the routine use of "kinetic" beds or continuous lateral rotational therapy (i.e., placing patients on beds that turn on their longitudinal axes intermittently or continuously) for prevention of nosocomial pneumonia in patients in the ICU, critically ill patients, or patients immobilized by illness and/or trauma.(372-377,703) *UNRESOLVED ISSUE*

Return to: Part I: Issues on Prevention of Nosocomial Pneumonia - Bacterial Pneumonia

Back to: Contents Page

DHQP Home | DHQP Index
CDC Home | CDC Search | CDC Health Topics A-Z

This page last reviewed March 26, 1996

Centers for Disease Control and Prevention
National Center for Infectious Diseases
Division of Healthcare Quality Promotion

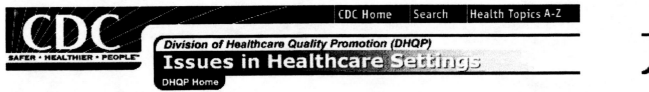

Back to: **Contents Page**

Legionnaires' Disease

Recommendations for Prevention of Nosocomial Legionnaires' Disease

---

I. STAFF EDUCATION AND INFECTION SURVEILLANCE

A. Staff Education

Educate (1) physicians to heighten their suspicion for cases of nosocomial Legionnaires' disease and to use appropriate methods for its diagnosis, and (2) patient-care, infection-control, and engineering personnel about measures to control nosocomial legionellosis.(659-661) *CATEGORY IA*

B. Surveillance

1. Establish mechanism(s) to provide clinicians with appropriate laboratory tests for the diagnosis of Legionnaires' disease. (386,414,415,419,704) *CATEGORY IA*

2. Maintain a high index of suspicion for the diagnosis of nosocomial Legionnaires' disease, especially in patients who are at high-risk of acquiring the disease (patients who are immunosuppressed, including organ-transplant patients, patients with AIDS, and patients receiving systemic steroids; are ≥65 years of age; or have chronic underlying disease such as diabetes mellitus, congestive heart failure, and chronic obstructive lung disease).(385,386,400,402-406,412) Refer to the accompanying background document for definition of nosocomial legionellosis. *CATEGORY II*

3. *No Recommendation* for routinely culturing water systems for *Legionella* spp.(271,385,429,433,435,436,438-440,456,705) *UNRESOLVED ISSUE*

II. Interruption of Transmission of *Legionella* Spp.

A. Primary Prevention (Preventing Nosocomial Legionnaires' Disease When No Cases Have Been Documented)

1. Nebulization and other devices

a. (1) Use sterile (not distilled, nonsterile) water for rinsing nebulization devices and other semicritical respiratory-care equipment after they have been cleaned and/or disinfected.(258,271,706) *CATEGORY IB*

(2) *No Recommendation* for using tap water as an alternative to sterile water to rinse reusable semicritical equipment and devices used on the respiratory tract, after they have been subjected to high-level disinfection, whether or not rinsing is followed by drying with or without the use of alcohol. *UNRESOLVED ISSUE*

b. Use only sterile (not distilled, nonsterile) water to fill reservoirs of devices used for nebulization.(241,252,258,271,706) *CATEGORY IA*

c. Do not use large-volume room-air humidifiers that create aerosols (eg, by venturi principle, ultrasound, or spinning disk) and thus are really nebulizers, unless they can be sterilized or subjected to high-level disinfection daily and filled only with sterile water.(252,706) *CATEGORY IA*

2. Cooling towers

a. When a new hospital building is constructed, place cooling tower(s) in such a way that the tower drift is directed away from the hospital's air-intake system, and design the cooling towers such that the volume of aerosol drift is minimized.(422,707) *CATEGORY IB*

http://www.cdc.gov/ncidod/hip/pneumonia/2_legion.htm

b. For operational cooling towers, install drift eliminators, regularly use an effective biocide, maintain the tower according to manufacturers' recommendations, and keep adequate maintenance records. (See Appendix D.) (422,464,708) *CATEGORY IB*

3. Water-Distribution System

a. *No Recommendation* for routinely maintaining potable water at the outlet at => 50°C or <20°c, or chlorinating heated water to achieve 1-2 mg/L free residual chlorine at the tap.(385,429,440,447-450) *UNRESOLVED ISSUE*

b. *No Recommendation* for treatment of water with ozone, ultraviolet light, or heavy-metal ions.(391,460-463,466) *UNRESOLVED ISSUE*

B. Secondary Prevention (Response to Identification of Laboratory-Confirmed Nosocomial Legionellosis)

When a single case of laboratory-confirmed, **definite** nosocomial Legionnaires' disease is identified, OR if two or more cases of laboratory-confirmed, **possible** nosocomial Legionnaires' disease occur within 6 months of each other (refer to background document for definition of definite and possible nosocomial Legionnaires' disease.):

1. Contact the local or state health department or the CDC if the disease is reportable in the state or if assistance is needed. *CATEGORY IB*

2. If a case is identified in a severely immunocompromised patient such as an organ-transplant recipient, OR if the hospital houses severely immunocompromised patients, conduct a combined epidemiologic and environmental investigation (as outlined from II-B-3-b-1 through II-B-5, below) to determine the source(s) of *Legionella* spp. *CATEGORY IB*

3. If the hospital does not house severely immunocompromised patients, conduct an epidemiologic investigation via a retrospective review of microbiologic, serologic, and postmortem data to identify previous cases, and begin an intensive prospective surveillance for additional cases of nosocomial Legionnaires' disease. *CATEGORY IB*

a. **If there is no evidence of continued nosocomial transmission,** continue the intensive prospective surveillance (as in II-B-3, above) for at least 2 months after surveillance was begun. *CATEGORY II*

b. **If there is evidence of continued transmission:**

(1) Conduct an environmental investigation to determine the source(s) of *Legionella* spp. by collecting water samples from potential sources of aerosolized water, following the methods described in Appendix C and saving and subtyping isolates of *Legionella* spp. obtained from patients and environment.(241,258,422-428,452,454) *CATEGORY IB*

(2) If a source is not identified, continue surveillance for new cases for at least 2 months, and, depending on the scope of the outbreak, decide on either deferring decontamination pending identification of the source(s) of *Legionella* spp., or proceeding with decontamination of the hospital's water distribution system, with special attention to the specific hospital areas involved in the outbreak. *CATEGORY II*

(3) If a source of infection is identified by epidemiologic and environmental investigation, promptly decontaminate it.(466) *CATEGORY IB*

(a) **If the heated-water system is implicated:**

i. Decontaminate the heated-water system either by superheating (flushing for at least 5 minutes each distal outlet of the system with water at 65şC), OR by hyperchlorination (flushing for at least 5 minutes all outlets of the system with water containing > or = 10 mg/L free residual chlorine).(450,452,456,457) Post warning signs at each outlet being flushed to prevent scald injury to patients, staff, or visitors. *CATEGORY IB*

ii. Depending on local and state regulations regarding potable water temperature in public buildings,(458) maintain potable water at the outlet at 50şC or <20şC, or chlorinate heated water to achieve 1-2 mg/L free residual chlorine at the tap in hospitals housing patients who are at high risk of acquiring nosocomial legionellosis (eg, immunocompromised patients).(385,429,440,447-450) (See Appendix B.) *CATEGORY II*

iii. *No Recommendation* for treatment of water with ozone, ultraviolet light, or heavy-metal ions.(391,460,461,463) *UNRESOLVED ISSUE*

iv. Clean hot-water storage tanks and waterheaters to remove accumulated scale and sediment.(393) *CATEGORY IB*

v. Restrict immunocompromised patients from taking showers, and use only sterile water for their oral consumption until *Legionella* spp. becomes undetectable by culture in the hospital water.(430) *CATEGORY II*

http://www.cdc.gov/ncidod/hip/pneumonia/2_legion.htm

(b) If cooling towers or evaporative condensers are implicated, decontaminate the cooling-tower system using the protocol outlined in Appendix D.(464) *CATEGORY IB*

(4) Assess the efficacy of implemented measures in reducing or eliminating *Legionella* spp. by collecting specimens for culture at 2-week intervals for 3 months. *CATEGORY II*

(a) If *Legionella* spp. are not detected in cultures during 3 months of monitoring, collect cultures monthly for another 3 months. *CATEGORY II*

(b) If *Legionella* spp. are detected in one or more cultures, reassess the implemented control measures, modify them accordingly, and repeat decontamination procedures. Options for repeat decontamination include the intensive use of the same technique utilized for initial decontamination, or a combination of superheating and hyperchlorination. *CATEGORY II*

(5) Keep adequate records of all infection control measures, including maintenance procedures, and of environmental test results for cooling towers and potable-water systems. *CATEGORY II*

Return to:Part I: Issues on Prevention of Nosocomial Pneumonia - Legionnaires' Disease

Back to: Contents Page

DHQP Home | DHQP Index
CDC Home | CDC Search | CDC Health Topics A-Z

This page last reviewed March 26, 1996

Centers for Disease Control and Prevention
National Center for Infectious Diseases
Division of Healthcare Quality Promotion

http://www.cdc.gov/ncidod/hip/pneumonia/2_legion.htm
204

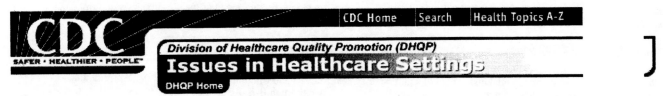

Back to: Contents Page

Nosocomial Pulmonary Aspergillosis

Recommendations for Prevention of Nosocomial Pulmonary Aspergillosis

---

I. STAFF EDUCATION AND INFECTION SURVEILLANCE

A. Staff Education

Educate healthcare workers regarding nosocomial pulmonary aspergillosis especially in immunocompromised patients, and about infection control procedures to decrease its occurrence.(659-661) *CATEGORY IA*

B. Surveillance

1. Maintain a high index of suspicion for the diagnosis of nosocomial pulmonary aspergillosis in high-risk patients, i.e., patients with prolonged, severe granulocytopenia (<1,000 polymorphonuclear cells/mm3 for 2 weeks or <100 polymorphonuclear cells/mm(3) for 1 week), most notably bone-marrow transplant recipients.(512,513,709) Consider solid-organ transplant recipients and patients with hematologic malignancies who are receiving chemotherapy also to be at high risk of developing the infection when they are severely granulocytopenic as defined above.(473,485,512,710) *CATEGORY IB*

2. Maintain surveillance for cases of nosocomial pulmonary aspergillosis by periodically reviewing the hospital's microbiologic, histopathologic, and postmortem data. *CATEGORY IB*

3. *No Recommendation* for performing routine, periodic cultures of the nasopharynx of high-risk patients, or devices, air samples, dust, ventilation ducts, and filters in rooms occupied by high-risk patients.(457,478,487,488,521-523) *UNRESOLVED ISSUE*

II. Interruption of Transmission of *Aspergillus* Spp. Spores

A. Planning New Specialized-Care Units for High-Risk Patients

1. When constructing new specialized-care units for high-risk patients, ensure that patient rooms have adequate capacity to minimize fungal spore counts via maintenance of (a) high-efficiency air filtration, (b) directed room airflow, (c) positive air pressure in patient's room in relation to the corridor, (d) properly sealed room, and (e) high rates of room-air changes.(474,529-531,534,538,711,712) *CATEGORY IB*

a. **Air filtration.** Install high efficiency particulate air (HEPA) filters that are 99.97% efficient in filtering 0.3 *u*-sized particles, either centrally or at the point of use, i.e., at the room-air intake site.(474,529-531,534,538,711,712) *CATEGORY IB*

b. **Directed room airflow.** Place air-intake and exhaust ports such that room air comes in from one side of the room, flows across the patient's bed, and exits on the opposite side of the room.(530,531) *CATEGORY IB*

c. **Well-sealed room.** Construct windows, doors, and intake and exhaust ports to achieve complete sealing of the room against air leaks. (530,531) *CATEGORY IB*

d. **Room-air pressure.** Ensure that room-air pressure can be maintained continuously above that of corridor, eg, as can be demonstrated by performance of the smoke-tube test, unless there are clinical-care or infection-control contraindications to doing so.(530,531) *CATEGORY IB*

(1) To maintain positive room-air pressure in relation to the corridor, supply room air at a rate that is 10-20% more than the rate of exhausting air from the room.(530,531) *CATEGORY IB*

(2) For placement of patients at high risk of aspergillosis who also have an infection (eg, varicella or infectious tuberculosis) requiring

negative room-air pressure in relation to the corridor, provide optimal conditions to prevent the spread of the airborne infection from and acquisition of aspergillosis by the patient, eg, by providing anterooms with an independent exhaust.(530) *CATEGORY II*

e. **Room-air changes.** Maintain room-air changes at >= 12 per hour.(1,530,536,537) *CATEGORY II*

2. *No Recommendation* for the preferential installation of a particular system, such as one with ultra-high air change rates (100-400 per hour), eg, laminar airflow, over other systems that meet the conditions in II-A-1-a through II-A-1-e above.(474,29-531,534,538,711,712) *UNRESOLVED ISSUE*

3. Formulate hospital policies to minimize exposures of high-risk patients to potential sources of *Aspergillus* spp., such as hospital construction and renovation, cleaning activities, carpets, food, potted plants, and flower arrangements.(467,487,523,528,713-715) *CATEGORY IB*

4. *No Recommendation* for prophylactic use of copper-8-quinolinolate biocide in fireproofing material.(467,477,531,538) *UNRESOLVED ISSUE*

B. In Existing Facilities with No Cases of Nosocomial Aspergillosis

1. Place high-risk patients in protected environment that meets the conditions outlined in Section II-A-1-a through II-A-1-e above. (474,487,529,538,711,712,716) *CATEGORY IB*

2. Routinely inspect air-handling systems in high-risk patient-care areas, maintain adequate air exchanges and pressure differentials, and eliminate air leakages. Coordinate repairs of the system with relocation of high-risk patients to other areas with optimal air-handling capabilities.(467,478,487) *CATEGORY IB*

3. Minimize the time high-risk patients spend outside their rooms for diagnostic procedures and other activities; and when high-risk patients leave their rooms, require them to wear well-fitting masks capable of filtering *Aspergillus* spp. spores. *CATEGORY IB*

4. Prevent dust accumulation by daily damp-dusting horizontal surfaces, regularly cleaning ceiling tiles and air-duct grates when the rooms are not occupied by patients, and maintaining adequate seals on windows to prevent room infiltration by outside air, especially in areas occupied by patients at high-risk for developing aspergillosis.(487) *CATEGORY IB*

5. Systematically review and coordinate infection-control strategies with personnel in charge of hospital engineering, maintenance, central supply and distribution, and catering.(467,523) *CATEGORY IB*

6. When planning hospital construction and renovation activities, assess whether patients at high-risk for aspergillosis are likely to be exposed to high ambient-air spore counts of *Aspergillus* spp. from construction and renovation sites, and develop a plan to prevent such exposures.(467,523) *CATEGORY IB*

7. During construction or renovation activities:

(a) Construct barriers between patient-care and construction areas to prevent dust from entering patient-care areas; these barriers, (eg, plastic or drywall) should be impermeable to *Aspergillus* spp.(467,478,522,523) *CATEGORY IB*

(b) In construction/renovation areas inside the hospital, create and maintain negative pressure relative to that in adjacent patient-care areas if there are no contraindications for such pressure differential, eg, there are patients with infectious tuberculosis in the adjacent patient-care areas.(467,478,522,523,538) *CATEGORY II*

(c) Direct pedestrian traffic from construction areas away from patient-care areas to limit opening and closing of doors (or other barriers) that may cause dust dispersion, entry of contaminated air, or tracking of dust into patient areas.(467,478,522,523) *CATEGORY IB*

(d) Clean newly constructed areas before allowing patients to enter the areas.(467,523) *CATEGORY IB*

8. Eliminate exposures of patients at high-risk for aspergillosis to activities, such as floor or carpet vacuuming, that may cause spores of *Aspergillus* spp. and other fungi to be aerosolized.(467,487,523) *CATEGORY IB*

9. Eliminate exposures of patients at high-risk for aspergillosis to potential environmental sources of *Aspergillus* spp., such as *Aspergillus*-contaminated food, potted plants, or flower arrangements.(467,487,523,713-715) *CATEGORY II*

10. Prevent birds from gaining access to hospital air-intake ducts.(524) *CATEGORY IB*

http://www.cdc.gov/ncidod/hip/pneumonia/2_asper.htm

C. When A Case of Nosocomial Aspergillosis Occurs

1. Begin a prospective search for additional cases in hospitalized patients and an intensified retrospective review of the hospital's microbiologic, histopathologic, and postmortem records. *CATEGORY IB*

2. If there is no evidence of continuing transmission, continue routine maintenance procedures to prevent nosocomial aspergillosis, as in Section II-B-1 through II-B-10 above. *CATEGORY IB*

3. If evidence of continuing *Aspergillus* spp. infection exists, conduct an environmental investigation to determine and eliminate the source. If assistance is needed, contact the local or state health department.(474,477,478,522,534,538) *CATEGORY IB*

a. Collect environmental samples from potential sources of *Aspergillus* spp., especially those sources implicated in the epidemiologic investigation, by using appropriate methods,(474,477,478,522,534,538,717) eg, use of a high-volume air sampler rather than settle plates. (474) *CATEGORY IB*

b. Perform molecular subtyping of *Aspergillus* spp. obtained from patients and the environment to establish strain identity, depending on test availability.(526,527) *CATEGORY IB*

c. If air-handling systems supplying high-risk patient-care areas are not optimal, consider temporary deployment of portable HEPA filters until rooms with optimal air-handling systems are available for all patients at high risk of invasive aspergillosis. *CATEGORY II*

d. If an environmental source is identified, perform corrective measures as needed to eliminate the source from the high-risk patients' environment. *CATEGORY IB*

e. If an environmental source is not identified, review existing infection-control measures, including engineering aspects, to identify potential areas that can be corrected or improved. *CATEGORY IB*

III. MODIFYING HOST RISK FOR INFECTION

A. Administer cytokines, including granulocyte colony-stimulating factor and granulocyte-macrophage stimulating factor, to increase host resistance to aspergillosis by decreasing the duration and severity of chemotherapy-induced granulocytopenia.(514,515) *CATEGORY II*

B. *No Recommendation* for administration of intranasal amphotericin B or oral antifungal agents (including amphotericin B and triazole compounds) in high-risk patients for prophylaxis against aspergillosis.(516,517,718) *UNRESOLVED ISSUE*

Return to: Part I: Issues on Prevention of Nosocomial Pneumonia - Aspergillosis

Back to: Contents Page

DHQP Home | DHQP Index
CDC Home | CDC Search | CDC Health Topics A-Z

This page last reviewed March 26, 1996

Centers for Disease Control and Prevention
National Center for Infectious Diseases
Division of Healthcare Quality Promotion

http://www.cdc.gov/ncidod/hip/pneumonia/2_asper.htm

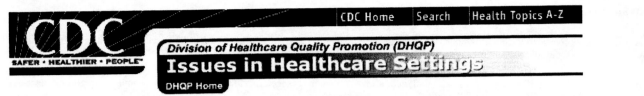

Back to: Contents Page

Respiratory Syncytial Virus Infection

Recommendations for Prevention of Nosocomial RSV Infection

I. Staff Education and Infection Surveillance

A. Staff education

Educate personnel about the epidemiology, modes of transmission and means of preventing spread of respiratory syncytial virus (RSV). (226,659-661) *CATEGORY IA*

B. Surveillance

1. Establish mechanism(s) by which the appropriate hospital personnel are promptly alerted to any increase in RSV activity in the local community. *CATEGORY IB*

2. During periods of increased prevalence of RSV in the community (and during December-March), attempt prompt diagnosis of RSV infection by using rapid diagnostic techniques as clinically indicated in pediatric patients, especially infants, and in immunocompromised adults admitted to the hospital with respiratory illness.(593,597) *CATEGORY IB*

II. Interruption of Transmission of RSV

A. Prevention of Person-to-Person Transmission

1. Primary measures for contact isolation

a. Handwashing

Wash hands after contact with a patient, or after touching respiratory secretions or fomites potentially contaminated with respiratory secretions, whether or not gloves are worn.(218,231,554,584-586,595) *CATEGORY IA*

b. Gloving

(1) Wear gloves for handling patients or respiratory secretions of patients with proven or suspected RSV infection, or fomites potentially contaminated with patient secretions.(226,554,584,585,591,597) *CATEGORY IA*

(2) Change gloves between patients, or after handling respiratory secretions or fomites contaminated with secretions from one patient before contact with another patient.(226,228) Wash hands after removing gloves. (See II-A-1-a, above.) *CATEGORY IA*

c. Gowning

Wear a gown when soiling with respiratory secretions from a patient is anticipated, eg, when handling infants with RSV infection or other viral respiratory illness, and change the gown after such contact and before caring for another patient.(226,590,592,597) *CATEGORY IB*

d. Staffing

Restrict health-care workers in the acute stages of an upper respiratory illness, i.e., those who are sneezing and/or coughing) from taking care of infants and other patients at high risk for complications from RSV infection (eg, children with severe underlying cardio-pulmonary conditions, children receiving chemotherapy for malignancy, premature infants, and patients who are otherwise immunocompromised).

http://www.cdc.gov/ncidod/hip/pneumonia/2_rsv.htm

(595,597) *CATEGORY IB*

e. Limiting visitors

Do not allow persons with symptoms of respiratory infection to visit uninfected pediatric, immunosuppressed, and cardiac patients.(591) *CATEGORY II*

2. Control of RSV outbreaks

a. Use of private room, cohorting, and patient-screening

To control ongoing RSV transmission in the hospital, admit young children with symptoms of viral respiratory illness to single rooms when possible, OR perform RSV-screening diagnostic tests on young children upon admission and cohort them according to their RSV-infection status. (591,593,595,597) *CATEGORY II*

b. Personnel cohorting

During an outbreak of nosocomial RSV, cohort personnel as much as practical, i.e., restrict personnel who give care to infected patients from giving care to uninfected patients, and vice-versa.(591,595,597) *CATEGORY II*

c. Postponing patient admission

During outbreaks of nosocomial RSV, postpone elective admission of uninfected patients at high risk of complications from RSV infection. *CATEGORY II*

d. Wearing eye-nose goggles

No Recommendation for wearing eye-nose goggles for close contact with an RSV-infected patient.(594,598) *UNRESOLVED ISSUE*

Return to:Part 1: Issues on Prevention of Nosocomial Pneumonia - RSV Infection

Back to: Contents Page

DHQP Home | DHQP Index
CDC Home | CDC Search | CDC Health Topics A-Z

This page last reviewed March 26, 1996

Centers for Disease Control and Prevention
National Center for Infectious Diseases
Division of Healthcare Quality Promotion

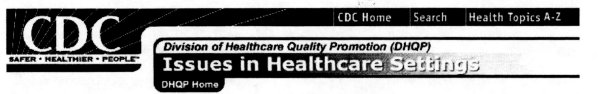

Influenza

Recommendations for the Prevention of Nosocomial Influenza

I. Staff Education and Infection Surveillance

A. Staff Education

Educate personnel about the epidemiology, modes of transmission, and means of preventing the spread of influenza.(659-661,719,720) *CATEGORY IA*

B. Surveillance

1. Establish mechanism(s) by which the appropriate hospital personnel are promptly alerted of any increase in influenza activity in the local community. *CATEGORY IB*

2. Arrange for laboratory tests to be available to clinicians, for use when clinically indicated, to promptly confirm the diagnosis of influenza and other acute viral respiratory illnesses, especially during November-April.(620-625) *CATEGORY IB*

II. Modifying Host Risk to Infection

A. Vaccination

1. Patients

Offer vaccine to outpatients and inpatients at high risk of complications from influenza, beginning in September and continuing until influenza activity has begun to decline.(628,631,648,721-723) Patients at high risk of complications from influenza include those > or = 65 years of age; in long-term-care units; with chronic disorders of the pulmonary or cardiovascular systems, diabetes mellitus, renal dysfunction, hemoglobinopathies, or immunosuppression; and children 6 months-18 years of age who are receiving long-term aspirin therapy.(628) In addition, consider patients with musculo-skeletal disorders that impede adequate respiration to be at risk of complications from influenza. *CATEGORY IA*

2. Personnel

Vaccinate health-care workers before the influenza season each year, preferably between mid-October and mid-November. Until influenza activity declines, continue to make vaccine available to newly hired personnel and to those who initially refuse vaccination. If vaccine supply is limited, give highest priority to staff caring for patients at greatest risk of severe complications from influenza infection, as listed in Section II-A-1 above.(628) *CATEGORY IB*

B. Use of Antiviral Agents (See Section IV below, Control of Influenza Outbreaks)

III. Interruption of (Person-to-Person) Transmission

A. Keep a patient for whom influenza is suspected or diagnosed in a private room, or in a room with other patients with proven influenza, unless there are medical contraindications to doing so. *CATEGORY IB*

B. As much as feasible, maintain negative air pressure in rooms of patients for whom influenza is suspected or diagnosed, or place together persons with influenza-like illness in a hospital area with an independent air-supply and exhaust system.(614,615,724) *CATEGORY II*

http://www.cdc.gov/ncidod/hip/pneumonia/2_flu.htm

C. Institute masking of individuals (except those immune to the infecting strain) who enter the room of a patient with influenza. (614,615,724) *CATEGORY IB*

D. As much as possible during periods of influenza activity in the community, have the hospital's employee health service evaluate patient-care staff who have symptoms of febrile upper respiratory tract infection suggestive of influenza for possible removal from duties that involve direct patient contact. Use more stringent guidelines for staff working in certain patient-care areas, eg, ICUs, nurseries, and units with severely immunosuppressed patients.(649,725) *CATEGORY II*

E. When community and/or nosocomial outbreaks occur, especially if they are characterized by high attack rates and severe illness:

1. Restrict hospital visitors who have a febrile respiratory·illness. *CATEGORY IB*

2. Curtail or eliminate elective medical and surgical admissions as necessary. *CATEGORY IB*

3. Restrict cardiovascular and pulmonary surgery to only emergency cases. *CATEGORY IB*

IV. Control of Influenza Outbreaks

A. Determining the Outbreak Strain

Early in the outbreak, obtain nasopharyngeal-swab or nasal-wash specimens from patients with recent-onset symptoms suggestive of influenza for influenza virus culture or antigen detection. *CATEGORY IB*

B. Vaccination of Patients and Personnel

Administer current influenza vaccine to unvaccinated patients and staff, especially if the outbreak occurs early in the influenza season. (610,628) *CATEGORY IB*

C. Amantadine or Rimantadine Administration

1. When a nosocomial outbreak of influenza A is suspected or recognized:

a. Administer amantadine or rimantadine for prophylaxis to all uninfected patients in the involved unit for whom it is not contraindicated. Do not delay administration of amantadine or rimantadine unless the results of diagnostic tests to identify the infecting strain(s) can be obtained within 12 to 24 hours after specimen collection.(634,642) *CATEGORY IB*

b. Administer amantadine or rimantadine for prophylaxis to unvaccinated staff members for whom it is not medically contraindicated, and who are in the involved unit or taking care of high-risk patients.(642) *CATEGORY II*

2. Discontinue amantadine or rimantadine if laboratory tests confirm or strongly suggest that influenza type A is not the cause of the outbreak.(632) *CATEGORY IA*

3. If the cause of the outbreak is confirmed or believed to be influenza type A AND vaccine has been administered only recently to susceptible patients and personnel, continue amantadine or rimantadine prophylaxis until 2 weeks after the vaccination.(726) *CATEGORY IB*

4. To the extent possible, do not allow contact between those at high risk of complications from influenza and patients or staff who are taking amantadine or rimantadine for treatment of acute respiratory illness; prevent contact during and for two days after the latter discontinue treatment.(633,643-647) *CATEGORY IB*

D. Interruption of (Person-to-Person) Transmission of Microorganisms (See Section III, A-E above.)

Return to: Part I: Issues on Prevention of Nosocomal Pneumonia - Influenza

Back to: Contents Page

Please note: An erratum has been published for this issue. To view the erratum, please click here.

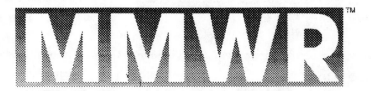

Morbidity and Mortality Weekly Report

Recommendations and Reports   August 9, 2002 / Vol. 51 / No. RR-10

Guidelines for the Prevention of Intravascular Catheter-Related Infections

CENTERS FOR DISEASE CONTROL AND PREVENTION
SAFER • HEALTHIER • PEOPLE™

The *MMWR* series of publications is published by the Epidemiology Program Office, Centers for Disease Control and Prevention (CDC), U.S. Department of Health and Human Services, Atlanta, GA 30333.

Centers for Disease Control and Prevention

Julie L. Gerberding, M.D., M.P.H.
Director

David W. Fleming, M.D.
Deputy Director for Science and Public Health

Dixie E. Snider, Jr., M.D., M.P.H.
Associate Director for Science

Epidemiology Program Office

Stephen B. Thacker, M.D., M.Sc.
Director

Office of Scientific and Health Communications

John W. Ward, M.D.
Director
Editor, MMWR Series

Suzanne M. Hewitt, M.P.A.
Managing Editor

Teresa F. Rutledge
Rachel J. Wilson
Project Editors

Malbea A. Heilman
Beverly J. Holland
Visual Information Specialists

Quang M. Doan
Erica R. Shaver
Information Technology Specialists

CONTENTS

Guidelines for the Prevention of Intravascular Catheter-Related Infections

Prepared by
Naomi P. O'Grady, M.D.[1]
Mary Alexander[2]
E. Patchen Dellinger, M.D.[3]
Julie L. Gerberding, M.D., M.P.H.[4]
Stephen O. Heard, M.D.[5]
Dennis G. Maki, M.D.[6]
Henry Masur, M.D.[1]
Rita D. McCormick, M.D.[7]
Leonard A. Mermel, D.O.[8]
Michele L. Pearson, M.D.[9]
Issam I. Raad, M.D.[10]
Adrienne Randolph, M.D., M.Sc.[11]
Robert A. Weinstein, M.D.[12]

[1]National Institutes of Health, Bethesda, Maryland
[2]Infusion Nurses Society, Cambridge, Massachusetts
[3]University of Washington, Seattle, Washington
[4]Office of the Director, CDC, Atlanta, Georgia
[5]University of Massachusetts Medical School, Worcester, Massachusetts
[6]University of Wisconsin Medical School, Madison, Wisconsin
[7]University of Wisconsin Hospital and Clinics, Madison, Wisconsin
[8]Rhode Island Hospital and Brown University School of Medicine, Providence, Rhode Island
[9]Division of Healthcare Quality Promotion, National Center for Infectious Diseases, CDC, Atlanta, Georgia
[10]MD Anderson Cancer Center, Houston, Texas
[11]The Children's Hospital, Boston, Massachusetts
[12]Cook County Hospital and Rush Medical College, Chicago, Illinois

Summary

These guidelines have been developed for practitioners who insert catheters and for persons responsible for surveillance and control of infections in hospital, outpatient, and home health-care settings. This report was prepared by a working group comprising members from professional organizations representing the disciplines of critical care medicine, infectious diseases, health-care infection control, surgery, anesthesiology, interventional radiology, pulmonary medicine, pediatric medicine, and nursing. The working group was led by the Society of Critical Care Medicine (SCCM), in collaboration with the Infectious Disease Society of America (IDSA), Society for Healthcare Epidemiology of America (SHEA), Surgical Infection Society (SIS), American College of Chest Physicians (ACCP), American Thoracic Society (ATS), American Society of Critical Care Anesthesiologists (ASCCA), Association for Professionals in Infection Control and Epidemiology (APIC), Infusion Nurses Society (INS), Oncology Nursing Society (ONS), Society of Cardiovascular and Interventional Radiology (SCVIR), American Academy of Pediatrics (AAP), and the Healthcare Infection Control Practices Advisory Committee (HICPAC) of the Centers for Disease Control and Prevention (CDC) and is intended to replace the Guideline for Prevention of Intravascular Device-Related Infections published in 1996. These guidelines are intended to provide evidence-based recommendations for preventing catheter-related infections. Major areas of emphasis include 1) educating and training health-care providers who insert and maintain catheters; 2) using maximal sterile barrier precautions during central venous catheter insertion; 3) using a 2% chlorhexidine preparation for skin antisepsis; 4) avoiding routine replacement of central venous catheters as a strategy to prevent infection; and 5) using antiseptic/antibiotic impregnated short-term central venous catheters if the rate of infection is high despite adherence to other strategies (i.e., education and training, maximal sterile barrier precautions, and 2% chlorhexidine for skin antisepsis). These guidelines also identify performance indicators that can be used locally by health-care institutions or organizations to monitor their success in implementing these evidence-based recommendations.

The material in this report was prepared for publication by the National Center for Infectious Diseases, James M. Hughes, M.D., Director; Division of Healthcare Quality Promotion, Steven L. Solomon, M.D., Acting Director.

Introduction

This report provides health-care practitioners with background information and specific recommendations to reduce the incidence of intravascular catheter-related bloodstream infections (CRBSI). These guidelines replace the *Guideline for Prevention of Intravascular Device-Related Infections*, which was published in 1996 (*1*).

The *Guidelines for the Prevention of Intravascular Catheter-Related Infections* have been developed for practitioners who insert catheters and for persons who are responsible for surveillance and control of infections in hospital, outpatient, and home health-care settings. This report was prepared by a working group composed of professionals representing the disciplines of critical care medicine, infectious diseases, health-care infection control, surgery, anesthesiology, interventional radiology, pulmonary medicine, pediatrics, and nursing. The working group was led by the Society of Critical Care Medicine (SCCM), in collaboration with Infectious Disease Society of America (IDSA), Society for Healthcare Epidemiology of America (SHEA), Surgical Infection Society (SIS), American College of Chest Physicians (ACCP), American Thoracic Society (ATS), American Society of Critical Care Anesthesiologists (ASCCA), Association for Professionals in Infection Control and Epidemiology (APIC), Infusion Nurses Society (INS), Oncology Nursing Society (ONS), Society of Cardiovascular and Interventional Radiology (SCVIR), American Academy of Pediatrics (AAP), and the Healthcare Infection Control Practices Advisory Committee (HICPAC) of the Centers for Disease Control and Prevention (CDC). The recommendations presented in this report reflect consensus of HICPAC and other professional organizations.

Intravascular Catheter-Related Infections in Adult and Pediatric Patients: An Overview

Background

Intravascular catheters are indispensable in modern-day medical practice, particularly in intensive care units (ICUs). Although such catheters provide necessary vascular access, their use puts patients at risk for local and systemic infectious complications, including local site infection, CRBSI, septic thrombophlebitis, endocarditis, and other metastatic infections (e.g., lung abscess, brain abscess, osteomyelitis, and endophthalmitis).

Health-care institutions purchase millions of intravascular catheters each year. The incidence of CRBSI varies considerably by type of catheter, frequency of catheter manipulation, and patient-related factors (e.g., underlying disease and acuity of illness). Peripheral venous catheters are the devices most frequently used for vascular access. Although the incidence of local or bloodstream infections (BSIs) associated with peripheral venous catheters is usually low, serious infectious complications produce considerable annual morbidity because of the frequency with which such catheters are used. However, the majority of serious catheter-related infections are associated with central venous catheters (CVCs), especially those that are placed in patients in ICUs. In the ICU setting, the incidence of infection is often higher than in the less acute in-patient or ambulatory setting. In the ICU, central venous access might be needed for extended periods of time; patients can be colonized with hospital-acquired organisms; and the catheter can be manipulated multiple times per day for the administration of fluids, drugs, and blood products. Moreover, some catheters can be inserted in urgent situations, during which optimal attention to aseptic technique might not be feasible. Certain catheters (e.g., pulmonary artery catheters and peripheral arterial catheters) can be accessed multiple times per day for hemodynamic measurements or to obtain samples for laboratory analysis, augmenting the potential for contamination and subsequent clinical infection.

The magnitude of the potential for CVCs to cause morbidity and mortality resulting from infectious complications has been estimated in several studies (*2*). In the United States, 15 million CVC days (i.e., the total number of days of exposure to CVCs by all patients in the selected population during the selected time period) occur in ICUs each year (*2*). If the average rate of CVC-associated BSIs is 5.3 per 1,000 catheter days in the ICU (*3*), approximately 80,000 CVC-associated BSIs occur in ICUs each year in the United States. The attributable mortality for these BSIs has ranged from no increase in mortality in studies that controlled for severity of illness (*4–6*), to 35% increase in mortality in prospective studies that did not use this control (*7,8*). Thus, the attributable mortality remains unclear. The attributable cost per infection is an estimated $34,508–$56,000 (*5,9*), and the annual cost of caring for patients with CVC-associated BSIs ranges from $296 million to $2.3 billion (*10*).

A total of 250,000 cases of CVC-associated BSIs have been estimated to occur annually if entire hospitals are assessed rather than ICUs exclusively (*11*). In this case, attributable mortality is an estimated 12%–25% for each infection, and the marginal cost to the health-care system is $25,000 per episode (*11*).

Therefore, by several analyses, the cost of CVC-associated BSI is substantial, both in terms of morbidity and in terms of financial resources expended. To improve patient outcome and reduce health-care costs, strategies should be implemented to reduce the incidence of these infections. This effort should be multidisciplinary, involving health-care professionals who insert and maintain intravascular catheters, health-care managers who allocate resources, and patients who are capable of assisting in the care of their catheters. Although several individual strategies have been studied and shown to be effective in reducing CRBSI, studies using multiple strategies have not been conducted. Thus, it is not known whether implementing multiple strategies will have an additive effect in reducing CRBSI, but it is logical to use multiple strategies concomitantly.

Terminology and Estimates of Risk

The terminology used to identify different types of catheters is confusing, because many clinicians and researchers use different aspects of the catheter for informal reference. A catheter can be designated by the type of vessel it occupies (e.g., peripheral venous, central venous, or arterial); its intended life span (e.g., temporary or short-term versus permanent or long-term); its site of insertion (e.g., subclavian, femoral, internal jugular, peripheral, and peripherally inserted central catheter [PICC]); its pathway from skin to vessel (e.g., tunneled versus nontunneled); its physical length (e.g., long versus short); or some special characteristic of the catheter (e.g., presence or absence of a cuff, impregnation with heparin, antibiotics or antiseptics, and the number of lumens). To accurately define a specific type of catheter, all of these aspects should be described (Table 1).

The rate of all catheter-related infections (including local infections and systemic infections) is difficult to determine. Although CRBSI is an ideal parameter because it represents the most serious form of catheter-related infection, the rate of such infection depends on how CRBSI is defined.

Health-care professionals should recognize the difference between surveillance definitions and clinical definitions. The surveillance definitions for catheter-associated BSI includes all BSIs that occur in patients with CVCs, when other sites of infection have been excluded (Appendix A). That is, the surveillance definition overestimates the true incidence of CRBSI because not all BSIs originate from a catheter. Some bacteremias are secondary BSIs from undocumented sources (e.g., postoperative surgical sites, intra-abdominal infections, and hospital-associated pneumonia or urinary tract infections). Thus, surveillance definitions are really definitions for

TABLE 1. Catheters used for venous and arterial access

Catheter type	Entry site	Length	Comments
Peripheral venous catheters (short)	Usually inserted in veins of forearm or hand	<3 inches; rarely associated with bloodstream infection	Phlebitis with prolonged use; rarely associated with bloodstream infection
Peripheral arterial catheters	Usually inserted in radial artery; can be placed in femoral, axillary, brachial, posterior tibial arteries	<3 inches; associated with bloodstream infection	Low infection risk; rarely associated with bloodstream infection
Midline catheters	Inserted via the antecubital fossa into the proximal basilic or cephalic veins; does not enter central veins, peripheral catheters	3 to 8 inches	Anaphylactoid reactions have been reported with catheters made of elastomeric hydrogel; lower rates of phlebitis than short peripheral catheters
Nontunneled central venous catheters	Percutaneously inserted into central veins (subclavian, internal jugular, or femoral)	≥8 cm depending on patient size	Account for majority of CRBSI
Pulmonary artery catheters	Inserted through a Teflon® introducer in a central vein (subclavian, internal jugular, or femoral)	≥30 cm depending on patient size	Usually heparin bonded; similar rates of bloodstream infection as CVCs; subclavian site preferred to reduce infection risk
Peripherally inserted central venous catheters (PICC)	Inserted into basilic, cephalic, or brachial veins and enter the superior vena cava	≥20 cm depending on patient size	Lower rate of infection than nontunneled CVCs
Tunneled central venous catheters	Implanted into subclavian, internal jugular, or femoral veins	≥8 cm depending on patient size	Cuff inhibits migration of organisms into catheter tract; lower rate of infection than nontunneled CVC
Totally implantable	Tunneled beneath skin and have subcutaneous port accessed with a needle; implanted in subclavian or internal jugular vein	≥8 cm depending on patient size	Lowest risk for CRBSI; improved patient self-image; no need for local catheter-site care; surgery required for catheter removal
Umbilical catheters	Inserted into either umbilical vein or umbilical artery	≤6 cm depending on patient size	Risk for CRBSI similar with catheters placed in umbilical vein versus artery

catheter-associated BSIs. A more rigorous definition might include only those BSIs for which other sources were excluded by careful examination of the patient record, and where a culture of the catheter tip demonstrated substantial colonies of an organism identical to those found in the bloodstream. Such a clinical definition would focus on catheter-related BSIs. Therefore, to accurately compare a health-care facility's infection rate to published data, comparable definitions also should be used.

CDC and the Joint Commission on Accreditation of Healthcare Organizations (JCAHO) recommend that the rate of catheter-associated BSIs be expressed as the number of catheter associated BSIs per 1,000 CVC days (12,13). This parameter is more useful than the rate expressed as the number of catheter-associated infections per 100 catheters (or percentage of catheters studied), because it accounts for BSIs over time and therefore adjusts risk for the number of days the catheter is in use.

Epidemiology and Microbiology

Since 1970, CDC's National Nosocomial Infection Surveillance System (NNIS) has been collecting data on the incidence and etiologies of hospital-acquired infections, including CVC-associated BSIs in a group of nearly 300 U.S. hospitals. The majority of hospital-acquired BSIs are associated with the use of a CVC, with BSI rates being substantially higher among patients with CVCs than among those without CVCs. Rates of CVC-associated BSI vary considerably by hospital size, hospital service/unit, and type of CVC. During 1992–2001, NNIS hospitals reported ICU rates of CVC-associated BSI ranging from 2.9 (in a cardiothoracic ICU) to 11.3 (in a neonatal nursery for infants weighing <1,000 g) BSIs per 1,000 CVC days (Table 2) (14).

The relative risk of catheter-associated BSI also has been assessed in a meta-analysis of 223 prospective studies of adult patients (11). Relative risk of infection was best determined by analyzing rates of infection both by BSIs per 100 catheters and BSIs per 1,000 catheter days. These rates, and the NNIS-derived data, can be used as benchmarks by individual hospitals to estimate how their rates compare with other institutions. Rates are influenced by patient-related parameters, such as severity of illness and type of illness (e.g., third-degree burns versus postcardiac surgery), and by catheter-related parameters, such as the condition under which the catheter was placed (e.g., elective versus urgent) and catheter type (e.g., tunneled versus nontunneled or subclavian versus jugular).

Types of organisms that most commonly cause hospital-acquired BSIs change over time. During 1986–1989, coagulase-negative staphylococci, followed by *Staphylococcus aureus*, were the most frequently reported causes of BSIs, accounting for

TABLE 2. Pooled means of the distribution of central venous catheter-associated bloodstream infection rates in hospitals reporting to the National Nosocomial Infection Surveillance System, January 1992–June 2001 (issued August 2001)

Type of intensive care unit	No.	Catheter days	Pool mean/1,000 catheter-days
Coronary	102	252,325	4.5
Cardiothoracic	64	419,674	2.9
Medical	135	671,632	5.9
Medical/surgical			
Major teaching	123	579,704	5.3
All others	180	863,757	3.8
Neurosurgical	47	123,780	4.7
Nursery, high risk (HRN)			
<1,000 g	138	438,261	11.3
1,001–1,500 g	136	213,351	6.9
1,501–2,500 g	132	163,697	4.0
>2,500 g	133	231,573	3.8
Pediatric	74	291,831	7.6
Surgical	153	900,948	5.3
Trauma	25	116,709	7.9
Burn	18	43,196	9.7
Respiratory	7	21,265	3.4

27% and 16% of BSIs, respectively (Table 3) (15). Pooled data from 1992 through 1999 indicate that coagulase-negative staphylococci, followed by enterococci, are now the most frequently isolated causes of hospital-acquired BSIs (12). Coagulase-negative staphylococci account for 37% (12) and *S. aureus* account for 12.6% of reported hospital-acquired BSIs (12). Also notable was the susceptibility pattern of *S. aureus* isolates. In 1999, for the first time since NNIS has been reporting susceptibilities, >50% of all *S. aureus* isolates from ICUs were resistant to oxacillin (12).

In 1999, enterococci accounted for 13.5% of BSIs, an increase from 8% reported to NNIS during 1986–1989. The percentage of enterococcal ICU isolates resistant to vancomycin also is increasing, escalating from 0.5% in 1989 to 25.9% in 1999 (12).

Candida spp. caused 8% of hospital-acquired BSIs reported to NNIS during 1986–1989 (15,16), and during 1992–1999 (12,17,18). Resistance of *Candida* spp. to commonly used

TABLE 3. Most common pathogens isolated from hospital acquired bloodstream infections

Pathogen	1986–1989 (%)	1992–1999 (%)
Coagulase-negative staphylococci	27	37
Staphylococcus aureus	16	13
Enterococcus	8	13
Gram-negative rods	19	14
Escherichia coli	6	2
Enterobacter	5	5
Pseudomonas aeruginosa	4	4
Klebsiella pneumoniae	4	3
Candida spp.	8	8

antifungal agents is increasing. Although NNIS has not reported the percentage of BSIs caused by nonalbicans species or fluconazole susceptibility data, other epidemiologic and clinical data document that fluconazole resistance is an increasingly relevant consideration when designing empiric therapeutic regimens for CRBSIs caused by yeast. Data from the Surveillance and Control of Pathogens of Epidemiologic Importance (SCOPE) Program documented that 10% of *C. albicans* bloodstream isolates from hospitalized patients were resistant to fluconazole (*17*). Additionally, 48% of *Candida* BSIs were caused by nonalbicans species, including *C. glabrata* and *C. krusei*, which are more likely than *C. albicans* to demonstrate resistance to fluconazole and itraconazole (*18,19*).

Gram-negative bacilli accounted for 19% of catheter-associated BSIs during 1986–1989 (*15*) compared with 14% of catheter-associated BSIs during 1992–1999 (*12*). An increasing percentage of ICU-related isolates are caused by *Enterobacteriaceae* that produce extended-spectrum ß-lactamases (ESBLs), particularly *Klebsiella pneumoniae* (*20*). Such organisms not only are resistant to extended-spectrum cephalosporins, but also to frequently used, broad spectrum antimicrobial agents.

Pathogenesis

Migration of skin organisms at the insertion site into the cutaneous catheter tract with colonization of the catheter tip is the most common route of infection for peripherally inserted, short-term catheters (*21,22*). Contamination of the catheter hub contributes substantially to intraluminal colonization of long-term catheters (*23–25*). Occasionally, catheters might become hematogenously seeded from another focus of infection. Rarely, infusate contamination leads to CRBSI (*26*).

Important pathogenic determinants of catheter-related infection are 1) the material of which the device is made and 2) the intrinsic virulence factors of the infecting organism. In vitro studies demonstrate that catheters made of polyvinyl chloride or polyethylene are likely less resistant to the adherence of microorganisms than are catheters made of Teflon®, silicone elastomer, or polyurethane (*27,28*). Therefore, the majority of catheters sold in the United States are no longer made of polyvinyl chloride or polyethylene. Some catheter materials also have surface irregularities that enhance the microbial adherence of certain species (e.g., coagulase-negative staphylococci, *Acinetobacter calcoaceticus*, and *Pseudomonas aeruginosa*) (*29–31*); catheters made of these materials are especially vulnerable to microbial colonization and subsequent infection. Additionally, certain catheter materials are more thrombogenic than others, a characteristic that also might predispose to catheter colonization and catheter-related

infection (*31,32*). This association has led to emphasis on preventing catheter-related thrombus as an additional mechanism for reducing CRBSI.

The adherence properties of a given microorganism also are important in the pathogenesis of catheter-related infection. For example, *S. aureus* can adhere to host proteins (e.g., fibronectin) commonly present on catheters (*33,34*). Also, coagulase-negative staphylococci adhere to polymer surfaces more readily than do other pathogens (e.g., *Escherichia coli* or *S. aureus*). Additionally, certain strains of coagulase-negative staphylococci produce an extracellular polysaccharide often referred to as "slime" (*35,36*). In the presence of catheters, this slime potentiates the pathogenicity of coagulase-negative staphylococci by allowing them to withstand host defense mechanisms (e.g., acting as a barrier to engulfment and killing by polymorphonuclear leukocytes) or by making them less susceptible to antimicrobial agents (e.g., forming a matrix that binds antimicrobials before their contact with the organism cell wall) (*37*). Certain *Candida* spp., in the presence of glucose-containing fluids, might produce slime similar to that of their bacterial counterparts, potentially explaining the increased proportion of BSIs caused by fungal pathogens among patients receiving parenteral nutrition fluids (*38*).

Strategies for Prevention of Catheter-Related Infections in Adult and Pediatric Patients

Quality Assurance and Continuing Education

Measures to minimize the risk for infection associated with intravascular therapy should strike a balance between patient safety and cost effectiveness. As knowledge, technology, and health-care settings change, infection control and prevention measures also should change. Well-organized programs that enable health-care providers to provide, monitor, and evaluate care and to become educated are critical to the success of this effort. Reports spanning the past two decades have consistently demonstrated that risk for infection declines following standardization of aseptic care (*39–43*), and that insertion and maintenance of intravascular catheters by inexperienced staff might increase the risk for catheter colonization and CRBSI (*43,44*). Specialized "IV teams" have shown unequivocal effectiveness in reducing the incidence of catheter-related infections and associated complications and costs (*45–47*). Additionally, infection risk increases with nursing staff reductions below a critical level (*48*).

Site of Catheter Insertion

The site at which a catheter is placed influences the subsequent risk for catheter-related infection and phlebitis. The influence of site on the risk for catheter infections is related in part to the risk for thrombophlebitis and density of local skin flora.

Phlebitis has long been recognized as a risk for infection. For adults, lower extremity insertion sites are associated with a higher risk for infection than are upper extremity sites (49–51). In addition, hand veins have a lower risk for phlebitis than do veins on the wrist or upper arm (52).

The density of skin flora at the catheter insertion site is a major risk factor for CRBSI. Authorities recommend that CVCs be placed in a subclavian site instead of a jugular or femoral site to reduce the risk for infection. No randomized trial satisfactorily has compared infection rates for catheters placed in jugular, subclavian, and femoral sites. Catheters inserted into an internal jugular vein have been associated with higher risk for infection than those inserted into a subclavian or femoral vein (22,53,54).

Femoral catheters have been demonstrated to have relatively high colonization rates when used in adults (55). Femoral catheters should be avoided, when possible, because they are associated with a higher risk for deep venous thrombosis than are internal jugular or subclavian catheters (56–60) and because of a presumption that such catheters are more likely to become infected. However, studies in pediatric patients have demonstrated that femoral catheters have a low incidence of mechanical complications and might have an equivalent infection rate to that of nonfemoral catheters (61–63). Thus, in adult patients, a subclavian site is preferred for infection control purposes, although other factors (e.g., the potential for mechanical complications, risk for subclavian vein stenosis, and catheter-operator skill) should be considered when deciding where to place the catheter. In a meta-analysis of eight studies, the use of bedside ultrasound for the placement of CVCs substantially reduced mechanical complications compared with the standard landmark placement technique (relative risk [RR] = 0.22; 95% confidence interval [CI] = 0.10–0.45) (64). Consideration of comfort, security, and maintenance of asepsis as well as patient-specific factors (e.g., preexisting catheters, anatomic deformity, and bleeding diathesis), relative risk of mechanical complications (e.g., bleeding and pneumothorax), the availability of bedside ultrasound, and the risk for infection should guide site selection.

Type of Catheter Material

Teflon® or polyurethane catheters have been associated with fewer infectious complications than catheters made of polyvinyl chloride or polyethylene (27,65,66). Steel needles used as an alternative to catheters for peripheral venous access have the same rate of infectious complications as do Teflon® catheters (67,68). However, the use of steel needles frequently is complicated by infiltration of intravenous (IV) fluids into the subcutaneous tissues, a potentially serious complication if the infused fluid is a vesicant (68).

Hand Hygiene and Aseptic Technique

For short peripheral catheters, good hand hygiene before catheter insertion or maintenance, combined with proper aseptic technique during catheter manipulation, provides protection against infection. Good hand hygiene can be achieved through the use of either a waterless, alcohol-based product (69) or an antibacterial soap and water with adequate rinsing (70). Appropriate aseptic technique does not necessarily require sterile gloves; a new pair of disposable nonsterile gloves can be used in conjunction with a "no-touch" technique for the insertion of peripheral venous catheters. However, gloves are required by the Occupational Safety and Health Administration as standard precautions for the prevention of bloodborne pathogen exposure.

Compared with peripheral venous catheters, CVCs carry a substantially greater risk for infection; therefore, the level of barrier precautions needed to prevent infection during insertion of CVCs should be more stringent. Maximal sterile barrier precautions (e.g., cap, mask, sterile gown, sterile gloves, and large sterile drape) during the insertion of CVCs substantially reduces the incidence of CRBSI compared with standard precautions (e.g., sterile gloves and small drapes) (22,71). Although the efficacy of such precautions for insertion of PICCs and midline catheters has not been studied, the use of maximal barrier precautions also is probably applicable to PICCs.

Skin Antisepsis

In the United States, povidone iodine has been the most widely used antiseptic for cleansing arterial catheter and CVC-insertion sites (72). However, in one study, preparation of central venous and arterial sites with a 2% aqueous chlorhexidine gluconate lowered BSI rates compared with site preparation with 10% povidone-iodine or 70% alcohol (73). Commercially available products containing chlorhexidine have not been available until recently; in July 2000, the U.S. Food and Drug Administration (FDA) approved a 2% tincture of chlorhexidine preparation for skin antisepsis. Other preparations of chlorhexidine might not be as effective. Tincture of chlorhexidine gluconate 0.5% is no more effective in preventing CRBSI or CVC colonization than 10% povidone iodine, as demonstrated by a prospective, randomized study of adults

(74). However, in a study involving neonates, 0.5% chlorhexidine reduced peripheral IV colonization compared with povidone iodine (20/418 versus 38/408 catheters; p = 0.01) (75). This study, which did not include CVCs, had an insufficient number of participants to assess differences in BSI rates. A 1% tincture of chlorhexidine preparation is available in Canada and Australia, but not yet in the United States. No published trials have compared a 1% chlorhexidine preparation to povidone-iodine.

Catheter Site Dressing Regimens

Transparent, semipermeable polyurethane dressings have become a popular means of dressing catheter insertion sites. Transparent dressings reliably secure the device, permit continuous visual inspection of the catheter site, permit patients to bathe and shower without saturating the dressing, and require less frequent changes than do standard gauze and tape dressings; the use of these dressings saves personnel time.

In the largest controlled trial of dressing regimens on peripheral catheters, the infectious morbidity associated with the use of transparent dressings on approximately 2,000 peripheral catheters was examined (65). Data from this study suggest that the rate of colonization among catheters dressed with transparent dressings (5.7%) is comparable to that of those dressed with gauze (4.6%) and that no clinically substantial differences exist in either the incidences of catheter-site colonization or phlebitis. Furthermore, these data suggest that transparent dressings can be safely left on peripheral venous catheters for the duration of catheter insertion without increasing the risk for thrombophlebitis (65).

A meta-analysis has assessed studies that compared the risk for catheter-related BSIs for groups using transparent dressings versus groups using gauze dressing (76). The risk for CRBSIs did not differ between the groups. The choice of dressing can be a matter of preference. If blood is oozing from the catheter insertion site, gauze dressing might be preferred.

In a multi-center study, a chlorhexidine-impregnated sponge (Biopatch™) placed over the site of short-term arterial and CVCs reduced the risk for catheter colonization and CRBSI (77). No adverse systemic effects resulted from use of this device.

Catheter Securement Devices

Sutureless securement devices can be advantageous over suture in preventing catheter-related BSIs. One study, which involved only a limited number of patients and was underpowered, compared a sutureless device with suture for the securement of PICCS; in this study, CRBSI was reduced in the group of patients that received the sutureless device (78).

In-Line Filters

In-line filters reduce the incidence of infusion-related phlebitis (79,80). No data support their efficacy in preventing infections associated with intravascular catheters and infusion systems. Proponents of filters cite several potential benefits to using these filters, including 1) reducing the risk for infection from contaminated infusate or proximal contamination (i.e., introduced proximal to the filter); 2) reducing the risk for phlebitis in patients who require high doses of medication or in those in whom infusion-related phlebitis already has occurred; 3) removing particulate matter that might contaminate IV fluids (81); and 4) filtering endotoxin produced by gram-negative organisms in contaminated infusate (82). These theoretical advantages should be tempered by the knowledge that infusate-related BSI is rare and that filtration of medications or infusates in the pharmacy is a more practical and less costly way to remove the majority of particulates. Furthermore, in-line filters might become blocked, especially with certain solutions (e.g., dextran, lipids, and mannitol), thereby increasing the number of line manipulations and decreasing the availability of administered drugs (83). Thus, for reducing the risk for CRBSI, no strong recommendation can be made in favor of using in-line filters.

Antimicrobial/Antiseptic Impregnated Catheters and Cuffs

Certain catheters and cuffs that are coated or impregnated with antimicrobial or antiseptic agents can decrease the risk for CRBSI and potentially decrease hospital costs associated with treating CRBSIs, despite the additional acquisition cost of an antimicrobial/antiseptic impregnated catheter (84). All of the studies involving antimicrobial/antiseptic impregnated catheters have been conducted using triple-lumen, noncuffed catheters in adult patients whose catheters remained in place <30 days. Although all of the studies have been conducted in adults, these catheters have been approved by FDA for use in patients weighing ≥3 kg. No antiseptic or antimicrobial impregnated catheters currently are available for use in weighing <3 kg.

Chlorhexidine/Silver sulfadiazine. Catheters coated with chlorhexidine/silver sulfadiazine only on the external luminal surface have been studied as a means to reduce CRBSI. Two meta-analyses (2,85) demonstrated that such catheters reduced the risk for CRBSI compared with standard noncoated catheters. The mean duration of catheter placement in one meta-analysis ranged from 5.1 to 11.2 days (86). The half-life of antimicrobial activity against *S. epidermidis* is 3 days in vitro for catheters coated with chlorhexidine/silver sulfadiazine; this antimicrobial activity decreases over time (87). The benefit for the patients who receive these catheters will be realized within the first 14 days (86). A second-generation catheter is now available with chlorhexidine coating both the internal and external luminal surfaces. The external surface has three times the amount of chlorhexidine and extended release of the surface bound antiseptics than that in the first generation catheters. The external surface coating of chlorhexidine is combined with silver-sulfadiazine, and the internal surface is coated with chlorhexidine alone. Preliminary studies indicate that prolonged anti-infective activity provides improved efficacy in preventing infections (88). Although rare, anaphylaxis has been reported with the use of these chlorhexidine/silver sulfadiazine catheters in Japan (89). Whether patients will become colonized or infected with organisms resistant to chlorhexidine/silver sulfadiazine has not been determined (86).

Chlorhexidine/silver sulfadiazine catheters are more expensive than standard catheters. However, one analysis has suggested that the use of chlorhexidine/silver sulfadiazine catheters should lead to a cost savings of $68 to $391 per catheter (90) in settings in which the risk for CRBSI is high despite adherence to other preventive strategies (e.g., maximal barrier precautions and aseptic techniques). Use of these catheters might be cost effective in ICU patients, burn patients, neutropenic patients, and other patient populations in which the rate of infection exceeds 3.3 per 1,000 catheter days (86).

Minocycline/Rifampin. In a multicenter randomized trial, CVCs impregnated on both the external and internal surfaces with minocycline/rifampin were associated with lower rates of CRBSI when compared with the first-generation chlorhexidine-silver sulfadiazine impregnated catheters (91). The beneficial effect began after day 6 of catheterization. None of the catheters were evaluated beyond 30 days. No minocycline/rifampin-resistant organisms were reported. However, in vitro data indicate that these impregnated catheters could increase the incidence of minocycline and rifampin resistance among pathogens, especially staphylococci. The half-life of antimicrobial activity against S. epidermidis is 25 days with catheters coated with minocycline/rifampin, compared with 3 days for the first-generation catheters coated with chlorhexidine/silver sulfadiazine in vitro (87). In vivo, the duration of antimicrobial activity of the minocycline/rifampin catheter is longer than that of the first-generation chlorhexidine/silver sulfadiazine catheter (91). No comparative studies have been published using the second-generation chlorhexidine/silver sulfadiazine catheter. Studies are needed to evaluated whether the improved performance of the minocycline/rifampin catheters results from the antimicrobial agents used or from the coating of both the internal and external surfaces. As with chlorhexidine/silver sulfadiazine catheters, some clinicians have recommended that the minocycline/rifampin catheters be

considered in patient populations when the rate of CRBSI exceeds 3.3 per 1,000 catheter days (86). Others suggest that reducing all rates of CRBSI should be the goal (92). The decision to use chlorhexidine/silver sulfadiazine or minocycline/rifampin impregnated catheters should be based on the need to enhance prevention of CRBSI after standard procedures have been implemented (e.g., educating personnel, using maximal sterile barrier precautions, and using 2% chlorhexidine skin antisepsis) and then balanced against the concern for emergence of resistant pathogens and the cost of implementing this strategy.

Platinum/Silver. Ionic metals have broad antimicrobial activity and are being used in catheters and cuffs to prevent CRBSI. A combination platinum/silver impregnated catheter is available in Europe and has recently been approved by FDA for use in the United States. Although these catheters are being marketed for their antimicrobial properties, no published studies have been presented to support an antimicrobial effect.

Silver cuffs. Ionic silver has been used in subcutaneous collagen cuffs attached to CVCs (93). The ionic silver provides antimicrobial activity and the cuff provides a mechanical barrier to the migration of microorganisms along the external surface of the catheter. In studies of catheters left in place >20 days, the cuff failed to reduce the incidence of CRBSI (94,95). Two other studies of short-term catheters could not demonstrate efficacy because of the minimal number of CRBSIs observed (93,96).

Systemic Antibiotic Prophylaxis

No studies have demonstrated that oral or parenteral antibacterial or antifungal drugs might reduce the incidence of CRBSI among adults (97–99). However, among low birth weight infants, two studies have assessed vancomycin prophylaxis; both demonstrated a reduction in CRBSI but no reduction in mortality (100,101). Because the prophylactic use of vancomycin is an independent risk factor for the acquisition of vancomycin-resistant enterococcus (VRE) (102), the risk for acquiring VRE likely outweighs the benefit of using prophylactic vancomycin.

Antibiotic/Antiseptic Ointments

Povidone-iodine ointment applied at the insertion site of hemodialysis catheters has been studied as a prophylactic intervention to reduce the incidence of catheter-related infections. One randomized study of 129 hemodialysis catheters demonstrated a reduction in the incidence of exit-site infections, catheter-tip colonization, and BSIs with the routine use of povidone-iodine ointment at the catheter insertion site compared with no ointment at the insertion site (103).

Several studies have evaluated the effectiveness of mupirocin ointment applied at the insertion sites of CVCs as a means to prevent CRBSI (104–106). Although mupirocin reduced the risk for CRBSI (106), mupirocin ointment also has been associated with mupirocin resistance (107,108), and might adversely affect the integrity of polyurethane catheters (109,110).

Nasal carriers of S. aureus have a higher risk for acquiring CRBSI than do noncarriers (103,111). Mupirocin ointment has been used intranasally to decrease nasal carriage of S. aureus and lessen the risk for CRBSI. However, resistance to mupirocin develops in both S. aureus and coagulase-negative staphylococci soon after routine use of mupirocin is instituted (107,108).

Other antibiotic ointments applied to the catheter insertion site also have been studied and have yielded conflicting results (112–114). In addition, rates of catheter colonization with Candida spp. might be increased with the use of antibiotic ointments that have no fungicidal activity (112,114). To avoid compromising the integrity of the catheter, any ointment that is applied to the catheter insertion site should be checked against the catheter and ointment manufacturers' recommendations regarding compatibility.

Antibiotic Lock Prophylaxis

To prevent CRBSI, antibiotic lock prophylaxis has been attempted by flushing and filling the lumen of the catheter with an antibiotic solution and leaving the solution to dwell in the lumen of the catheter. Three studies have demonstrated the usefulness of such prophylaxis in neutropenic patients with long-term catheters (115–117). In two of the studies, patients received either heparin alone (10 U/ml) or heparin plus 25 micrograms/ml of vancomycin. The third study compared vancomycin/ciprofloxacin/heparin (VCH) to vancomycin/ heparin (VH) and then to heparin alone. The rate of CRBSI with vancomycin-susceptible organisms was significantly lower (VCH p = 0.022; VH p = 0.028) and the time to the first episode of bacteremia with vancomycin-susceptible organisms was substantially longer (VCH p = 0.036; VH p = 0.011) in patients receiving either vancomycin/ciprofloxacin/heparin or vancomycin/heparin compared with heparin alone (115–117). One study involving a limited number of children revealed no difference in rates of CRBSI between children receiving a heparin flush compared with those receiving heparin and vancomycin (118). However, because the use of vancomycin is an independent risk factor for the acquisition of VRE (102), this practice is not recommended routinely.

An anticoagulant/antimicrobial combination comprising minocycline and ethylenediaminetetraraacetic acid (EDTA) has been proposed as a lock solution because it has antibiofilm and antimicrobial activity against gram-positive, gram-negative, and Candida organisms (119), as well as anticoagulant properties. However, no controlled or randomized trials have demonstrated its efficacy.

Anticoagulants

Anticoagulant flush solutions are used widely to prevent catheter thrombosis. Because thrombi and fibrin deposits on catheters might serve as a nidus for microbial colonization of intravascular catheters (120,121), the use of anticoagulants might have a role in the prevention of CRBSI.

In a meta-analysis evaluating the benefit of heparin prophylaxis (3 U/ml in TPN, 5,000 U every 6 or 12 hours flush, or 2,500 U low molecular weight heparin subcutaneously) in patients with short-term CVCs, the risk for catheter-related central venous thrombosis was reduced with the use of prophylactic heparin (122). However, no substantial difference in the rate for CRBSI was observed. Because the majority of heparin solutions contain preservatives with antimicrobial activity, whether any decrease in the rate of CRBSI is a result of the reduced thrombus formation, the preservative, or both is unclear.

The majority of pulmonary artery, umbilical, and central venous catheters are available with a heparin-bonded coating. The majority are heparin-bonded with benzalkonium chloride, which provides the catheters with antimicrobial activity (123) and provides an anti-thrombotic effect (124).

Warfarin also has been evaluated as a means for reducing CRBSI by reducing thrombus formation on catheters (125,126). In patients with long-term CVCs, low-dose warfarin (i.e., 1 mg/day) reduced the incidence of catheter thrombus. No data demonstrate that warfarin reduces the incidence of CRBSI.

Replacement of Catheters
Peripheral Venous Catheters

Scheduled replacement of intravascular catheters has been proposed as a method to prevent phlebitis and catheter-related infections. Studies of short peripheral venous catheters indicate that the incidence of thrombophlebitis and bacterial colonization of catheters increases when catheters are left in place >72 hours (66,67,127). However, rates of phlebitis are not substantially different in peripheral catheters left in place 72 hours compared with 96 hours (128). Because phlebitis and catheter colonization have been associated with an increased risk for catheter-related infection, short peripheral catheter sites commonly are rotated at 72–96-hour intervals to reduce both the risk for infection and patient discomfort associated with phlebitis.

Midline Catheters

Midline catheters have been associated with lower rates of phlebitis than short peripheral catheters and with lower rates of infection than CVCs (129–131). In one prospective study of 140 midline catheters, their use was associated with a BSI rate of 0.8 per 1,000 catheter-days (131). No specific risk factors, including duration of catheterization, were associated with infection. Midline catheters were in place a median of 7 days, but for as long as 49 days. Although the findings of this study suggested that midline catheters can be changed only when there is a specific indication, no prospective, randomized studies have assessed the benefit of routine replacement as a strategy to prevent CRBSI associated with midline catheters.

CVCs, Including PICCs and Hemodialysis Catheters

Catheter replacement at scheduled time intervals as a method to reduce CRBSI has not lowered rates. Two trials have assessed a strategy of changing the catheter every 7 days compared with a strategy of changing catheters as needed (132,133). One of these studies involved 112 surgical ICU patients needing CVCs, pulmonary artery catheters, or peripheral arterial catheters (132), whereas the other study involved only subclavian hemodialysis catheters (133). In both studies, no difference in CRBSI was observed in patients undergoing scheduled catheter replacement every 7 days compared with patients whose catheters were replaced as needed.

Scheduled guidewire exchanges of CVCs is another proposed strategy for preventing CRBSI. The results of a meta-analysis of 12 randomized controlled trials assessing CVC management failed to prove any reduction of CRBSI rates through routine replacement of CVCs by guidewire exchange compared with catheter replacement on an as-needed basis (134). Thus, routine replacement of CVCs is not necessary for catheters that are functioning and have no evidence of causing local or systemic complications.

Catheter replacement over a guidewire has become an accepted technique for replacing a malfunctioning catheter or exchanging a pulmonary artery catheter for a CVC when invasive monitoring no longer is needed. Catheter insertion over a guidewire is associated with less discomfort and a significantly lower rate of mechanical complications than are those percutaneously inserted at a new site (135); in addition, this technique provides a means of preserving limited venous access in some patients. Replacement of temporary catheters over a guidewire in the presence of bacteremia is not an acceptable replacement strategy, because the source of infection is usually colonization of the skin tract from the insertion site to the vein (22,135). However, in selected patients with tunneled hemodialysis catheters and bacteremia, catheter exchange over a guidewire, in combination with antibiotic therapy, might be an alternative as a salvage strategy in patients with limited venous access (136–139).

Hemodialysis Catheters

The use of catheters for hemodialysis is the most common factor contributing to bacteremia in dialysis patients (140,141). The relative risk for bacteremia in patients with dialysis catheters is sevenfold the risk for patients with primary arteriovenous fistulas (142). Despite the National Kidney Foundation's effort to reduce the number of hemodialysis patients maintained with catheter access, catheter use increased from 12.7% in 1995 to 22.2% in 1999 (143). Rates for bacteremia per 100 patient months were 0.2 for arteriovenous fistulas, 0.5 for grafts, 5.0 for cuffed catheters, and 8.5 for noncuffed catheters (CDC, unpublished data, 1999).

To reduce the rate of infection, hemodialysis catheters should be avoided in favor of arteriovenous fistulas and grafts. If temporary access is needed for dialysis, a cuffed catheter is preferable to a noncuffed catheter, even in the ICU setting, if the catheter is expected to stay in place for >3 weeks (11,144).

Pulmonary Artery Catheters

Pulmonary artery catheters are inserted through a Teflon® introducer and typically remain in place an average of 3 days. The majority of pulmonary artery catheters are heparin bonded, which reduces not only catheter thrombosis but also microbial adherence to the catheter (145). Meta-analysis indicates that standard nonheparin-bonded pulmonary artery catheter rates of CRBSI are 5.5 per 1,000 catheter days; for heparin-bonded pulmonary artery catheters, this rate is 2.6 per 1,000 catheter days (11). Because the majority of pulmonary artery catheters are heparin-bonded, the relative risk of infection with these catheters is similar to that of CVC (2.6 versus 2.3 per 1,000 catheter days) (11).

A prospective study of 442 pulmonary artery catheters demonstrated an increased risk for CRBSI after 5 days (0/442 CRBSI before 5 days versus 5/442 CSBSI after 5 days; p < 0.001) (146). A prospective observational study of 71 pulmonary artery catheters demonstrated higher infection rates in catheters left in place longer than 7 days (2% before 7 days versus 16% after 7 days; p = 0.056) (147). However, no studies indicate that catheter replacement at scheduled time intervals is an effective method to reduce CRBSI (132,135). In patients who continue to require hemodynamic monitoring, pulmonary artery catheters do not need to be changed more frequently than every 7 days. No specific recommendation can be made regarding routine replacement of catheters that need to be in place for >7 days.

Pulmonary artery catheters are usually packaged with a thin plastic sleeve that prevents touch contamination when placed over the catheter. In a study of 166 catheters, patients who were randomly assigned to have their catheters self-contained within this sleeve had a reduced risk for CRBSI compared with those who had a pulmonary artery catheter placed without the sleeve (p = 0.002) (148).

Peripheral Arterial Catheters

Peripheral arterial catheters are usually inserted into the radial or femoral artery and permit continuous blood pressure monitoring and blood gas measurements. The rate of CRBSI is comparable to that of temporary CVCs (2.9 versus 2.3 per 1,000 catheter days) (11). One study of peripheral arterial catheters demonstrated no difference in infection rates between changing catheters at scheduled times and changing arterial catheters on an as-needed basis (132). One observational study of 71 arterial catheters revealed that 10 local infections and four CRBSIs occurred in patients who had peripheral arterial catheters in place for >4 days compared with one local infection and no CRBSIs in patients whose catheters were in place ≤4 days (p < 0.05) (147). Because the risk for CRBSI is likely similar to that of short-term CVCs, arterial catheters can be approached in a similar way. No specific recommendation can be made regarding replacement of catheters that need to be in place for >5 days.

Replacement of Administration Sets

The optimal interval for routine replacement of IV administration sets has been examined in three well-controlled studies. Data from each of these studies reveal that replacing administration sets no more frequently than 72 hours after initiation of use is safe and cost-effective (149–151). Data from a more recent study demonstrated that rates of phlebitis were not substantially different if administration sets were left in place 96 hours compared with 72 hours (128). When a fluid that enhances microbial growth is infused (e.g., lipid emulsions and blood products), more frequent changes of administration sets are indicated, because these products have been identified as independent risk factors for CRBSI (152–158).

Stopcocks (used for injection of medications, administration of IV infusions, and collection of blood samples) represent a potential portal of entry for microorganisms into vascular access catheters and IV fluids. Stopcock contamination is common, occurring in 45% and 50% in the majority of series.

Whether such contamination is a substantial entry point of CRBSI has been difficult to prove.

"Piggyback" systems are used as an alternative to stopcocks. However, they also pose a risk for contamination of the intravascular fluid if the device entering the rubber membrane of an injection port is exposed to air or comes into direct contact with nonsterile tape used to fix the needle to the port. Modified piggyback systems have the potential to prevent contamination at these sites (159).

Needleless Intravascular Catheter Systems

Attempts to reduce the incidence of sharp injuries and the resultant risk for transmission of bloodborne infections to health-care workers have led to the design and introduction of needleless infusion systems. When the devices are used according to manufacturers' recommendations, they do not substantially affect the incidence of CRBSI (160–167).

Multidose Parenteral Medication Vials

Parenteral medications commonly are dispensed in multidose, parenteral medication vials that might be used for prolonged periods for one or more patients. Although the overall risk for extrinsic contamination of multidose vials is likely minimal (168), the consequences of contamination might result in life-threatening infection (169,170). Single-use vials are frequently preservative-free and might pose a risk for contamination if they are punctured several times.

Special Considerations for Intravascular Catheter-Related Infections in Pediatric Patients

Prevention of CRBSI in children requires additional considerations, although only certain studies have been performed specifically in children. Pediatric data have been derived largely from studies in neonatal or pediatric ICUs and pediatric oncology patients.

Epidemiology

As in adults, the majority of BSIs in children are associated with the use of an intravascular catheter. From 1995 through 2000, the pooled mean catheter-associated BSI rate for all pediatric ICUs reporting data to NNIS was 7.7 per 1,000 catheter days (171,172). Umbilical catheter and CVC-associated BSI rates for neonatal ICUs ranged from 11.3 per 1,000 catheter days in children with birth weight <1,000 g to 4.0 per 1,000 catheter days in children whose birth weight was

>2,500 g (171). Catheter utilization rates were comparable in adult and pediatric ICUs (172,173).

Microbiology

As in adults, the majority of CRBSIs in children are caused by coagulase-negative staphylococci. During 1992–1999, these bacteria accounted for 37.7% of BSIs in pediatric ICUs reporting to NNIS (12). Exposure to lipids has been identified as an independent risk factor for development of coagulase-negative staphylococcal bacteremia in very low birth weight infants (i.e., those weighing <1,000 g) (odds ratio [OR] = 9.4; 95% CI = 1.2–74.2) (155), as well as candidemia in the neonatal ICU (OR = 5.33; 95% CI = 1.23–48.4) (154). Gram-negative bacteria accounted for 25% of BSIs reported in pediatric ICUs (172), whereas enterococci and *Candida* spp. accounted for 10% and 9%, respectively (172).

Peripheral Venous Catheters

As in adults, the use of peripheral venous catheters in pediatric patients might be complicated by phlebitis, infusion extravasation, and catheter infection (174). Catheter location, infusion of parenteral nutritional fluids with continuous IV lipid emulsions, and length of ICU stay before catheter insertion have all increased pediatric patients' risk for phlebitis. However, contrary to the risk in adults, the risk for phlebitis in children has not increased with the duration of catheterization (174,175).

Peripheral Arterial Catheters

In a prospective study of 340 peripheral arterial catheters in children, the following two risk factors for catheter-related infection were identified: 1) use of an arterial system that permitted backflow of blood into the pressure tubing and 2) duration of catheterization (176). Although a correlation was found between duration of arterial catheterization and risk for catheter colonization, the risk remained constant for 2–20 days at 6.2% (176).

Umbilical Catheters

Although the umbilical stump becomes heavily colonized soon after birth, umbilical-vessel catheterization often is used for vascular access in newborn infants. Umbilical vessels can be cannulated easily and permit both collection of blood samples and measurement of hemodynamic status. The incidences of catheter colonization and BSI are similar for umbilical vein catheters and umbilical artery catheters. In several studies, an estimated 40%–55% of umbilical artery catheters were colonized and 5% resulted in CRBSI; umbilical

vein catheters were associated with colonization in 22%–59% of cases (177–179) and with CRBSI in 3%–8% of cases (178). Although CRBSI rates are similar for umbilical catheters in the high position (i.e., above the diaphragm) compared with the low position (i.e., below the diaphragm and above the aortic bifurcation), catheters placed in the high position result in a lower incidence of vascular complications without an increase in adverse sequelae (178).

Risk factors for infection differ for umbilical artery and umbilical vein catheters. In one study, neonates with very low birth weight who also received antibiotics for ≥10 days were at increased risk for umbilical artery CRBSIs (178). In comparison, those with higher birth weight and receipt of parenteral nutrition fluids were at increased risk for umbilical vein CRBSI. Duration of catheterization was not an independent risk factor for infection of either type of umbilical catheter.

CVCs

Because of the limited vascular sites in children, attention should be given to the frequency with which catheters are replaced in these patients. In a study in which survival analysis techniques were used to examine the relation between the duration of central venous catheterization and complications in pediatric ICU patients, all of the patients studied (n = 397) remained uninfected for a median of 23.7 days (180). In addition, no relation was found between duration of catheterization and the daily probability of infection (r = 0.21; p > 0.1), suggesting that routine replacement of CVCs likely does not reduce the incidence of catheter-related infection (180).

Catheter Site Care

Although data regarding the use of the chlorhexidine-impregnated sponge (Biopatch™) in children are limited, one randomized, controlled study involving 705 neonates reported a substantial decrease in colonized catheter tips in infants in the Biopatch™ group compared with the group that had standard dressings (15% versus 24%; RR = 0.6; 95% CI = 0.5–0.9), but no difference in the rates of CRBSI or BSI without a source. Biopatch™ was associated with localized contact dermatitis in infants of very low birth weight. Of 98 neonates with very low birth weight, 15 (15%) developed localized contact dermatitis; four (1.5%) of 237 neonates weighing >1,000 g developed this reaction (p < 0.0001). Infants with gestational age <26 weeks who had CVCs placed at age ≤8 days were at increased risk for having localized contact dermatitis, whereas no infants in the control group developed this local reaction (181).

Performance Indicators

Performance indicators for reducing CRBSI are 1) implementation of educational programs that include didactic and interactive components for those who insert and maintain catheters; 2) use of maximal sterile barrier precautions during catheter placement; 3) use of chlorhexidine for skin antisepsis; and 4) rates of catheter discontinuation when the catheter is no longer essential for medical management. The impact these recommendations will have on individual institutions should be evaluated using specific performance indicators.

Recommendations for Placement of Intravascular Catheters in Adults and Children

These recommendations are designed to reduce the infectious complications associated with intravascular catheter use. Recommendations should be considered in the context of the institution's experience with catheter-related infections, experience with other adverse catheter-related complications (e.g., thrombosis, hemorrhage, and pneumothorax), and availability of personnel skilled in the placement of intravascular devices. Recommendations are provided for 1) intravascular-catheter use in general; 2) specific devices; and 3) special circumstances (i.e., intravascular-device use in pediatric patients and CVC use for parenteral nutrition and hemodialysis access). Recommendations regarding the frequency of replacing catheters, dressings, administration sets, and fluids also are provided (Appendix B).

As in previous guidelines issued by CDC and HICPAC, each recommendation is categorized on the basis of existing scientific data, theoretical rationale, applicability, and economic impact. The CDC/HICPAC system for categorizing recommendations is as follows:

Category IA. Strongly recommended for implementation and strongly supported by well-designed experimental, clinical, or epidemiologic studies.

Category IB. Strongly recommended for implementation and supported by some experimental, clinical, or epidemiologic studies, and a strong theoretical rationale.

Category IC. Required by state or federal regulations, rules, or standards.

Category II. Suggested for implementation and supported by suggestive clinical or epidemiologic studies or a theoretical rationale.

Unresolved issue. Represents an unresolved issue for which evidence is insufficient or no consensus regarding efficacy exists.

I. Health-care worker education and training
  A. Educate health-care workers regarding the indications for intravascular catheter use, proper procedures for the insertion and maintenance of intravascular catheters, and appropriate infection-control measures to prevent intravascular catheter-related infections (*39,43,45–47,182–187*). **Category IA**
  B. Assess knowledge of and adherence to guidelines periodically for all persons who insert and manage intravascular catheters (*39,43,46,182,188*). **Category IA**
  C. Ensure appropriate nursing staff levels in ICUs to minimize the incidence of CRBSIs (*48,189,190*). **Category IB**

II. Surveillance
  A. Monitor the catheter sites visually or by palpation through the intact dressing on a regular basis, depending on the clinical situation of individual patients. If patients have tenderness at the insertion site, fever without obvious source, or other manifestations suggesting local or BSI, the dressing should be removed to allow thorough examination of the site (*1,191–193*). **Category IB**
  B. Encourage patients to report to their health-care provider any changes in their catheter site or any new discomfort. **Category II**
  C. Record the operator, date, and time of catheter insertion and removal, and dressing changes on a standardized form. **Category II**
  D. Do not routinely culture catheter tips (*8,194,195*). **Category IA**

III. Hand hygiene
  A. Observe proper hand-hygiene procedures either by washing hands with conventional antiseptic-containing soap and water or with waterless alcohol-based gels or foams. Observe hand hygiene before and after palpating catheter insertion sites, as well as before and after inserting, replacing, accessing, repairing, or dressing an intravascular catheter. Palpation of the insertion site should not be performed after the application of antiseptic, unless aseptic technique is maintained (*43,70,196–200*). **Category IA**
  B. Use of gloves does not obviate the need for hand hygiene (*43,198,199*). **Category IA**

IV. Aseptic technique during catheter insertion and care
  A. Maintain aseptic technique for the insertion and care of intravascular catheters (*22,71,201,202*). **Category IA**

B. Wear clean or sterile gloves when inserting an intravascular catheter as required by the Occupational Safety and Health Administration Bloodborne Pathogens Standard. **Category IC**. Wearing clean gloves rather than sterile gloves is acceptable for the insertion of peripheral intravascular catheters if the access site is not touched after the application of skin antiseptics. Sterile gloves should be worn for the insertion of arterial and central catheters (*201,203*). **Category IA**

C. Wear clean or sterile gloves when changing the dressing on intravascular catheters. **Category IC**

V. Catheter insertion

Do not routinely use arterial or venous cutdown procedures as a method to insert catheters (*204–206*). **Category IA**

VI. Catheter site care

A. Cutaneous antisepsis

1. Disinfect clean skin with an appropriate antiseptic before catheter insertion and during dressing changes. Although a 2% chlorhexidine-based preparation is preferred, tincture of iodine, an iodophor, or 70% alcohol can be used (*73,75,207,208*). **Category IA**

2. No recommendation can be made for the use of chlorhexidine in infants aged <2 months. **Unresolved issue**

3. Allow the antiseptic to remain on the insertion site and to air dry before catheter insertion. Allow povidone iodine to remain on the skin for at least 2 minutes, or longer if it is not yet dry before insertion (*73,75,207,208*). **Category IB**

4. Do not apply organic solvents (e.g., acetone and ether) to the skin before insertion of catheters or during dressing changes (*209*). **Category IA**

VII. Catheter-site dressing regimens

A. Use either sterile gauze or sterile, transparent, semipermeable dressing to cover the catheter site (*146,210–212*). **Category IA**

B. Tunneled CVC sites that are well healed might not require dressings. **Category II**

C. If the patient is diaphoretic, or if the site is bleeding or oozing, a gauze dressing is preferable to a transparent, semi-permeable dressing (*146,210–212*). **Category II**

D. Replace catheter-site dressing if the dressing becomes damp, loosened, or visibly soiled (*146,210*). **Category IB**

E. Change dressings at least weekly for adult and adolescent patients depending on the circumstances of the individual patient (*211*). **Category II**

F. Do not use topical antibiotic ointment or creams on insertion sites (except when using dialysis catheters) because of their potential to promote fungal infections and antimicrobial resistance (*107,213*). **Category IA** (See Central Venous Catheters, Including PICCs, Hemodialysis, and Pulmonary Artery Catheters, in Adult and Pediatric Patients, Section II.I.)

G. Do not submerge the catheter under water. Showering should be permitted if precautions can be taken to reduce the likelihood of introducing organisms into the catheter (e.g., if the catheter and connecting device are protected with an impermeable cover during the shower (*214,215*). **Category II**

VIII. Selection and replacement of intravascular catheters

A. Select the catheter, insertion technique, and insertion site with the lowest risk for complications (infectious and noninfectious) for the anticipated type and duration of IV therapy (*22,55,59, 216–218*). **Category IA**

B. Promptly remove any intravascular catheter that is no longer essential (*219,220*). **Category IA**

C. Do not routinely replace central venous or arterial catheters solely for the purposes of reducing the incidence of infection (*134,135,221*). **Category IB**

D. Replace peripheral venous catheters at least every 72–96 hours in adults to prevent phlebitis (*128*). Leave peripheral venous catheters in place in children until IV therapy is completed, unless complications (e.g., phlebitis and infiltration) occur (*174,175,222,223*). **Category IB**

E. When adherence to aseptic technique cannot be ensured (i.e., when catheters are inserted during a medical emergency), replace all catheters as soon as possible and after no longer than 48 hours (*22,71,201,202*). **Category II**

F. Use clinical judgment to determine when to replace a catheter that could be a source of infection (e.g., do not routinely replace catheters in patients whose only indication of infection is fever). Do not routinely replace venous catheters in patients who are bacteremic or fungemic if the source of infection is unlikely to be the catheter (*224*). **Category II**

G. Replace any short-term CVC if purulence is observed at the insertion site, which indicates infection (*224,225*). **Category IB**

H. Replace all CVCs if the patient is hemodynamically unstable and CRBSI is suspected (*224,225*). **Category II**

I. Do not use guidewire techniques to replace catheters in patients suspected of having catheter-related infection (*134,135*). **Category IB**

IX. Replacement of administration sets*, needleless systems, and parenteral fluids

A. Administration sets

1. Replace administration sets, including secondary sets and add-on devices, no more frequently than at 72-hour intervals, unless catheter-related infection is suspected or documented (*23, 149–151*). **Category IA**

2. Replace tubing used to administer blood, blood products, or lipid emulsions (those combined with amino acids and glucose in a 3-in-1 admixture or infused separately) within 24 hours of initiating the infusion (*158,226–229*). **Category IB**. If the solution contains only dextrose and amino acids, the administration set does not need to be replaced more frequently than every 72 hours (*226*). **Category II**

3. Replace tubing used to administer propofol infusions every 6 or 12 hours, depending on its use, per the manufacturer's recommendation (*230*). **Category IA**

B. Needleless intravascular devices

1. Change the needleless components at least as frequently as the administration set (*160–162, 164–167*). **Category II**

2. Change caps no more frequently than every 72 hours or according to manufacturers' recommendations (*160,162,165,166*). **Category II**

3. Ensure that all components of the system are compatible to minimize leaks and breaks in the system (*163*). **Category II**

4. Minimize contamination risk by wiping the access port with an appropriate antiseptic and accessing the port only with sterile devices (*162,163,165*). **Category IB**

C. Parenteral fluids

1. Complete the infusion of lipid-containing solutions (e.g., 3-in-1 solutions) within 24 hours of hanging the solution (*156–158,226,229*). **Category IB**

2. Complete the infusion of lipid emulsions alone within 12 hours of hanging the emulsion. If volume considerations require more time, the infusion should be completed within 24 hours (*156–158*). **Category IB**

3. Complete infusions of blood or other blood products within 4 hours of hanging the blood (*231–234*). **Category II**

4. No recommendation can be made for the hang time of other parenteral fluids. **Unresolved issue**

X. IV-injection ports

A. Clean injection ports with 70% alcohol or an iodophor before accessing the system (*164,235,236*). **Category IA**

B. Cap all stopcocks when not in use (*235*). **Category IB**

XI. Preparation and quality control of IV admixtures

A. Admix all routine parenteral fluids in the pharmacy in a laminar-flow hood using aseptic technique (*237,238*). **Category IB**

B. Do not use any container of parenteral fluid that has visible turbidity, leaks, cracks, or particulate matter or if the manufacturer's expiration date has passed (*237*). **Category IB**

C. Use single-dose vials for parenteral additives or medications when possible (*237,239*). **Category II**

D. Do not combine the leftover content of single-use vials for later use (*237,239*). **Category IA**

E. If multidose vials are used

1. Refrigerate multidose vials after they are opened if recommended by the manufacturer. **Category II**

2. Cleanse the access diaphragm of multidose vials with 70% alcohol before inserting a device into the vial (*236*). **Category IA**

3. Use a sterile device to access a multidose vial and avoid touch contamination of the device before penetrating the access diaphragm (*235,240*). **Category IA**

4. Discard multidose vial if sterility is compromised (*235,240*). **Category IA**

XII. In-line filters

Do not use filters routinely for infection-control purposes (*80,241*). **Category IA**

XIII. IV-therapy personnel

Designate trained personnel for the insertion and maintenance of intravascular catheters (*46,47,210,242*). **Category IA**

---

* Administration sets include the area from the spike of tubing entering the fluid container to the hub of the vascular access device. However, a short extension tube might be connected to the catheter and might be considered a portion of the catheter to facilitate aseptic technique when changing administration sets.

XIV. Prophylactic antimicrobials

Do not administer intranasal or systemic antimicrobial prophylaxis routinely before insertion or during use of an intravascular catheter to prevent catheter colonization or BSI (*97,98,108,243*). **Category IA**

Peripheral Venous Catheters, Including Midline Catheters, in Adult and Pediatric Patients

I. Selection of peripheral catheter
   A. Select catheters on the basis of the intended purpose and duration of use, known complications (e.g., phlebitis and infiltration), and experience of individual catheter operators (*67,68,244*). **Category IB**
   B. Avoid the use of steel needles for the administration of fluids and medication that might cause tissue necrosis if extravasation occurs (*67,68*). **Category IA**
   C. Use a midline catheter or PICC when the duration of IV therapy will likely exceed 6 days (*244*). **Category IB**

II. Selection of peripheral-catheter insertion site
   A. In adults, use an upper- instead of a lower-extremity site for catheter insertion. Replace a catheter inserted in a lower-extremity site to an upper-extremity site as soon as possible (*67,245*). **Category IA**
   B. In pediatric patients, the hand, the dorsum of the foot, or the scalp can be used as the catheter insertion site. **Category II**
   C. Replacement of catheter
      1. Evaluate the catheter insertion site daily, by palpation through the dressing to discern tenderness and by inspection if a transparent dressing is in use. Gauze and opaque dressings should not be removed if the patient has no clinical signs infection. If the patient has local tenderness or other signs of possible CRBSI, an opaque dressing should be removed and the site inspected visually. **Category II**
      2. Remove peripheral venous catheters if the patient develops signs of phlebitis (e.g., warmth, tenderness, erythema, and palpable venous cord), infection, or a malfunctioning catheter (*66*). **Category IB**
      3. In adults, replace short, peripheral venous catheters at least 72–96 hours to reduce the risk for phlebitis. If sites for venous access are limited and no evidence of phlebitis or infection is present, peripheral venous catheters can be left in place for longer periods, although the patient and the

insertion sites should be closely monitored (*66,128,246*). **Category IB**
      4. Do not routinely replace midline catheters to reduce the risk for infection (*131*). **Category IB**
      5. In pediatric patients, leave peripheral venous catheters in place until IV therapy is completed, unless a complication (e.g., phlebitis and infiltration) occurs (*174,175,222,223*). **Category IB**

III. Catheter and catheter-site care

Do not routinely apply prophylactic topical antimicrobial or antiseptic ointment or cream to the insertion site of peripheral venous catheters (*107,213*). **Category IA**

Central Venous Catheters, Including PICCs, Hemodialysis, and Pulmonary Artery Catheters, in Adult and Pediatric Patients

I. Surveillance
   A. Conduct surveillance in ICUs and other patient populations to determine CRBSI rates, monitor trends in those rates, and assist in identifying lapses in infection-control practices (*3,12,16,247–250*). **Category IA**
   B. Express ICU data as the number of catheter-associated BSIs per 1,000 catheter-days for both adults and children and stratify by birth weight categories for neonatal ICUs to facilitate comparisons with national data in comparable patient populations and health-care settings (*3,12,16,247–250*). **Category IB**
   C. Investigate events leading to unexpected life-threatening or fatal outcomes. This includes any process variation for which a recurrence would likely present an adverse outcome (*13*). **Category IC**

II. General principles
   A. Use a CVC with the minimum number of ports or lumens essential for the management of the patient (*251–254*). **Category IB**
   B. Use an antimicrobial or antiseptic-impregnated CVC in adults whose catheter is expected to remain in place >5 days if, after implementing a comprehensive strategy to reduce rates of CRBSI, the CRBSI rate remains above the goal set by the individual institution based on benchmark rates (Table 2) and local factors. The comprehensive strategy should include the following three components: educating persons who insert and maintain catheters, use of maximal sterile barrier precautions, and a 2% chlorhexidine preparation for skin antisepsis during CVC insertion (*84–86,90,91,255*). **Category IB**

C. No recommendation can be made for the use of impregnated catheters in children. **Unresolved issue**

D. Designate personnel who have been trained and exhibit competency in the insertion of catheters to supervise trainees who perform catheter insertion (*39,43,46,182,187,188*). **Category IA**

E. Use totally implantable access devices for patients who require long-term, intermittent vascular access. For patients requiring frequent or continuous access, a PICC or tunneled CVC is preferable (*256,257*). **Category II**

F. Use a cuffed CVC for dialysis if the period of temporary access is anticipated to be prolonged (e.g., >3 weeks) (*144,258*). **Category IB**

G. Use a fistula or graft instead of a CVC for permanent access for dialysis (*142*). **Category IB**

H. Do not use hemodialysis catheters for blood drawing or applications other than hemodialysis except during dialysis or under emergency circumstances. **Category II**

I. Use povidone-iodine antiseptic ointment at the hemodialysis catheter exit site after catheter insertion and at the end of each dialysis session only if this ointment does not interact with the material of the hemodialysis catheter per manufacturer's recommendation (*103,114,144*). **Category II**

III. Selection of catheter insertion site

A. Weigh the risk and benefits of placing a device at a recommended site to reduce infectious complications against the risk for mechanical complications (e.g., pneumothorax, subclavian artery puncture, subclavian vein laceration, subclavian vein stenosis, hemothorax, thrombosis, air embolism, and catheter misplacement) (*22,55,59,218*). **Category IA**

B. Use a subclavian site (rather than a jugular or a femoral site) in adult patients to minimize infection risk for nontunneled CVC placement (*22,55,59,60*). **Category IA**

C. No recommendation can be made for a preferred site of insertion to minimize infection risk for a nontunneled CVC (*61–63*). **Unresolved issue**

D. Place catheters used for hemodialysis and pheresis in a jugular or femoral vein rather than a subclavian vein to avoid venous stenosis if catheter access is needed (*259–263*). **Category IA**

IV. Maximal sterile barrier precautions during catheter insertion

A. Use aseptic technique including the use of a cap, mask, sterile gown, sterile gloves, and a large sterile sheet, for the insertion of CVCs (including PICCS) or guidewire exchange (*22,71*). **Category IA**

B. Use a sterile sleeve to protect pulmonary artery catheters during insertion (*148*). **Category IB**

V. Replacement of catheter

A. Do not routinely replace CVCs, PICCs, hemodialysis catheters, or pulmonary artery catheters to prevent catheter-related infections (*132,134,135*). **Category IB**

B. Do not remove CVCs or PICCs on the basis of fever alone. Use clinical judgment regarding the appropriateness of removing the catheter if infection is evidenced elsewhere or if a noninfectious cause of fever is suspected (*224,264*). **Category II**

C. Guidewire exchange

1. Do not use guidewire exchanges routinely for nontunneled catheters to prevent infection (*135,265*). **Category IB**

2. Use a guidewire exchange to replace a malfunctioning nontunneled catheter if no evidence of infection is present (*135,265*). **Category IB**

3. Use a new set of sterile gloves before handling the new catheter when guidewire exchanges are performed (*22,71*). **Category II**

VI. Catheter and catheter-site care

A. General measures

Designate one port exclusively for hyperalimentation if a multilumen catheter is used to administer parenteral nutrition (*266*). **Category II**

B. Antibiotic lock solutions

Do not routinely use antibiotic lock solutions to prevent CRBSI. Use prophylactic antibiotic lock solution only in special circumstances (e.g., in treating a patient with a long-term cuffed or tunneled catheter or port who has a history of multiple CRBSIs despite optimal maximal adherence to aseptic technique) (*115,116,267,268*). **Category II**

C. Catheter-site dressing regimens

1. Replace the catheter-site dressing when it becomes damp, loosened, or soiled or when inspection of the site is necessary (*65,146,211*). **Category IA**

2. Replace dressings used on short-term CVC sites every 2 days for gauze dressings and at least every 7 days for transparent dressings, except in those pediatric patients in which the risk for dislodging the catheter outweighs the benefit of changing the dressing (*211*). **Category IB**

3. Replace dressings used on tunneled or implanted CVC sites no more than once per week, until the insertion site has healed (*211*). **Category IB**

4. No recommendation can be made regarding the necessity for any dressing on well-healed exit sites of long-term cuffed and tunneled CVCs. **Unresolved issue**

D. No recommendation can be made for the use of chlorhexidine sponge dressings to reduce the incidence of infection. **Unresolved issue**

E. Do not use chlorhexidine sponge dressings in neonates aged <7 days or of gestational age <26 weeks (*181*). **Category II**

F. No recommendation can be made for the use of sutureless securement devices. **Unresolved issue**

G. Ensure that catheter-site care is compatible with the catheter material (*109,110*). **Category IB**

H. Use a sterile sleeve for all pulmonary artery catheters (*148*). **Category IB**

Additional Recommendations for Peripheral Arterial Catheters and Pressure Monitoring Devices for Adult and Pediatric Patients

I. Selection of pressure monitoring system
    Use disposable, rather than reusable, transducer assemblies when possible (*269–273*). **Category IB**

II. Replacement of catheter and pressure monitoring system
  A. Do not routinely replace peripheral arterial catheters to prevent catheter-related infections (*132,147, 221,274*). **Category II**
  B. Replace disposable or reusable transducers at 96-hour intervals. Replace other components of the system (including the tubing, continuous-flush device, and flush solution) at the time the transducer is replaced (*22,270*). **Category IB**

III. Care of pressure monitoring systems
  A. General measures
    1. Keep all components of the pressure monitoring system (including calibration devices and flush solution) sterile (*269,275–277*). **Category IA**
    2. Minimize the number of manipulations of and entries into the pressure monitoring system. Use a closed-flush system (i.e., continuous flush), rather than an open system (i.e., one that requires a syringe and stopcock), to maintain the patency of the pressure monitoring catheters (*272,278*). **Category II**
    3. When the pressure monitoring system is accessed through a diaphragm rather than a stopcock, wipe the diaphragm with an appropriate antiseptic before accessing the system (*272*). **Category IA**

4. Do not administer dextrose-containing solutions or parenteral nutrition fluids through the pressure monitoring circuit (*272,279,280*). **Category IA**

B. Sterilization or disinfection of pressure monitoring systems
  1. Use disposable transducers (*272,279–282*). **Category IB**
  2. Sterilize reusable transducers according to the manufacturers' instructions if the use of disposable transducers is not feasible (*272,279–282*). **Category IA**

Recommendations for Umbilical Catheters

I. Replacement of catheters
  A. Remove and do not replace umbilical artery catheters if any signs of CRBSI, vascular insufficiency, or thrombosis are present (*283*). **Category II**
  B. Remove and do not replace umbilical venous catheters if any signs of CRBSI or thrombosis are present (*283*). **Category II**
  C. No recommendation can be made for treating through an umbilical venous catheter suspected of being infected. **Unresolved issue**
  D. Replace umbilical venous catheters only if the catheter malfunctions. **Category II**

II. Catheter-site care
  A. Cleanse the umbilical insertion site with an antiseptic before catheter insertion. Avoid tincture of iodine because of the potential effect on the neonatal thyroid. Other iodine-containing products (e.g., povidone-iodine) can be used (*75,177,178,284,285*). **Category IB**
  B. Do not use topical antibiotic ointment or creams on umbilical catheter insertion sites because of the potential to promote fungal infections and antimicrobial resistance (*107,213*). **Category IA**
  C. Add low doses of heparin (0.25–1.0 F/ml) to the fluid infused through umbilical arterial catheters (*286–288*). **Category IB**
  D. Remove umbilical catheters as soon as possible when no longer needed or when any sign of vascular insufficiency to the lower extremities is observed. Optimally, umbilical artery catheters should not be left in place >5 days (*283,289*). **Category II**
  E. Umbilical venous catheters should be removed as soon as possible when no longer needed but can be used up to 14 days if managed aseptically (*290,291*). **Category II**

Appendix A

Examples of Clinical Definitions for Catheter-Related Infections

Localized Catheter Colonization

Significant growth of a microorganism (>15 CFU) from the catheter tip, subcutaneous segment of the catheter, or catheter hub

Exit Site Infection

Erythema or induration within 2 cm of the catheter exit site, in the absence of concomitant bloodstream infection (BSI) and without concomitant purulence

Clinical Exit Site Infection (Or Tunnel Infection)

Tenderness, erythema, or site induration >2 cm from the catheter site along the subcutaneous tract of a tunneled (e.g., Hickman or Broviac) catheter, in the absence of concomitant BSI

Pocket Infection

Purulent fluid in the subcutaneous pocket of a totally implanted intravascular catheter that might or might not be associated with spontaneous rupture and drainage or necrosis of the overlaying skin, in the absence of concomitant BSI

Infusate-Related BSI

Concordant growth of the same organism from the infusate and blood cultures (preferably percutaneously drawn) with no other identifiable source of infection

Catheter-Related BSI

Bacteremia/fungemia in a patient with an intravascular catheter with at least one positive blood culture obtained from a peripheral vein, clinical manifestations of infections (i.e., fever, chills, and/or hypotension), and no apparent source for the BSI except the catheter. One of the following should be present: a positive semiquantitative (>15 CFU/catheter segment) or quantitative (>10³ CFU/catheter segment catheter) culture whereby the same organism (species and antibiogram) is isolated from the catheter segment and peripheral blood; simultaneous quantitative blood cultures with a ≥5:1 ratio CVC versus peripheral; differential period of CVC culture versus peripheral blood culture positivity of >2 hours.

Surveillance Definitions for Primary BSIs, National Nosocomial Infections Surveillance System

Laboratory-Confirmed BSI

Should meet at least one of the following criteria:

Criterion 1: Patient has a recognized pathogen cultured from one or more blood cultures, and the pathogen cultured from the blood is not related to an infection at another site.

Criterion 2: Patient has at least one of the following signs or symptoms: fever (>100.4° F [>38° C]), chills, or hypotension, and at least one of the following:

1. Common skin contaminant (e.g., diphtheroids, *Bacillus* spp., *Propionibacterium* spp., coagulase-negative staphylococci, or micrococci) cultured from two or more blood cultures drawn on separate occasions.
2. Common skin contaminant (e.g., diphtheroids, *Bacillus* spp., *Propionibacterium* spp., coagulase-negative staphylococci, or micrococci) cultured from at least one blood culture from a patient with an intravenous line, and the physician institutes appropriate antimicrobial therapy.
3. Positive antigen test on blood (e.g., *Hemophilus influenzae, Streptococcus pneumoniae, Neisseria meningitides,* or group B streptococcus).

and signs and symptoms with positive laboratory results are not related to an infection at another site.

Criterion 3: Patient aged <1 year has at least one of the following signs or symptoms: fever (>100.4° F [>38° C]), hypothermia (<98.6° F [<37° C]), apnea, or bradycardia, and at least one of the following:

1. Common skin contaminant (e.g., diphtheroids, *Bacillus* spp., *Propionibacterium* spp., coagulase-negative staphylococci, or micrococci) cultured from two or more blood cultures drawn on separate occasions.
2. Common skin contaminant (e.g., diphtheroids, *Bacillus* spp., *Propionibacterium* spp., coagulase-negative staphylococci, or micrococci) cultured from at least one blood culture from a patient with an intravenous line, and the physician institutes appropriate antimicrobial therapy.
3. Positive antigen test on blood (e.g., *Hemophilus influenzae, Streptococcus pneumoniae, Neisseria meningitides,* or group B streptococcus).

and signs and symptoms with positive laboratory results are not related to an infection at another site.

Clinical Sepsis

Should meet at least one of the following criteria:

Criterion 1: Patient has at least one of the following clinical signs with no other recognized cause: fever (>100.4° F [>38° C]), hypotension (systolic pressure <90 mm Hg), or oliguria (<20 mL/hr), and blood culture not done or no organisms or antigen detected in blood and no apparent infection at another site, and physician institutes treatment for sepsis.

Criterion 2: Patient aged <1 year has at least one of the following clinical signs or symptoms with no other recognized cause: fever (>100.4° F [>38° C]), hypothermia (<98.6° F [<37° C]), apnea, or bradycardia, and blood culture not done or no organisms or antigen detected in blood and no apparent infection at another site, and physician institutes treatment for sepsis.

Catheter-Associated BSI

Defined by the following:

- Vascular access device that terminates at or close to the heart or one of the great vessels. An umbilical artery or vein catheter is considered a central line.
- BSI is considered to be associated with a central line if the line was in use during the 48-hour period before development of the BSI. If the time interval between onset of infection and device use is >48 hours, there should be compelling evidence that the infection is related to the central line.

Arterial or Venous Infection

Included are arteriovenous graft, shunt, fistula, or intravenous cannulation. Should meet at least one of the following criteria:

Criterion 1: Patient has organisms cultured from arteries or veins removed during a surgical operation and blood culture not done or no organisms cultured from blood.

Criterion 2: Patient has evidence of arterial or venous infection seen during a surgical operation or histopathologic examination.

Criterion 3: Patient has at least one of the following signs or symptoms with no other recognized cause: fever (>100.4° F [>38° C]), pain, erythema, or heat at involved vascular site and >15 CFUs cultured from an intravascular cannula tip using a semiquantitative culture method and blood culture not done or no organisms cultured from blood.

Criterion 4: Patient has purulent drainage at the involved vascular site and blood culture not done or no organisms cultured from blood.

Criterion 5: Patient aged <1 year has at least one of the following signs or symptoms with no other recognized cause: fever (>100.4° F [>38° C]), hypothermia (<98.6° F [<37° C]), apnea, bradycardia, lethargy, or pain, erythema or heat at involved vascular site and >15 colonies cultured from intravascular cannula tip using semiquantitative method and blood culture not done or no organisms cultured from blood.

Appendix B

Summary of Recommended Frequency of Replacements for Catheters, Dressings, Administration Sets, and Fluids

Catheter	Replacement and relocation of device	Replacement of catheter site dressing	Replacement of administration sets	Hang time for parenteral fluids
Peripheral venous catheters	Replacement and relocation of device	Replace dressing when the catheter is removed or replaced, or when the dressing becomes damp, loosened, or soiled. Replace dressings more frequently in diaphoretic patients. In patients who have large bulky dressings that prevent palpation or direct visualization of the catheter insertion site, remove the dressing and visually inspect the catheter at least daily and apply a new dressing.	Replace intravenous tubing, including add-on devices, no more frequently than at 72-hour intervals unless clinically indicated. Replace tubing used to administer blood, blood products, or lipid emulsions within 24 hours of initiating the infusion. *No recommendation* for replacement of tubing used for intermittent infusions. Consider short extension tubing connected to the catheter to be a portion of the device. Replace such extension tubing when the catheter is changed.	*No recommendation* for the hang time of intravenous fluids, including nonlipid-containing parenteral nutrition fluids. Complete infusion of lipid-containing parenteral nutrition fluids (e.g., 3-in-1 solutions) within 24 hours of hanging the fluid. Complete infusion of lipid emulsions alone within 12 hours of hanging the fluid. Complete infusions of blood products within 4 hours of hanging the product.
Midline catheters	In *adults*, replace catheter and rotate site no more frequently than every 72–96 hours. Replace catheters inserted under emergency basis and insert a new catheter at a different site within 48 hours. In *pediatric* patients, do not replace peripheral catheters unless clinically indicated.	As above.	As above.	As above.
Peripheral arterial catheters	*No recommendation* for the frequency of the catheter replacement.	Replace dressing when the catheter is replaced, or when the dressing becomes damp, loosened, or soiled, or when inspection of the site is necessary.	Replace the intravenous tubing at the time the transducer is replaced (i.e., 72-hour intervals).	Replace the flush solution at the time the transducer is replaced (i.e., 72-hour intervals).
Central venous catheters including peripherally inserted central catheters and hemodialysis catheters	In *adults*, do not replace catheters routinely to prevent catheter-related infection. In *pediatric* patients, *no recommendation* for the frequency of catheter replacement. Replace disposable or reusable transducers at 72-hour intervals. Replace continuous flush device at the time the transducer is replaced.	Replace gauze dressings every 2 days and transparent dressings every 7 days on short-term catheters. Replace the dressing when the catheter is replaced, or when the dressing becomes damp, loosened, or soiled, or when inspection of the site is necessary.	Replace intravenous tubing and add-on devices no more frequently than at 72-hour intervals. Replace tubing used to administer blood products or lipid emulsions within 24 hours of initiating the infusion.	*No recommendation* for the hang time of intravenous fluids, including nonlipid-containing parenteral nutrition fluids. Complete infusions of lipid-containing fluids within 24 hours of hanging the fluid.
Pulmonary artery catheters	Do not routinely replace catheters.	As above.	As above.	As above.
Umbilical catheters	Do not replace catheter to prevent catheter-related infection. Do not routinely replace catheters.	Not applicable.	Replace intravenous tubing and add-on devices no more frequently than at 72-hour intervals. Replace tubing used to administer blood products or lipid emulsions within 24 hours of initiating the infusion.	*No recommendation* for the hang time of intravenous fluids, including nonlipid-containing parenteral nutrition fluids. Complete infusion of lipid-containing fluids within 24 hours of hanging the fluid. Includes nontunneled catheters, tunneled catheters, and totally *implanted* devices.

Appendix B

Summary of Recommended Frequency of Replacements for Catheters, Dressings, Administration Sets, and Fluids

Catheter	Replacement and relocation of device	Replacement of catheter site dressing	Replacement of administration sets	Hang time for parenteral fluids
Peripheral venous catheters	Replacement and relocation of device	Replace dressing when the catheter is removed or replaced, or when the dressing becomes damp, loosened, or soiled. Replace dressings more frequently in diaphoretic patients. In patients who have large bulky dressings that prevent palpation or direct visualization of the catheter insertion site, remove the dressing and visually inspect the catheter at least daily and apply a new dressing.	Replace intravenous tubing, including add-on devices, no more frequently than at 72-hour intervals unless clinically indicated. Replace tubing used to administer blood, blood products, or lipid emulsions within 24 hours of initiating the infusion. *No recommendation* for replacement of tubing used for intermittent infusions. Consider short extension tubing connected to the catheter to be a portion of the device. Replace such extension tubing when the catheter is changed.	*No recommendation* for the hang time of intravenous fluids, including nonlipid-containing parenteral nutrition fluids. Complete infusion of lipid-containing parenteral nutrition fluids (e.g., 3-in-1 solutions) within 24 hours of hanging the fluid. Complete infusion of lipid emulsions alone within 12 hours of hanging the fluid. Complete infusions of blood products within 4 hours of hanging the product.
Midline catheters	In *adults* replace catheter and rotate site no more frequently than every 72–96 hours. Replace catheters inserted under emergency basis and insert a new catheter at a different site within 48 hours. In *pediatric* patients, do not replace peripheral catheters unless clinically indicated.	As above.	As above.	As above.
Peripheral arterial catheters	*No recommendation* for the frequency of the catheter replacement.	Replace dressing when the catheter is replaced, or when the dressing becomes damp, loosened, or soiled, or when inspection of the site is necessary.	Replace the intravenous tubing at the time the transducer is replaced (i.e., 72-hour intervals).	Replace the flush solution at the time the transducer is replaced (i.e., 72-hour intervals).
Central venous catheters including peripherally inserted central catheters and hemodialysis catheters	In *adults*, do not replace catheters routinely to prevent catheter-related infection. In *pediatric* patients, *no recommendation* for the frequency of catheter replacement. Replace disposable or reusable transducers at 72-hour intervals. Replace continuous flush device at the time the transducer is replaced.	Replace gauze dressings every 2 days and transparent dressings every 7 days on short-term catheters. Replace the dressing when the catheter is replaced, or when the dressing becomes damp, loosened, or soiled, or when inspection of the site is necessary.	Replace intravenous tubing and add-on devices no more frequently than at 72-hour intervals. Replace tubing used to administer blood products or lipid emulsions within 24 hours of initiating the infusion.	*No recommendation* for the hang time of intravenous fluids, including nonlipid-containing parenteral nutrition fluids. Complete infusions of lipid-containing fluids within 24 hours of hanging the fluid.
Pulmonary artery catheters	Do not routinely replace catheters.	As above.	As above.	As above.
Umbilical catheters	Do not replace catheter to prevent catheter-related infection. Do not routinely replace catheters.	Not applicable.	Replace intravenous tubing and add-on devices no more frequently than at 72-hour intervals. Replace tubing used to administer blood products or lipid emulsions within 24 hours of initiating the infusion.	*No recommendation* for the hang time of intravenous fluids, including nonlipid-containing parenteral nutrition fluids. Complete infusion of lipid-containing fluids within 24 hours of hanging the fluid. Includes nontunneled catheters, tunneled catheters, and totally implanted devices.

GUIDELINE FOR PREVENTION OF SURGICAL SITE INFECTION, 1999

Alicia J. Mangram, MD; Teresa C. Horan, MPH, CIC; Michele L. Pearson, MD; Leah Christine Silver, BS; William R. Jarvis, MD; The Hospital Infection Control Practices Advisory Committee

Hospital Infections Program
National Center for Infectious Diseases
Centers for Disease Control and Prevention
Public Health Service
US Department of Health and Human Services

Hospital Infection Control Practices Advisory Committee Membership List, January 1999

CHAIRMAN
Elaine L. Larson, RN, PhD, FAAN, CIC
Columbia University School of Nursing
New York, New York

EXECUTIVE SECRETARY
Michele L. Pearson, MD
Centers for Disease Control and Prevention
Atlanta, Georgia

SURGICAL SITE INFECTION GUIDELINE SPONSOR
James T. Lee, MD, PhD, FACS
University of Minnesota
Minneapolis, Minnesota

MEMBERS

Audrey B. Adams, RN, MPH
Montefiore Medical Center
Bronx, New York

Raymond Y. W. Chinn, MD
Sharp Memorial Hospital
San Diego, California

Alfred DeMaria, Jr, MD
Massachusetts Department of
 Public Health
Jamaica Plain, Massachusetts

Susan W. Forlenza, MD
New York City Health Department
New York, New York

Ramon E. Moncada, MD
Coronado Physician's Medical Center
Coronado, California

William E. Scheckler, MD
University of Wisconsin Medical
 School
Madison, Wisconsin

Jane D. Siegel, MD
University of Texas Southwestern
 Medical Center
Dallas, Texas

Marjorie A. Underwood, RN, BSN, CIC
Mt. Diablo Medical Center
Concord, California

Robert A. Weinstein, MD
Cook County Hospital
Chicago, Illinois

Table of Contents

Special Report

Guideline for Prevention of Surgical Site Infection, 1999

Alicia J. Mangram, MD; Teresa C. Horan, MPH, CIC; Michele L. Pearson, MD; Leah Christine Silver, BS; William R. Jarvis, MD;
The Hospital Infection Control Practices Advisory Committee

EXECUTIVE SUMMARY

The "Guideline for Prevention of Surgical Site Infection, 1999" presents the Centers for Disease Control and Prevention (CDC)'s recommendations for the prevention of surgical site infections (SSIs), formerly called surgical wound infections. This two-part guideline updates and replaces previous guidelines.[1,2]

Part I, "Surgical Site Infection: An Overview," describes the epidemiology, definitions, microbiology, pathogenesis, and surveillance of SSIs. Included is a detailed discussion of the pre-, intra-, and postoperative issues relevant to SSI genesis.

Part II, "Recommendations for Prevention of Surgical Site Infection," represents the consensus of the Hospital Infection Control Practices Advisory Committee (HICPAC) regarding strategies for the prevention of SSIs.[3] Whenever possible, the recommendations in Part II are based on data from well-designed scientific studies. However, there are a limited number of studies that clearly validate risk factors and prevention measures for SSI. By necessity, available studies have often been conducted in narrowly defined patient populations or for specific kinds of operations, making generalization of their findings to all specialties and types of operations potentially problematic. This is especially true regarding the implementation of SSI prevention measures. Finally, some of the infection control practices routinely used by surgical teams cannot be rigorously studied for ethical or logistical reasons (e.g., wearing vs not wearing gloves). Thus, some of the recommendations in Part II are based on a strong theoretical rationale and suggestive evidence in the absence of confirmatory scientific knowledge.

It has been estimated that approximately 75% of all operations in the United States will be performed in "ambulatory," "same-day," or "outpatient" operating rooms by the turn of the century.[4] In recommending various SSI prevention methods, this document makes no distinction between surgical care delivered in such settings and that provided in conventional inpatient operating rooms. This document is primarily intended for use by surgeons, operating room nurses, postoperative inpatient and clinic nurses, infection control professionals, anesthesiologists, healthcare epidemiologists, and other personnel directly responsible for the prevention of nosocomial infections.

This document does *not*:

● Specifically address issues unique to burns, trauma, transplant procedures, or transmission of bloodborne pathogens from healthcare worker to patient, nor does it specifically address details of SSI prevention in pediatric surgical practice. It has been recently shown in a multicenter study of pediatric surgical patients that characteristics related to the operations are more important than those related to the physiologic status of the patients.[5] In general, all SSI prevention measures effective in adult surgical care are indicated in pediatric surgical care.

● Specifically address procedures performed outside of the operating room (e.g., endoscopic procedures), nor does it provide guidance for infection prevention for invasive procedures such as cardiac catheterization or interventional radiology. Nonetheless, it is likely that many SSI prevention strategies also could be applied or adapted to reduce infectious complications associated with these procedures.

● Specifically recommend SSI prevention methods

From the Hospital Infections Program, National Center for Infectious Diseases, Centers for Disease Control and Prevention, Public Health Service, US Department of Health and Human Services, Atlanta, Georgia.

The Hospital Infection Control Practices Committee thanks the following subject-matter experts for reviewing a preliminary draft of this guideline: Carol Applegeet, RN, MSN, CNOR, CNAA, FAAN; Ona Baker, RN, MSHA; Philip Barie, MD, FACS; Arnold Berry, MD; Col. Nancy Bjerke, BSN, MPH, CIC; John Bohnen, MD, FRCSC, FACS; Robert Condon, MS, MD, FACS; E. Patchen Dellinger, MD, FACS; Terrie Lee, RN, MS, MPH, CIC; Judith Mathias, RN; Anne Matlow, MD, MS, FRCPC; C. Glen Mayhall, MD; Rita McCormick, RN, CIC; Ronald Nichols, MD, FACS; Barbara Pankratz, RN; William Rutala, PhD, MPH, CIC; Julie Wagner, RN; Samuel Wilson, MD, FACS. The opinions of all the reviewers might not be reflected in all the recommendations contained in this document.

The authors thank Connie Alfred, Estella Cormier, Karen Friend, Charlene Gibson, and Geraldine Jones for providing invaluable assistance.

Dr. Mangram is currently affiliated with the University of Texas Medical Center, Houston, Texas.

Published simultaneously in Infection Control and Hospital Epidemiology, the American Journal of Infection Control, and the Journal of Surgical Outcomes.

This document is not copyright-protected and may be photocopied.

Address reprint requests to SSI Guideline, Hospital Infections Program, Mailstop E69, Centers for Disease Control and Prevention, 1600 Clifton Rd, Atlanta, GA 30333.

The "Guideline for Prevention of Surgical Site Infection, 1999" is available online at www.cdc.gov/ncidod/hip.

99-SR-024. Mangram AJ, Horan TC, Pearson ML, Silver LC, Jarvis WR, the Hospital Infection Control Practices Advisory Committee. Guideline for the prevention of surgical site infection, 1999. Infect Control Hosp Epidemiol 1999;20:247-280.

unique to minimally invasive operations (i.e., laparoscopic surgery). Available SSI surveillance data indicate that laparoscopic operations generally have a lower or comparable SSI risk when contrasted to open operations.[6-11] SSI prevention measures applicable in open operations (e.g., open cholecystectomy) are indicated for their laparoscopic counterparts (e.g., laparoscopic cholecystectomy).

• Recommend specific antiseptic agents for patient preoperative skin preparations or for healthcare worker hand/forearm antisepsis. Hospitals should choose from products recommended for these activities in the latest Food and Drug Administration (FDA) monograph.[12]

I. SURGICAL SITE INFECTION (SSI): AN OVERVIEW

A. INTRODUCTION

Before the mid-19th century, surgical patients commonly developed postoperative "irritative fever," followed by purulent drainage from their incisions, overwhelming sepsis, and often death. It was not until the late 1860s, after Joseph Lister introduced the principles of antisepsis, that postoperative infectious morbidity decreased substantially. Lister's work radically changed surgery from an activity associated with infection and death to a discipline that could eliminate suffering and prolong life.

Currently, in the United States alone, an estimated 27 million surgical procedures are performed each year.[13] The CDC's National Nosocomial Infections Surveillance (NNIS) system, established in 1970, monitors reported trends in nosocomial infections in U.S. acute-care hospitals. Based on NNIS system reports, SSIs are the third most frequently reported nosocomial infection, accounting for 14% to 16% of all nosocomial infections among hospitalized patients.[14] During 1986 to 1996, hospitals conducting SSI surveillance in the NNIS system reported 15,523 SSIs following 593,344 operations (CDC, unpublished data). Among surgical patients, SSIs were the most common nosocomial infection, accounting for 38% of all such infections. Of these SSIs, two thirds were confined to the incision, and one third involved organs or spaces accessed during the operation. When surgical patients with nosocomial SSI died, 77% of the deaths were reported to be related to the infection, and the majority (93%) were serious infections involving organs or spaces accessed during the operation.

In 1980, Cruse estimated that an SSI increased a patient's hospital stay by approximately 10 days and cost an additional $2,000.[15,16] A 1992 analysis showed that each SSI resulted in 7.3 additional postoperative hospital days, adding $3,152 in extra charges.[17] Other studies corroborate that increased length of hospital stay and cost are associated with SSIs.[18,19] Deep SSIs involving organs or spaces, as compared to SSIs confined to the incision, are associated with even greater increases in hospital stays and costs.[20,21]

Advances in infection control practices include improved operating room ventilation, sterilization methods, barriers, surgical technique, and availability of antimicrobial prophylaxis. Despite these activities, SSIs remain a

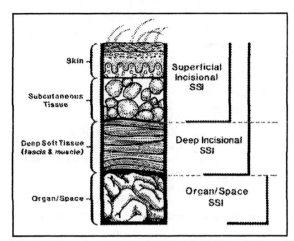

FIGURE. Cross-section of abdominal wall depicting CDC classifications of surgical site infection.[22]

substantial cause of morbidity and mortality among hospitalized patients. This may be partially explained by the emergence of antimicrobial-resistant pathogens and the increased numbers of surgical patients who are elderly and/or have a wide variety of chronic, debilitating, or immunocompromising underlying diseases. There also are increased numbers of prosthetic implant and organ transplant operations performed. Thus, to reduce the risk of SSI, a systematic but realistic approach must be applied with the awareness that this risk is influenced by characteristics of the patient, operation, personnel, and hospital.

B. KEY TERMS USED IN THE GUIDELINE
1. Criteria for Defining SSIs

The identification of SSI involves interpretation of clinical and laboratory findings, and it is crucial that a surveillance program use definitions that are consistent and standardized; otherwise, inaccurate or uninterpretable SSI rates will be computed and reported. The CDC's NNIS system has developed standardized surveillance criteria for defining SSIs (Table 1).[22] By these criteria, SSIs are classified as being either incisional or organ/space. Incisional SSIs are further divided into those involving only skin and subcutaneous tissue (superficial incisional SSI) and those involving deeper soft tissues of the incision (deep incisional SSI). Organ/space SSIs involve any part of the anatomy (e.g., organ or space) other than incised body wall layers, that was opened or manipulated during an operation (Figure). Table 2 lists site-specific classifications used to differentiate organ/space SSIs. For example, in a patient who had an appendectomy and subsequently developed an intra-abdominal abscess not draining through the incision, the infection would be reported as an organ/space SSI at the intra-abdominal site. Failure to use objective criteria to define SSIs has been shown to substantially affect reported SSI rates.[23,24] The CDC NNIS definitions of SSIs have been applied consistently by surveillance and surgical personnel in many settings and currently are a de facto national standard.[22,25]

TABLE 1
CRITERIA FOR DEFINING A SURGICAL SITE INFECTION (SSI)*

Superficial Incisional SSI

Infection occurs within 30 days after the operation

and

infection involves only skin or subcutaneous tissue of the incision

and at least *one* of the following:

    1. Purulent drainage, with or without laboratory confirmation, from the superficial incision.

    2. Organisms isolated from an aseptically obtained culture of fluid or tissue from the superficial incision.

    3. At least one of the following signs or symptoms of infection: pain or tenderness, localized swelling, redness, or heat *and* superficial incision
       is deliberately opened by surgeon, *unless* incision is culture-negative.

    4. Diagnosis of superficial incisional SSI by the surgeon or attending physician.

Do *not* report the following conditions as SSI:

    1. Stitch abscess (minimal inflammation and discharge confined to the points of suture penetration).

    2. Infection of an episiotomy or newborn circumcision site.

    3. Infected burn wound.

    4. Incisional SSI that extends into the fascial and muscle layers (see deep incisional SSI).

Note: Specific criteria are used for identifying infected episiotomy and circumcision sites and burn wounds.[433]

Deep Incisional SSI

Infection occurs within 30 days after the operation if no implant[†] is left in place or within 1 year if implant is in place and the infection appears to
be related to the operation

and

infection involves deep soft tissues (e.g., fascial and muscle layers) of the incision

and at least *one* of the following:

    1. Purulent drainage from the deep incision but not from the organ/space component of the surgical site.

    2. A deep incision spontaneously dehisces or is deliberately opened by a surgeon when the patient has at least one of the following signs or
       symptoms: fever (>38°C), localized pain, or tenderness, unless site is culture-negative.

    3. An abscess or other evidence of infection involving the deep incision is found on direct examination, during reoperation, or by histopatholog
       ic or radiologic examination.

    4. Diagnosis of a deep incisional SSI by a surgeon or attending physician.

Notes:

    1. Report infection that involves both superficial and deep incision sites as deep incisional SSI.

    2. Report an organ/space SSI that drains through the incision as a deep incisional SSI.

Organ/Space SSI

Infection occurs within 30 days after the operation if no implant[†] is left in place or within 1 year if implant is in place and the infection appears to
be related to the operation

and

infection involves any part of the anatomy (e.g., organs or spaces), other than the incision, which was opened or manipulated during an operation

and at least *one* of the following:

    1. Purulent drainage from a drain that is placed through a stab wound[‡] into the organ/space.

    2. Organisms isolated from an aseptically obtained culture of fluid or tissue in the organ/space.

    3. An abscess or other evidence of infection involving the organ/space that is found on direct examination, during reoperation, or by
       histopathologic or radiologic examination.

    4. Diagnosis of an organ/space SSI by a surgeon or attending physician.

* Horan TC et al.[22]
† National Nosocomial Infection Surveillance definition: a nonhuman-derived implantable foreign body (e.g., prosthetic heart valve, nonhuman vascular graft, mechanical heart, or hip prosthesis) that
is permanently placed in a patient during surgery.
‡ If the area around a stab wound becomes infected, it is not an SSI. It is considered a skin or soft tissue infection, depending on its depth.

2. Operating Suite

A physically separate area that comprises operating rooms and their interconnecting hallways and ancillary work areas such as scrub sink rooms. No distinction is made between operating suites located in conventional inpatient hospitals and those used for "same-day" surgical care, whether in a hospital or a free-standing facility.

3. Operating Room

A room in an operating suite where operations are performed.

4. Surgical Personnel

Any healthcare worker who provides care to surgical patients during the pre-, intra-, or postoperative periods.

5. Surgical Team Member

Any healthcare worker in an operating room during the operation who has a surgical care role. Members of the surgical team may be "scrubbed" or not; scrubbed members have direct contact with the sterile operating field or sterile instruments or supplies used in the field (refer to "Preoperative Hand/Forearm Antisepsis" section).

C. MICROBIOLOGY

According to data from the NNIS system, the distribution of pathogens isolated from SSIs has not changed markedly during the last decade (Table 3).[26,27] *Staphylococcus aureus,* coagulase-negative staphylococci, *Enterococcus* spp., and *Escherichia coli* remain the most frequently isolated pathogens. An increasing proportion of SSIs are caused by antimicrobial-resistant pathogens, such as methicillin-resistant *S. aureus* (MRSA),[28,29] or by *Candida albicans.*[30] From 1991 to 1995, the incidence of fungal SSIs among patients at NNIS hospitals increased from 0.1 to 0.3 per 1,000 discharges.[30] The increased proportion of SSIs caused by resistant pathogens and *Candida* spp. may reflect increasing numbers of severely ill and immunocompromised surgical patients and the impact of widespread use of broad-spectrum antimicrobial agents.

Outbreaks or clusters of SSIs have also been caused by unusual pathogens, such as *Rhizopus oryzae, Clostridium perfringens, Rhodococcus bronchialis, Nocardia farcinica, Legionella pneumophila* and *Legionella dumoffii,* and *Pseudomonas multivorans.* These rare outbreaks have been traced to contaminated adhesive dressings,[31] elastic bandages,[32] colonized surgical personnel,[33,34] tap water,[35] or contaminated disinfectant solutions.[36] When a cluster of SSIs involves an unusual organism, a formal epidemiologic investigation should be conducted.

D. PATHOGENESIS

Microbial contamination of the surgical site is a necessary precursor of SSI. The risk of SSI can be conceptualized according to the following relationship[37,38]:

$$\frac{\text{Dose of bacterial contamination} \times \text{virulence}}{\text{Resistance of the host patient}} = \text{Risk of surgical site infection}$$

Quantitatively, it has been shown that if a surgical site is contaminated with >10⁵ microorganisms per gram of tissue, the risk of SSI is markedly increased.[39] However, the dose of contaminating microorganisms required to produce infection may be much lower when foreign material is present at the site (i.e., 100 staphylococci per gram of tissue introduced on silk sutures).[40-42]

Microorganisms may contain or produce toxins and other substances that increase their ability to invade a host, produce damage within the host, or survive on or in host tissue. For example, many gram-negative bacteria produce

TABLE 2

SITE-SPECIFIC CLASSIFICATIONS OF ORGAN/SPACE SURGICAL SITE INFECTION*

Arterial or venous infection
Breast abscess or mastitis
Disc space
Ear, mastoid
Endocarditis
Endometritis
Eye, other than conjunctivitis
Gastrointestinal tract
Intra-abdominal, not specified elsewhere
Intracranial, brain abscess or dura
Joint or bursa
Mediastinitis
Meningitis or ventriculitis
Myocarditis or pericarditis
Oral cavity (mouth, tongue, or gums)
Osteomyelitis
Other infections of the lower respiratory tract (e.g., abscess or empyema)
Other male or female reproductive tract
Sinusitis
Spinal abscess without meningitis
Upper respiratory tract
Vaginal cuff

* Horan TC et al.[22]

endotoxin, which stimulates cytokine production. In turn, cytokines can trigger the systemic inflammatory response syndrome that sometimes leads to multiple system organ failure.[43-45] One of the most common causes of multiple system organ failure in modern surgical care is intra-abdominal infection.[46,47] Some bacterial surface components, notably polysaccharide capsules, inhibit phagocytosis,[48] a critical and early host defense response to microbial contamination. Certain strains of clostridia and streptococci produce potent exotoxins that disrupt cell membranes or alter cellular metabolism.[49] A variety of microorganisms, including gram-positive bacteria such as coagulase-negative staphylococci, produce glycocalyx and an associated component called "slime,"[50-55] which physically shields bacteria from phagocytes or inhibits the binding or penetration of antimicrobial agents.[56] Although these and other virulence factors are well defined, their mechanistic relationship to SSI development has not been fully determined.

For most SSIs, the source of pathogens is the endogenous flora of the patient's skin, mucous membranes, or hollow viscera.[57] When mucous membranes or skin is incised, the exposed tissues are at risk for contamination with endogenous flora.[58] These organisms are usually aerobic gram-positive cocci (e.g., staphylococci), but may include fecal flora (e.g., anaerobic bacteria and gram-negative aerobes) when incisions are made near the perineum or groin. When a gastrointestinal organ is opened

TABLE 3
DISTRIBUTION OF PATHOGENS ISOLATED* FROM SURGICAL SITE INFECTIONS, NATIONAL NOSOCOMIAL INFECTIONS SURVEILLANCE SYSTEM, 1986 TO 1996

	Percentage of Isolates	
	1986-1989[179]	1990-1996[28]
Pathogen	(N=16,727)	(N=17,671)
Staphylococcus aureus	17	20
Coagulase-negative staphylococci	12	14
Enterococcus spp.	13	12
Escherichia coli	10	8
Pseudomonas aeruginosa	8	8
Enterobacter spp.	8	7
Proteus mirabilis	4	3
Klebsiella pneumoniae	3	3
Other *Streptococcus* spp.	3	3
Candida albicans	2	3
Group D streptococci (non-enterococci)	—	2
Other gram-positive aerobes	—	2
Bacteroides fragilis	—	2

*Pathogens representing less than 2% of isolates are excluded.

during an operation and is the source of pathogens, gram-negative bacilli (e.g., *E. coli*), gram-positive organisms (e.g., enterococci), and sometimes anaerobes (e.g., *Bacillus fragilis*) are the typical SSI isolates. Table 4 lists operations and the likely SSI pathogens associated with them. Seeding of the operative site from a distant focus of infection can be another source of SSI pathogens,[59-68] particularly in patients who have a prosthesis or other implant placed during the operation. Such devices provide a nidus for attachment of the organism.[50,69-73]

Exogenous sources of SSI pathogens include surgical personnel (especially members of the surgical team),[74-78] the operating room environment (including air), and all tools, instruments, and materials brought to the sterile field during an operation (refer to "Intraoperative Issues" section). Exogenous flora are primarily aerobes, especially gram-positive organisms (e.g., staphylococci and streptococci). Fungi from endogenous and exogenous sources rarely cause SSIs, and their pathogenesis is not well understood.[79]

E. RISK AND PREVENTION

The term *risk factor* has a particular meaning in epidemiology and, in the context of SSI pathophysiology and prevention, strictly refers to a variable that has a significant, independent association with the development of SSI after a specific operation. Risk factors are identified by multivariate analyses in epidemiologic studies. Unfortunately, the term risk factor often is used in the surgical literature in a broad sense to include patient or operation features which, although associated with SSI development in univariate analysis, are not necessarily independent predictors.[80] The literature cited in the sections that follow includes risk factors identified by both univariate and multivariate analyses.

Table 5 lists patient and operation characteristics that may influence the risk of SSI development. These characteristics are useful in two ways: (1) they allow stratification of operations, making surveillance data more comprehensible; and, (2) knowledge of risk factors before certain operations may allow for targeted prevention measures. For example, if it is known that a patient has a remote site infection, the surgical team may reduce SSI risk by scheduling an operation after the infection has resolved.

An SSI prevention measure can be defined as an action or set of actions intentionally taken to reduce the risk of an SSI. Many such techniques are directed at reducing opportunities for microbial contamination of the patient's tissues or sterile surgical instruments; others are adjunctive, such as using antimicrobial prophylaxis or avoiding unnecessary traumatic tissue dissection. Optimum application of SSI prevention measures requires that a variety of patient and operation characteristics be carefully considered.

1. Patient Characteristics

In certain kinds of operations, patient characteristics possibly associated with an increased risk of an SSI include coincident remote site infections[59-68] or colonization,[81-83] diabetes,[84-87] cigarette smoking,[85,88-92] systemic steroid use,[84,87,93] obesity (>20% ideal body weight),[85-87,94-97] extremes of age,[92,98-102] poor nutritional status,[85,94,98,103-105] and perioperative transfusion of certain blood products.[106-109]

a. Diabetes

The contribution of diabetes to SSI risk is controversial,[84-86,98,110] because the independent contribution of diabetes to SSI risk has not typically been assessed after controlling for potential confounding factors. Recent preliminary findings from a study of patients who underwent coronary artery bypass graft showed a significant relationship between increasing levels of HgA1c and SSI rates.[111] Also, increased glucose levels (>200 mg/dL) in the immediate postoperative period (≤48 hours) were associated with increased SSI risk.[112,113] More studies are needed to assess the efficacy of perioperative blood glucose control as a prevention measure.

b. Nicotine use

Nicotine use delays primary wound healing and may increase the risk of SSI.[85] In a large prospective study, current cigarette smoking was an independent risk factor for sternal and/or mediastinal SSI following cardiac surgery.[85] Other studies have corroborated cigarette smoking as an important SSI risk factor.[88-92] The limitation of these studies, however, is that terms like *current cigarette smoking* and *active smokers* are not always defined. To appropriately determine the contribution of tobacco use to SSI risk, standardized definitions of smoking history must be adopted and used in studies designed to control for confounding variables.

c. Steroid use

Patients who are receiving steroids or other immuno-

TABLE 4
OPERATIONS, LIKELY SURGICAL SITE INFECTION (SSI) PATHOGENS, AND REFERENCES ON USE OF ANTIMICROBIAL PROPHYLAXIS*

Operations	Likely Pathogens[†‡]	References
Placement of all grafts, prostheses, or implants	*Staphylococcus aureus;* coagulase-negative staphylococci	269,282-284,290
Cardiac	*S. aureus;* coagulase-negative staphylococci	251-253,462,463
Neurosurgery	*S. aureus;* coagulase-negative staphylococci	241,249,258,259,261,464,465
Breast	*S. aureus;* coagulase-negative staphylococci	242,248
Ophthalmic	*S. aureus;* coagulase-negative staphylococci; streptococci; gram-negative bacilli	466
Limited data; however, commonly used in procedures such as anterior segment resection, vitrectomy, and scleral buckles		
Orthopedic	*S. aureus;* coagulase-negative staphylococci; gram-negative bacilli	60,243-246,254,255,467-473
Total joint replacement		
Closed fractures/use of nails, bone plates, other internal fixation devices		
Functional repair without implant/device		
Trauma		
Noncardiac thoracic	*S. aureus;* coagulase-negative staphylococci; *Streptococcus pneumoniae;* gram-negative bacilli	240,247,474,475
Thoracic (lobectomy, pneumonectomy, wedge resection, other noncardiac mediastinal procedures)		
Closed tube thoracostomy		
Vascular	*S. aureus;* coagulase-negative staphylococci	250,463,476,477
Appendectomy	Gram-negative bacilli; anaerobes	263,452,478
Biliary tract	Gram-negative bacilli; anaerobes	260,262,479-484
Colorectal	Gram-negative bacilli; anaerobes	200,239,256,287-289,485-490
Gastroduodenal	Gram-negative bacilli; streptococci; oropharyngeal anaerobes (e.g., peptostreptococci)	256,257,491-493
Head and neck (major procedures with incision through oropharyngeal mucosa)	*S. aureus;* streptococci; oropharyngeal anaerobes (e.g., peptostreptococci)	494-497
Obstetric and gynecologic	Gram-negative bacilli; enterococci; group B streptococci; anaerobes	270-280,435
Urologic	Gram-negative bacilli	267
May not be beneficial if urine is sterile		

* Refer to "Antimicrobial prophylaxis in surgery." *The Medical Letter,* 1997.[266] for current recommendations of antimicrobial agents and doses.
† Likely pathogens from both endogenous and exogenous sources.
‡ Staphylococci will be associated with SSI following all types of operations.

suppressive drugs preoperatively may be predisposed to developing SSI,[84,87] but the data supporting this relationship are contradictory. In a study of long-term steroid use in patients with Crohn's disease, SSI developed significantly more often in patients receiving preoperative steroids (12.5%) than in patients without steroid use (6.7%).[93] In contrast, other investigations have not found a relationship between steroid use and SSI risk.[98,114,115]

d. Malnutrition

For some types of operations, severe protein-calorie malnutrition is crudely associated with postoperative nosocomial infections, impaired wound healing dynamics, or death.[116-124] The National Academy of Sciences/National Research Council (NAS/NRC),[94] Study on the Efficacy of Infection Control (SENIC),[125] and NNIS[126] schemes for SSI risk stratification do not explicitly incorporate nutritional status as a predictor variable, although it may be represented indirectly in the latter two. In a widely quoted 1987

study of 404 high-risk general surgery operations, Christou and coworkers derived an SSI probability index in which final predictor variables were patient age, operation duration, serum albumin level, delayed hypersensitivity test score, and intrinsic wound contamination level.[117] Although this index predicted SSI risk satisfactorily for 404 subsequent patients and was generally received as a significant advance in SSI risk stratification, it is not widely used in SSI surveillance data analysis, surgical infection research, or analytic epidemiology.

Theoretical arguments can be made for a belief that severe preoperative malnutrition should increase the risk of both incisional and organ/space SSI. However, an epidemiologic association between incisional SSI and malnutrition is difficult to demonstrate consistently for all surgical subspecialties.[118-120,124,127-131] Multivariate logistic regression modeling has shown that preoperative protein-calorie malnutrition is not an independent predictor of

TABLE 5
PATIENT AND OPERATION CHARACTERISTICS THAT MAY INFLUENCE
THE RISK OF SURGICAL SITE INFECTION DEVELOPMENT

Patient
    Age
    Nutritional status
    Diabetes
    Smoking
    Obesity
    Coexistent infections at a remote body site
    Colonization with microorganisms
    Altered immune response
    Length of preoperative stay
Operation
    Duration of surgical scrub
    Skin antisepsis
    Preoperative shaving
    Preoperative skin prep
    Duration of operation
    Antimicrobial prophylaxis
    Operating room ventilation
    Inadequate sterilization of instruments
    Foreign material in the surgical site
    Surgical drains
    Surgical technique
        Poor hemostasis
        Failure to obliterate dead space
        Tissue trauma

Adapted from references 25, 37.

mediastinitis after cardiac bypass operations.[85,132]

In the modern era, total parenteral nutrition (TPN) and total enteral alimentation (TEA) have enthusiastic acceptance by surgeons and critical care specialists.[118,133-137] However, the benefits of preoperative nutritional repletion of malnourished patients in reducing SSI risk are unproven. In two randomized clinical trials, preoperative "nutritional therapy" did not reduce incisional and organ/space SSI risk.[138-141] In a recent study of high-risk pancreatectomy patients with cancer, the provision of TPN preoperatively had no beneficial effect on SSI risk.[142] A randomized prospective trial involving 395 general and thoracic surgery patients compared outcomes for malnourished patients preoperatively receiving either a 7- to 15-day TPN regimen or a regular preoperative hospital diet. All patients were followed for 90 days postoperatively. There was no detectable benefit of TPN administration on the incidence of incisional or organ/space SSI.[143] Administering TPN or TEA may be indicated in a number of circumstances, but such repletion cannot be viewed narrowly as a prevention measure for organ/space or incisional SSI risk. When a major elective operation is necessary in a severely malnourished patient, experienced surgeons often use both pre- and postoperative nutritional support in consideration of the major morbidity associated with numerous potential complications, only one of which is organ/space SSI.[118,124,130,133,137,138,144-149] In addition, postoperative nutritional support is important for certain major oncologic operations,[135,136] after many operations on major trauma victims,[134] or in patients suffering a variety of catastrophic surgical complications that preclude eating or that trigger a hypermetabolic state. Randomized clinical trials will be necessary to determine if nutritional support alters SSI risk in specific patient-operation combinations.

e. Prolonged preoperative hospital stay

Prolonged preoperative hospital stay is frequently suggested as a patient characteristic associated with increased SSI risk. However, length of preoperative stay is likely a surrogate for severity of illness and co-morbid conditions requiring inpatient work-up and/or therapy before the operation.[16,26,65,85,94,100,150,151]

f. Preoperative nares colonization with *Staphylococcus aureus*

S. aureus is a frequent SSI isolate. This pathogen is carried in the nares of 20% to 30% of healthy humans.[81] It has been known for years that the development of SSI involving *S. aureus* is definitely associated with preoperative nares carriage of the organism in surgical patients.[81] A recent multivariate analysis demonstrated that such carriage was the most powerful independent risk factor for SSI following cardiothoracic operations.[82]

Mupirocin ointment is effective as a topical agent for eradicating *S. aureus* from the nares of colonized patients or healthcare workers. A recent report by Kluytmans and coworkers suggested that SSI risk was reduced in patients who had cardiothoracic operations when mupirocin was applied preoperatively to their nares, regardless of carrier status.[152] In this study, SSI rates for 752 mupirocin-treated patients were compared with those previously observed for an untreated group of 928 historical control patients, and the significant SSI rate reduction was attributed to the mupirocin treatment. Concerns have been raised regarding the comparability of the two patient groups.[153] Additionally, there is concern that mupirocin resistance may emerge, although this seems unlikely when treatment courses are brief.[81] A prospective, randomized clinical trial will be necessary to establish definitively that eradication of nasal carriage of *S. aureus* is an effective SSI prevention method in cardiac surgery. Such a trial has recently been completed on 3,909 patients in Iowa.[83] Five types of operations in two facilities were observed. Preliminary analysis showed a significant association between nasal carriage of *S. aureus* and subsequent SSI development. The effect of mupirocin on reducing SSI risk is yet to be determined.

g. Perioperative transfusion

It has been reported that perioperative transfusion of leukocyte-containing allogeneic blood components is an apparent risk factor for the development of postoperative bacterial infections, including SSI.[106] In three of five randomized trials conducted in patients undergoing elective colon resection for cancer, the risk of SSI was at least doubled in patients receiving blood transfusions.[107-109] However, on the basis of detailed epidemiologic reconsid-

TABLE 6
MECHANISM AND SPECTRUM OF ACTIVITY OF ANTISEPTIC AGENTS COMMONLY USED FOR PREOPERATIVE SKIN PREPARATION AND SURGICAL SCRUBS

Agent	Mechanism of Action	Gram-Positive Bacteria	Gram-Negative Bacteria	Mtb	Fungi	Virus	Rapidity of Action	Residual Activity	Toxicity	Uses
Alcohol	Denature proteins	E	E	G	G	G	Most rapid	None	Drying, volatile	SP, SS
Chlorhexidine	Disrupt cell membrane	E	G	P	F	G	Intermediate	E	Ototoxicity, keratitis	SP, SS
Iodine/Iodophors	Oxidation/substitution by free iodine	E	G	G	G	G	Intermediate	Minimal	Absorption from skin with possible toxicity, skin irritation	SP, SS
PCMX	Disrupt cell wall	G	F*	F	F	F	Intermediate	G	More data needed	SS
Triclosan	Disrupt cell wall	G	G	G	P	U	Intermediate	E	More data needed	SS

Abbreviations: E, excellent; F, fair; G, good; Mtb, *Mycobacterium tuberculosis*; P, poor; PCMX, para-chloro-meta-xylenol; SP, skin preparation; SS, surgical scrubs; U, unknown.
Data from Larson E.[176]
* Fair, except for *Pseudomonas* spp.; activity improved by addition of chelating agent such as EDTA.

erations, as many as 12 confounding variables may have influenced the reported association, and any effect of transfusion on SSI risk may be either small or nonexistent.[106] Because of methodologic problems, including the timing of transfusion, and use of nonstandardized SSI definitions, interpretation of the available data is limited. A meta-analysis of published trials will probably be required for resolution of the controversy.[154] There is currently no scientific basis for withholding necessary blood products from surgical patients as a means of either incisional or organ/space SSI risk reduction.

2. Operative Characteristics: Preoperative Issues
a. Preoperative antiseptic showering
A preoperative antiseptic shower or bath decreases skin microbial colony counts. In a study of >700 patients who received two preoperative antiseptic showers, chlorhexidine reduced bacterial colony counts ninefold (2.8×10^2 to 0.3), while povidone-iodine or triclocarban-medicated soap reduced colony counts by 1.3- and 1.9-fold, respectively.[155] Other studies corroborate these findings.[156,157] Chlorhexidine gluconate-containing products require several applications to attain maximum antimicrobial benefit, so repeated antiseptic showers are usually indicated.[158] Even though preoperative showers reduce the skin's microbial colony counts, they have not definitively been shown to reduce SSI rates.[159-165]

b. Preoperative hair removal
Preoperative shaving of the surgical site the night before an operation is associated with a significantly higher SSI risk than either the use of depilatory agents or no hair removal.[16,100,166-169] In one study, SSI rates were 5.6% in patients who had hair removed by razor shave compared to a 0.6% rate among those who had hair removed by depilatory or who had no hair removed.[166] The increased SSI risk associated with shaving has been attributed to microscopic cuts in the skin that later serve as foci for bacterial multi-

plication. Shaving immediately before the operation compared to shaving within 24 hours preoperatively was associated with decreased SSI rates (3.1% vs 7.1%); if shaving was performed >24 hours prior to operation, the SSI rate exceeded 20%.[166] Clipping hair immediately before an operation also has been associated with a lower risk of SSI than shaving or clipping the night before an operation (SSI rates immediately before = 1.8% vs night before = 4.0%).[170-173] Although the use of depilatories has been associated with a lower SSI risk than shaving or clipping,[166,167] depilatories sometimes produce hypersensitivity reactions.[166] Other studies showed that preoperative hair removal by any means was associated with increased SSI rates and suggested that no hair be removed.[100,174,175]

c. Patient skin preparation in the operating room
Several antiseptic agents are available for preoperative preparation of skin at the incision site (Table 6). The iodophors (e.g., povidone-iodine), alcohol-containing products, and chlorhexidine gluconate are the most commonly used agents. No studies have adequately assessed the comparative effects of these preoperative skin antiseptics on SSI risk in well-controlled, operation-specific studies.

Alcohol is defined by the FDA as having one of the following active ingredients: ethyl alcohol, 60% to 95% by volume in an aqueous solution, or isopropyl alcohol, 50% to 91.3% by volume in an aqueous solution.[12] Alcohol is readily available, inexpensive, and remains the most effective and rapid-acting skin antiseptic.[176] Aqueous 70% to 92% alcohol solutions have germicidal activity against bacteria, fungi, and viruses, but spores can be resistant.[176,177] One potential disadvantage of the use of alcohol in the operating room is its flammability.[176-178]

Both chlorhexidine gluconate and iodophors have broad spectra of antimicrobial activity.[177,179-181] In some comparisons of the two antiseptics when used as preoperative hand scrubs, chlorhexidine gluconate achieved greater reductions in skin microflora than did povidone-iodine and also had greater residual activity after a single application.[182-184] Further, chlorhexidine gluconate is not inactivated by blood or serum proteins.[176,179,185,186] Iodophors may be inactivated by blood or serum proteins, but exert a bacteriostatic effect as long as they are present on the skin.[178,179]

Before the skin preparation of a patient is initiated, the skin should be free of gross contamination (i.e., dirt, soil, or any other debris).[187] The patient's skin is prepared by applying an antiseptic in concentric circles, beginning in the area of the proposed incision. The prepared area should be large enough to extend the incision or create new incisions or drain sites, if necessary.[1,177,187] The application of the skin preparation may need to be modified, depending on the condition of the skin (e.g., burns) or location of the incision site (e.g., face).

There are reports of modifications to the procedure for preoperative skin preparation which include: (1) removing or wiping off the skin preparation antiseptic agent after application, (2) using an antiseptic-impregnated adhesive drape, (3) merely painting the skin with an antiseptic in lieu of the skin preparation procedure described above, or (4) using a "clean" versus a "sterile" surgical skin preparation kit.[188-191] However, none of these modifications has been shown to represent an advantage.

d. Preoperative hand/forearm antisepsis

Members of the surgical team who have direct contact with the sterile operating field or sterile instruments or supplies used in the field wash their hands and forearms by performing a traditional procedure known as scrubbing (or the surgical scrub) immediately before donning sterile gowns and gloves. Ideally, the optimum antiseptic used for the scrub should have a broad spectrum of activity, be fast-acting, and have a persistent effect.[1,192,193] Antiseptic agents commercially available in the United States for this purpose contain alcohol, chlorhexidine, iodine/iodophors, para-chloro-meta-xylenol, or triclosan (Table 6).[176,177,179,194,195] Alcohol is considered the gold standard for surgical hand preparation in several European countries.[196-199] Alcohol-containing products are used less frequently in the United States than in Europe, possibly because of concerns about flammability and skin irritation. Povidone-iodine and chlorhexidine gluconate are the current agents of choice for most U.S. surgical team members.[177] However, when 7.5% povidone-iodine or 4% chlorhexidine gluconate was compared to alcoholic chlorhexidine (60% isopropanol and 0.5% chlorhexidine gluconate in 70% isopropanol), alcoholic chlorhexidine was found to have greater residual antimicrobial activity.[200,201] No agent is ideal for every situation, and a major factor, aside from the efficacy of any product, is its acceptability by operating room personnel after repeated use. Unfortunately, most studies evaluating surgical scrub antiseptics have focused on measuring hand bacterial colony counts. No clinical trials have evaluated the impact of scrub agent choice on SSI risk.[195,202-206]

Factors other than the choice of antiseptic agent influence the effectiveness of the surgical scrub. Scrubbing technique, the duration of the scrub, the condition of the hands, or the techniques used for drying and gloving are examples of such factors. Recent studies suggest that scrubbing for at least 2 minutes is as effective as the traditional 10-minute scrub in reducing hand bacterial colony counts,[207-211] but the optimum duration of scrubbing is not known. The first scrub of the day should include a thorough cleaning underneath fingernails (usually with a brush).[180,194,212] It is not clear that such cleaning is a necessary part of subsequent scrubs during the day. After performing the surgical scrub, hands should be kept up and away from the body (elbows in flexed position) so that water runs from the tips of the fingers toward the elbows. Sterile towels should be used for drying the hands and forearms before the donning of a sterile gown and gloves.[212]

A surgical team member who wears artificial nails may have increased bacterial and fungal colonization of the hands despite performing an adequate hand scrub.[212,213] Hand carriage of gram-negative organisms has been shown to be greater among wearers of artificial nails than among non-wearers.[213] An outbreak of *Serratia marcescens* SSIs in cardiovascular surgery patients was found to be associated with a surgical nurse who wore artificial nails.[214] While the relationship between nail length and SSI risk is unknown, long nails—artificial or natural—may be associated with tears in surgical gloves.[177,180,212] The relationship between the wearing of nail polish or jewelry by surgical team members and SSI risk has not been adequately studied.[194,212,215-217]

e. Management of infected or colonized surgical personnel

Surgical personnel who have active infections or are colonized with certain microorganisms have been linked to outbreaks or clusters of SSIs.[33,34,76,218-237] Thus, it is important that healthcare organizations implement policies to prevent transmission of microorganisms from personnel to patients. These policies should address management of job-related illnesses, provision of postexposure prophylaxis after job-related exposures and, when necessary, exclusion of ill personnel from work or patient contact. While work exclusion policies should be enforceable and include a statement of authority to exclude ill personnel, they should also be designed to encourage personnel to report their illnesses and exposures and not penalize personnel with loss of wages, benefits, or job status.[238]

f. Antimicrobial prophylaxis

Surgical antimicrobial prophylaxis (AMP) refers to a very brief course of an antimicrobial agent initiated just before an operation begins.[239-265] AMP is not an attempt to sterilize tissues, but a critically timed adjunct used to reduce the microbial burden of intraoperative contamination to a level that cannot overwhelm host defenses. AMP does not pertain to prevention of SSI caused by postoperative contamination.[265] Intravenous infusion is the mode of AMP delivery used most often in modern surgical practice.[20,26,242,266-281] Essentially all confirmed AMP indications pertain to elective operations in which skin incisions are closed in the operating room.

TABLE 7
SURGICAL WOUND CLASSIFICATION

Class I/Clean: An uninfected operative wound in which no inflammation is encountered and the respiratory, alimentary, genital, or uninfected urinary tract is not entered. In addition, clean wounds are primarily closed and, if necessary, drained with closed drainage. Operative incisional wounds that follow nonpenetrating (blunt) trauma should be included in this category if they meet the criteria.

Class II/Clean-Contaminated: An operative wound in which the respiratory, alimentary, genital, or urinary tracts are entered under controlled conditions and without unusual contamination. Specifically, operations involving the biliary tract, appendix, vagina, and oropharynx are included in this category, provided no evidence of infection or major break in technique is encountered.

Class III/Contaminated: Open, fresh, accidental wounds. In addition, operations with major breaks in sterile technique (e.g., open cardiac massage) or gross spillage from the gastrointestinal tract, and incisions in which acute, nonpurulent inflammation is encountered are included in this category.

Class IV/Dirty-Infected: Old traumatic wounds with retained devitalized tissue and those that involve existing clinical infection or perforated viscera. This definition suggests that the organisms causing postoperative infection were present in the operative field before the operation.

Garner JS[1] and Simmons BP.[2]

Four principles must be followed to maximize the benefits of AMP:

- Use an AMP agent for all operations or classes of operations in which its use has been shown to reduce SSI rates based on evidence from clinical trials or for those operations after which incisional or organ/space SSI would represent a catastrophe.[266,268,269,282-284]

- Use an AMP agent that is safe, inexpensive, and bactericidal with an in vitro spectrum that covers the most probable intraoperative contaminants for the operation.

- Time the infusion of the initial dose of antimicrobial agent so that a bactericidal concentration of the drug is established in serum and tissues by the time the skin is incised.[285]

- Maintain therapeutic levels of the antimicrobial agent in both serum and tissues throughout the operation and until, at most, a few hours after the incision is closed in the operating room.[179,266-268,282,284,286] Because clotted blood is present in all surgical wounds, therapeutic serum levels of AMP agents are logically important in addition to therapeutic tissue levels. Fibrin-enmeshed bacteria may be resistant to phagocytosis or to contact with antimicrobial agents that diffuse from the wound space.

Table 4 summarizes typical SSI pathogens according to operation type and cites studies that establish AMP efficacy for these operations. A simple way to organize AMP indications is based on using the surgical wound classification scheme shown in Table 7, which employs descriptive case features to *postoperatively* grade the degree of intraoperative microbial contamination. A surgeon makes the decision to use AMP by anticipating *preoperatively* the surgical wound class for a given operation.

AMP is indicated for all operations that entail entry into a hollow viscus under controlled conditions. The most frequent SSI pathogens for such clean-contaminated operations are listed in Table 4. Certain clean-contaminated operations, such as elective colon resection, low anterior resection of the rectum, and abdominoperineal resection of the rectum, also require an additional preoperative protective maneuver called "preparation of the colon," to empty the bowel of its contents and to reduce the levels of live microorganisms.[200,239,256,268,284,287] This maneuver includes the administration of enemas and cathartic agents followed by the oral administration of nonabsorbable antimicrobial agents in divided doses the day before the operation.[200,288,289]

AMP is sometimes indicated for operations that entail incisions through normal tissue and in which no viscus is entered and no inflammation or infection is encountered. Two well-recognized AMP indications for such clean operations are: (1) when any intravascular prosthetic material or a prosthetic joint will be inserted, and (2) for any operation in which an incisional or organ/space SSI would pose catastrophic risk. Examples are all cardiac operations, including cardiac pacemaker placement,[290] vascular operations involving prosthetic arterial graft placement at any site or the revascularization of the lower extremity, and most neurosurgical operations (Table 4). Some have advocated use of AMP during all operations on the breast.[80,242,264]

By definition, AMP is not indicated for an operation classified in Table 7 as contaminated or dirty. In such operations, patients are frequently receiving therapeutic antimicrobial agents perioperatively for established infections.

Cephalosporins are the most thoroughly studied AMP agents.[284] These drugs are effective against many gram-positive and gram-negative microorganisms. They also share the features of demonstrated safety, acceptable pharmacokinetics, and a reasonable cost per dose.[242] In particular, cefazolin is widely used and generally viewed as the AMP agent of first choice for clean operations.[266] If a patient is unable to receive a cephalosporin because of penicillin allergy, an alternative for gram-positive bacterial coverage is either clindamycin or vancomycin.

Cefazolin provides adequate coverage for many clean-contaminated operations,[268,291] but AMP for operations on the distal intestinal tract mandates use of an agent such as cefoxitin (or some other second-generation cephalosporin) that provides anaerobic coverage. If a patient cannot safely receive a cephalosporin because of allergy, a reasonable alternative for gram-negative cover-

TABLE 8
PARAMETERS FOR OPERATING ROOM VENTILATION, AMERICAN
INSTITUTE OF ARCHITECTS, 1996

Temperature	68-73°F, depending on normal ambient temperatures
Relative humidity	30%-60%
Air movement	From "clean to less clean" areas
Air changes	Minimum 15 total air changes per hour
	Minimum 3 air changes of outdoor air per hour

American Institute of Architects.[299]

age is aztreonam. However, an agent such as clindamycin or metronidazole should also be included to ensure anaerobic coverage.

The aminoglycosides are seldom recommended as first choices for AMP, either as single drugs or as components of combination regimens.[242,264] References cited in Table 4 provide many details regarding AMP choices and dosages, antimicrobial spectra and properties, and other practical clinical information.

The routine use of vancomycin in AMP is not recommended for any kind of operation.[242,266,283,292] However, vancomycin may be the AMP agent of choice in certain clinical circumstances, such as when a cluster of MRSA mediastinitis or incisional SSI due to methicillin-resistant coagulase-negative staphylococci has been detected. A threshold has not been scientifically defined that can support the decision to use vancomycin in AMP. The decision should involve consideration of local frequencies of MRSA isolates, SSI rates for particular operations, review of infection prevention practices for compliance, and consultation between surgeons and infectious disease experts. An effective SSI surveillance program must be operational, with careful and timely culturing of SSI isolates to determine species and AMP agent susceptibilities.[80]

Agents most commonly used for AMP (i.e., cephalosporins) exhibit time-dependent bactericidal action. The therapeutic effects of such agents are probably maximized when their levels continuously exceed a threshold value best approximated by the minimal bactericidal concentration value observed for the target pathogens in vitro. When the duration of an operation is expected to exceed the time in which therapeutic levels of the AMP agent can be maintained, additional AMP agent should be infused. That time point for cefazolin is estimated as 3 to 4 hours. In general, the timing of a second (or third, etc.) dose of any AMP drug is estimated from three parameters: tissue levels achieved in normal patients by a standard therapeutic dose, the approximate serum half-life of the drug, and awareness of approximate MIC_{90} values for anticipated SSI pathogens. References in Table 6 should be consulted for these details and important properties of antimicrobial agents used for AMP in various specialties.

Basic "rules of thumb" guide decisions about AMP dose sizes and timing. For example, it is believed that a full

therapeutic dose of cefazolin (1-2 g) should be given to adult patients no more than 30 minutes before the skin is incised.[242,285] There are a few exceptions to this basic guide. With respect to dosing, it has been demonstrated that larger doses of AMP agents are necessary to achieve optimum effect in morbidly obese patients.[293] With respect to timing, an exception occurs for patients undergoing cesarean section in whom AMP is indicated: the initial dose is administered immediately after the umbilical cord is clamped.[266,272,273] If vancomycin is used, an infusion period of approximately 1 hour is required for a typical dose. Clearly, the concept of "on-call" infusion of AMP is flawed simply because delays in transport or schedule changes can mean that suboptimal tissue and serum levels may be present when the operation starts.[242,294] Simple protocols of AMP timing and oversight responsibility should be locally designed to be practical and effective.

3. Operative characteristics: Intraoperative issues
a. Operating room environment
(1) Ventilation

Operating room air may contain microbial-laden dust, lint, skin squames, or respiratory droplets. The microbial level in operating room air is directly proportional to the number of people moving about in the room.[295] Therefore, efforts should be made to minimize personnel traffic during operations. Outbreaks of SSIs caused by group A beta-hemolytic streptococci have been traced to airborne transmission of the organism from colonized operating room personnel to patients.[233,237,296,297] In these outbreaks, the strain causing the outbreak was recovered from the air in the operating room.[237,296] It has been demonstrated that exercising and changing of clothing can lead to airborne dissemination of group A streptococci from vaginal or rectal carriage.[233,234,237,297]

Operating rooms should be maintained at positive pressure with respect to corridors and adjacent areas.[298] Positive pressure prevents airflow from less clean areas into more clean areas. All ventilation or air conditioning systems in hospitals, including those in operating rooms, should have two filter beds in series, with the efficiency of the first filter bed being ≥30% and that of the second filter bed being ≥90%.[299] Conventional operating room ventilation systems produce a minimum of about 15 air changes of filtered air per hour, three (20%) of which must be fresh air.[299,300] Air should be introduced at the ceiling and exhausted near the floor.[300,301] Detailed ventilation parameters for operating rooms have been published by the American Institute of Architects in collaboration with the U.S. Department of Health and Human Services (Table 8).[299]

Laminar airflow and use of UV radiation have been suggested as additional measures to reduce SSI risk for certain operations. Laminar airflow is designed to move particle-free air (called "ultraclean air") over the aseptic operating field at a uniform velocity (0.3 to 0.5 μm/sec), sweeping away particles in its path. Laminar airflow can be directed vertically or horizontally, and recirculated air is usually passed through a high efficiency particulate air (HEPA) filter.[302,303] HEPA filters remove particles $\geq$0.3μm in diameter with an efficiency of 99.97%.[64,300,302,304] Most of the studies examining the efficacy of ultraclean air involve only orthopedic operations.[298,305-311] Charnley and Eftaknan studied vertical laminar airflow systems and exhaust-ventilated clothing and found that their use decreased the SSI rate from 9% to 1%.[305] However, other variables (i.e., surgeon experience and surgical technique) changed at the same time as the type of ventilation, which may have confounded the associations. In a multicenter study examining 8,000 total hip and knee replacements, Lidwell et al. compared the effects of ultraclean air alone, antimicrobial prophylaxis alone, and ultraclean air in combination with antimicrobial prophylaxis on the rate of deep SSIs.[307] The SSI rate following operations in which ultraclean air alone was used decreased from 3.4% to 1.6%, whereas the rate for those who received only antimicrobial prophylaxis decreased from 3.4% to 0.8%. When both interventions were used in combination, the SSI rate decreased from 3.4% to 0.7%. These findings suggest that both ultraclean air and antimicrobial prophylaxis can reduce the incidence of SSI following orthopedic implant operations, but antimicrobial prophylaxis is more beneficial than ultraclean air. Intraoperative UV radiation has not been shown to decrease overall SSI risk.[94,312]

(2) Environmental surfaces

Environmental surfaces in U.S. operating rooms (e.g., tables, floors, walls, ceilings, lights) are rarely implicated as the sources of pathogens important in the development of SSIs. Nevertheless, it is important to perform routine cleaning of these surfaces to reestablish a clean environment after each operation.[180,212,300,302] There are no data to support routine disinfecting of environmental surfaces or equipment between operations in the absence of contamination or visible soiling. When visible soiling of surfaces or equipment occurs during an operation, an Environmental Protection Agency (EPA)-approved hospital disinfectant should be used to decontaminate the affected areas before the next operation.[180,212,300-302,313-315] This is in keeping with the Occupational Safety and Health Administration (OSHA) requirement that all equipment and environmental surfaces be cleaned and decontaminated after contact with blood or other potentially infectious materials.[315] Wet-vacuuming of the floor with an EPA-approved hospital disinfectant is performed routinely after the last operation of the day or night. Care should be taken to ensure that medical equipment left in the operating room be covered so that solutions used during cleaning and disinfecting do not contact sterile devices or equipment.[316] There are no data to support special cleaning procedures or closing of an operating room after a contaminated or dirty operation has been performed.[300,301]

Tacky mats placed outside the entrance to an operating room/suite have not been shown to reduce the number of organisms on shoes or stretcher wheels, nor do they reduce the risk of SSI.[1,179,295,301]

(3) Microbiologic sampling

Because there are no standardized parameters by which to compare microbial levels obtained from cultures

of ambient air or environmental surfaces in the operating room, routine microbiologic sampling cannot be justified. Such environmental sampling should only be performed as part of an epidemiologic investigation.

(4) Conventional sterilization of surgical instruments

Inadequate sterilization of surgical instruments has resulted in SSI outbreaks.[302,317,318] Surgical instruments can be sterilized by steam under pressure, dry heat, ethylene oxide, or other approved methods. The importance of routinely monitoring the quality of sterilization procedures has been established.[1,180,212,299] Microbial monitoring of steam autoclave performance is necessary and can be accomplished by use of a biological indicator.[212,314,319] Detailed recommendations for sterilization of surgical instruments have been published.[212,314,320,321]

(5) Flash sterilization of surgical instruments

The Association for the Advancement of Medical Instrumentation defines flash sterilization as "the process designated for the steam sterilization of patient care items for immediate use."[321] During any operation, the need for emergency sterilization of equipment may arise (e.g., to reprocess an inadvertently dropped instrument). However, flash sterilization is not intended to be used for either reasons of convenience or as an alternative to purchasing additional instrument sets or to save time. Also, flash sterilization is not recommended for implantable devices(*) because of the potential for serious infections.[314,320,321]

Flash sterilization is not recommended as a routine sterilization method because of the lack of timely biologic indicators to monitor performance, absence of protective packaging following sterilization, possibility for contamination of processed items during transportation to operating rooms, and use of minimal sterilization cycle parameters (i.e., time, temperature, pressure).[319] To address some of these concerns, many hospitals have placed equipment for flash sterilization in close proximity to operating rooms and new biologic indicators that provide results in 1 to 3 hours are now available for flash-sterilized items.[322-325] Nevertheless, flash sterilization should be restricted to its intended purpose until studies are performed that can demonstrate comparability with conventional sterilization methods regarding risk of SSI. Sterilization cycle parameters for flash sterilization are shown in Table 9.

b. Surgical attire and drapes

In this section the term *surgical attire* refers to scrub suits, caps/hoods, shoe covers, masks, gloves, and gowns. Although experimental data show that live microorganisms are shed from hair, exposed skin, and mucous membranes of operating room personnel,[75,181,326-330] few controlled clinical studies have evaluated the relationship between the use of surgical attire and SSI risk. Nevertheless, the use of barriers seems prudent to minimize a patient's exposure to the skin, mucous membranes, or hair of surgical team mem-

---

* According to the FDA, an implantable device is a "device that is placed into a surgically or naturally formed cavity of the human body if it is intended to remain there for a period of 30 days or more."[321]

TABLE 9
PARAMETERS FOR FLASH STERILIZATION CYCLES, ASSOCIATION FOR THE ADVANCEMENT OF MEDICAL INSTRUMENTATION

Gravity-Displacement	Minimum Exposure Time and Temperature	
	Nonporous items	3 min at 132°C (270°F)
	Nonporous and porous items	10 min at 132°C (270°F)
Prevacuum	**Minimum Exposure Time and Temperature**	
	Nonporous items	3 min at 132°C (270°F)
	Nonporous and porous items	4 min at 132°C (270°F)

Association for the Advancement of Medical Instrumentation.[321]

bers, as well as to protect surgical team members from exposure to blood and bloodborne pathogens (e.g., human immunodeficiency virus and hepatitis viruses).

(1) Scrub suits

Surgical team members often wear a uniform called a "scrub suit" that consists of pants and a shirt. Policies for laundering, wearing, covering, and changing scrub suits vary greatly. Some policies restrict the laundering of scrub suits to the facility, while other facilities have policies that allow laundering by employees. There are no well-controlled studies evaluating scrub suit laundering as an SSI risk factor.[331] Some facilities have policies that restrict the wearing of scrub suits to the operating suite, while other facilities allow the wearing of cover gowns over scrub suits when personnel leave the suite. The Association of Operating Room Nurses recommends that scrub suits be changed after they become visibly soiled and that they be laundered only in an approved and monitored laundry facility.[212] Additionally, OSHA regulations require that "if a garment(s) is penetrated by blood or other potentially infectious materials, the garment(s) shall be removed immediately or as soon as feasible."[315]

(2) Masks

The wearing of surgical masks during operations to prevent potential microbial contamination of incisions is a longstanding surgical tradition. However, some studies have raised questions about the efficacy and cost-benefit of surgical masks in reducing SSI risk.[328,332-338] Nevertheless, wearing a mask can be beneficial since it protects the wearer's nose and mouth from inadvertent exposures (i.e., splashes) to blood and other body fluids. OSHA regulations require that masks in combination with protective eyewear, such as goggles or glasses with solid shields, or chin-length face shields be worn whenever splashes, spray, spatter, or droplets of blood or other potentially infectious material may be generated and eye, nose, or mouth contamination can be reasonably anticipated.[315] In addition, a respirator certified by the National Institute for Occupational Safety and Health with protection factor N95 or higher is required when the patient has or is suspected of having infectious tuberculosis.[339]

(3) Surgical caps/hoods and shoe covers

Surgical caps/hoods are inexpensive and reduce contamination of the surgical field by organisms shed from the hair and scalp. SSI outbreaks have occasionally been traced to organisms isolated from the hair or scalp (*S. aureus* and group A *Streptococcus*),[75,76] even when caps were worn by personnel during the operation and in the operating suites.

The use of shoe covers has never been shown to decrease SSI risk or to decrease bacteria counts on the operating room floor.[340,341] Shoe covers may, however, protect surgical team members from exposure to blood and other body fluids during an operation. OSHA regulations require that surgical caps or hoods and shoe covers or boots be worn in situations when gross contamination can reasonably be anticipated (e.g., orthopedic operations, penetrating trauma cases).[315]

(4) Sterile gloves

Sterile gloves are put on after donning sterile gowns. A strong theoretical rationale supports the wearing of sterile gloves by all scrubbed members of the surgical team. Sterile gloves are worn to minimize transmission of microorganisms from the hands of team members to patients and to prevent contamination of team members' hands with patients' blood and body fluids. If the integrity of a glove is compromised (e.g., punctured), it should be changed as promptly as safety permits.[315,342,343] Wearing two pairs of gloves (double-gloving) has been shown to reduce hand contact with patients' blood and body fluids when compared to wearing only a single pair.[344,345]

(5) Gowns and drapes

Sterile surgical gowns and drapes are used to create a barrier between the surgical field and potential sources of bacteria. Gowns are worn by all scrubbed surgical team members and drapes are placed over the patient. There are limited data that can be used to understand the relationship of gown or drape characteristics with SSI risk. The wide variation in the products and study designs make interpretation of the literature difficult.[329,346-350]

Gowns and drapes are classified as disposable (single use) or reusable (multiple use). Regardless of the material used to manufacture gowns and drapes, these items should be impermeable to liquids and viruses.[351,352] In general, only gowns reinforced with films, coatings, or membranes appear to meet standards developed by the American Society for Testing and Materials.[351-353] However, such "liquid-proof" gowns may be uncomfortable because they also inhibit heat loss and the evaporation of sweat from the wearer's body. These factors should be considered when selecting gowns.[353,354] A discussion of the role of gowns and drapes in preventing the transmission of bloodborne pathogens is beyond the scope of this document.[355]

c. Asepsis and surgical technique

(1) Asepsis

Rigorous adherence to the principles of asepsis by all scrubbed personnel is the foundation of surgical site infection prevention. Others who work in close proximity to the sterile surgical field, such as anesthesia personnel who are separated from the field only by a drape barrier, also must abide by these principles. SSIs have occurred in which anesthesia personnel were implicated as the source of the pathogen.[34,231,234,356-358] Anesthesiologists and nurse anesthetists perform a variety of invasive procedures such as placement of intravascular devices and endotracheal tubes, and administration of intravenous drugs and solutions. Lack of adherence to the principles of asepsis during such procedures,[359] including use of common syringes[360,361] and contaminated infusion pumps,[359,362-364] and the assembly of equipment and solutions in advance of procedures,[316,360] have been associated with outbreaks of postoperative infections, including SSI. Recommendations for infection control practices in anesthesiology have been published.[212,365-367]

(2) Surgical technique

Excellent surgical technique is widely believed to reduce the risk of SSI.[26,49,179,180,368,369] Such techniques include maintaining effective hemostasis while preserving adequate blood supply, preventing hypothermia, gently handling tissues, avoiding inadvertent entries into a hollow viscus, removing devitalized (e.g., necrotic or charred) tissues, using drains and suture material appropriately, eradicating dead space, and appropriately managing the postoperative incision.

Any foreign body, including suture material, a prosthesis, or drain, may promote inflammation at the surgical site[94] and may increase the probability of SSI after otherwise benign levels of tissue contamination. Extensive research compares different types of suture material and their presumed relationships to SSI risk.[370-379] In general, monofilament sutures appear to have the lowest infection-promoting effects.[3,94,179,180]

A discussion of appropriate surgical drain use and details of drain placement exceed the scope of this document, but general points should be briefly noted. Drains placed through an operative incision increase incisional SSI risk.[380] Many authorities suggest placing drains through a separate incision distant from the operative incision.[283,381] It appears that SSI risk also decreases when closed suction drains are used rather than open drains.[174] Closed suction drains can effectively evacuate postoperative hematomas or seromas, but timing of drain removal is important. Bacterial colonization of initially sterile drain tracts increases with the duration of time the drain is left in place.[382]

Hypothermia in surgical patients, defined as a core body temperature below 36°C, may result from general anesthesia, exposure to cold, or intentional cooling such as

is done to protect the myocardium and central nervous system during cardiac operations.[302,383,384] In one study of patients undergoing colorectal operations, hypothermia was associated with an increased SSI risk.[385] Mild hypothermia appears to increase incisional SSI risk by causing vasoconstriction, decreased delivery of oxygen to the wound space, and subsequent impairment of function of phagocytic leukocytes (i.e., neutrophils).[386-390] In animal models, supplemental oxygen administration has been shown to reverse the dysfunction of phagocytes in fresh incisions.[391] In recent human experiments, controlled local heating of incisions with an electrically powered bandage has been shown to improve tissue oxygenation.[392] Randomized clinical trials are needed to establish that measures which improve wound space oxygenation can reduce SSI risk.

4. Operative Characteristics: Postoperative Issues

a. Incision care

The type of postoperative incision care is determined by whether the incision is closed primarily (i.e., the skin edges are re-approximated at the end of the operation), left open to be closed later, or left open to heal by second intention. When a surgical incision is closed primarily, as most are, the incision is usually covered with a sterile dressing for 24 to 48 hours.[393,394] Beyond 48 hours, it is unclear whether an incision must be covered by a dressing or whether showering or bathing is detrimental to healing. When a surgical incision is left open at the skin level for a few days before it is closed (delayed primary closure), a surgeon has determined that it is likely to be contaminated or that the patient's condition prevents primary closure (e.g., edema at the site). When such is the case, the incision is packed with a sterile dressing. When a surgical incision is left open to heal by second intention, it is also packed with sterile moist gauze and covered with a sterile dressing. The American College of Surgeons, CDC, and others have recommended using sterile gloves and equipment (sterile technique) when changing dressings on any type of surgical incision.[180,395-397]

b. Discharge planning

In current practice, many patients are discharged very soon after their operation, before surgical incisions have fully healed.[398] The lack of optimum protocols for home incision care dictates that much of what is done at home by the patient, family, or home care agency practitioners must be individualized. The intent of discharge planning is to maintain integrity of the healing incision, educate the patient about the signs and symptoms of infection, and advise the patient about whom to contact to report any problems.

F. SSI SURVEILLANCE

Surveillance of SSI with feedback of appropriate data to surgeons has been shown to be an important component of strategies to reduce SSI risk.[16,399,400] A successful surveillance program includes the use of epidemiologically sound infection definitions (Tables 1 and 2) and effective

TABLE 10
PHYSICAL STATUS CLASSIFICATION, AMERICAN SOCIETY OF ANESTHESIOLOGISTS*

Code	Patient's Preoperative Physical Status
1	Normally healthy patient
2	Patient with mild systemic disease
3	Patient with severe systemic disease that is not incapacitating
4	Patient with an incapacitating systemic disease that is a constant threat to life
5	Moribund patient who is not expected to survive for 24 hours with or without operation

* Reference 406.
Note: The above is the version of the ASA Physical Status Classification System that was current at the time of development of, and still is used in, the NNIS Risk Index. Meanwhile, the American Society of Anesthesiologists has revised their classification system; the most recent version is available at http://www.asahq.org/profinfo/physicalstatus.html.

surveillance methods, stratification of SSI rates according to risk factors associated with SSI development, and data feedback.[25]

1. SSI Risk Stratification
a. Concepts

Three categories of variables have proven to be reliable predictors of SSI risk: (1) those that estimate the intrinsic degree of microbial contamination of the surgical site, (2) those that measure the duration of an operation, and (3) those that serve as markers for host susceptibility.[25] A widely accepted scheme for classifying the degree of intrinsic microbial contamination of a surgical site was developed by the 1964 NAS/NRC Cooperative Research Study and modified in 1982 by CDC for use in SSI surveillance (Table 7).[2,94] In this scheme, a member of the surgical team classifies the patient's wound at the completion of the operation. Because of its ease of use and wide availability, the surgical wound classification has been used to predict SSI risk.[16,94,126,401-405] Some researchers have suggested that surgeons compare clean wound SSI rates with those of other surgeons.[16,399] However, two CDC efforts—the SENIC Project and the NNIS system—incorporated other predictor variables into SSI risk indices. These showed that even within the category of clean wounds, the SSI risk varied by risk category from 1.1% to 15.8% (SENIC) and from 1.0% to 5.4% (NNIS).[125,126] In addition, sometimes an incision is incorrectly classified by a surgical team member or not classified at all, calling into question the reliability of the classification. Therefore, reporting SSI rates stratified by wound class alone is not recommended.

Data on 10 variables collected in the SENIC Project were analyzed by using logistic regression modeling to develop a simple additive SSI risk index.[125] Four of these were found to be independently associated with SSI risk: (1) an abdominal operation, (2) an operation lasting >2 hours, (3) a surgical site with a wound classification of either contaminated or dirty/infected, and (4) an operation performed on a patient having ≥3 discharge diagnoses. Each of these equally weighted factors contributes a point when present, such that the risk index values range from 0 to 4. By using these factors, the SENIC index predicted SSI risk twice as well as the traditional wound classification scheme alone.

The NNIS risk index is operation-specific and applied to prospectively collected surveillance data. The index values range from 0 to 3 points and are defined by three independent and equally weighted variables. One point is scored for each of the following when present: (1) American Society of Anesthesiologists (ASA) Physical Status Classification of >2 (Table 10), (2) either contaminated or dirty/infected wound classification (Table 7), and (3) length of operation >T hours, where T is the approximate 75th percentile of the duration of the specific operation being performed.[126] The ASA class replaced discharge diagnoses of the SENIC risk index as a surrogate for the patient's underlying severity of illness (host susceptibility)[406,407] and has the advantage of being readily available in the chart during the patient's hospital stay. Unlike SENIC's constant 2-hour cut-point for duration of operation, the operation-specific cut-points used in the NNIS risk index increase its discriminatory power compared to the SENIC index.[126]

b. Issues

Adjustment for variables known to confound rate estimates is critical if valid comparisons of SSI rates are to be made between surgeons or hospitals.[408] Risk stratification, as described above, has proven useful for this purpose, but relies on the ability of surveillance personnel to find and record data consistently and correctly. For the three variables used in the NNIS risk index, only one study has focused on how accurately any of them are recorded. Cardo et al. found that surgical team members' accuracy in assessing wound classification for general and trauma surgery was 88% (95% CI: 82%-94%).[409] However, there are sufficient ambiguities in the wound class definitions themselves to warrant concern about the reproducibility of Cardo's results. The accuracy of recording the duration of operation (i.e., time from skin incision to skin closure) and the ASA class has not been studied. In an unpublished report from the NNIS system, there was evidence that overreporting of high ASA class existed in some hospitals. Further validation of the reliability of the recorded risk index variables is needed.

Additionally, the NNIS risk index does not adequately discriminate the SSI risk for all types of operations.[27,410] It seems likely that a combination of risk factors specific to patients undergoing an operation will be more predictive. A few studies have been performed to develop procedure-specific risk indices[218,411-414] and research in this area continues within CDC's NNIS system.

2. SSI Surveillance Methods

SSI surveillance methods used in both the SENIC Project and the NNIS system were designed for monitoring inpatients at acute-care hospitals. Over the past decade, the shift from inpatient to outpatient surgical care (also called ambulatory or day surgery) has been dramatic. It has been estimated that 75% of all operations in the United States will be performed in outpatient settings by the year 2000.[4] While it may be appropriate to use common definitions of SSI for inpatients and outpatients,[415] the types of operations monitored, the risk factors assessed, and the case-finding methods used may differ. New predictor variables may emerge from analyses of SSIs among outpatient surgery patients, which may lead to different ways of estimating SSI risk in this population.

The choice of which operations to monitor should be made jointly by surgeons and infection control personnel. Most hospitals do not have the resources to monitor all surgical patients all the time, nor is it likely that the same intensity of surveillance is necessary for certain low-risk procedures. Instead, hospitals should target surveillance efforts toward high-risk procedures.[416]

a. Inpatient SSI surveillance

Two methods, alone or together, have been used to identify inpatients with SSIs: (1) direct observation of the surgical site by the surgeon, trained nurse surveyor, or infection control personnel[16,97,399,402,409,417-420] and (2) indirect detection by infection control personnel through review of laboratory reports, patient records, and discussions with primary care providers.[15,84,399,402,404,409,418,421-427] The surgical literature suggests that direct observation of surgical sites is the most accurate method to detect SSIs, although sensitivity data are lacking.[16,399,402,417,418] Much of the SSI data reported in the infection control literature has been generated by indirect case-finding methods,[125,126,422,425,426,428-430] but some studies of direct methods also have been conducted.[97,409] Some studies use both methods of detection.[84,409,424,427,431] A study that focused solely on the sensitivity and specificity of SSIs detected by indirect methods found a sensitivity of 83.8% (95% CI: 75.7%-91.9%) and a specificity of 99.8% (95% CI: 99%-100%).[409] Another study showed that chart review triggered by a computer-generated report of antibiotic orders for post-cesarean section patients had a sensitivity of 89% for detecting endometritis.[432]

Indirect SSI detection can readily be performed by infection control personnel during surveillance rounds. The work includes gathering demographic, infection, surgical, and laboratory data on patients who have undergone operations of interest.[433] These data can be obtained from patients' medical records, including microbiology, histopathology, laboratory, and pharmacy data; radiology reports; and records from the operating room. Additionally, inpatient admissions, emergency room, and clinic visit records are sources of data for those postdischarge surgical patients who are readmitted or seek follow-up care.

The optimum frequency of SSI case-finding by either method is unknown and varies from daily to ≤3 times per week, continuing until the patient is discharged from the hospital. Because duration of hospitalization is often very short, postdischarge SSI surveillance has become increasingly important to obtain accurate SSI rates (refer to "Postdischarge SSI Surveillance" section).

To calculate meaningful SSI rates, data must be collected on all patients undergoing the operations of interest (i.e., the population at risk). Because one of its purposes is to develop strategies for risk stratification, the NNIS system collects the following data on all surgical patients surveyed: operation date; NNIS operative procedure category;[434] surgeon identifier; patient identifier; age and sex; duration of operation; wound class; use of general anesthesia; ASA class; emergency; trauma; multiple procedures; endoscopic approach; and discharge date.[433] With the exception of discharge date, these data can be obtained manually from operating room logs or be electronically downloaded into surveillance software, thereby substantially reducing manual transcription and data entry errors.[433] Depending on the needs for risk-stratified SSI rates by personnel in infection control, surgery, and quality assurance, not all data elements may be pertinent for every type of operation. At minimum, however, variables found to be predictive of increased SSI risk should be collected (refer to "SSI Risk Stratification" section).

b. Postdischarge SSI surveillance

Between 12% and 84% of SSIs are detected after patients are discharged from the hospital.[98,337,402,428,435-454] At least two studies have shown that most SSIs become evident within 21 days after operation.[446,447] Since the length of postoperative hospitalization continues to decrease, many SSIs may not be detected for several weeks after discharge and may not require readmission to the operating hospital. Dependence solely on inpatient case-finding will result in underestimates of SSI rates for some operations (e.g., coronary artery bypass graft) (CDC/NNIS system, unpublished data, 1998). Any comparison of SSI rates must take into account whether case-finding included SSIs detected after discharge. For comparisons to be valid, even in the same institution over time, the postdischarge surveillance methods must be the same.

Postdischarge surveillance methods have been used with varying degrees of success for different procedures and among hospitals and include (1) direct examination of patients' wounds during follow-up visits to either surgery clinics or physicians' offices,[150,399,402,404,430,436,440,441,447,452,455] (2) review of medical records of surgery clinic patients,[404,430,439] (3) patient surveys by mail or telephone,[435,437,438,441,442,444,445,448,449,455-457] or (4) surgeon surveys by mail or telephone.[98,428,430,437-439,443,444,446,448,450,451,455] One study found that patients have difficulty assessing their own wounds for infection (52% specificity, 26% positive predictive value),[458] suggesting that data obtained by patient questionnaire may inaccurately represent actual SSI rates.

Recently, Sands et al. performed a computerized search of three databases to determine which best identified SSIs: ambulatory encounter records for diagnostic, testing, and treatment codes; pharmacy records for specific antimicrobial prescriptions; and administrative records for rehospitalizations and emergency room visits.[446] This study found that pharmacy records indicating a patient had received antimicrobial agents commonly used to treat soft tissue infections had the highest sensitivity (50%) and positive predictive value (19%), although even this approach alone was not very effective.

As integrated health information systems expand, tracking surgical patients through the entire course of care may become more feasible, practical, and effective. At this time, no consensus exists on which postdischarge surveillance methods are the most sensitive, specific, and practical. Methods chosen will necessarily reflect the hospital's unique mix of operations, personnel resources, and data needs.

c. Outpatient SSI surveillance

Both direct and indirect methods have been used to detect SSIs that complicate outpatient operations. One 8-year study of operations for hernia and varicose veins used home visits by district health nurses combined with a survey completed by the surgeon at the patient's 2-week postoperative clinic visit to identify SSIs.[459] While ascertainment was essentially 100%, this method is impractical for widespread implementation. High response rates have been obtained from questionnaires mailed to surgeons (72%->90%).[443,444,446,455,459-461] Response rates from telephone questionnaires administered to patients were more variable (38%,[444] 81%,[457] and 85%[455]), and response rates from questionnaires mailed to patients were quite low (15%[455] and 33%[446]). At this time, no single detection method can be recommended. Available resources and data needs determine which method(s) should be used and which operations should be monitored. Regardless of which detection method is used, it is recommended that the CDC NNIS definitions of SSI (Tables 1 and 2) be used without modification in the outpatient setting.

G. GUIDELINE EVALUATION PROCESS

The value of the HICPAC guidelines is determined by those who use them. To help assess that value, HICPAC is developing an evaluation tool to learn how guidelines meet user expectations, and how and when these guidelines are disseminated and implemented.

II. RECOMMENDATIONS FOR PREVENTION OF SURGICAL SITE INFECTION

A. RATIONALE

The Guideline for Prevention of Surgical Site Infection, 1999, provides recommendations concerning reduction of surgical site infection risk. Each recommendation is categorized on the basis of existing scientific data, theoretical rationale, and applicability. However, the previous CDC system for categorizing recommendations has been modified slightly.

Category I recommendations, including IA and IB, are those recommendations that are viewed as effective by HICPAC and experts in the fields of surgery, infectious diseases, and infection control. Both Category IA and IB recommendations are applicable for, and should be adopted by, all healthcare facilities; IA and IB recommendations differ only in the strength of the supporting scientific evidence.

Category II recommendations are supported by less scientific data than Category I recommendations; such recommendations may be appropriate for addressing specific nosocomial problems or specific patient populations.

No recommendation is offered for some practices, either because there is a lack of consensus regarding their efficacy or because the available scientific evidence is insufficient to support their adoption. For such unresolved issues, practitioners should use judgement to determine a policy regarding these practices within their organization. Recommendations that are based on federal regulation are denoted with an asterisk.

B. RANKINGS

Category IA. Strongly recommended for implementation and supported by well-designed experimental, clinical, or epidemiological studies.

Category IB. Strongly recommended for implementation and supported by some experimental, clinical, or epidemiological studies and strong theoretical rationale.

Category II. Suggested for implementation and supported by suggestive clinical or epidemiological studies or theoretical rationale.

No recommendation; unresolved issue. Practices for which insufficient evidence or no consensus regarding efficacy exists.

Practices required by federal regulation are denoted with an asterisk (*).

C. RECOMMENDATIONS

1. Preoperative

a. Preparation of the patient

1. Whenever possible, identify and treat all infections remote to the surgical site before elective operation and postpone elective operations on patients with remote site infections until the infection has resolved. *Category IA*

2. Do not remove hair preoperatively unless the hair at or around the incision site will interfere with the operation. *Category IA*

3. If hair is removed, remove immediately before the operation, preferably with electric clippers. *Category IA*

4. Adequately control serum blood glucose levels in all diabetic patients and particularly avoid hyperglycemia perioperatively. *Category IB*

5. Encourage tobacco cessation. At minimum, instruct patients to abstain for at least 30 days before elective operation from smoking cigarettes, cigars, pipes, or any other form of tobacco consumption (e.g., chewing/dipping). *Category IB*

6. Do not withhold necessary blood products from surgical patients as a means to prevent SSI. *Category IB*

7. Require patients to shower or bathe with an antiseptic agent on at least the night before the operative day. *Category IB*

8. Thoroughly wash and clean at and around the incision site to remove gross contamination before performing antiseptic skin preparation. *Category IB*

9. Use an appropriate antiseptic agent for skin preparation (Table 6). *Category IB*

10. Apply preoperative antiseptic skin preparation in concentric circles moving toward the periphery. The prepared area must be large enough to extend the incision or create new incisions or drain sites, if necessary. *Category II*

11. Keep preoperative hospital stay as short as possible while allowing for adequate preoperative preparation of the patient. *Category II*

12. No recommendation to taper or discontinue systemic steroid use (when medically permissible) before elective operation. *Unresolved issue*

13. No recommendation to enhance nutritional support for surgical patients solely as a means to prevent SSI. *Unresolved issue*

14. No recommendation to preoperatively apply mupirocin to nares to prevent SSI. *Unresolved issue*

15. No recommendation to provide measures that enhance wound space oxygenation to prevent SSI. *Unresolved issue*

b. Hand/forearm antisepsis for surgical team members

1. Keep nails short and do not wear artificial nails. *Category IB*

2. Perform a preoperative surgical scrub for at least 2 to 5 minutes using an appropriate antiseptic (Table 6). Scrub the hands and forearms up to the elbows. *Category IB*

3. After performing the surgical scrub, keep hands up and away from the body (elbows in flexed position) so that water runs from the tips of the fingers toward the elbows. Dry hands with a sterile towel and don a sterile gown and gloves. *Category IB*

4. Clean underneath each fingernail prior to performing the first surgical scrub of the day. *Category II*

5. Do not wear hand or arm jewelry. *Category II*

6. No recommendation on wearing nail polish. *Unresolved Issue*

c. Management of infected or colonized surgical personnel

1. Educate and encourage surgical personnel who have signs and symptoms of a transmissible infectious illness to report conditions promptly to their supervisory and occupational health service personnel. *Category IB*

2. Develop well-defined policies concerning patient-care responsibilities when personnel have potentially transmissible infectious conditions. These policies should govern (a) personnel responsibility in using the health service and reporting illness, (b) work restrictions, and (c) clearance to resume work after an illness that required work restriction. The policies also should identify persons who have the authority to remove personnel from duty. *Category IB*

3. Obtain appropriate cultures from, and exclude from duty, surgical personnel who have draining skin lesions until infection has been ruled out or personnel have received adequate therapy and infection has resolved. *Category IB*

4. Do not routinely exclude surgical personnel who are colonized with organisms such as *S. aureus* (nose, hands, or other body site) or group A *Streptococcus,* unless such personnel have been linked epidemiologically to dissemination of the organism in the healthcare setting. *Category IB*

d. Antimicrobial prophylaxis

1. Administer a prophylactic antimicrobial agent only when indicated, and select it based on its efficacy against the most common pathogens causing SSI for a specific operation (Table 4) and published recommendations.[266,268,269,282-284] *Category IA*

2. Administer by the intravenous route the initial dose of prophylactic antimicrobial agent, timed such that a bactericidal concentration of the drug is established in serum and tissues when the incision is made. Maintain therapeutic levels of the agent in serum and tissues throughout the operation and until, at most, a few hours after the incision is closed in the operating room. *Category IA*

3. Before elective colorectal operations in addition to d2 above, mechanically prepare the colon by use of enemas and cathartic agents. Administer nonabsorbable oral antimicrobial agents in divided doses on the day before the operation. *Category IA*

4. For high-risk cesarean section, administer the prophylactic antimicrobial agent immediately after the umbilical cord is clamped. *Category IA*

5. Do not routinely use vancomycin for antimicrobial prophylaxis. *Category IB*

2. Intraoperative

a. Ventilation

1. Maintain positive-pressure ventilation in the operating room with respect to the corridors and adjacent areas. *Category IB*

2. Maintain a minimum of 15 air changes per hour, of which at least 3 should be fresh air. *Category IB*

3. Filter all air, recirculated and fresh, through the appropriate filters per the American Institute of Architects' recommendations.[299] *Category IB*

4. Introduce all air at the ceiling, and exhaust near the floor. *Category IB*

5. Do not use UV radiation in the operating room to prevent SSI. *Category IB*

6. Keep operating room doors closed except as needed for passage of equipment, personnel, and the patient. *Category IB*

7. Consider performing orthopedic implant operations in operating rooms supplied with ultraclean air. *Category II*

8. Limit the number of personnel entering the operating room to necessary personnel. *Category II*

b. Cleaning and disinfection of environmental surfaces

1. When visible soiling or contamination with blood or other body fluids of surfaces or equipment occurs during an operation, use an EPA-approved hospital disinfectant to clean the affected areas before the next operation. *Category IB**

2. Do not perform special cleaning or closing of operating rooms after contaminated or dirty operations. *Category IB*

3. Do not use tacky mats at the entrance to the operating room suite or individual operating rooms for infection control. *Category IB*

4. Wet vacuum the operating room floor after the last operation of the day or night with an EPA-approved hospital disinfectant. *Category II*

5. No recommendation on disinfecting environmental surfaces or equipment used in operating rooms between operations in the absence of visible soiling. *Unresolved issue*

c. Microbiologic sampling

1. Do not perform routine environmental sampling of the operating room. Perform microbiologic sampling of operating room environmental surfaces or air only as part of an epidemiologic investigation. *Category IB*

d. Sterilization of surgical instruments

1. Sterilize all surgical instruments according to published guidelines.[212,299,314,321] *Category IB*

2. Perform flash sterilization only for patient care items that will be used immediately (e.g., to reprocess an inadvertently dropped instrument). Do not use flash sterilization for reasons of convenience, as an alternative to purchasing additional instrument sets, or to save time. *Category IB*

e. Surgical attire and drapes

1. Wear a surgical mask that fully covers the mouth and nose when entering the operating room if an operation is about to begin or already under way, or if sterile instruments are exposed. Wear the mask throughout the operation. *Category IB**

2. Wear a cap or hood to fully cover hair on the head and face when entering the operating room. *Category IB**

3. Do not wear shoe covers for the prevention of SSI. *Category IB**

4. Wear sterile gloves if a scrubbed surgical team member. Put on gloves after donning a sterile gown. *Category IB**

5. Use surgical gowns and drapes that are effective barriers when wet (i.e., materials that resist liquid penetration). *Category IB*

6. Change scrub suits that are visibly soiled, contaminated, and/or penetrated by blood or other potentially infectious materials. *Category IB**

7. No recommendations on how or where to launder scrub suits, on restricting use of scrub suits to the operating suite, or for covering scrub suits when out of the operating suite. *Unresolved issue*

f. Asepsis and surgical technique

1. Adhere to principles of asepsis when placing

* Federal regulation: OSHA.

intravascular devices (e.g., central venous catheters), spinal or epidural anesthesia catheters, or when dispensing and administering intravenous drugs. *Category IA*

2. Assemble sterile equipment and solutions immediately prior to use. *Category II*

3. Handle tissue gently, maintain effective hemostasis, minimize devitalized tissue and foreign bodies (i.e., sutures, charred tissues, necrotic debris), and eradicate dead space at the surgical site. *Category IB*

4. Use delayed primary skin closure or leave an incision open to heal by second intention if the surgeon considers the surgical site to be heavily contaminated (e.g., Class III and Class IV). *Category IB*

5. If drainage is necessary, use a closed suction drain. Place a drain through a separate incision distant from the operative incision. Remove the drain as soon as possible. *Category IB*

3. Postoperative incision care

a. Protect with a sterile dressing for 24 to 48 hours postoperatively an incision that has been closed primarily. *Category IB*

b. Wash hands before and after dressing changes and any contact with the surgical site. *Category IB*

c. When an incision dressing must be changed, use sterile technique. *Category II*

d. Educate the patient and family regarding proper incision care, symptoms of SSI, and the need to report such symptoms. *Category II*

e. No recommendation to cover an incision closed primarily beyond 48 hours, nor on the appropriate time to shower or bathe with an uncovered incision. *Unresolved issue*

4. Surveillance

a. Use CDC definitions of SSI (Table 1) without modification for identifying SSI among surgical inpatients and outpatients. *Category IB*

b. For inpatient case-finding (including readmissions), use direct prospective observation, indirect prospective detection, or a combination of both direct and indirect methods for the duration of the patient's hospitalization. *Category IB*

c. When postdischarge surveillance is performed for detecting SSI following certain operations (e.g., coronary artery bypass graft), use a method that accommodates available resources and data needs. *Category II*

d. For outpatient case-finding, use a method that accommodates available resources and data needs. *Category IB*

e. Assign the surgical wound classification upon completion of an operation. A surgical team member should make the assignment. *Category II*

f. For each patient undergoing an operation chosen for surveillance, record those variables shown to be associated with increased SSI risk (e.g., surgical wound class, ASA class, and duration of operation). *Category IB*

g. Periodically calculate operation-specific SSI rates

stratified by variables shown to be associated with increased SSI risk (e.g., NNIS risk index). *Category IB*

h. Report appropriately stratified, operation-specific SSI rates to surgical team members. The optimum frequency and format for such rate computations will be determined by stratified case-load sizes (denominators) and the objectives of local, continuous quality improvement initiatives. *Category IB*

i. No recommendation to make available to the infection control committee coded surgeon-specific data. *Unresolved issue*

REFERENCES

1. Garner JS. CDC guideline for prevention of surgical wound infections, 1985. Supercedes guideline for prevention of surgical wound infections published in 1982. (Originally published in 1995). Revised. *Infect Control* 1986;7(3):193-200.
2. Simmons BP. Guideline for prevention of surgical wound infections. *Infect Control* 1982;3:185-196.
3. Garner JS. The CDC Hospital Infection Control Practices Advisory Committee. *Am J Infect Control* 1993;21:160-2.
4. Hecht AD. Creating greater efficiency in ambulatory surgery. *J Clin Anesth* 1995;7:581-4.
5. Horwitz JR, Chwals WJ, Doski JJ, Suescun EA, Cheu HW, Lally KP. Pediatric wound infections: a prospective multicenter study. *Ann Surg* 1998;227:553-8.
6. Golub R, Siddiqui F, Pohl D. Laparoscopic versus open appendectomy: a metaanalysis. *J Am Coll Surg* 1998;186:545-53.
7. Mayol J, Garcia-Aguilar J, Ortiz-Oshiro E, De-Diego Carmona JA, Ferndandez-Represa JA. Risks of the minimal access approach for laparoscopic surgery: multivariate analysis of morbidity related to umbilical trocar insertion. *World J Surg* 1997;21:529-33.
8. Lacy AM, Garcia-Valdecasas JC, Delgado S, Grande L, Fuster J, Tabet J, et al. Postoperative complications of laparoscopic-assisted colectomy. *Surg Endosc* 1997;11:119-22.
9. Pagni S, Salloum EJ, Tobin GR, VanHimbergen DJ, Spence PA. Serious wound infections after minimally invasive coronary bypass procedures. *Ann Thorac Surg* 1998;66:92-4.
10. The Southern Surgeons Club. A prospective analysis of 1518 laparoscopic cholecystectomies. *N Engl J Med* 1991;324:1073-8.
11. Centers for Disease Control and Prevention. National Nosocomial Infections Surveillance (NNIS) report, data summary from October 1986-April 1997, issued May 1997. *Am J Infect Control* 1997;25:477-87.
12. Food and Drug Administration. Topical antimicrobial drug products for over-the-counter human use: tentative final monograph for health-care antiseptic drug products—proposed rule (21 CFR Parts 333 and 369). *Federal Register* 1994;59:31441-52.
13. Centers for Disease Control and Prevention, National Center for Health Statistics. *Vital and Health Statistics, Detailed Diagnoses and Procedures, National Hospital Discharge Survey, 1994.* Vol 127. Hyattsville, Maryland: DHHS Publication; 1997.
14. Emori TG, Gaynes RP. An overview of nosocomial infections, including the role of the microbiology laboratory. *Clin Microbiol Rev* 1993;6(4):428-42.
15. Cruse P. Wound infection surveillance. *Rev Infect Dis* 1981;4(3):734-7.
16. Cruse PJ, Foord R. The epidemiology of wound infection: a 10-year prospective study of 62,939 wounds. *Surg Clin North Am* 1980;60(1):27-40.
17. Martone WJ, Jarvis WR, Culver DH, Haley RW. Incidence and nature of endemic and epidemic nosocomial infections. In: Bennett JV, Brachman PS, eds. *Hospital Infections.* 3rd ed. Boston: Little, Brown and Co; 1992. p. 577-96.
18. Boyce JM, Potter-Bynoe G, Dziobek L. Hospital reimbursement patterns among patients with surgical wound infections following open heart surgery. *Infect Control Hosp Epidemiol* 1990;11(2):89-93.
19. Poulsen KB, Bremmelgaard A, Sorensen AI, Raahave D, Petersen JV. Estimated costs of postoperative wound infections. A case-control study of marginal hospital and social security costs. *Epidemiol Infect* 1994;113(2):283-95.
20. Vegas AA, Jodra VM, Garcia ML. Nosocomial infection in surgery wards: a controlled study of increased duration of hospital stays and direct cost of hospitalization. *Eur J Epidemiol* 1993;9(5):504-10.
21. Albers BA, Patka P, Haarman HJ, Kostense PJ. Cost effectiveness of preventive antibiotic administration for lowering risk of infection by 0.25%. [German]. *Unfallchirurg* 1994;97(12):625-8.
22. Horan TC, Gaynes RP, Martone WJ, Jarvis WR, Emori TG. CDC definitions of nosocomial surgical site infections, 1992: a modification of CDC definitions of surgical wound infections. *Infect Control Hosp Epidemiol* 1992;13(10):606-8.
23. Ehrenkranz NJ, Richter EI, Phillips PM, Shultz JM. An apparent excess of operative site infections: analyses to evaluate false-positive diagnoses. *Infect Control Hosp Epidemiol* 1995;16(12):712-6.
24. Taylor G, McKenzie M, Kirkland T, Wiens R. Effect of surgeon's diagnosis on surgical wound infection rates. *Am J Infect Control* 1990;18(5):295-9.
25. SHEA, APIC, CDC, SIS. Consensus paper on the surveillance of surgical wound infections. *Infect Control Hosp Epidemiol* 1992;13(10):599-605.
26. Nooyen SM, Overbeek BP, Brutel de la Riviere A, Storm AJ, Langemeyer JM. Prospective randomised comparison of single-dose versus multiple-dose cefuroxime for prophylaxis in coronary artery bypass grafting. *Eur J Clin Microbiol Infect Dis* 1994;13:1033-7.
27. Centers for Disease Control and Prevention. National Nosocomial Infections Surveillance (NNIS) report, data summary from October 1986-April 1996, issued May 1996. A report from the National Nosocomial Infections Surveillance (NNIS) System. *Am J Infect Control* 1996;24:380-8.
28. Schaberg DR. Resistant gram-positive organisms. *Ann Emerg Med* 1994;24(3):462-4.
29. Schaberg DR, Culver DH, Gaynes RP. Major trends in the microbial etiology of nosocomial infection. *Am J Med* 1991;91(3B):72S-5S.
30. Jarvis WR. Epidemiology of nosocomial fungal infections, with emphasis on *Candida* species. *Clin Infect Dis* 1995;20:1526-30.
31. Centers for Disease Control. Nosocomial outbreak of *Rhizopus* infections associated with Elastoplast wound dressings—Minnesota. *MMWR* 1978;27:33-4.
32. Pearson RD, Valenti WM, Steigbigel RT. *Clostridium perfringens* wound infections associated with elastic bandages. *JAMA* 1980;244:1128-30.
33. Richet HM, Craven PC, Brown JM, Lasker BA, Cox CD, McNeil MM, et al. A cluster of *Rhodococcus (Gordona) bronchialis* sternal-wound infections after coronary-artery bypass surgery. *N Engl J Med* 1991;324:104-9.
34. Wenger PN, Brown JM, McNeil MM, Jarvis WR. *Nocardia farcinica* sternotomy site infections in patients following open heart surgery. *J Infect Dis* 1998;178:1539-43.
35. Lowry PW, Blankenship RJ, Gridley W, Troup NJ, Tompkins LS. A cluster of *Legionella* sternal-wound infections due to postoperative topical exposure to contaminated tap water. *N Engl J Med* 1991;324:109-13.
36. Bassett DC, Stokes KJ, Thomas WR. Wound infection with *Pseudomonas multivorans:* a water-borne contaminant of disinfectant solutions. *Lancet* 1970;1:1188-91.
37. Cruse PJ. Surgical wound infection. In: Wonsiewicz MJ, ed. *Infectious Diseases.* Philadelphia: W.B. Saunders Co; 1992. p. 758-64.
38. Altemeier WA, Culbertson WR. Surgical infection. In: Moyer CA, Rhoads JE, Allen JG, Harkins HN, eds. *Surgery, principles and practice.* 3rd ed. Philadelphia: JB Lippincott; 1965. p. 51-77.
39. Krizek TJ, Robson MC. Evolution of quantitative bacteriology in wound management. *Am J Surg* 1975;130:579-84.
40. Elek SD, Conen PE. The virulence of *Staphylococcus pyogenes* for man: a study of problems with wound infection. *Br J Exp Pathol* 1957;38:573-86.
41. Noble WC. The production of subcutaneous staphylococcal skin lesions in mice. *Br J Exp Pathol* 1965;46:254-62.
42. James RC, MacLeod CJ. Induction of staphylococcal infections in mice with small inocula introduced on sutures. *Br J Exp Pathol* 1961;42:266-77.
43. Henderson B, Poole S, Wilson M. Microbial/host interactions in health and disease: who controls the cytokine network? *Immunopharmacology* 1996;35:1-21.
44. Morrison DC, Ryan JL. Endotoxins and disease mechanisms. *Ann Rev Med* 1987;38:417-32.
45. Demling R, LaLonde C, Saldinger P, Knox J. Multiple-organ dysfunction in the surgical patient: pathophysiology, prevention, and treatment. *Curr Probl Surg* 1993;30:345-414.
46. Eiseman B, Beart R, Norton L. Multiple organ failure. *Surg Gynecol Obstet* 1977;14:323-6.
47. Fry DE, Pearlstein L, Fulton RL, Polk HC, Jr. Multiple system organ failure: the role of uncontrolled infection. *Arch Surg* 1980;115:136-40.
48. Kasper DL. Bacterial capsule—old dogmas and new tricks. *J Infect Dis* 1986;153:407-15.
49. Dellinger EP. Surgical infections and choice of antibiotics. In: Sabiston DC, ed. *Textbook of Surgery. The Biological Basis of Modern Surgical Practice.* 15th ed. Philadelphia: W.B. Saunders Co; 1997. p. 264-80.
50. Goeau-Brissonniere O, Leport C, Guidoin R, Lebrault C, Pechere JC,

Walter E. Stamm, M.D.
Assistant Professor of Medicine
University of Washington
School of Medicine
Harborview Medical Center
Seattle, Washington
U.S. DEPARTMENT OF HEALTH & HUMAN SERVICES
Public Health Service

Guideline for Prevention of Catheter-associated Urinary Tract Infections

INTRODUCTION

The urinary tract is the most common site of nosocomial infection, accounting for more than 40% of the total number reported by acute-care hospitals and affecting an estimated 600,000 patients per year *(1)*.

Most of these infections--66% to 86%--follow instrumentation of the urinary tract, mainly urinary catheterization *(2)*. Although not all catheter-associated urinary tract infections can be prevented, it is believed that a large number could be avoided by the proper management of the indwelling catheter. The following recommendations were developed for the care of patients with temporary indwelling urethral catheters. Patients who require chronic indwelling catheters or individuals who can be managed with intermittent catheterization may have different needs. Determination of the optimal catheter care for these and other patients with different drainage systems requires separate evaluation.

EPIDEMIOLOGY

The risk of acquiring a urinary tract infection depends on the method and duration of catheterization, the quality of catheter care, and host susceptibility. Reported infection rates vary widely, ranging from 1%-5% after a single brief catheterization *(3)* to virtually 100% for patients with indwelling urethral catheters draining into an open system for longer than 4 days *(4)*. Adoption of the closed method of urinary drainage has markedly reduced the risk of acquiring a catheter-associated infection, but the risk is still substantial. As recent studies have shown, over 20% of patients catheterized and maintained on closed drainage on busy hospital wards may be expected to become infected *(5, 6)*. In these studies, errors in maintaining sterile closed drainage were common and predisposed patients to infection. Host factors which appear to increase the risk of acquiring catheter-associated urinary tract infections include advanced age, debilitation, and the postpartum state *(7,8)*.

Catheter-associated urinary tract infections are generally assumed to be benign. Such infection in otherwise healthy patients is often asymptomatic and is likely to resolve spontaneously with the removal of the catheter. Occasionally, infection persists and leads to such complications as prostatitis, epididymitis, cystitis, pyelonephritis, and gram-negative bacteremia, particularly in high-risk patients *(8)*. The last complication is serious since it is associated with a significant mortality, but fortunately occurs in fewer than 1% of catheterized patients *(9,10)*. The natural history of catheter-associated urinary tract infections has been largely unstudied.

Catheter-associated urinary tract infections are caused by a variety of pathogens, including *Escherichia coli*, *Klebsiella*, *Proteus*, enterococcus, *Pseudomonas*, *Enterobacter*, *Serratia*, and *Candida*. Many of these microorganisms are part of the patient's endogenous bowel flora, but they can also be acquired by cross-contamination from other patients or hospital personnel or by exposure to contaminated solutions or non-sterile equipment *(11,12)*. Urinary tract pathogens such as *Serratia marcescens* and *Pseudomonas cepacia* have special epidemiologic significance. Since these microorganisms do not commonly reside in the gastrointestinal tract, their isolation from catheterized patients suggests acquisition from an exogenous source *(13,14)*.

Whether from endogenous or exogenous sources, infecting microorganisms gain access to the urinary tract by several routes. Microorganisms that inhabit the meatus or distal urethra can be introduced directly into the bladder when the catheter is inserted. Generally, however, low rates of infection have been reported after single brief catheterization *(4)*, suggesting that microorganisms introduced by this method are usually removed from healthy individuals by voiding or by antibacterial mechanisms of the bladder mucosa *(15)*. With indwelling catheters, infecting microorganisms can migrate to the bladder along the outside of the catheter in the periurethral mucous sheath *(16,17)* or along the internal lumen of the catheter after the collection bag or catheter-drainage tube junction has been contaminated *(5, 6)*. The importance of intraluminal ascension is suggested by the substantial reduction in infections that has been achieved through the use of the closed urinary drainage system. However, if sterile closed drainage can be maintained, extraluminal migration of microorganisms in the periurethral space becomes a relatively more important pathway of entry into the bladder *(17)*.

CONTROL MEASURES

An estimated 4 million patients are subjected yearly to urinary catheterization and, therefore, are at risk for catheter-associated infection and its related sequelae. One of the most important infection control measures is to limit the use of urinary catheters to carefully selected patients, thereby reducing the size of the population at risk. Generally, urinary catheterization is indicated 1) to relieve urinary tract obstruction, 2) to permit urinary drainage in patients with neurogenic bladder dysfunction and urinary retention, 3) to aid in urologic surgery or other surgery on contiguous structures, and 4) to obtain accurate measurements of urinary output in critically ill patients. Specifically, urinary catheterization should be discouraged as a means of obtaining urine for culture or certain diagnostic tests such as urinary electrolytes when the patient can voluntarily void or as a substitute for nursing care in the incontinent patient.

In selected populations, other methods of urinary drainage exist as possible alternatives to the use of the indwelling urethral catheter. Condom catheter drainage may be useful for incontinent male patients without outlet obstruction and with an intact voiding reflex. Its use, however, requires meticulous nursing care if local complications such as skin maceration or phimosis are to be avoided. In addition, frequent manipulation of the condom catheter drainage system (e.g., by agitated patients) has been associated with an increased risk of urinary tract infection (18). Another alternative, suprapubic catheter drainage, is most frequently used in patients on urologic or gynecologic services. Although preliminary data on the risk of infection are encouraging (19,20), the benefit of the suprapubic catheter with regard to infection control has not been proven by controlled clinical studies. For certain types of patients with bladder-emptying dysfunction, such as those with spinal cord injuries or children with meningomyelocele, a third alternative, intermittent catheterization, is commonly employed. The "no-touch" method of intermittent catheterization advocated by Guttmann (21) is generally reserved for patients hospitalized during the acute phase of their spinal cord injury, while the clean, nonsterile method of Lapides (22) is frequently used by ambulatory patients for whom the practice of aseptic catheter insertion is difficult to maintain. As with suprapubic catheterization, however, well-designed clinical trials comparing the efficacy of intermittent catheterization by either method to indwelling catheterization in minimizing the risk of infection are lacking.

For patients who require indwelling urethral catheterization, adherence to the sterile continuously closed system of urinary drainage is the cornerstone of infection control. For short-term catheterization, this measure alone can reduce the rate of infection from an inevitable 100% when open drainage is employed to less than 25% (5). All other interventions can be viewed as adjunctive measures since none have proven to be as effective in reducing the frequency of catheter-associated urinary tract infections.

Efforts have been made to improve the design of the closed urinary drainage system by modifying or adding to the basic unit introduced and widely adopted in the 1960s. Two modifications, the addition of a urine sampling port in the drainage tubing and the preconnected catheter/collecting tube system seem to have been logical advances since they discourage or prevent opening the closed system which has been well-documented to predispose patients to infection (6). Other alterations have included the insertion of air vents, drip chambers, and one-way valves that were designed to prevent the reflux of contaminated urine. Although these modifications have some theoretical basis, none have been shown to be effective in reducing the frequency of catheter-associated infections. Additionally, overly complex drainage systems can affect the ease of operation or more easily malfunction (5). These latter factors can influence the acceptance of different systems by hospital personnel and ultimately affect infection control.

Other efforts to reduce the incidence of catheter-associated infections have been directed toward 1) preventing microorganisms at the meatus from entering the bladder and 2) eradicating microorganisms that gain entry into the urinary tract before they can proliferate (23). Measures directed toward the first objective include aseptic catheter insertion, daily meatal cleansing, and daily application of antimicrobial ointments or solutions. On the basis of recent studies that have shown that catheterized patients colonized at the meatus with gram-negative bacilli or enterococci are at increased risk for subsequent infection (17,24), these measures have some theoretical value and can be expected to delay or prevent the onset of infection. Generally, clinical trials that have attempted to demonstrate their efficacy have not been well designed or did not include the use of the closed system of urinary drainage. However, 2 recent prospective, controlled studies conducted by the same research group have shown that meatal care as it is currently commonly practiced (either twice-a-day cleansing with povidone-iodine solution followed by povidone-iodine ointment or daily cleansing with soap and water) was ineffective in reducing the frequency of catheter-associated infections in patients on closed urinary drainage (25, 26). The value of different regimens (e.g., more frequent application, other concentrations, or other antimicrobial agents) is not known and requires further evaluation.

Infection control measures for purposes of eradicating microorganisms in the urinary tract before they can proliferate and cause infection include irrigation of the bladder and the use of prophylactic systemic antibiotics. In one controlled study, continuous irrigation of the bladder with nonabsorbable antibiotics was associated with frequent interruption of the closed drainage system and did not bring about a reduction in the frequency of catheter-associated infections (27). It is not known, however, whether such irrigation would be effective if the integrity of the closed drainage system could be maintained. Several recent studies have shown that prophylactic systemic antibiotics delay the emergence of catheter-related infection (6,28), but this protective effect was transient and was associated with the selection of antibiotic-resistant microorganisms. Thus, controversy regarding the value of prophylactic systemic antibiotics remains.

When cross-infection is likely to be responsible for the spread of catheter-associated infections, additional measures have been proposed (29). In several outbreaks of nosocomial urinary tract infections, catheterized patients with asymptomatic infections served as unrecognized reservoirs of infecting organisms, and the mechanism of transmission appeared to be carriage on the hands of patient-care personnel (13,14). In these outbreaks, the implementation of control measures to prevent cross-infection, including renewed emphasis on handwashing and spatial separation of catheterized patients, particularly infected from uninfected ones, effectively ended the outbreak. In the absence of epidemic spread or frequent cross-infection, spatial separation of catheterized patients is probably less effective in controlling catheter-associated infections.

Regular bacteriologic monitoring of catheterized patients has been advocated to ensure early diagnosis and treatment of urinary tract infections (8). Its possible value as an infection measure lies in its potential usefulness in detecting and initiating treatment of clinically inapparent infections, which may serve as reservoirs of hospital pathogens, and thus, reducing the likelihood of cross-infection. However, the potential benefit of bacteriologic monitoring for such a purpose has not been adequately investigated.

RECOMMENDATIONS

1. Personnel

a. Only persons (e.g., hospital personnel, family members, or patients themselves) who know the correct technique of aseptic insertion and maintenance of the catheter should handle catheters *(5, 6, 8)*. *Category I*

b. Hospital personnel and others who take care of catheters should be given periodic in-service training stressing the correct techniques and potential complications of urinary catheterization. *Category II*

2. Catheter Use

a. Urinary catheters should be inserted only when necessary and left in place only for as long as necessary. They should not be used solely for the convenience of patient-care personnel. *Category I*

b. For selected patients, other methods of urinary drainage such as condom catheter drainage, suprapubic catheterization, and intermittent urethral catheterization can be useful alternatives to indwelling urethral catheterization *(8,19, 21, 22)*. *Category III*

3. Handwashing

Handwashing should be done immediately before and after any manipulation of the catheter site or apparatus *(14,30)*. *Category I*

4. Catheter Insertion

a. Catheters should be inserted using aseptic technique and sterile equipment *(8,16,31)*. *Category I*

b. Gloves, drape, sponges, an appropriate antiseptic solution for periurethral cleaning, and a single-use packet of lubricant jelly should be used for insertion. *Category II*

c. As small a catheter as possible, consistent with good drainage, should be used to minimize urethral trauma *(8)*. *Category II*

d. Indwelling catheters should be properly secured after insertion to prevent movement and urethral traction *(31)*. *Category I*

5. Closed Sterile Drainage

a. A sterile, continuously closed drainage system should be maintained *(5,6,27)*. *Category I*

b. The catheter and drainage tube should not be disconnected unless the catheter must be irrigated (see Irrigation Recommendation 6). *Category I*

c. If breaks in aseptic technique, disconnection, or leakage occur, the collecting system should be replaced using aseptic technique after disinfecting the catheter-tubing junction. *Category III*

6. Irrigation

a. Irrigation should be avoided unless obstruction is anticipated (e.g., as might occur with bleeding after prostatic or bladder surgery); closed continuous irrigation may be used to prevent obstruction. To relieve obstruction due to clots, mucus, or other causes, an intermittent method of irrigation may be used. Continuous irrigation of the bladder with antimicrobials has not proven to be useful *(28)* and should not be performed as a routine infection prevention measure. *Category II*

b. The catheter-tubing junction should be disinfected before disconnection. *Category II*

c. A large-volume sterile syringe and sterile irrigant should be used and then discarded. The person performing irrigation should use aseptic technique. *Category I*

d. If the catheter becomes obstructed and can be kept open only by frequent irrigation, the catheter should be changed if it is likely that the catheter itself is contributing to the obstruction (e.g., formation of concretions). *Category II*

7. Specimen Collection

a. If small volumes of fresh urine are needed for examination. the distal end of the catheter, or preferably the sampling port if present, should be cleansed with a disinfectant, and urine then aspirated with a sterile needle and syringe *(5,8)*. *Category I*

b. Larger volumes of urine for special analyses should be obtained aseptically from the drainage bag. *Category I*

8. Urinary Flow

a. Unobstructed flow should be maintained *(6,8)*. *Category I* (Occasionally, it is necessary to temporarily obstruct the catheter for specimen collection or other medical purposes.)

b. To achieve free flow of urine 1) the catheter and collecting tube should be kept from kinking; 2) the collecting bag should be emptied regularly using a separate collecting container for each patient (the draining spigot and nonsterile collecting container should never come in contact) *(33)*; 3) poorly functioning or obstructed catheters should be irrigated (see Irrigation Recommendation 6) or if necessary, replaced; and 4) collecting bags should always be kept below the level of the bladder. *Category I*

9. Meatal Care

Twice daily cleansing with povidone-iodine solution and daily cleansing with soap and water have been shown in 2 recent studies not to reduce catheter-associated urinary tract infection *(25,26)*. Thus, at this time, daily meatal care with either of these 2 regimens cannot be endorsed. *Category II*

10. Catheter Change Interval

Indwelling catheters should not be changed at arbitrary fixed intervals *(34)*. *Category II*

11. Spatial Separation of Catheterized Patients

To minimize the chances of cross-infection, infected and uninfected patients with indwelling catheters should not share the same room or adjacent beds *(29)*. *Category III*

12. Bacteriologic Monitoring

The value of regular bacteriologic monitoring of catheterized patients as an infection control measure has not been established and is not recommended *(35)*. *Category III*

Summary of Major Recommendations

Category I. Strongly Recommended for Adoption*

- Educate personnel in correct techniques of catheter insertion and care.
- Catheterize only when necessary.
- Emphasize handwashing.
- Insert catheter using aseptic technique and sterile equipment.
- Secure catheter properly.
- Maintain closed sterile drainage.
- Obtain urine samples aseptically.
- Maintain unobstructed urine flow.

Category II. Moderately Recommended for Adoption

- Periodically re-educate personnel in catheter care.
- Use smallest suitable bore catheter.

- Avoid irrigation unless needed to prevent or relieve obstruction.
- Refrain from daily meatal care with either of the regimens discussed in text.
- Do not change catheters at arbitrary fixed intervals.

Category III. Weakly Recommended for Adoption

- Consider alternative techniques of urinary drainage before using an indwelling urethral catheter.
- Replace the collecting system when sterile closed drainage has been violated.
- Spatially separate infected and uninfected patients with indwelling catheters.
- Avoid routine bacteriologic monitoring.

*Refer to Introduction of manual for full explanation of the ranking scheme for recommendations.

REFERENCES

1. Center for Disease Control. National Nosocomial Infections Study Report, Atlanta: Center for Disease Control, November 1979: 2-14.
2. Martin CM, Bookrajian EN. Bacteriuria prevention after indwelling urinary catheterization. Arch Intern Med 1962;110:703-11.
3. Turck M, Goffe B, Petersdorf RG. The urethral catheters and urinary tract infection. J Urol 1962;88:834-7.
4. Kass EH. Asymptomatic infections of the urinary tract. Trans Assoc Am Physicians 1956;69:56-63.
5. Kunin CM, McCormack RC. Prevention of catheter-induced urinary tract infections by sterile closed drainage. N Engl J Med 1966;274:1155-62.
6. Garibaldi RA, Burke JP, Dickman ML, Smith CB. Factors predisposing to bacteriuria during indwelling urethral catheterization. N Engl J Med 1974;291:215-8.
7. Brumfitt W, Davies BL, Rosser E. The urethral catheter as a cause of urinary tract infection in pregnancy and puerperium. Lancet 1961;2:1059-61.
8. Kunin CM. Detection, prevention, and management of urinary tract infections. 3rd ed. Philadelphia: Lea and Febiger, 1979.
9. Steere AC, Stamm WE, Martin SM, Bennett JV. Gram-negative rod bacteremia. In: Bennett JV, Brachman PS, eds. Hospital infections. Boston: Little, Brown and Company. 1979:507-18.
10. Kreger BE, Craven DE. McCabe WR. Gram-negative bacteremia IV. Re-evaluation of clinical features and treatment in 612 patients. Am J Med 1980,68:344-55.
11. Selden R, Lee S, Wang WLL, et al. Nosocomial *Klebsiella* infections: intestinal colonization as a reservoir. Ann Intern Med 1971;74:657-64.
12. McLeod JW. The hospital urine bottle and bedpan as reservoirs of infection by *Pseudomonas*. Lancet 1958;1:394-5.
13. Maki DG, Hennekens CH, Bennett JV, et al. Nosocomial urinary tract infection with *Serratia marcesens*: an epidemiologic study. 1973; J Infect Dis 128:579-87.
14. Kaslow RA, Lindsey JO, Bisno AL, Price A. Nosocomial infection with highly resistant *Proteus rettgeri*. Report of an epidemic. Am J Epidemiol 1976; 104:278-86.
15. Norden CW, Green GM, Kass EH. Antibacterial mechanisms of the urinary bladder. J Clin Invest 1968;47:2689-700.
16. Kass EH, Schneiderman LJ. Entry of bacteria into the urinary tract of patients with inlying catheters. N Engl J Med 1957;256:556-7.
17. Garibaldi RA, Burke JP, Britt MR, Miller WA, Smith CB. Meatal colonization and catheter-associated bacteriuria. N Engl J Med 1980;303:316-8.
18. Hirsh DD, Fainstein V, Musher DM. Do condom catheter collecting systems cause urinary tract infection? JAMA 1979;242:340-1.
19. Hodgkinson CP, Hodari AA. Trocar suprapubic cystostomy for postoperative bladder drainage in the female. J Obstet Gynecol 1966;96:773-83.
20. Marcus RT. Narrow-bore suprapubic bladder drainage in Uganda. Lancet 1967;1:748-50.
21. Guttman L, Frankel H. The value of intermittent catheterization in the early management of traumatic paraplegia and tetraplegia. Paraplegia 1966;4:63-83.
22. Lapides J, Diokno AC, Gould FR, Lowe. BS. Further observations on self-catheterization. J Urol 1976; 116:169-71.
23. Sanford JP. Hospital-acquired urinary tract infections. Ann Intern Med 1964;60:903-14.
24. Garibaldi RA, Britt MR, Miller WA, Steinmuller P, Burke JP. Evaluation of periurethral colonization as a risk factor for catheter-associated bacteriuria. In: Proceedings of the 16th Interscience Conference on Antimicrobial Agents and Chemotherapy, 1976;142.
25. Britt MR, Burke JP, Miller WA, Steinmiller P, Garibaldi RA. The non-effectiveness of daily meatal care in the prevention of catheter-associated bacteriuria. In: Proceedings of the 16th Interscience Conference on Antimicrobial Agents and Chemotherapy, 1976; 141.
26. Burke JP, Garibaldi RA, Britt MR, Jacobson JA, Conti M, Alling DW. Prevention of catheter-associated urinary tract infections. Efficacy of daily meatal care regimens. In: Proceedings of the 2nd International Conference on Nosocomial Infections. Atlanta, August 4-8, 1980. Am J Med 1981;70:655-8.
27. Warren JW, Platt R, Thomas KJ, Rosner B, Kass EH. Antibiotic irrigation and catheter-associated urinary tract infections. N Engl J Med 1978;299:570-73.
28. Britt MR, Garibaldi RA, Miller WA, Hebertson RM, Burke JP. Antimicrobial prophylaxis for catheter-associated bacteriuria . Antimicrob Agents Chemother 1977;11:240- 3.
29. Maki DG, Hennekens CH, Bennett JV. Prevention of catheter-associated urinary tract infection: an additional measure. JAMA 1972;221:1270-1.
30. Steere AC, Mallison GF. Handwashing practices for the prevention of nosocomial infections. Ann Intern Med 1975; 83:683-90.
31. Desautels RF, Walter CW, Graves RC. et al. Technical advances in the prevention of urinary tract infection. J Urol 1962;87:487-90.
32. Viant AC, Linton KB, Gillespie WA. Improved method for preventing movement of indwelling catheters in female patients. Lancet

SPECIAL COMMUNICATION

Infection prevention and control in the long-term–care facility

Philip W. Smith, MD
Patricia G. Rusnak, RN

More than 1.5 million residents reside in US nursing homes. In recent years, the acuity of illness of nursing home residents has increased. Long-term–care facility residents have a risk of developing nosocomial infection that is similar to acute-care hospital patients. A great deal of information has been published concerning infections in the long-term–care facility, and infection control programs are nearly universal.

This position paper reviews the literature on infections and infection control programs in the long-term–care facility, covering such topics as tuberculosis, bloodborne pathogens, epidemics, isolation systems, immunization, and antibiotic-resistant bacteria. Recommendations are developed for long-term–care infection control programs based on interpretation of currently available evidence. The recommendations cover the structure and function of the infection control program, including surveillance, isolation, outbreak control, resident care, and employee health. Infection control resources also are presented. (AJIC Am J Infect Control 1997;25:488-512)

INTRODUCTION

Hospital infection control is well established in the United States. Infection control committees (ICCs) began to appear in the 1960s in response to recognized institutional outbreaks of infectious diseases and increased regulatory pressures. Infection control programs now are mandated in acute-care facilities; virtually every hospital has an infection control practitioner (ICP), and many larger hospitals have a consulting hospital epidemiologist. The Study on the Efficacy of Nosocomial Infection Control (SENIC) documented the effectiveness of an in-fection control program that applies standard surveillance and control measures.[1]

The term "nosocomial" often is applied to the long-term–care facility (LTCF), as well as to the acute-care hospital. The major elements leading to a nosocomial (institutionally associated) infection are the infectious agent, a susceptible host, and a means of transmission. These elements are present in LTCFs, as well as in hospitals. It is not surprising, therefore, that almost as many nosocomial infections occur annually in LTCFs as in hospitals in the United States.[2]

The 1980s saw recognition of the problem of infections in LTCFs, with subsequent widespread development of LTCF infection control programs, and definition of the role of the ICP in LTCFs. Research studies delineated the descriptive epidemiology of nosocomial infections and infectious disease outbreaks in LTCFs (see below), and regulatory requirements significantly increased.[3] Nevertheless, there is as yet no SENIC-equivalent study documenting the efficacy of infection control in LTCFs, and virtually no controlled studies have analyzed the effectiveness of specific control measures in that setting.

Application of currently available hospital infection control guidelines to the LTCF may be

From the SHEA Long-Term–Care Committee and APIC Guidelines Committee.

Dr. Smith and Ms. Rusnak are affiliated with the Nebraska Health System in Omaha.

This 1997 version supersedes the 1991 guideline.

inappropriate and unrealistic in view of the different nature of infection control challenges that exist. Even so, regulators occasionally expect LTCFs to meet hospital standards. The problem is compounded by the varying levels of nursing intensity, as well as varying LTCF size and accessibility to physician input.

Although hospitals and LTCFs both have closed populations requiring nursing care, they are quite different. They differ with regard to payment systems, patient acuity, availability of laboratory and x-ray, and nurse-to-patient ratios. The LTCF must deal with a host whose resistance is declining, without the acute-care focus on recovery and high technology.[4]

This position paper provides basic infection control recommendations that could be widely applied to LTCFs with the expectation of minimizing nosocomial infections. The efficacy of these measures in the LTCF, in most cases, is not proved by prospective controlled studies, but is based on infection control logic, adaptation of hospital experience, LTCF studies, and field experience. Every effort will be made to address the unique concerns of LTCFs. Because facilities differ, the infection risk factors specific to the resident population, the nature of the facility, and the resources available should dictate the scope and focus of the infection control program.

In a number of instances, specific hospital-oriented guidelines have been published and are referenced (e.g. guidelines for prevention of intravascular-device–associated infections or vancomycin-resistant enterococci). These guidelines are relevant, at least in part, to the long-term–care setting, but must be adapted depending on facility size, resources, resident acuity, local regulations, local infection control issues, and so on. Reworking these guidelines to a form applicable to all LTCFs is not feasible.

Any discussion of these issues must be made in the context of the LTCF as a community. The LTCF is a home for residents, a home in which they usually reside for months or years; comfort and infection control principles both must be addressed.

BACKGROUND

Demography and definitions

The US population aged 65 to 85 years is increasing rapidly, and the population aged 85 years and older has doubled in the last 15 years. Currently, approximately 20% of the latter group

reside in LTCFs.[5] One of every four persons who reach the age of 65 can be expected to spend part of his or her life in a nursing home; more people currently occupy nursing home beds than acute-care hospital beds in the United States.[6] More than 1.5 million persons in the United States reside in a nursing home; there are approximately 19,000 nursing homes in this country.[7] Ninety percent of nursing home residents are over 65 years of age, and the mean age of residents is over 80 years.

A long-term–care facility is a residential institution for providing nursing care and related services to residents. It may be attached to a hospital (swing-bed) or free standing; the latter is often called a nursing home. A resident is a person living in the LTCF and receiving care, analogous to the patient in a hospital.

Scope of position paper

This position paper addresses all levels of care in the LTCF. The focus is specifically the LTCF, also known as the nursing home, caring for elderly or chronically ill residents. These recommendations generally also should apply to special extended-care situations (such as institutions for the mentally retarded, psychiatric hospitals, and rehabilitation hospitals). However, other extended-care facilities may have different populations (e.g. the residents of institutions for the mentally retarded are much younger than nursing home residents) or different disease risks (e.g. hepatitis B in psychiatric hospitals). Thus, the recommendations may need to be adapted for these special extended-care situations.

Changes from prior Guideline

This position paper is similar to the 1991 APIC guideline,[8] although the present version reflects an updating of research and experience in the field. Several specific areas of discussion are new or changed, including the elimination of the regulatory requirement for an infection control committee, the discussion of vancomycin-resistant enterococci, a new Centers for Disease Control and Prevention (CDC) isolation system, more extensive tuberculosis control requirements, and several new published infection control guidelines (e.g. for pneumonia, medical waste).

INFECTIONS IN THE LONG-TERM–CARE FACILITY

Epidemiology

It is well known that the elderly population has a substantially increased incidence and severity of many infectious diseases.[9-12] This vulnerability to infection is due partly to an age-related decline in immunologic function, specifically cell-mediated immunity and antibody response.[13,14] T-lymphocyte numbers and function decline with age, reflected in reactivation of latent infections in the elderly such as herpes zoster and tuberculosis. Antibody production declines with age as well.

The elderly have a variety of local host defense problems that predispose to infection. Examples are thinning of the skin (cellulitis), gastric achlorhydria (*Salmonella* gastroenteritis), urinary retention (urinary tract infection), and decreased mucociliary clearance of bacteria from the airways (pneumonia).[14]

Furthermore, a number of underlying diseases commonly seen in elderly persons (such as diabetes mellitus and malignancy) are known to increase the risk of infection. Depressed mental status from dementia may lead to either aspiration pneumonia or a pressure ulcer.

Elderly patients in the hospital and LTCF are particularly susceptible to infection.[15,16] In addition to the generic susceptibility to infection in the elderly population, the LTCF resident is a more susceptible host on the basis of severity of underlying diseases, medications that affect resistance to infection (such as steroids and antibiotics), impaired mental status (predisposing to pressure ulcers and aspiration pneumonia), incontinence, indwelling urinary catheters, and other factors. Garibaldi and coworkers[17] noted that LTCF residents had an average of 3.3 underlying conditions recorded in the medical record, and 12% had indwelling urinary catheters. Many residents are demented or incontinent of stool or urine. Jackson et al.[18] found a mean age of 82 years and a mean length of stay of 166 days.

An additional problem is the increasing severity of illness in LTCF residents. This is due in part to more rapid transfer of hospitalized patients following implementation of the diagnosis-related group-based hospital reimbursement system[19] and in part to the fact that LTCFs are sharing in the burden of caring for persons with acquired immunodeficiency syndrome (AIDS). LTCFs now occasionally have residents with tracheostomies, indwelling central venous lines, or ventilator dependence, once exclusively the province of hospitals.

There are many reservoirs for infectious agents in LTCFs. Most infections are thought to be endogenous, resulting from the resident's own flora of the perineum, skin, or nasopharynx. Infected or colonized residents may serve as reservoirs for certain infectious agents (such as methicillin-resistant *Staphylococcus aureus* [MRSA]); visitors and staff also are important reservoirs (e.g. for influenza).

Transmission is most frequently by direct contact (for example, by hands), but airborne, vehicle, and vectorborne spread may occur. As in the hospital, healthcare providers go from person to person, serving as important sources for transmission by the contact route. Vehicle transmission occurs through items such as food and water, whereas airborne spread occurs by dissemination of droplet nuclei or particles in the air. A unique problem facing LTCFs is that of an ambulatory resident who may be incontinent or coughing and serves as a potential means for spread of infectious agents. Transmission in the LTCF may be accentuated by lack of conveniently placed handwashing facilities, absence of private rooms, or deficiencies in ventilation systems.

Nosocomial infections—magnitude of the problem

Nosocomial infections are those that develop after admission to the LTCF. Infections that are incubating at the time of admission, or develop within 48 to 72 hours of admission, usually are community-acquired, or hospital-associated if the resident was transferred from an acute-care setting. Because of the long length of stay in the LTCF, the vast majority of infections will be nosocomial. Classification of an infection as nosocomial does not imply that the LTCF caused the infection, that the infecting organism was acquired in the LTCF, or that it was preventable, but simply that it occurred in the LTCF.

The CDC estimates that 1.5 million nosocomial infections occur in LTCF residents per year; this translates to an average of one infection per resident per year.[2] Approximately 20 surveys (most of them prevalence studies) of LTCF nosocomial infections have been done, using a variety of surveillance techniques and infection definitions. The studies found nosocomial infection prevalence rates ranging from 2.7% to 32.7% and incidence rates ranging from 10.7% to 20.1%, or 2.6 to 7.1 infections per 1,000 resident days.[17,18, 20-37] The most common infections found in LTCF surveys are urinary tract infections (UTIs), respiratory infections (influenza, pneumonia), infected pressure ulcers, gastroenteritis, and conjunctivitis. There is an association between pneumonia and increased mortality in the LTCF,[18,37] but the morbidity and mortality of infections in this setting have not been well defined.

SPECIFIC NOSOCOMIAL INFECTIONS IN THE LONG-TERM–CARE FACILITY

Urinary tract infections

In most surveys, the leading nosocomial infection in LTCFs is UTI, generally related to an indwelling urinary catheter.[38] External catheters also appear to be a risk factor for UTIs in male residents.[39] A high percentage of LTCF residents are incontinent of urine or feces, which contributes to the risk of UTI.[40] Bacteriuria is associated with incontinence and dementia, but may not by itself adversely affect survival.[41]

Several surveys reveal that the prevalence of urethral catheters in the LTCF is 7% to 10%.[42-44] Catheterization predisposes to clinical UTI, and the urinary tract is a frequent source of bacteremia in the LTCF.[45] Long-term catheterization may be associated with increased mortality.[43]

The symptoms of urinary tract infection are dysuria and frequency (cystitis) or fever and flank pain (pyelonephritis). The elderly often have atypical symptoms. The diagnosis of urinary tract infection requires demonstration of white blood cells in the urine (pyuria) or a positive quantitative urine culture. The latter is obtained by the clean-catch voided technique (often difficult in the LTCF setting) or by aspiration through a catheter system sampling port.

The vast majority of residents with indwelling urinary catheters in the LTCF are colonized with more than 50,000 colony-forming units of bacteria per mL of urine,[46] and the bacteria found generally are more resistant to oral antibiotics than the corresponding bacteria found in elderly persons in the community.[24,47] Although residents with newly placed catheters have quantitatively less bacteriuria, routine catheter changes may not alter the course of bacteriuria or culture results and are not advocated. Catheter-related bacteriuria is ever-changing and not amenable to prophylactic antibiotics.[48] These factors make it inappropriate to screen asymptomatic residents for bacteriuria or to treat asymptomatic bacteriuria.

Guidelines were published for prevention of catheter-associated UTIs in hospitalized patients,[49] and the recommendations generally are applicable to catheterized residents in LTCFs. Recommended measures include limiting use of catheters, inser-

tion of catheters aseptically by trained personnel, use of as small a catheter as possible, handwashing before and after catheter manipulation, maintenance of a closed catheter system, avoiding irrigation unless the catheter is obstructed, keeping the collecting bag below the bladder, and maintaining good hydration in residents.

The CDC guideline[49] briefly discusses care of condom catheters and suprapubic catheters, but no guideline for leg bags is available. Leg bags allow for improved ambulation of residents, but probably increase the risk of UTI, because opening of the system and reflux of urine from the bag to the bladder occur more frequently than with a standard closed system. Suggestions for care of leg bags include using aseptic technique when disconnecting and reconnecting, disinfecting connections with alcohol, changing bags at regular intervals, rinsing with diluted vinegar, and drying between uses.[50] A 1:3 dilution of white vinegar has been recommended for leg bag disinfection.[51] The role of suprapubic catheters in prevention of urinary tract infections in long-term catheter situations has not been determined.

Respiratory tract infections

Because of the impaired immunity of elderly persons, viral upper respiratory infections that generally are mild in other populations may cause significant disease in the institutionalized elderly patient.[52] Examples include rhinoviruses, parainfluenza, respiratory syncytial virus, and adenoviruses.

Pneumonia

Pneumonia is a frequent infection in the LTCF. The elderly person is predisposed to pneumonia by virtue of decreased clearance of bacteria from the airways and altered throat flora.[53] Underlying diseases, such as chronic obstructive pulmonary disease and heart disease, further increase the risk of pneumonia in this population.[54] The clinical presentation of pneumonia in the elderly often is atypical. The diagnosis of pneumonia in the LTCF is hampered by lack of x-ray facilities and the difficulty of getting good sputum specimens from elderly residents. *Streptococcus pneumoniae* appears to be the most common etiologic agent.[55,56] However, the elderly LTCF resident, with frequent underlying medical diseases such as chronic obstructive pulmonary disease, is more likely than the community-dwelling elderly to develop pneumonia due to *Klebsiella pneumoniae* or *S. aureus*, pneumonias with higher mortality rates.[53] *Legionella* pneumonia also is a concern in the LTCF.

Aspiration pneumonia is important in this setting. Nursing home residents commonly have conditions that predispose to aspiration, including mental status abnormalities, swallowing disorders, and feeding tubes. The mortality rate for LTCF-acquired pneumonia is significantly higher than for community-acquired pneumonia in the elderly population.[57]

The CDC guideline for prevention of pneumonia[58] is oriented toward acute-care hospitals but covers a number of points relevant to the LTCF, including respiratory therapy equipment, suctioning techniques, tracheostomy care, prevention of aspiration with enteral feedings, and immunizations. Examples of relevant recommendations for the LTCF include handwashing after contact with respiratory secretions, wearing gloves for suctioning, elevating the head of the bed 30 to 45 degrees during tube feeding and for at least 1 hour after to decrease aspiration, and vaccination of high-risk residents with pneumococcal vaccine.[58] The evidence for the efficacy of pneumococcal vaccine in high-risk populations, including the elderly population, is debated.[59,60] However, the vaccine is safe, relatively inexpensive, and recommended for routine use in individuals over the age of 65 years.[61] It is an important vaccine in the LTCF setting.

Influenza

Influenza is an acute respiratory disease signaled by the acute onset of fever, cough, chills, and headache. It is a major threat to LTCF residents, who are among the high-risk groups deserving preventive measures.[62] Influenza is very contagious, and outbreaks in LTCFs are common and often severe. Clinical attack rates range from 25% to 70%, and case fatality rates average over 10%.[63-66]

A killed virus vaccine is available, but must be given annually. Influenza vaccine in the elderly is approximately 40% effective at preventing hospitalization for pneumonia and approximately 50% effective at preventing hospital deaths from pneumonia.[67] Although concern has been expressed regarding the efficacy of the influenza vaccine in institutionalized elderly patients, most authors feel that the influenza vaccine is effective and indicated for all residents and caregivers.[65-70] Amantadine or rimantadine prophylaxis may be an effective adjunctive measure for influenza A, especially during an outbreak in an institution with a high percentage of unvaccinated elderly persons.[69] It is given orally, usually for 2 weeks following influenza vaccine administration, when protective antibodies develop. Central nervous system side effects (such as insomnia, nervous-

ness, and confusion), more common in the elderly population, require careful medical management and dosage adjustment of amantadine. Amantadine-resistant influenza has caused nursing home outbreaks.[71]

Other measures recommended during an outbreak of influenza include restricting admissions or visitors and cohorting of residents with influenza.[63,72,73] It may be advisable to confine residents to their rooms during an outbreak[73]; ill staff should not work.

Tuberculosis

Tuberculosis (TB) also has caused extensive outbreaks in LTCFs, generally traced to a single ambulatory resident. Large numbers of staff and residents may be involved.[74-76] Price and Rutala[77] found 8.1% of new employees and 6.4% of new residents to be positive by the purified protein derivative of tuberculin method in their North Carolina survey, with significant 5-year skin-test conversion rates in both groups.

The diagnosis of TB in the LTCF is problematic. Clinical signs (fever, cough, weight loss) are nonspecific. Chest radiographs, when obtained, often show characteristic pulmonary infiltrates (eg., cavities in the upper lung fields). Infection with TB usually causes a positive tuberculin skin test, although occasional false positives and false negatives are seen. The most specific diagnostic test is a sputum culture for TB, but a good specimen can be difficult to obtain.

Guidelines discussing standards for control of TB in institutions are available.[78-89] A CDC guideline discusses skin testing, isolation, preventive therapy, and contact investigation.[79] There appears to be a consensus that TB skin testing of residents and personnel in the LTCF should be undertaken on a regular basis,[81] although many LTCFs have inadequate TB screening programs.[82] The cost-effectiveness of using a two-step TB skin test to survey for the booster effect is not demonstrable for all populations,[83] but the two-step skin test is recommended by the CDC for initial screening of employees[80] and residents.[79]

Recent advances in microbiology have facilitated the diagnosis of TB greatly. The nucleic acid amplification technique has shortened the time for identification of *Mycobacterium tuberculosis* to several days on smear-positive cases, although susceptibility testing requires several weeks.

There was a resurgence of TB in the United States in the mid-1980s; multidrug-resistant cases of TB have been seen, and nosocomial spread is a concern.[84] In response to this, guidelines have been promulgated by the CDC and the Occupational Safety and Health Administration (OSHA) that address a hierarchy of TB controls in the hospital: administrative control measures (eg, education of personnel), ventilation (e.g. negative air pressure with at least six air exchanges per hour), and personal protective respirators.[80] The necessity and cost-effectiveness of these measures are the object of debate even in hospitals,[85] and the applicability to LTCFs remains to be determined. The CDC guideline states that LTCFs should follow the hospital recommendations.[86] In an LTCF that does not have a negative-pressure room, residents with suspected active TB should be transferred to an appropriate acute-care facility for evaluation. There should be a referral agreement with that facility.

Skin and soft-tissue infections, infestations

Pressure ulcers (also termed decubitus ulcers) occur in up to 20% of residents in LTCFs and are associated with increased mortality.[86,87] Infected pressure ulcers often are deep soft-tissue infections and may have underlying osteomyelitis; secondary bacteremic infections have a 50% mortality rate.[88] They require aggressive medical and surgical therapy.

Medical factors predisposing to pressure ulcers have been delineated[86] and include immobility, pressure, friction, shear, moisture, incontinence, steroids, malnutrition, and infection. Several of these factors may be partially preventable (such as malnutrition and fecal incontinence). Prevention of pressure ulcers involves developing a plan for turning, positioning, eliminating focal pressure, reducing shearing forces, and keeping skin dry.

Many physical and chemical products are available for the purpose of skin protection, debridement, and packing, although controlled studies are lacking in the area of pressure ulcer prevention and healing.[89] A variety of products may be used to relieve or distribute pressure (such as special mattresses, kinetic beds, or foam protectors) or to protect the skin (such as transparent dressings or hydrogels). Nursing measures such as regular turning are essential as well. A pressure-ulcer flow sheet is a useful tool in detecting and monitoring pressure ulcers: recording information such as ulcer location, depth, size, stage, and signs of inflammation, as well as the timing of care measures.

Because all pressure ulcers, like the skin, are colonized with bacteria, antibiotic therapy is not appropriate for a positive surface-swab culture without signs and symptoms of infection.

True infection of a pressure ulcer (cellulitis, osteomyelitis, sepsis) is a serious condition, generally requiring broad-spectrum parenteral antibiotics and surgical debridement in an acute-care facility.

Cellulitis (infection of the skin and soft tissues) can occur either at the site of a previous skin break (pressure ulcer) or spontaneously. Skin infections generally are caused by Group A streptococci or *S. aureus*. Outbreaks of Group A streptococcal infections have been described, presenting as cellulitis, pharyngitis, pneumonia, or septicemia.[90,91]

Scabies is a contagious skin infection caused by a mite. Lesions usually are very pruritic. Scabies causes large outbreaks in long-term–care institutions.[92] Diagnosis in an individual with a rash requires a high index of suspicion, in order to recognize the need for diagnostic skin scrapings. The presence of a proven case should prompt a thorough search for secondary cases. A single treatment with permethrin or lindane usually is effective, but repeated treatment or treatment of all LTCF residents, personnel, and families occasionally is necessary.[93] Therapy of rashes without confirming the diagnosis of scabies unnecessarily exposes residents to the toxic effects of the topical agents. Because scabies can be transmitted by linen and clothing, the environment should be cleaned thoroughly. This includes cleaning inanimate surfaces, hot-cycle washing of washable items (clothing, sheets, towels, etc), and vacuuming the carpet.

Other infections

Viral gastroenteritis,[94] salmonellosis, and *Clostridium perfringens* food poisoning are well-known causes of diarrhea outbreaks in LTCFs. *Escherichia coli* O157:H7, *Clostridium difficile*, and *Giardia lamblia* have been added to the long list of enteric pathogens in the LTCF.[95-99]

The elderly are at increased risk of infectious gastroenteritis due to age-related decrease in gastric acid. In a population with a high prevalence of incontinence, the risk of cross-infection is substantial. Person-to-person spread plays a role in viral gastroenteritis and in *Shigella* and *C. difficile* diarrhea.[100] Foodborne disease outbreaks also are very common in this setting,[101] most often caused by *Salmonella* or *S. aureus*. *E. coli* O157:H7 and *Giardia* also may cause foodborne outbreaks, underscoring the importance of proper food preparation and storage.

Bacteremia[102] in the LTCF, although rarely documented, may be primary or secondary to an

TABLE 1

Common Long-Term–Care Facility Epidemics

Respiratory
   Influenza
   Other respiratory viruses
   Tuberculosis
Gastrointestinal
   Salmonellosis
   Viral gastroenteritis
   Escherichia coli O157:H7 colitis
Other infections
   Scabies
   Conjunctivitis
   Group A streptococcal infections
   Methicillin-resistant *Staphylococcus aureus* infections

infection at another site (pneumonia, UTI). The most common source of secondary bacteremia is the urinary tract.[103] As the acuity of illness in LTCF residents has risen, the prevalence of IV devices and related bacteremic complications appear to have increased. The CDC guideline for prevention of IV infections is a useful resource and generally applicable to the LTCF.[104] Relevant points include aseptic insertion of the IV cannula, daily inspection of the IV for complications such as phlebitis, and quality control of IV fluids and administration sets.

Conjunctivitis in the adult presents as ocular pain, redness, and discharge. In the LTCF, cases may be sporadic or outbreak-associated.[17] Many cases are nonspecific or of viral origin; *S. aureus* appears to be the most frequent bacterial isolate.[105] Epidemic conjunctivitis may spread rapidly through the LTCF. Transmission may occur by contaminated eye drops or hand cross-contamination. Gloves should be worn for contact with eyes or ocular secretions, with handwashing performed immediately after removing gloves.

Many additional infections have been encountered in the LTCF, including herpes zoster, herpes simplex, endocarditis, viral hepatitis, septic arthritis, and abdominal infections. There has been a resurgence of "pediatric" infections in the LTCF (e.g. pertussis, respiratory syncytial virus, and *Haemophilus influenzae* respiratory tract infections), reflecting the decline of the host's immunologic memory with aging.

The elderly nursing home resident is known to have a blunted febrile response to infections.[11] This parallels other age-related immunologic abnormalities. A notable fever in this population often signals a treatable infection, such as urinary tract infection or aspiration pneumonia.

Epidemic nosocomial infections in the long-term–care facility

Most LTCF nosocomial infections are sporadic, but epidemic clustering of infectious diseases can occur. An epidemic, or outbreak, implies the occurrence of cases in excess of the expected number. For TB, this may be a single case. Outbreaks in LTCFs account for a substantial proportion of reported epidemics[196] (Table 1). Garibaldi and coworkers[17] noted clustering of upper respiratory tract infections, diarrhea, conjunctivitis, and multiply antibiotic-resistant bacteriuria. Major outbreaks of infection also have been ascribed to *E. coli*,[95,96] *Streptococcus pyogenes*,[90,91] *C. difficile*,[97,98] respiratory viruses,[52] gastrointestinal viruses,[94] and many other infectious agents. These outbreaks underscore the vulnerability of the elderly to infection, as well as the role of cross-infection in epidemics.[107]

As discussed above, large outbreaks of influenza and TB are well documented. Influenza outbreaks can spread rapidly through the LTCF and result in significant mortality.[52] TB outbreaks are caused by single cases of infected residents and may infect large numbers of residents and staff by the airborne route before detection.[74,81]

During a 12-year period, nursing homes accounted for 2% of all foodborne disease outbreaks reported to the CDC and 19% of outbreak-associated deaths. Salmonellosis was the most frequently reported cause, accounting for 52% of the LTCF outbreaks and 81% of the deaths. The most commonly implicated food vehicles were eggs or egg products. The next most commonly identified cause was *S. aureus*.[101]

Other epidemics are frequent, including scabies and conjunctivitis. Group A streptococcal infections[91] are spread by cross-infection and can cause significant morbidity in residents.

Antibiotic-resistant bacteria

Finally, antibiotic-resistant bacteria, such as MRSA and multiply resistant gram-negative bacteria, are not simply a problem confined to hospitals but cause colonization and infection in LTCFs.[108-113] Both infected and colonized residents may serve as sources for the spread of MRSA in the LTCF.[114] Vancomycin-resistant enterococci (VRE) is a major problem in hospitals and already has spilled over into LTCFs.[115] MRSA in the LTCF poses a particular problem for several reasons. Elderly and disabled residents are at increased risk for colonization with MRSA, and colonized residents tend to carry MRSA for long periods of time.[113] When MRSA becomes endemic within a facility, elimination is unlikely. Spread usually is by the hands of personnel.[114]

The treatment of MRSA infections is limited to vancomycin, a parenteral drug that is more toxic and expensive than beta-lactam antibiotics. Eradication of the MRSA carrier state by oral or topical medications often is impossible. Multi-drug-resistant TB has been seen in hospitals and may spread to nursing homes as well. Long-term–care facilities can expect outbreaks of highly resistant organisms to be a continuing problem. The isolation of residents colonized or infected by resistant organisms is discussed under "Antibiotic Use and Resistance" (below).

THE INFECTION CONTROL PROGRAM

Evolution of programs

The 1980s saw a dramatic increase in LTCF infection control activities, stimulated by federal and state regulations. Several studies provide insight into the extent of program development. A 1981 survey of Utah LTCFs[17] noted that all facilities had regular infection control meetings, but none performed systematic surveillance for infections or conducted regular infection control training. All LTCFs had policies regarding the maintenance and care of urinary catheters, although the policies were not uniform. Price and associates[21] surveyed 12 North Carolina LTCFs in 1985 and found that, although all 12 had a designated ICP, none of the ICPs had received special training in this area. Also noted were deficiencies in isolation facilities, particularly an insufficient number of sinks and recirculated, inadequately filtered air.

In a 1985 survey of Minnesota LTCFs, Crossley and colleagues[116] found that the majority had an ICC and a designated ICP, although substantial deficiencies in resident and employee health programs occurred. For instance, only 61% offered the influenza vaccine to residents, and one third did not screen new employees for a history of infectious disease problems. A 1988 Maryland survey[117] found that one third of nursing homes still performed routine environmental cultures, and many lacked proper isolation policies. In 1990, a survey of Connecticut LTCFs found that most ICPs had received some training in infection control.[118,119] Most LTCFs performed surveillance at least weekly, and most used written criteria to determine nosocomial infections.

A more recent survey[120] noted increasing infection control activity in Maryland nursing homes

in 1994. The mean time spent on infection control activities by the infection control staff was 9 hours per week, of which approximately half was spent on surveillance. Seventy-eight percent of the LTCFs reported a systematic surveillance system, and 59% calculated infection rates. All facilities reportedly used Universal Precautions in caring for their residents.

From these surveys, one can develop a composite picture of the LTCF ICP as an individual who spends 8 to 57 hours per month on infection control activities, depending on facility size, resident acuity, and facility commitment to infection control. The ICP frequently has other duties such as general duty nursing, nursing supervision, in-service education, employee health, and quality assurance.[3]

Regulatory aspects

Long-term–care facilities are covered by federal, state, and voluntary-agency guidelines.[121,122] Skilled nursing facilities are required by the Omnibus Budget Reconciliation Act of 1987 (OBRA) to have an infection control program.[123] The Health Care Financing Administration (HCFA) has published requirements for LTCFs[124] that apply to LTCFs accepting Medicare or Medicaid residents. HCFA regulations address the need for an infection control program, surveillance of infections, isolation, employee health, and handwashing.[124,125] For example, the LTCF is required to have an infection control program to investigate, control, and prevent infections in the facility. An infection control committee per se no longer is required. Interpretive guidelines for surveyors further discuss definitions of infection, risk assessment, outbreak control, antibiotic monitoring, and assessment of compliance with infection control policies.[126]

Because the LTCF is an employer of healthcare workers, it must comply with federal and state OSHA guidelines. Standards[127,128] deal primarily with protection of workers from exposure to bloodborne pathogens such as human immunodeficiency virus (HIV) and hepatitis B virus (HBV) and from TB exposure.[80] Adherence of LTCFs to infection control standards is an OSHA priority.

Other standards that apply to LTCFs include the federal minimum requirements for construction and equipment[129] and the Joint Commission on Accreditation of Healthcare Organizations' (JCAHO) Long-Term Care Standards.[130] The 1996 JCAHO standards for long-term care require a coordinated infection control process with clinical, nursing, and administrative oversight; it deals

TABLE 2

Long-Term–Care Facility Infection Control Elements

Oversight Committee, which directs the
Infection Control Practitioner, who directs the
Infection Control Functions
    Surveillance
    Outbreak control
    Isolation and precautions
    Policies and procedures
    Education
    Resident health program
    Employee health program
    Antibiotic review
    Disease reporting
    Other functions

with sick employees, handwashing, surveillance, and control issues.[130] In addition, many states have statutory requirements for LTCFs that vary widely.[131]

The LTCF administrative staff should be knowledgeable about the federal, state, and local regulations dealing with infection control in order to conduct a program in compliance with these regulations. The LTCF ICP ideally should be involved in the formation and revision of regulations, through local and national infection control and long-term–care organizations, to help assure the scientific validity of the regulations.

Components of an Infection Prevention and Control Program

Overview

Several authors have discussed the components of an infection control program in the LTCF.[3,16,50,122,132,133] These components generally are drawn from regulatory requirements, current nursing home practices, and extrapolations from hospital programs. The limited resources of most LTCFs affect the type and extent of programs developed.[16] Most authors feel that an infection control program should include some form of surveillance for infections, an epidemic control program, education of employees in infection control methods, policy and procedure formation and review, an employee health program, a resident health program, and monitoring of resident-care practices. The program also may be involved in quality management (QM), environmental review, antibiotic monitoring, product review and evaluation, and reporting of diseases to public health authorities. The elements of an infection control program are shown in Table 2.

An ICP is an essential component of an effective infection control program and is the person designated by the facility to be responsible for infection control. The regulatory requirement for a nursing home ICC was dropped by OBRA at the federal level, but some states still require them.[124] The ICP should be familiar with state regulations. This committee frequently has been less active than the corresponding ICC in the hospital setting, in part because of decreased physician availability. A small working group consisting of the ICP, the administrator, and the medical director may efficiently make most of the infection control decisions. The ICC functions may be merged with the quality management committee, but infection control must remain identifiable as a distinct program. Whatever group is selected to oversee the infection control program, it should meet regularly to review infection control data, review policies, and monitor program goals and activities. Records of meetings should be kept.

The ICP usually is a staff nurse, a background that is helpful for resident assessment and chart review. The ICP most commonly is a registered nurse. Because of size and staffing limitations, the vast majority of LTCF ICPs have other duties, such as assistant director of nursing, charge nurse, in-service coordinator, employee health, or quality management. The number of LTCF beds justifying a full-time ICP is unknown and usually depends on the acuity level of residents and the level of care provided. A LTCF with more than 250 to 300 beds may need a full-time ICP. The LTCF ICP, like the hospital ICP, requires specific training in infection control, well-defined support from administration, and the ability to interact tactfully with personnel, physicians, and residents.

The LTCF administrative staff should support the ICP with appropriate educational opportunities and resources, including expert consultation in infectious diseases and infection control as needed. Participation of a physician with training or experience in infectious diseases and infection control should be considered on at least a consultative basis. Information may be obtained from the Society for Healthcare Epidemiology of America (SHEA; 609-845-1636). The local health department may have useful information, and local ICPs are another valuable source of information.[134]

A few courses are available. The Association for Professionals in Infection Control and Epidemiology offers a training course for hospital and LTCF infection control professionals (202-

296-2742). The Nebraska Infection Control Network offers regular 2-day basic training courses specifically for LTCF infection control ICPs (402-552-2360), and other local courses are available. SHEA offers courses in hospital infection control for physicians (609-845-1636).

Surveillance. Infection surveillance in the LTCF involves the collection of data on nosocomial infections. Traditionally, outcome measures (such as "number of UTIs") are used, rather than process measures (such as "Was correct catheter-care procedure followed?"). Quality improvement methods focusing on process (such as antibiotic appropriateness studies) often are quite useful and may measure process variation. Surveillance data are used primarily to plan control activities and educational programs and to prevent epidemics, but surveillance also may detect infections that require therapeutic action.

The feasibility of routine surveillance in LTCFs has been demonstrated, and data have been used to provide a basis for continuing education.[30] Surveillance needs to be simple and pragmatic, particularly because the ICP may be able to spend only a few hours per week on infection control activities.

Surveillance requires objective, valid definitions of infections. Most hospital surveillance definitions are based on the National Nosocomial Infections Surveillance (NNIS) System criteria,[135] but no such standard exists for long-term care. NNIS definitions depend heavily on laboratory data and recorded clinical observations. In the LTCF, radiology and microbiology data are less available, and written physician notes and nursing assessments in the medical record usually are brief. Timely detection of nosocomial infections in the LTCF often depends on recognition of clues to infection by nurses' aides and reporting of these findings to the licensed nursing staff.[136] Positive cultures do not necessarily signify infection.

Modified LTCF-specific surveillance criteria were developed by a Canadian consensus conference.[137] These definitions were designed in light of some of the unique limitations of nursing home surveillance mentioned previously. They are used widely, although they have not yet been validated in the field.[138]

The surveillance process consists of collecting data on individual cases and determining whether or not a nosocomial infection is present by comparing collected data to standard written definitions (criteria) of infections. One recommended data-collection method in the LTCF is "walking rounds."[134] This is a means of collecting concurrent and prospective infection data that are necessary to make infection control decisions. Surveillance should be done on a timely basis, probably at least weekly.[137] During rounds, the ICP may use house reports from nursing staff, chart review, laboratory or radiology reports, treatment review, and clinical observations as sources of information. Monthly computer printouts of antibiotic use may be available from pharmacies, and monthly computer printouts of cultures and susceptibilities may be available from medical laboratories.

Published LTCF surveys have been either incidence or prevalence studies. Prevalence studies detect the number of existing (old and new) cases in a population at a given time, whereas incidence studies find new cases during a defined time period. The latter is preferred, because more current information can be collected by an incidence study if data are collected with regularity.

Analysis and reporting of infection case data usually are done monthly, quarterly, and annually to detect trends. This process is facilitated by an individual infection report form, samples of which have been published.[50,122,132]

Analysis of absolute numbers of infections is misleading; calculation of rates provides the most accurate information. Rates may be calculated by using resident days or average resident census for the surveillance period (such as month, quarter, or year) as the denominator. The average daily census is not an accurate denominator for hospitals; however, it can be used by LTCFs, because the facility usually is full, and resident turnover is less than in acute-care facilities.

For example, if in a 30-day month an LTCF with an average census of 200 has 15 new nosocomial infections:

Infection (incidence) rate =

$$\frac{\text{Number of new nosocomial infections}}{\text{Number of resident days in the month}} \times 1,000 =$$

$$\frac{15}{(30)(200)} \times 1,000 =$$

2.5 infections per 1,000 resident days

The preferred rate is infections per 1,000 resident days. Infection control data, including rates, then need to be displayed and distributed to appropriate committees and personnel (including administration) and used in planning infection control efforts. The data should lead to specific educational and control programs. To compare rates within a facility or to other facilities, the method of calculation must be identical (including the denominator). Even when calculation methods are consistent, infection rates may vary between facilities because of differences in resident risk factors and disease severity, and comparisons may not be valid.

Although facility-wide surveillance is useful for calculating baseline rates and detecting outbreaks, a more detailed analysis could include examination of infection rates in residents who are at risk for certain kinds of infection (such as aspiration pneumonia in residents receiving tube feedings or UTI in nonambulatory residents). Facility-wide surveillance is useful for establishing an infection control "presence" in the LTCF and may be required as a part of local or state regulatory programs. To establish baseline infection rates, track progress, determine trends, and detect outbreaks, site-specific rates should be calculated. Routine analysis should try to explain the variation in site-specific rates. For example, a change in the rate might be related to a change in the resident population. Focused or high-risk resident surveillance may permit conservation of resources.

Published studies of LTCF infections have yet to describe adequately the specific risk factors (eg, device use) for site-specific infections. When such data become available, appropriate risk stratification of infection rates might be a worthwhile objective for this field of practice. This also could lead to focusing resources on those residents at highest risk for developing infections. Also needed are methods that are simple and appropriate for the comparison of site-specific data within an LTCF over time, to establish endemic levels of infection and to recognize potential outbreaks.

The statistics used in analysis of data need not be complex. Computerization for sorting and analysis of data may be time-saving for larger programs, and software for use on a personal computer is available. Graphs and charts facilitate presentation and understanding of infection control data and also may be facilitated by computer programs. The commercially available programs may help with analysis of surveillance data, but manual data collection is still necessary.

Outbreak control. An important reason to collect and analyze surveillance data is for the early detection and prevention of infectious disease outbreaks. The leading causes of LTCF outbreaks are discussed above and listed in Table 1. When the number of cases exceeds the normal baseline, an outbreak should be considered. Even a single new case of an infection such as TB or MRSA should trigger an evaluation.

The approach to investigation of an outbreak involves a number of steps, including (1) determining if an outbreak has occurred, (2) developing a case definition, (3) analyzing the outbreak, (4) formulating a hypothesis, (5) designating control measures, (6) evaluating control measures, and (7) making a report. Concurrently, the potential for spread of disease is evaluated and addressed.[139]

The LTCF may have difficulty responding to an epidemic with appropriate therapeutic measures (such as mass vaccination or administration of amantadine in an influenza outbreak) if consent needs to be obtained on short notice from a resident's relatives or the primary physician. One way to circumvent this problem is to develop a policy for obtaining prospective consent that gives the medical director or administrator the power to act in an infectious disease emergency. Ultimately, outbreak prevention depends on key prevention strategies (such as influenza and pneumococcal vaccination), and the LTCF can obtain consent for pneumococcal vaccine and yearly influenza vaccine on admission.

Isolation and precautions. An isolation and precautions system is an important means of preventing cross-infection. The use of barrier precautions in LTCFs has been handicapped by lack of adequate handwashing facilities, private rooms, and appropriate ventilation systems.[23]

Two traditional systems for implementing barrier precautions in the hospital were developed by the CDC.[140] The Category-Specific System listed seven categories of isolation or precautions based on means of disease transmission: strict isolation, contact isolation, respiratory isolation, TB isolation, enteric precautions, drainage and secretion precautions, and blood and body fluid precautions. The Disease-Specific System listed all relevant contagious diseases and the recommended barrier method. In general, the Category-Specific System was simpler to use, but the Disease-Specific System consumed fewer resources, because precautions were tailored to the specific disease. A third isolation system, Body Substance Isolation, was a generic precautions system that emphasized isolation of all moist and potentially infectious body substances from all residents, primarily through glove use.[141]

The human immunodeficiency virus profoundly affected institutional isolation issues. Subsequent CDC guidelines and OSHA regulations mandate the concept of Universal Precautions (UP) designed to protect the healthcare worker from bloodborne pathogens, including HIV and

HBV.[127,128,142,143] In this system, all blood and certain body fluids are potentially infectious. Education, provision of needle-disposal units, provision of protective equipment (such as gloves, gowns, and protective eye wear), and monitoring compliance are part of UP. UP by itself is not a complete isolation system.

The newest CDC isolation guideline is an attempt to integrate and update the four systems above.[144] This two-tiered system consists of basic Standard Precautions, to be applied to all patients, which are designed to reduce the risk of transmission of infectious agents in moist body secretions. Standard Precautions emphasize handwashing, gloves (when touching body fluids), masks, eye protection, and gowns (when splashing of body fluids is likely), as well as avoidance of needlestick and other sharps injuries. There are additional Transmission-Based Precautions for patients with documented or suspected contagious pathogens. These include Airborne Precautions (eg, for varicella and TB), Droplet Precautions (eg, for influenza and streptococcal pneumonia), and Contact Precautions (eg, for MRSA infection and Salmonella diarrhea). The guideline lists specific symptoms that are highly suspicious for infection and suggests using Transmission-Based Precautions temporarily until a diagnosis is made.

The CDC guideline was developed for hospitals but states that some of the recommendations are applicable to LTCFs.[144] This two-tiered system is a reasonable basis on which to build an LTCF isolation system; each LTCF needs to adapt the aspects of the CDC isolation system that apply to its needs. Isolation and precautions policies need to define authority. The nurse should have the authority to initiate precautions without a physician's order in an emergency, and a policy for this should be developed.

Handwashing appears to be the most important infection control measure in the LTCF, as well as in the hospital. Unfortunately, inadequate handwashing has been noted in LTCFs, as in other settings.[145,146] Several published guidelines for handwashing and choice of antiseptic agents are applicable.[147,148] In general, handwashing with bar or liquid soap is adequate in the LTCF. Handwashing with an antiseptic agent is recommended before invasive procedures such as placement of an intravenous or urinary catheter. Alcohol-based handrubs are recommended only when handwashing facilities are not accessible.

Several conditions, such as TB and major wound infections caused by *S aureus*, require use of a private room, if the LTCF has adequate isolation facilities. For certain infections that have significant implications for the LTCF (such as TB, MRSA, and VRE), the facility should assess its isolation needs and capabilities before facing admission of a case. Tuberculosis cases, for example, require a negative–air-pressure room with at least six air exchanges per hour and special masks.[80] The air should not be recirculated unless it passes through a high-efficiency filter.

Infections are an important reason for transfer of LTCF residents to acute-care hospitals.[149] LTCF-hospital transfers result in a dynamic microbiological equilibrium, making interinstitutional epidemics a concern. Minimizing spread of hazardous organisms requires open and honest communication between hospital and LTCF ICPs.

Resident health. Resident health programs are believed to be important in prevention of nosocomial infections,[138] but comprehensive programs often are lacking in LTCFs.[21] One of the major functions of a resident health program is the immunization of the elderly resident.[61,62,150] In addition to the basic childhood vaccines, residents benefit from tetanus, diphtheria, pneumococcal, and influenza immunizations. The elderly are underserved in terms of immunization to tetanus,[151] as well as pneumococcal and influenza vaccines.[152] The elderly should receive pneumococcal vaccine at age 65, when they are relatively immunologically responsive, rather than at age 80 to 85 when entering the LTCF. The influenza vaccine should be given annually in the fall.

It is required that residents receive a TB skin test on admission[79] and undergo chest radiograph if skin-test positive or symptomatic. Other resident-care practices that should be addressed include prevention of aspiration, skin care, prevention of UTIs, and oral hygiene.

Employee health. Published information on infection control in hospital personnel is available.[153,154] Employee infection control considerations in the LTCF are somewhat different than in the hospital (eg, hepatitis B and measles are lesser concerns), but these articles generally apply to the LTCF. LTCFs are required to prohibit employees with communicable diseases or infected skin lesions from direct contact with residents and to prohibit employees with potentially infectious skin lesions from contact with residents' food.[124] Also, OSHA regulations concerning protection of employees from bloodborne pathogens apply to the LTCF.[127,143] The LTCF should be able to provide chemoprophylaxis to employees exposed to HIV in the workplace.[155]

Initial assessment of employees and education in infection control also are important, as is a reasonable sick-leave policy.[116] Ill employees may cause significant outbreaks in the LTCF.[94] Tuberculosis is a primary concern in initial employee screening.[79,80] Employee health policies and procedures also should address postexposure follow-up or prophylaxis for certain infections, such as HIV, HBV, TB, and scabies. Employee vaccinations include tetanus, diphtheria, influenza, and HBV (if exposure to blood or body fluids occurs). Varicella vaccine is indicated if an employee is not immune, and hepatitis A vaccine may be appropriate in certain circumstances (especially psychiatric facilities and facilities for the mentally impaired).

Education. The value of education of the LTCF ICP has long been recognized, and surveys of personnel confirm this need.[156] The importance of ICP education is accentuated by the great turnover in LTCF personnel. While the benefits of ICP training are widely assumed, one study analyzed the effects of a 2-day, intensive basic training program on 266 ICPs.[157,158] Trainees not only demonstrated an increase in postcourse knowledge but, at 3- and 12-month follow-up, had a significant increase in implementation of key infection control practices. Practices included performance of surveillance, using infection definitions, calculating infection rates, and giving employees and residents TB skin tests and influenza vaccine.

One of the most important roles of the ICP is education of LTCF personnel in basic infection control principles. Education should focus on new personnel and nursing aides.[122] Surveillance data are an excellent starting point for infection control training, and walking rounds provides an opportunity for the ICP to provide timely, informal education to personnel. Infection control content should include information on disease transmission, handwashing, barrier precautions, and basic hygiene.[157] In addition, all individuals with direct resident-care responsibility need education in early problem or symptom recognition. The teaching methods used need to be sensitive to language, cultural background, and educational level. A coordinated, effective educational program will result in improved infection control activities.[158]

Antibiotic use and resistance. Antibiotic-resistant bacteria pose a significant hazard in the LTCF, and this resistance develops largely as a consequence of antibiotic use. Antibiotics are given to approximately 7% to 10% of residents in LTCFs, frequently for lengthy periods of time.[159-161] Several studies have questioned the appropriateness of this practice.[159-161] A common problem is the confusion of infection with colonization (such as a positive swab culture of a pressure ulcer or a urine culture showing bacteriuria without signs or symptoms of infection) and the treatment of the colonization with antibiotics. In addition, antibiotics often are prescribed over the telephone in this setting.[162] A recent position paper published by SHEA encourages inclusion of antimicrobial review in the LTCF infection control program and discusses appropriate choices for various clinical situations.[163]

Approaches to isolation of MRSA in the LTCF vary. Transfer of MRSA patients between hospitals and nursing homes often is problematic, which led a number of states to develop MRSA guidelines. Barrier precautions are necessary to prevent cross-infection with known resistant microorganisms (such as MRSA and VRE). General guidelines for control of MRSA[114] and VRE[164] are published, but emphasize hospital settings. These guidelines serve as an appropriate starting point for adapting an LTCF approach. A SHEA position paper on antimicrobial resistance, focused on the LTCF,[165] discusses prescreening admissions for resistant bacteria, surveillance for resistant bacteria, and endemic resistance. It is not recommended that the LTCF refuse MRSA or VRE cases, but rather develop an institutional strategy for control of the resistant organisms based on local considerations.[113,114,165]

HIV-related issues. The increasing burden of care for persons with AIDS is being shared by the LTCF, especially for individuals who are too ill to reside at home but do not require acute-hospital care.

Guidelines for dealing with HIV infection in the healthcare setting are incorporated widely in hospitals but also apply in the LTCF.[142,143,166] Information is available that discusses HIV infection and AIDS in the LTCF.[167] Issues to be considered include development of policies for acceptance of residents with HIV infection, protection of employees (such as needle-disposal units), education of employees, HIV-positive employees, confidentiality issues, cost of care, and social concerns. For example, needle-stick injuries do occur in the LTCF and usually are related to needle recapping.[168]

Residents infected with HIV do not require any isolation or precautions beyond those previously discussed unless they have certain contagious secondary infections, such as pulmonary TB (see

TABLE 3

Classification of the Strength and Quality of Evidence of Each Recommendation

Category	Definition
Categories reflecting the strength of the recommendation	
A	Good evidence to support the recommendation
B	Moderate evidence to support the recommendation
C	Poor evidence to support the recommendation
Categories reflecting the quality of evidence for the recommendation	
I	Evidence from at least one properly randomized, controlled trial.
II	Evidence from at least one well-designed clinical trial without randomization, from cohort or case-controlled analytic studies (preferably from more than one center), from multiple time-series studies, or from dramatic results in uncontrolled experiments.
III	Evidence from opinions of respected authorities, based on clinical experience, descriptive studies, or reports of expert committees.

"Isolation and Precautions"). The institution should develop plans for HIV-related issues. At least one survey has suggested the need for education in the LTCF regarding AIDS-related attitudes,[169] and such education is required by OSHA regulations.[127]

Other aspects of the program. An important aspect of infection control programs is the development and updating of infection control policies and procedures. Resources are available on the writing of policies and procedures in general,[125,170] dietetic service policies,[125] laundry policies,[171] physical therapy policies,[125,172,173] and handwashing.[147,148] Respiratory therapy issues may be relevant to the LTCF, including cleaning of humidifiers, respiratory therapy equipment, suctioning technique, and tracheotomy care.[56] Pharmacy and medication issues include use of multidose medication vials.

No policy or procedure is more important than that of addressing handwashing. The policy details specific indications for handwashing (including when coming on duty; whenever hands are soiled; after personal use of toilet; after blowing or wiping nose; after contact with resident blood or body secretions; before per-

forming any invasive procedures on a resident; after leaving an isolation room; after handling items such as dressings, bedpans, catheters, or urinals; after removing gloves; before eating; and on completion of duty), and the procedure lists explicit steps in the handwashing process. A 10-second handwash usually is recommended.[50,148] When handwashing facilities are inadequate or inaccessible, alcohol-based handrubs should be made available. Handwashing compliance should be monitored.

The ICP is concerned with the environment in the facility. While routine environmental cultures are not cost-effective, periodic environmental rounds are recommended.[122] Sources are available suggesting specific environmental measures such as dishwasher and laundry cleaning temperatures,[122,174] although limited data exist.

Selection of proper disinfectants and antiseptics is difficult and requires the input of the ICP. The participation of the ICP also is essential in evaluating sterilization and disinfection methods, such as monitoring reuse of disposable equipment. Resources are available.[175]

The ICP should be asked to give advice on additional and new products that affect infection prevention, such as urinary catheter systems, gloves, and disposable diapers. Quality, efficacy, and cost issues need to be weighed in product selection.[176]

Medical waste issues are controversial, and there is a disparity between Environmental Protection Agency regulations and CDC recommendations.[177] The ICP may be involved in medical waste issues relevant to the LTCF, and several resources are available.[125,174,177,178]

Another important function of the infection control program is *disease reporting* to public health authorities. State health departments provide a list of reportable diseases.

Finally, the increased emphasis on *QM* in health care is becoming evident in long-term care. A quality assessment and assurance committee is required.[124] Infection control is an important form of QM, and the ICP's skills are well suited to addressing QM measurement issues.[179] The QM process focuses on adverse events and assesses functions of the system.[180,181] In the course of performing control activities such as surveillance, the ICP is able to monitor compliance with policies and procedures and to provide informal infection control education to correct observed problems. Examples of appropriate quality indicators for longitudinal study include percentage of employees vaccinated for influenza, number of employee TB skin-test conversions, and employee handwashing compliance.

RESOURCES

A few resources for the ICP are listed below:

1.   Smith PW, ed. Infection Control in Long-Term Care Facilities. 2nd ed. Albany, NY: Delmar Publishers, Inc (800-347-7707); 1994. Cost, $38.95.

2.   APIC Infection Control in Long-Term Care Facilities Newsletter. Available from the Association for Professionals in Infection Control and Epidemiology (202-296-2742). Cost for nonmembers, $15.

3.   Strausbaugh, LJ, Joseph C. Epidemiology and prevention of infections in residents of long-term care facilities. In: Mayhall CG, ed. Hospital Epidemiology and Infection Control. Baltimore, MD: Williams & Wilkins (800-638-0672); 1996. Cost, $160.

4.   Duma RJ, ed. Recognition and Management of Nursing Home Infections. Bethesda, MD: National Foundation for Infectious Diseases (301-656- 0003); 1992.

Cost, $6.

5.   Benenson AS, ed. Control of Communicable Diseases in Man.16th ed. Washington, DC: American Public Health Association. Cost, $22.

RECOMMENDATIONS (See Table 3 for scoring scheme)

A. Infection Control Program

1. An active, effective, facility-wide infection control program should be established in the LTCF to help prevent the development and spread of infectious diseases (Category BIII). Comment: LTCF infection control programs developed in response to studies of LTCF infections and regulations. The elements of a program generally include the following:

   a. Surveillance based on systematic data collection to identify infections in residents

   b. A system for detection, investigation, and control of institutional outbreaks of infectious diseases

   c. An isolation and precautions system to reduce the risk of transmission of infectious agents

   d. Infection control policies and procedures

   e. Continuing education in infection prevention and control

   f. A resident health program

   g. An employee health program

   h. A system for antibiotic review and control

   i. Disease reporting to public health authorities

2. The infection control program must be in compliance with federal, state, and local regulations.

B. Infection Control Administrative Structure

1. Oversight of the infection control program should include participation of the ICP, administration, nursing staff, and physician staff (Category BIII).

Comment: A committee, traditionally the ICC, may oversee the infection control program for the facility. ICC members often include the ICP, the medical director, and representatives from nursing, administration, and pharmacy. Participation of other departments, such as dietary, housekeeping, and physical therapy, should be considered on an ad hoc basis. Administrative structures other than an ICC may provide oversight to the infection control program. One example of an infection control oversight committee is a small group consisting of the LTCF administrator, the ICP, and the medical director. Alternatively, the quality management committee and the ICC may be combined, but it is important to maintain the identity of the infection control program. The duties of the ICC should be delegated appropriately if no formal ICC exists. Consultation may be obtained from an infectious disease physician with expertise in infection control.

2. Management of the infection control program involves establishing policies and procedures for investigating, controlling, and preventing infection transmission in the facility. Other functions include review of infection control data, approval of policies and procedures, monitoring program activities, and recommending policy to the facility administration (Category BIII).

Comment: Those responsible for infection control program oversight should meet on a regular basis and as needed for emergent situations and should keep written minutes of all meetings. The minutes should reflect problem identification and follow-up action.

C. Infection Control Practitioner

1. One person, the ICP, should be assigned the responsibility of directing infection control activities in the LTCF. The ICP should be someone familiar with LTCF resident-care problems (Category BIII).

2. The ICP should have a written job description of infection control duties (Category BIII).

3. The ICP is responsible for implementing, monitoring, and evaluating the infection control program for the LTCF (Category BIII).

4. The ICP requires the support of administration in order to function effectively (Category BIII).

5. The ICP should be guaranteed sufficient time to direct the infection control program (Category BIII).

6. The ICP (or another appropriate individual, such as the medical director) should have written authority to institute infection control measures (such as isolation or visitor restrictions) in emergency situations (Category BIII).

Comment: The ICP should have a sufficient infection control knowledge base to carry out responsibilities appropriately. A background in infectious diseases, microbiology, geriatrics, and educational methods is advisable. Management and teaching skills also are helpful. Continuing education is essential for the

ICP (eg, meetings, courses, journals). The ICP should know the federal, state, and local regulations dealing with infection control in the LTCF.

Communication is an important part of infection control. The ICP should communicate with relevant facility committees and personnel. The ICP should communicate openly with hospital ICPs about residents transferred into or out of the LTCF, to ensure appropriate isolation and collection of surveillance information.

D. Surveillance

1. The LTCF should have a system for ongoing collection of data on infections in the institution (Category BIII).

2. A documented surveillance procedure should be used, including written definitions of infections (Category BIII).

Comment: Concurrent surveillance is preferable to retrospective surveillance. The frequency of surveillance for nosocomial infections should be based on factors such as acuity level of the resident population. Surveillance at least once a week generally is needed to collect timely data.

Surveillance data should be collected primarily from communication with staff; this may be during walking rounds in the LTCF. Medical progress notes in the chart, laboratory or radiology reports, nursing notes, treatment records, medication records, physical assessment, environmental observations, and follow-up information from transfers to acute-care hospitals provide clues to the presence of infections.

3. The ICP should review surveillance data frequently and recommend infection control measures, as appropriate, in response to identified problems (Category BIII).

Comment: Analysis of surveillance data should include at least the following elements on each infection to detect clusters and trends: type of infection, date of onset, location in the facility, and appropriate culture information. An infection surveillance report form facilitates recording of data on residents with nosocomial infections.

4. Infection rates should be calculated periodically, recorded, analyzed, and reported to the administration and the ICC (Category BIII).

Comment: Infection rates usually are calculated monthly, quarterly, and annually. Nosocomial infection rates are calculated preferably as nosocomial infections per 1,000 resident days. A standard infection report form facilitates reporting of surveillance information. Tables, graphs, and charts may be used, and facilitate education of personnel.

5. Surveillance data should be used for planning infection control efforts, detecting epidemics, directing continuing education, and identifying individual resident problems for intervention (Category BIII).

Comment: In addition to collection of baseline infection rates, the ICP should perform problem-focused studies. Examples of special studies are evaluation of UTIs in catheterized residents, a study of the occurrence of influenza in vaccinated versus unvaccinated residents, or the prevalence of pressure ulcers in bed-bound residents.

E. Outbreak Control

1. Surveillance data should be used to detect and prevent outbreaks in the LTCF (Category BIII).

Comment: The occurrence of even a single verified case of a disease of epidemiological significance (such as nosocomial TB, influenza, or VRE infection) in the LTCF should prompt consideration of an outbreak, notification of appropriate individuals (such as the administrator or medical director), and a search for additional cases. A nosocomial case of TB in the facility should lead to TB skin testing and evaluation of residents and employees.

After the institution of isolation or precautions, assessment of exposed residents and personnel should be made in a timely fashion to detect other cases. Obtaining cultures of the environment or personnel is not recommended except as targeted by an epidemic investigation.

2. The facility should define authority for intervention during an outbreak (Category BIII).

Comment: The LTCF should have an administrative protocol for dealing with infectious disease epidemics, including the authority to relocate residents, confine residents to their rooms, restrict visitors, obtain cultures, isolate, and administer relevant prophylaxis or treatment (such as amantadine during an influenza outbreak).

In order to facilitate response to an outbreak, consent for appropriate diagnostic or therapeutic measures should be obtained from the resident, the resident's family, or the resident's primary physician on admission to the facility.

3. A TB control program should focus on detection of cases in residents, periodic

screening of employees, and isolation or transfer of residents with known or suspected TB disease (Category BIII).

Comment: TB control programs are mandated by OSHA.

F. The Facility

1. Handwashing facilities that are conveniently located with adequate supplies should be available for residents and staff (Category BIII).

2. Clean and dirty utility areas should be functionally separate and designated (Category BIII).

3. Appropriate ventilation and air filtration should be addressed by the LTCF (Category BIII).

Comment: Each LTCF should be able to provide a room with negative air pressure and direct exhaust of air to the outside if TB cases are handled in the LTCF. If TB cases cannot be handled, a system for transfer of suspected TB cases to an appropriate institution should be developed.

4. Housekeeping in the facility should be performed on a routine and consistent basis to provide for a safe and sanitary environment (Category BIII).

Comment: Cleaning schedules should be kept for all areas in the LTCF. Cleaning products should be approved by the ICP or the ICC and labeled appropriately; manufacturers' (or other authoritative) recommendations for use and dilution should be followed.

5. Measures should be instituted to correct unsafe and unsanitary practices (Category BIII).

Comment: Environmental cleanliness may be monitored by walking rounds with a checklist for each area of the LTCF. Nursing interventions may be monitored by direct observation during such rounds.

6. Areas in the LTCF with unique infection control concerns (eg, laundry, kitchen, physical therapy) should have appropriate policies and procedures developed (Category BIII).

Comment: Laundry policies and procedures should address the following: proper bagging of linen at the site of use, transporting linen in appropriate carts, cleaning of the carts on a regular basis, separation of clean and dirty linen, washing temperatures, covering of clean linen, protection of personnel handling dirty laundry, and handwashing after contact with dirty linen. Adequate supplies of clean linen should be available. Laundry regulations should be addressed if the facility does its own laundry. Dietetic-service–area policies and procedures should address the following: handling of uncooked foods, cooking of food, cleaning of food preparation areas, food storage, cooking and refrigeration temperatures, hygienic practices, dishwashing temperatures, cleaning of ice machines, handwashing indications, and employee health. Food and drink should be limited to specific areas.

Policies and procedures covering infection control aspects of physical therapy (including cleaning of hydrotherapy tanks) should be developed. It should include cleaning and disinfection of hydrotherapy equipment, handwashing indications, and cleaning of exercise equipment.

If pets are allowed, the LTCF should have a policy defining access, containment, cleanliness, and vaccination of pets.

7. Policies and procedures for disposal of infectious medical waste (including waste categorization, packaging, collection, transport, and disposal) should be developed in accordance with federal, state, and local regulations (Category BIII).

Comment: Examples of specific issues include types of waste disposal bags, cleaning of waste transportation carts, and types of waste storage containers. Policies for sharps disposal should be developed.

G. Isolation and Precautions

1. Isolation and precautions policies and procedures should be developed, evaluated, and updated. Compliance (eg, with handwashing) should be monitored (Category BIII).

2. Any isolation and precautions system used should include wearing of masks, eye protection, and gowns when contamination or splashing with blood or body fluids is likely (Category BIII).

3. Used needles and syringes should not be manually recapped, broken, or bent. They should be disposed of, with all sharps, in a puncture-resistant, leak-proof container (Category BIII).

4. Gloves are indicated for contact with blood or body fluids, contaminated items, mucous membranes, or nonintact skin (Category BIII).

5. Policies should be developed to deal with spills and personnel exposure to blood or body fluids. Employees should know how to respond to an exposure (eg, washing the skin in the event of a blood exposure) (Category BIII).

6. The facility should have infection control policies dealing with acceptance and transfer of residents with infectious diseases (Category BIII).

Comment: A variety of isolation systems may be appropriate to the LTCF. All should include the concept of UP for prevention of exposure to bloodborne pathogens. Masks, gowns, and gloves should be provided as appropriate. Private rooms used for isolation or precautions should have readily accessible toilet and handwashing facilities and should be identified by precautionary signs. A new CDC guideline[145] simplifies isolation by proposing a two-tiered system, Standard Precautions (similar to UP) and Transmission-Based Precautions.

H. Asepsis and Handwashing

1. Handwashing must be encouraged. Hands should be washed after contact with body fluids, after removing gloves, when soiled, and when otherwise indicated (Category AII).

Comment: Handwashing with plain soap is adequate for most situations in the LTCF.

2. A handwashing policy and procedure should be developed by the LTCF (Category BIII).

Comment: Issues such as indications for handwashing, selection of handwashing agent, cleaning of soap containers, hand lotion use, and use of alcohol-based antiseptic handrubs should be addressed. The institution should monitor handwashing compliance.

3. Policies and procedures for disinfection and sterilization should be developed (Category BIII).

Comment: These policies and procedures should address issues such as sterile supplies, reuse of disposable items, disinfection of equipment (such as thermometers), and cleaning of non-critical items. All items, other than disposables, should be cleaned, disinfected, or sterilized, following published guidelines and manufacturers' recommendations. The ICP should identify those resident-care procedures that require aseptic technique.

I. Resident Care

1. Resident rooms should have an accessible sink, with soap, water, towels, and toilet facilities (Category BIII).

Comment: Provision should be made for maintaining adequate resident personal hygiene and for instructing residents in hygiene and handwashing as appropriate to their functional status.

2. A resident skin-care program should be developed to maintain the skin as a barrier to infection (Category BIII).

Comment: Resident skin care should include

the following: routine frequent turning for those unable to do so themselves, keeping the residents clean and dry, inspecting all residents' skin on a routine basis, ensuring appropriate nutrition, and treating pressure ulcers. Turning schedules and pressure ulcer assessment forms may be useful.

3. A program to prevent UTIs should address catheter use, catheter insertion, closed drainage systems, irrigation of catheters, maintenance of urinary flow, and indications for changing the catheter (Category BIII). *Comment:* Adequate hydration should be maintained. If leg bags are used, the LTCF should develop policies and procedures for aseptic connection, cleaning, and storage of leg bags. Intermittent catheterization is an alternative to an indwelling urinary catheter.

4. A program to minimize the risk of pneumonia in the LTCF should address immunizations, reducing the potential for aspiration following feeding, minimizing atelectasis, and caring for respiratory therapy equipment (Category BIII).

5. Policies and procedures should be developed for prevention of infections associated with nasogastric and gastrostomy feeding tubes, including preparation, storage, refrigeration, and administration of feeding solutions (Category BIII).

6. Policies and procedures should be developed for prevention of IV infections, if IV devices are used (Category BIII). *Comment:* Policies should address indications for IV therapy, the type of dressing used to cover the IV exit site, cannula insertion, site maintenance, and changing fluids or tubing.

7. The LTCF should develop policies for dealing with HIV-infected residents (Category BIII).

J. Resident Health Program

1. Each resident should have an initial history (including important past and present infectious diseases), immunization status evaluation, recent physical examination, and intradermal (Mantoux) skin test (Category BIII). *Comment:* A recent chest radiograph is advisable if the skin test is positive.

2. All newly admitted residents should receive TB screening by the intradermal (Mantoux) tuberculin method unless a physician's statement is obtained that the resident had a past positive reaction to tuberculin. When new or active TB is suggested by a positive skin-test result or by symptoms, a chest radiograph and medical evaluation should be obtained (Category BIII).

Comment: A two-step booster technique may be used.

3. Follow-up skin testing for TB should be performed periodically or after discovery of a new case of TB in a resident or staff member. The intradermal Mantoux method should be used (Category BIII). *Comment:* The frequency of skin testing depends on the regional prevalence of TB, and federal, state, or local regulations.

4. Each resident should receive tetanus and diphtheria vaccine every 10 years. This should be recorded in the resident's chart (Category AII).

5. Each resident should receive the pneumococcal vaccine if indicated. This should be recorded in the resident's chart (Category BIII).

6. Each resident should receive the influenza vaccine annually in the fall, unless medically contraindicated. This should be recorded in the resident's chart (Category AII).

7. Policies and procedures addressing visitors should be developed to deal with introduction of community infections (such as influenza) into the LTCF (Category BIII).

K. Employee Health Program

1. All new employees should have a baseline health assessment, including immunization status and history of relevant past or present infectious diseases (Category BIII). *Comment:* The past history of infectious diseases should address diseases such as chickenpox, measles, hepatitis, skin boils, and bacterial diarrhea. Screening cultures of new employees rarely are indicated.

2. All new employees should receive TB screening by the intradermal (Mantoux) method unless a physician's statement is obtained that the employee had a positive reaction to tuberculin. When new or active TB is suggested by a positive skin-test result or by symptoms, a chest radiograph and medical evaluation should be obtained (Category BIII). *Comment:* A two-step booster technique may be used.

3. Follow-up skin testing for TB should be performed periodically or after discovery of a new case of TB in a resident or staff member. Skin-test–negative personnel should undergo repeat skin testing at regular intervals as determined by a risk assessment. The intradermal Mantoux method should be used (Category BIII).

Comment: The frequency of skin testing depends on the regional prevalence of TB and on federal, state, or local regulations.

4. All employees should have current immunizations, with documentation in the employee record, including tetanus and diphtheria vaccination every 10 years (Category BIII).

5. Employees with blood or body fluid contact should be offered HBV immunization (Category AII).

Comment: Refusal of this vaccine should be documented.

6. Employees should be offered the influenza vaccine annually in the fall (Category AII).

7. Each employee should be taught basic hygiene and handwashing and to consider blood and all body fluids as potentially infectious (Category BIII).

8. Employees with signs or symptoms of communicable diseases (eg, cough, rash, diarrhea) should not have contact with the residents or their food (Category BIII).

9. All employees should be educated to report any significant infectious illnesses to the staff member responsible for employee health (Category BIII).

Comment: Each employee record should include factors affecting immune status (such as steroid therapy, diabetes, HIV infection), illnesses, and incidents such as exposures to contagious diseases, needlesticks, injuries, and accidents.

10. The LTCF should develop protocols for managing employee illnesses and exposures (such as HBV, HIV, TB, scabies) (Category BIII).

Comment: An employee absentee policy that discourages the employee from working while ill should be developed. The LTCF should develop policies for dealing with the HIV-infected employee.

L. Education

1. Infection control education should be provided at the initiation of employment and regularly thereafter. Training should include all staff, especially those providing direct resident care (Category BIII).

2. All programs should be documented with the date, topic, names of attendees, and evaluations (Category C).

Comment: Program topics should be timely and relevant to infection prevention. Basic hygiene, handwashing, transmission of infectious diseases, employee health, prevention of TB, UP, and the susceptibility of residents to infectious diseases are topics that should be

included. The ICP may recommend topics. Surveillance data are of interest to staff and may be included as appropriate.

M. Policies and Procedures

1. Infection control policies and procedures should be approved, reviewed, and revised on a regular basis (Category BIII).

Comment: The ICP should assist in the development and updating of infection-related policies and procedures.

2. Employees should be made aware of infection control policies and procedures (Category BIII).

Comment: The ICP should develop a system for monitoring staff compliance with infection control policies and procedures.

N. Antibiotic Resistance and Monitoring[163,165]

1. The ICP should monitor antibiotic susceptibility results from cultures to detect clinically significant antibiotic-resistant bacteria (such as MRSA or VRE) in the institution. Changes in antibiotic-susceptibility trends should be communicated to appropriate individuals and committees (Category BIII).

2. The LTCF should have a policy dealing with resistant bacteria (such as MRSA or VRE) (Category BIII).

Comment: This policy deals with acceptance of colonized or infected patients into the facility, inquiring about colonization of admissions with resistant bacteria, isolation of residents with resistant bacteria, and surveillance for residents of the facility who are colonized or infected with resistant bacteria. Denial of admission to the LTCF solely on the basis of colonization or infection with a resistant organism is not appropriate.

3. Infection control programs in LTCFs should be encouraged to include a component of antimicrobial utilization review (Category BIII).

Comment: The LTCF should encourage prudent antimicrobial prescribing. In selected LTCFs, a more intensive antimicrobial utilization program may be developed, including review of antibiotic appropriateness.

O. Miscellaneous Aspects

1. There should be a system for reporting notifiable diseases to proper public health officials.

2. The ICP should communicate with the director of the QM program, if a formal program exists (Category BIII).

Comment: Infection control is an important component of QM, and the epidemiological techniques used in infection control will assist the QM program.

3. The ICP may be involved with the infection control implications of new products and the safety program as needed (Category C).

4. The ICP may be involved with other activities relevant to infection control, as compatible with program goals and time constraints (Category C).

References

1. Haley RW, Culver DH, White JW, et al. The efficacy of infection surveillance and control programs in preventing nosocomial infections in US hospitals. *Am J Epidemiol* 1985;121:182-205.
2. Haley RW, Culver DH, White JW, et al. The nationwide nosocomial infection rate—a new need for vital statistics. *Am J Epidemiol* 1985;121:159-167.
3. Smith PW, Daly P, Roccaforte JA. Current status of nosocomial infection control in extended care facilities. *Am J Med* 1991;91(suppl 3B):281-285.
4. Smith PW. Infection in long-term care facilities. *Infect Control* 1985;6:435-436.
5. US Senate Special Committee on Aging: *Aging America—Trends and Projections.* Washington, DC: US Department of Health and Human Services, 1988.
6. American Medical Association White Paper on Elderly Health. *Arch Intern Med* 1990;150:2459-2472.
7. Verghese A, Berk SL. Introduction and epidemiologic considerations. In: Verghese A, Berk SL, eds. *Infections in Nursing Homes and Long-Term Care Facilities.* Basel, Switzerland: Karger; 1990.
8. Smith PW, Rusnak PG. Guideline for infection prevention and control in the long-term care facility. *Am J Infect Control* 1991;19:198-215.
9. Schneider EL. Infectious diseases in the elderly. *Ann Intern Med* 1983;98:395-400.
10. Garibaldi RA, Nurse BA. Infections in the elderly. *Am J Med* 1986;81(suppl):53-58.
11. Yoshikawa TT. Geriatric infectious diseases: an emerging problem. *J Am Geriatr Soc* 1983;31:34-38.
12. Norman DC, Yoshikawa TT. Clinical features of infection and the significance of fever in the elderly nursing home patient. In: Verghese A, Berk SL, eds. *Infections in Nursing Homes and Long-Term Care Facilities.* Basel, Switzerland: Karger; 1990.
13. Saltzman RL, Peterson PK. Immunodeficiency of the elderly. *Reviews of Infectious Diseases* 1987;9:1127-1137.
14. Smith PW, Roccaforte JS, Daly PB. Infection and immune response in the elderly. *Ann Epidemiol* 1992;2:813-822.
15. Jackson MM, Fierer J. Infections and infection risk in residents of long-term care facilities: a review of the literature, 1970-1984. *Am J Infect Control* 1985;13:63-77.
16. Nicolle LE, Garibaldi RA. Infection control in long-term care facilities. *Infect Control Hosp Epidemiol* 1995;16:348-353.
17. Garibaldi RA, Brodine S, Matsumiya S. Infections among patients in nursing homes—policies, prevalence, and problems. *N Engl J Med* 1981;305:731-735.
18. Jackson MM, Fierer J, Barrett-Connor E, et al. Intensive surveillance for infections in a three-year study of nursing home patients. *Am J Epidemiol* 1992;135:685-696.
19. Sager MA, Easterling DV, Kindig DA, Anderson OW. Changes in the location of death after passage of Medicare's prospective payment system. *N Engl J Med* 1989;320:433-439.
20. Scheckler WE, Peterson PJ. Infections and infection control among residents of eight rural Wisconsin nursing homes. *Arch Intern Med* 1986;146:1981-1984.
21. Price LE, Sarubbi FA Jr, Rutala WA. Infection control programs in twelve North Carolina extended care facilities. *Infect Control* 1985;6:437-441.
22. Cohen ED, Hierholzer WJ, Schilling CR, Snydman DR. Nosocomial infections in skilled nursing facilities: a preliminary survey. *Public Health Rep* 1979;94:162-166.
23. Magnussen MH, Robb SS. Nosocomial infections in a long-term care facility. *Am J Infect Control* 1980;8:12-17.
24. Gambert SR, Duthie EH Jr, Priefer B, Rabinovitch RA. Bacterial infections in a hospital-based skilled nursing facility. *Journal of Chronic Diseases* 1982;35:781-786.
25. Farber BF, Brennen C, Puntereri AJ, Brody JP. A prospective study of nosocomial infections in a chronic care facility. *J Am Geriatr Soc* 1984;32:499-502.
26. Nicolle LE, McIntyre M, Zacharias H, MacDonell JA. Twelve month surveillance of infections in institutionalized elderly men. *J Am Geriatr Soc* 1984;32:513-519.
27. Standfast SJ, Michelsen PB, Baltch AL, et al. A prevalence survey of infections in a combined acute and long-term care hospital. *Infect Control* 1984;5:177-184.
28. Setia U, Serventi I, Lorenz P. Nosocomial infections among patients in a long-term care facility: spectrum, prevalence, and risk factors. *Am J Infect Control* 1985;13:57-62.
29. Franson TR, Duthie GH Jr, Cooper JE, Oudenhoven EV, Hoffmann RC. Prevalence survey of infections and their predisposing factors at a hospital-based nursing home care unit. *J Am Geriatr Soc* 1986;34:95-100.
30. Vlahov D, Tenney JH, Cervino KW, Shamer DK. Routine surveillance for infections in nursing homes: experience at two facilities. *Am J Infect Control* 1987;15:47-53.
31. Alvarez S, Shell CG, Woolley TW, Berk SL, Smith JK. Nosocomial infections in long-term facilities. *J Gerontol* 1988;43:M9-M17.
32. Hoffman N, Jenkins R, Putney K. Nosocomial infection rates during a one-year period in a nursing home care unit of a Veterans' Administration hospital. *Am J Infect Control* 1990;18:55-63.
33. Jacobson C, Strausbaugh LJ. Incidence and impact of infection in a nursing home care unit. *Am J Infect Control* 1990;18:151-159.
34. Darnowski SB, Gordon M, Simor AE. Two years of infection surveillance in a geriatric long-term care facility. *Am J Infect Control* 1991;19:185-190.
35. Magaziner J, Tenney JH, DeForge B, Hebel R, Muncie HL, Warren JW. Prevalence and characteristics of nursing home acquired infections in the aged. *J Am Geriatr Soc* 1991;39:1071-1078.
36. Steinmiller AM, Robb SS, Muder RR. Prevalence of nosocomial infection in long-term-care Veterans' Administration medical centers. *Am J Infect Control* 1991;19:143-146.
37. Beck-Sague C, Villarino E, Giuliano D, et al. Infectious diseases and death among nursing home residents: results of surveillance in 13 nursing homes. *Infect Control Hosp Epidemiol* 1994;15:494-496.
38. Warren JF. Catheter-associated bacteriuria in long-term care facilities. *Infect Control Hosp Epidemiol* 1994;15:557-562.

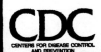

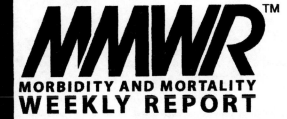

MORBIDITY AND MORTALITY
WEEKLY REPORT

June 29, 2001 / Vol. 50 / No. RR-11

*Recommendations
and
Reports*

Inside: Continuing Education Examination

Updated U.S. Public Health Service Guidelines for the Management of Occupational Exposures to HBV, HCV, and HIV and Recommendations for Postexposure Prophylaxis

U.S. DEPARTMENT OF HEALTH AND HUMAN SERVICES
Centers for Disease Control and Prevention (CDC)
Atlanta, GA 30333

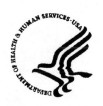

Contents

INTRODUCTION

Avoiding occupational blood exposures is the primary way to prevent transmission of hepatitis B virus (HBV), hepatitis C virus (HCV), and human immunodeficiency virus (HIV) in health-care settings (1). However, hepatitis B immunization and postexposure management are integral components of a complete program to prevent infection following bloodborne pathogen exposure and are important elements of workplace safety (2).

The U.S. Public Health Service (PHS) has published previous guidelines for the management of HIV exposures that included considerations for postexposure prophylaxis (PEP) (3–5). Since publication of the 1998 HIV exposure guidelines (5), several new antiretroviral agents have been approved by the Food and Drug Administration (FDA), and more information is available about the use and safety of HIV PEP (6–11). In addition, questions exist regarding considerations about PEP regimens when the source person's virus is known or suspected to be resistant to one or more of the antiretroviral agents that might be used for PEP. Concern also has arisen about the use of PEP when it is not warranted. Data indicate that some health-care personnel (HCP) take a full course of HIV PEP after exposures that do not confer an HIV transmission risk (10,11).

In September 1999, a meeting of a PHS interagency working group* and expert consultants was convened by CDC. The PHS working group decided to issue updated recommendations for the management of occupational exposure to HIV. In addition, the report was to include recommendations for the management of occupational HBV and HCV exposures so that a single document could comprehensively address the management of occupational exposures to bloodborne pathogens. This report updates and consolidates the previous PHS guidelines and recommendations for occupational HBV, HCV, and HIV exposure management for HCP. Specific practice recommendations for the management of occupational bloodborne pathogen exposures are outlined to assist health-care institutions with the implementation of these PHS guidelines (Appendices A and B). As relevant information becomes available, updates of these recommendations will be published. Recommendations for nonoccupational (e.g., sexual, pediatric, and perinatal) HBV, HCV, and HIV exposures are not addressed in these guidelines and can be found elsewhere (12–15).

Definition of Health-Care Personnel and Exposure

In this report, health-care personnel (HCP) are defined as persons (e.g., employees, students, contractors, attending clinicians, public-safety workers, or volunteers) whose activities involve contact with patients or with blood or other body fluids from patients in a health-care, laboratory, or public-safety setting. The potential exists for blood and body fluid exposure to other workers, and the same principles of exposure management could be applied to other settings.

---

*This interagency working group comprised representatives of CDC, the Food and Drug Administration (FDA), the Health Resources and Services Administration, and the National Institutes of Health. Information included in these recommendations may not represent FDA approval or approved labeling for the particular product or indications in question. Specifically, the terms "safe" and "effective" may not be synonymous with the FDA-defined legal standards for product approval.

Updated U.S. Public Health Service Guidelines for the Management of Occupational Exposures to HBV, HCV, and HIV and Recommendations for Postexposure Prophylaxis

Summary

This report updates and consolidates all previous U.S. Public Health Service recommendations for the management of health-care personnel (HCP) who have occupational exposure to blood and other body fluids that might contain hepatitis B virus (HBV), hepatitis C virus (HCV), or human immunodeficiency virus (HIV).

Recommendations for HBV postexposure management include initiation of the hepatitis B vaccine series to any susceptible, unvaccinated person who sustains an occupational blood or body fluid exposure. Postexposure prophylaxis (PEP) with hepatitis B immune globulin (HBIG) and/or hepatitis B vaccine series should be considered for occupational exposures after evaluation of the hepatitis B surface antigen status of the source and the vaccination and vaccine-response status of the exposed person. Guidance is provided to clinicians and exposed HCP for selecting the appropriate HBV PEP.

Immune globulin and antiviral agents (e.g., interferon with or without ribavirin) are not recommended for PEP of hepatitis C. For HCV postexposure management, the HCV status of the source and the exposed person should be determined, and for HCP exposed to an HCV positive source, follow-up HCV testing should be performed to determine if infection develops.

Recommendations for HIV PEP include a basic 4-week regimen of two drugs (zidovudine [ZDV] and lamivudine [3TC]; 3TC and stavudine [d4T]; or didanosine [ddI] and d4T) for most HIV exposures and an expanded regimen that includes the addition of a third drug for HIV exposures that pose an increased risk for transmission. When the source person's virus is known or suspected to be resistant to one or more of the drugs considered for the PEP regimen, the selection of drugs to which the source person's virus is unlikely to be resistant is recommended.

In addition, this report outlines several special circumstances (e.g., delayed exposure report, unknown source person, pregnancy in the exposed person, resistance of the source virus to antiretroviral agents, or toxicity of the PEP regimen) when consultation with local experts and/or the National Clinicians' Post-Exposure Prophylaxis Hotline ([PEPline] 1-888-448-4911) is advised.

Occupational exposures should be considered urgent medical concerns to ensure timely postexposure management and administration of HBIG, hepatitis B vaccine, and/or HIV PEP.

INTRODUCTION

Avoiding occupational blood exposures is the primary way to prevent transmission of hepatitis B virus (HBV), hepatitis C virus (HCV), and human immunodeficiency virus (HIV) in health-care settings (1). However, hepatitis B immunization and postexposure management are integral components of a complete program to prevent infection following bloodborne pathogen exposure and are important elements of workplace safety (2).

The U.S. Public Health Service (PHS) has published previous guidelines for the management of HIV exposures that included considerations for postexposure prophylaxis (PEP) (3–5). Since publication of the 1998 HIV exposure guidelines (5), several new antiretroviral agents have been approved by the Food and Drug Administration (FDA), and more information is available about the use and safety of HIV PEP (6–11). In addition, questions exist regarding considerations about PEP regimens when the source person's virus is known or suspected to be resistant to one or more of the antiretroviral agents that might be used for PEP. Concern also has arisen about the use of PEP when it is not warranted. Data indicate that some health-care personnel (HCP) take a full course of HIV PEP after exposures that do not confer an HIV transmission risk (10,11).

In September 1999, a meeting of a PHS interagency working group* and expert consultants was convened by CDC. The PHS working group decided to issue updated recommendations for the management of occupational exposure to HIV. In addition, the report was to include recommendations for the management of occupational HBV and HCV exposures so that a single document could comprehensively address the management of occupational exposures to bloodborne pathogens. This report updates and consolidates the previous PHS guidelines and recommendations for occupational HBV, HCV, and HIV exposure management for HCP. Specific practice recommendations for the management of occupational bloodborne pathogen exposures are outlined to assist health-care institutions with the implementation of these PHS guidelines (Appendices A and B). As relevant information becomes available, updates of these recommendations will be published. Recommendations for nonoccupational (e.g., sexual, pediatric, and perinatal) HBV, HCV, and HIV exposures are not addressed in these guidelines and can be found elsewhere (12–15).

Definition of Health-Care Personnel and Exposure

In this report, health-care personnel (HCP) are defined as persons (e.g., employees, students, contractors, attending clinicians, public-safety workers, or volunteers) whose activities involve contact with patients or with blood or other body fluids from patients in a health-care, laboratory, or public-safety setting. The potential exists for blood and body fluid exposure to other workers, and the same principles of exposure management could be applied to other settings.

---

*This interagency working group comprised representatives of CDC, the Food and Drug Administration (FDA), the Health Resources and Services Administration, and the National Institutes of Health. Information included in these recommendations may not represent FDA approval or approved labeling for the particular product or indications in question. Specifically, the terms "safe" and "effective" may not be synonymous with the FDA-defined legal standards for product approval.

An exposure that might place HCP at risk for HBV, HCV, or HIV infection is defined as a percutaneous injury (e.g., a needlestick or cut with a sharp object) or contact of mucous membrane or nonintact skin (e.g., exposed skin that is chapped, abraded, or afflicted with dermatitis) with blood, tissue, or other body fluids that are potentially infectious (16,17).

In addition to blood and body fluids containing visible blood, semen and vaginal secretions also are considered potentially infectious. Although semen and vaginal secretions have been implicated in the sexual transmission of HBV, HCV, and HIV, they have not been implicated in occupational transmission from patients to HCP. The following fluids also are considered potentially infectious: cerebrospinal fluid, synovial fluid, pleural fluid, peritoneal fluid, pericardial fluid, and amniotic fluid. The risk for transmission of HBV, HCV, and HIV infection from these fluids is unknown; the potential risk to HCP from occupational exposures has not been assessed by epidemiologic studies in health-care settings. Feces, nasal secretions, saliva, sputum, sweat, tears, urine, and vomitus are not considered potentially infectious unless they contain blood. The risk for transmission of HBV, HCV, and HIV infection from these fluids and materials is extremely low.

Any direct contact (i.e., contact without barrier protection) to concentrated virus in a research laboratory or production facility is considered an exposure that requires clinical evaluation. For human bites, the clinical evaluation must include the possibility that both the person bitten and the person who inflicted the bite were exposed to bloodborne pathogens. Transmission of HBV or HIV infection only rarely has been reported by this route (18–20) (CDC, unpublished data, 1998).

BACKGROUND

This section provides the rationale for the postexposure management and prophylaxis recommendations presented in this report. Additional details concerning the risk for occupational bloodborne pathogen transmission to HCP and management of occupational bloodborne pathogen exposures are available elsewhere (5,12,13,21-24).

Occupational Transmission of HBV

Risk for Occupational Transmission of HBV

HBV infection is a well recognized occupational risk for HCP (25). The risk of HBV infection is primarily related to the degree of contact with blood in the work place and also to the hepatitis B e antigen (HBeAg) status of the source person. In studies of HCP who sustained injuries from needles contaminated with blood containing HBV, the risk of developing clinical hepatitis if the blood was both hepatitis B surface antigen (HBsAg)- and HBeAg-positive was 22%–31%; the risk of developing serologic evidence of HBV infection was 37%–62%. By comparison, the risk of developing clinical hepatitis from a needle contaminated with HBsAg-positive, HBeAg-negative blood was 1%–6%, and the risk of developing serologic evidence of HBV infection, 23%–37% (26).

Although percutaneous injuries are among the most efficient modes of HBV transmission, these exposures probably account for only a minority of HBV infections among HCP. In several investigations of nosocomial hepatitis B outbreaks, most infected HCP could not recall an overt percutaneous injury (27,28), although in some studies, up to one third of infected HCP recalled caring for a patient who was HBsAg-positive (29,30). In addition, HBV has been demonstrated to survive in dried blood at room temperature on environmental surfaces for at least 1 week (*31*). Thus, HBV infections that occur in HCP with no history of nonoccupational exposure or occupational percutaneous injury might have resulted from direct or indirect blood or body fluid exposures that inoculated HBV into cutaneous scratches, abrasions, burns, other lesions, or on mucosal surfaces (*32–34*). The potential for HBV transmission through contact with environmental surfaces has been demonstrated in investigations of HBV outbreaks among patients and staff of hemodialysis units (*35–37*).

Blood contains the highest HBV titers of all body fluids and is the most important vehicle of transmission in the health-care setting. HBsAg is also found in several other body fluids, including breast milk, bile, cerebrospinal fluid, feces, nasopharyngeal washings, saliva, semen, sweat, and synovial fluid (*38*). However, the concentration of HBsAg in body fluids can be 100–1000—fold higher than the concentration of infectious HBV particles. Therefore, most body fluids are not efficient vehicles of transmission because they contain low quantities of infectious HBV, despite the presence of HBsAg.

In serologic studies conducted in the United States during the 1970s, HCP had a prevalence of HBV infection approximately 10 times higher than the general population (*39–42*). Because of the high risk of HBV infection among HCP, routine preexposure vaccination of HCP against hepatitis B and the use of standard precautions to prevent exposure to blood and other potentially infectious body fluids have been recommended since the early 1980s (*43*). Regulations issued by the Occupational Safety and Health Administration (OSHA) (*2*) have increased compliance with these recommendations. Since the implementation of these recommendations, a sharp decline has occurred in the incidence of HBV infection among HCP.

PEP for HBV

Efficacy of PEP for HBV. The effectiveness of hepatitis B immune globulin (HBIG) and/ or hepatitis B vaccine in various postexposure settings has been evaluated by prospective studies. For perinatal exposure to an HBsAg-, HBeAg-positive mother, a regimen combining HBIG and initiation of the hepatitis B vaccine series at birth is 85%–95% effective in preventing HBV infection (*44,45*). Regimens involving either multiple doses of HBIG alone or the hepatitis B vaccine series alone are 70%–75% effective in preventing HBV infection (*46*). In the occupational setting, multiple doses of HBIG initiated within 1 week following percutaneous exposure to HBsAg-positive blood provides an estimated 75% protection from HBV infection (*47–49*). Although the postexposure efficacy of the combination of HBIG and the hepatitis B vaccine series has not been evaluated in the occupational setting, the increased efficacy of this regimen observed in the perinatal setting, compared with HBIG alone, is presumed to apply to the occupational setting as well. In addition, because persons requiring PEP in the occupational setting are generally at continued risk for HBV exposure, they should receive the hepatitis B vaccine series.

Safety of PEP for HBV. Hepatitis B vaccines have been found to be safe when administered to infants, children, or adults (*12,50*). Through the year 2000, approximately 100 million persons have received hepatitis B vaccine in the United States. The most common side effects from hepatitis B vaccination are pain at the injection site and mild to moderate fever (*50–55*). Studies indicate that these side effects are reported no more frequently among persons vaccinated than among those receiving placebo (*51,52*).

Approximately 45 reports have been received by the Vaccine Adverse Event Reporting System (VAERS) of alopecia (hair loss) in children and adults after administration of plasma-derived and recombinant hepatitis B vaccine; four persons sustained hair loss following vaccination on more than one occasion (56). Hair loss was temporary for approximately two thirds of persons who experienced hair loss. An epidemiologic study conducted in the Vaccine Safety Datalink found no statistical association between alopecia and receipt of hepatitis B vaccine in children (CDC, unpublished data, 1998). A low rate of anaphylaxis has been observed in vaccine recipients based on reports to VAERS; the estimated incidence is 1 in 600,000 vaccine doses distributed. Although none of the persons who developed anaphylaxis died, anaphylactic reactions can be life-threatening; therefore, further vaccination with hepatitis B vaccine is contraindicated in persons with a history of anaphylaxis after a previous dose of vaccine.

Hepatitis B immunization programs conducted on a large scale in Taiwan, Alaska, and New Zealand have observed no association between vaccination and the occurrence of serious adverse events. Furthermore, in the United States, surveillance of adverse events following hepatitis B vaccination has demonstrated no association between hepatitis B vaccine and the occurrence of serious adverse events, including Guillain-Barré syndrome, transverse myelitis, multiple sclerosis, optic neuritis, and seizures (57–59) (CDC, unpublished data, 1991). However, several case reports and case series have claimed an association between hepatitis B vaccination and such syndromes and diseases as multiple sclerosis, optic neuritis, rheumatoid arthritis, and other autoimmune diseases (57,60–66). Most of these reported adverse events have occurred in adults, and no report has compared the frequency of the purported vaccine-associated syndrome/disease with the frequency in an unvaccinated population. In addition, recent case-control studies have demonstrated no association between hepatitis B vaccination and development or short-term risk of relapse of multiple sclerosis (67,68), and reviews by international panels of experts have concluded that available data do not demonstrate a causal association between hepatitis B vaccination and demyelinating diseases, including multiple sclerosis (69).

HBIG is prepared from human plasma known to contain a high titer of antibody to HBsAg (anti-HBs). The plasma from which HBIG is prepared is screened for HBsAg and antibodies to HIV and HCV. The process used to prepare HBIG inactivates and eliminates HIV from the final product. Since 1996, the final product has been free of HCV RNA as determined by the polymerase chain reaction (PCR), and, since 1999, all products available in the United States have been manufactured by methods that inactivate HCV and other viruses. No evidence exists that HBV, HCV, or HIV have ever been transmitted by HBIG commercially available in the United States (70,71).

Serious adverse effects from HBIG when administered as recommended have been rare. Local pain and tenderness at the injection site, urticaria and angioedema might occur; anaphylactic reactions, although rare, have been reported following the injection of human immune globulin (IG) preparations (72). Persons with a history of anaphylactic reaction to IG should not receive HBIG.

PEP for HBV During Pregnancy. No apparent risk exists for adverse effects to developing fetuses when hepatitis B vaccine is administered to pregnant women (CDC, unpublished data, 1990). The vaccine contains noninfectious HBsAg particles and should pose no risk to the fetus. HBV infection during pregnancy might result in severe disease for the mother and chronic infection for the newborn. Therefore, neither pregnancy nor lactation should be considered a contraindication to vaccination of women. HBIG is not contraindicated for pregnant or lactating women.

Occupational Transmission of HCV

Risk for Occupational Transmission of HCV

HCV is not transmitted efficiently through occupational exposures to blood. The average incidence of anti-HCV seroconversion after accidental percutaneous exposure from an HCV-positive source is 1.8% (range: 0%–7%) (73–76), with one study indicating that transmission occurred only from hollow-bore needles compared with other sharps (75). Transmission rarely occurs from mucous membrane exposures to blood, and no transmission in HCP has been documented from intact or nonintact skin exposures to blood (77,78). Data are limited on survival of HCV in the environment. In contrast to HBV, the epidemiologic data for HCV suggest that environmental contamination with blood containing HCV is not a significant risk for transmission in the health-care setting (79,80), with the possible exception of the hemodialysis setting where HCV transmission related to environmental contamination and poor infection-control practices have been implicated (81–84). The risk for transmission from exposure to fluids or tissues other than HCV-infected blood also has not been quantified but is expected to be low.

Postexposure Management for HCV

In several studies, researchers have attempted to assess the effectiveness of IG following possible exposure to non-A, non-B hepatitis. These studies have been difficult to interpret because they lack uniformity in diagnostic criteria and study design, and, in all but one study, the first dose of IG was administered before potential exposure (48,85,86). In an experiment designed to model HCV transmission by needlestick exposure in the health-care setting, high anti-HCV titer IG administered to chimpanzees 1 hour after exposure to HCV-positive blood did not prevent transmission of infection (87). In 1994, the Advisory Committee on Immunization Practices (ACIP) reviewed available data regarding the prevention of HCV infection with IG and concluded that using IG as PEP for hepatitis C was not supported (88). This conclusion was based on the following facts:

- No protective antibody response has been identified following HCV infection.

- Previous studies of IG use to prevent posttransfusion non-A, non-B hepatitis might not be relevant in making recommendations regarding PEP for hepatitis C.

- Experimental studies in chimpanzees with IG containing anti-HCV failed to prevent transmission of infection after exposure.

No clinical trials have been conducted to assess postexposure use of antiviral agents (e.g., interferon with or without ribavirin) to prevent HCV infection, and antivirals are not FDA-approved for this indication. Available data suggest that an established infection might need to be present before interferon can be an effective treatment. Kinetic studies suggest that the effect of interferon on chronic HCV infection occurs in two phases. During the first phase, interferon blocks the production or release of virus from infected cells. In the second phase, virus is eradicated from the infected cells (89); in this later phase, higher pretreatment alanine aminotransferase (ALT) levels correlate with an increasing decline in infected cells, and the rapidity of the decline correlates with viral clearance. In contrast, the effect of antiretrovirals when used for PEP after exposure to HIV is based on inhibition of HIV DNA synthesis early in the retroviral replicative cycle.

In the absence of PEP for HCV, recommendations for postexposure management are intended to achieve early identification of chronic disease and, if present, referral for evaluation of treatment options. However, a theoretical argument is that intervention with antivirals when HCV RNA first becomes detectable might prevent the development of chronic infection. Data from studies conducted outside the United States suggest that a short course of interferon started early in the course of acute hepatitis C is associated with a higher rate of resolved infection than that achieved when therapy is begun after chronic hepatitis C has been well established (*90–92*). These studies used various treatment regimens and included persons with acute disease whose peak ALT levels were 500–1,000 IU/L at the time therapy was initiated (2.6–4 months after exposure).

No studies have evaluated the treatment of acute infection in persons with no evidence of liver disease (i.e., HCV RNA-positive <6 months duration with normal ALT levels); among patients with chronic HCV infection, the efficacy of antivirals has been demonstrated only among patients who also had evidence of chronic liver disease (i.e., abnormal ALT levels). In addition, treatment started early in the course of chronic HCV infection (i.e., 6 months after onset of infection) might be as effective as treatment started during acute infection (*13*). Because 15%–25% of patients with acute HCV infection spontaneously resolve their infection (*93*), treatment of these patients during the acute phase could expose them unnecessarily to the discomfort and side effects of antiviral therapy.

Data upon which to base a recommendation for therapy of acute infection are insufficient because a) no data exist regarding the effect of treating patients with acute infection who have no evidence of disease, b) treatment started early in the course of chronic infection might be just as effective and would eliminate the need to treat persons who will spontaneously resolve their infection, and c) the appropriate regimen is unknown.

Occupational Transmission of HIV

Risk for Occupational Transmission of HIV

In prospective studies of HCP, the average risk of HIV transmission after a percutaneous exposure to HIV-infected blood has been estimated to be approximately 0.3% (95% confidence interval [CI] = 0.2%–0.5%) (*94*) and after a mucous membrane exposure, approximately 0.09% (95% CI = 0.006%–0.5%) (*95*). Although episodes of HIV transmission after nonintact skin exposure have been documented (*96*), the average risk for transmission by this route has not been precisely quantified but is estimated to be less than the risk for mucous membrane exposures (*97*). The risk for transmission after exposure to fluids or tissues other than HIV-infected blood also has not been quantified but is probably considerably lower than for blood exposures (*98*).

As of June 2000, CDC had received voluntary reports of 56 U.S. HCP with documented HIV seroconversion temporally associated with an occupational HIV exposure. An additional 138 episodes in HCP are considered possible occupational HIV transmissions. These workers had a history of occupational exposure to blood, other infectious body fluids, or laboratory solutions containing HIV, and no other risk for HIV infection was identified, but HIV seroconversion after a specific exposure was not documented (*99*).

Epidemiologic and laboratory studies suggest that several factors might affect the risk of HIV transmission after an occupational exposure. In a retrospective case-control study of HCP who had percutaneous exposure to HIV, the risk for HIV infection was found to be increased with exposure to a larger quantity of blood from the source person as indicated by a) a device visibly contaminated with the patient's blood, b) a procedure that involved a needle being placed directly in a vein or artery, or c) a deep injury (*100*). The risk also was increased for exposure to blood from source persons with terminal illness, possibly reflecting either the higher titer of HIV in blood late in the course of AIDS or other factors (e.g., the presence of syncytia-inducing strains of HIV). A laboratory study that demonstrated that more blood is transferred by deeper injuries and hollow-bore needles lends further support for the observed variation in risk related to blood quantity (*101*).

The use of source person viral load as a surrogate measure of viral titer for assessing transmission risk has not yet been established. Plasma viral load (e.g., HIV RNA) reflects only the level of cell-free virus in the peripheral blood; latently infected cells might transmit infection in the absence of viremia. Although a lower viral load (e.g., <1,500 RNA copies/mL) or one that is below the limits of detection probably indicates a lower titer exposure, it does not rule out the possibility of transmission.

Some evidence exists regarding host defenses possibly influencing the risk for HIV infection. A study of HIV-exposed but uninfected HCP demonstrated an HIV-specific cytotoxic T-lymphocyte (CTL) response when peripheral blood mononuclear cells were stimulated in vitro with HIV-specific antigens (*102*). Similar CTL responses have been observed in other groups who experienced repeated HIV exposure without resulting infection (*103–108*). Among several possible explanations for this observation is that the host immune response sometimes might prevent establishment of HIV infection after a percutaneous exposure; another is that the CTL response simply might be a marker for exposure. In a study of 20 HCP with occupational exposure to HIV, a comparison was made of HCP treated with zidovudine (ZDV) PEP and those not treated. The findings from this study suggest that ZDV blunted the HIV-specific CTL response and that PEP might inhibit early HIV replication (*109*).

Rationale for HIV PEP

Considerations that influence the rationale and recommendations for PEP include

- the pathogenesis of HIV infection, particularly the time course of early infection;

- the biological plausibility that infection can be prevented or ameliorated by using antiretroviral drugs;

- direct or indirect evidence of the efficacy of specific agents used for prophylaxis; and

- the risk and benefit of PEP to exposed HCP.

The following discussion considers each of these concerns.

Role of Pathogenesis in Considering Antiretroviral Prophylaxis. Information about primary HIV infection indicates that systemic infection does not occur immediately, leaving a brief window of opportunity during which postexposure antiretroviral intervention might modify or prevent viral replication. In a primate model of simian immunodeficiency virus (SIV) infection, infection of dendritic-like cells occurred at the site of inoculation during the first 24 hours following mucosal exposure to cell-free virus. Over the subsequent 24–48 hours, migration of these cells to regional lymph nodes occurred, and virus was detectable in the peripheral blood within 5 days (*110*). Theoretically, initiation of antiretroviral PEP soon after exposure might prevent or inhibit systemic infection by limiting the proliferation of virus in the initial target cells or lymph nodes.

Efficacy of Antiretrovirals for PEP in Animal Studies. Data from animal studies have been difficult to interpret, in part, because of problems identifying an animal model that is comparable to humans. In early studies, differences in controlled variables (e.g., choice of viral strain [based on the animal model used], inoculum size, route of inoculation, time of prophylaxis initiation, and drug regimen) made extrapolation of the results to humans difficult. Recently, refinements in methodology have facilitated more relevant studies; in particular, the viral inocula used in animal studies have been reduced to levels more analogous to human exposures but sufficient to cause infection in control animals (*111–113*). These studies provide encouraging evidence of postexposure chemoprophylactic efficacy.

Studies among primates and in murine and feline animal models have demonstrated that larger viral inocula decrease prophylactic efficacy (*114–117*). In addition, delaying initiation, shortening the duration, or decreasing the antiretroviral dose of PEP, individually or in combination, decreased prophylactic efficacy (*113,118–124*). For example, when (R)-9-(2-phosphonylmethoxypropyl) adenine (tenofovir) was administered 48 hours before, 4 hours after, or 24 hours after intravenous SIV inoculation to long-tailed macaques, a 4-week regimen prevented infection in all treated animals (*122*). A subsequent study confirmed the efficacy of tenofovir PEP when administered 24 hours after intravenous inoculation of a dose of SIV that uniformly results in infection in untreated macaques. In the same study, protection was incomplete if the tenofovir administration was delayed to 48 or 72 hours postexposure or if the total duration of treatment was curtailed to 3 or 10 days (*123*).

Efficacy of Antiretrovirals for PEP in Human Studies. Little information exists from which the efficacy of PEP in humans can be assessed. Seroconversion is infrequent following an occupational exposure to HIV-infected blood; therefore, several thousands of exposed HCP would need to enroll in a prospective trial to achieve the statistical power necessary to directly demonstrate PEP efficacy (*125*).

In the retrospective case-control study of HCP, after controlling for other risk factors for HIV transmission, use of ZDV as PEP was associated with a reduction in the risk of HIV infection by approximately 81% (95% CI = 43%–94%) (*100*). Although the results of this study suggest PEP efficacy, its limitations include the small number of cases studied and the use of cases and controls from different cohorts.

In a multicenter trial in which ZDV was administered to HIV-infected pregnant women and their infants, the administration of ZDV during pregnancy, labor, and delivery and to the infant reduced transmission by 67% (*126*). Only part of the protective effect of ZDV was explained by reduction of the HIV viral load in the maternal blood, suggesting that ZDV prophylaxis, in part, involves a mechanism other than the reduction of maternal viral burden (*127,128*). Since 1998, studies have highlighted the importance of PEP for prevention of perinatal HIV transmission. In Africa, the use of ZDV in combination with lamivudine (3TC) decreased perinatal HIV transmission by 50% when administered during pregnancy, labor, and for 1 week postpartum, and by 37% when started at the onset of labor and continued for 1 week postpartum (*129*). Studies in the United States and Uganda also have demonstrated that rates of perinatal HIV transmission have been reduced with the use of abbreviated PEP regimens started intrapartum or during the first 48–72 hours of life (*130–132*).

The limitations of all of these studies with animals and humans must be considered when reviewing evidence of PEP efficacy. The extent to which data from animal studies can be extrapolated to humans is largely unknown, and the exposure route for mother-to-infant HIV transmission is not similar to occupational exposures; therefore, these findings might not be directly applicable to PEP in HCP.

Reports of Failure of PEP. Failure of PEP to prevent HIV infection in HCP has been reported in at least 21 instances (*78,133–139*). In 16 of the cases, ZDV was used alone as a single agent; in two cases, ZDV and didanosine (ddl) were used in combination (*133,138*); and in three cases, ≥3 drugs were used for PEP (*137–139*). Thirteen of the source persons were known to have been treated with antiretroviral therapy before the exposure. Antiretroviral resistance testing of the virus from the source person was performed in seven instances, and in four, the HIV infection transmitted was found to have decreased sensitivity to ZDV and/or other drugs used for PEP. In addition to possible exposure to an antiretroviral-resistant strain of HIV, other factors that might have contributed to these apparent failures might include a high titer and/or large inoculum exposure, delayed initiation and/or short duration of PEP, and possible factors related to the host (e.g., cellular immune system responsiveness) and/or to the source person's virus (e.g., presence of syncytia-forming strains) (*133*). Details regarding the cases of PEP failure involving combinations of antiretroviral agents are included in this report (Table 1).

Antiretroviral Agents for PEP

Antiretroviral agents from three classes of drugs are available for the treatment of HIV infection. These agents include the nucleoside reverse transcriptase inhibitors (NRTIs), nonnucleoside reverse transcriptase inhibitors (NNRTIs), and protease inhibitors (PIs). Only antiretroviral agents that have been approved by FDA for treatment of HIV infection are discussed in these guidelines.

Determining which agents and how many to use or when to alter a PEP regimen is largely empiric. Guidelines for the treatment of HIV infection, a condition usually involving a high total body burden of HIV, include recommendations for the use of three drugs (*140*); however, the applicability of these recommendations to PEP remains unknown. In HIV-infected patients, combination regimens have proved superior to monotherapy regimens in reducing HIV viral load, reducing the incidence of opportunistic infections and death, and delaying onset of drug resistance (*141,142*). A combination of drugs with activity at different stages in the viral replication cycle (e.g., nucleoside analogues with a PI) theoretically could offer an additional preventive effect in PEP, particularly for occupational exposures that pose an increased risk of transmission. Although the use of a three-drug regimen might be justified for exposures that pose an increased risk of transmission, whether the potential added toxicity of a third drug is justified for lower-risk exposures is uncertain. Therefore, the recommendations at the end of this document provide guidance for two- and three-drug PEP regimens that are based on the level of risk for HIV transmission represented by the exposure.

NRTI combinations that can be considered for PEP include ZDV and 3TC, 3TC and stavudine (d4T), and ddl and d4T. In previous PHS guidelines, a combination of ZDV and 3TC was considered the first choice for PEP regimens (*3*). Because ZDV and 3TC are available in a combination formulation (Combivir™, manufactured by Glaxo Wellcome, Inc., Research Triangle Park, NC), the use of this combination might be more convenient for HCP. However, recent data suggest that mutations associated with ZDV and 3TC resistance might be common in some areas (*143*). Thus, individual clinicians might prefer other NRTIs or combinations based on local knowledge and experience in treating HIV infection and disease.

TABLE 1. Reported instances of failure of combination drug postexposure prophylaxis to prevent HIV infection in health-care personnel exposed to HIV-infected blood

Report no.	Source of injury	Regimen*	Hours to first dose	Days to onset of retroviral illness	Days to seroconversions[†]	Source patient on antiretrovirals
1[§]	Biopsy needle	ZDV, ddl	0.50	23	23	yes
2[¶]	Hollow needle	ZDV, ddl**	1.50	45	97	no
3[§]	Large-bore hollow needle	3-drugs[††]	1.50	40	55	yes[§§]
4[¶]	Hollow needle	ZDV, 3TC ddl, IDV	0.67	70	83	yes***
5[†††]	Unknown sharp	ddl, d4T NVP[§§§]	2.00	42	100	yes***

* ZDV = zidovudine, ddl = didanosine, 3TC = lamivudine, IDV = indinavir, d4T = stavudine, and NVP = nevirapine

[†] By enzyme immunoassay for HIV-1 antibody and Western blot.

[§] Jochimsen EM. Failures of zidovudine postexposure prophylaxis. Am J Med 1997;102(suppl 5B):52–5.

[¶] Lot F, Abiteboul D. Occupational HIV infection in France [Abstract WP-25]. In: Keynote addresses and abstracts of the 4th ICOH International Conference on Occupational Health for Health Care Workers. Montreal, Canada, 1999.

** Report 2: ZDV and ddl taken for 48 hours then changed to ZDV alone.

[††] Report 3: ZDV, 3TC, and IDV taken for 48 hours then changed to d4T, 3TC, and IDV.

[§§] HIV isolate tested and determined to be sensitive to antiretroviral agent(s).

[¶] Perdue B, Wolderufael D, Mellors J, Quinn T, Margolick J. HIV-1 transmission by a needlestick injury despite rapid initiation of four-drug postexposure prophylaxis [Abstract 210]. In: Program and abstracts of the 6th Conference on Retroviruses and Opportunistic Infections. Chicago, IL: Foundation for Retrovirology and Human Health in scientific collaboration with the National Institute of Allergy and Infectious Diseases and CDC, 1999:107.

*** HIV isolate tested and determined to be resistant to antiretroviral agent(s).

[†††] Beltrami EM, Luo C-C, Dela Torre N, Cardo DM. HIV transmission after an occupational exposure despite postexposure prophylaxis with a combination drug regimen [Abstract P-S2-62]. In: Program and abstracts of the 4th Decennial International Conference on Nosocomial and Healthcare-Associated Infections in conjunction with the 10th Annual Meeting of SHEA. Atlanta, GA: CDC, 2000:125–6.

[§§§] Report 5: ZDV and 3TC taken for one dose then changed to ddl, d4T, and NVP; ddl was discontinued after 3 days because of severe vomiting.

The addition of a third drug for PEP following high-risk exposures is based on demonstrated effectiveness in reducing viral burden in HIV-infected persons. Previously, indinavir (IDV) or nelfinavir (NFV) were recommended as first-choice agents for inclusion in an expanded PEP regimen (5). Since the publication of the 1998 PEP guidelines, efavirenz (EFV), an NNRTI; abacavir (ABC), a potent NRTI; and Kaletra™, a PI, have been approved by FDA. Although side effects might be common with the NNRTIs, EFV might be considered for expanded PEP regimens, especially when resistance to PIs in the source person's virus is known or suspected. ABC has been associated with dangerous hypersensitivity reactions but, with careful monitoring, may be considered as a third drug for PEP. Kaletra, a combination of lopinavir and ritonavir, is a potent HIV inhibitor that, with expert consultation, may be considered in an expanded PEP regimen.

Toxicity and Drug Interactions of Antiretroviral Agents. When administering PEP, an important goal is completion of a 4-week PEP regimen when PEP is indicated. Therefore, the toxicity profile of antiretroviral agents, including the frequency, severity, duration, and reversibility of side effects, is a relevant consideration. All of the antiretroviral agents have been associated with side effects (Table 2). However, studies of adverse events have been conducted primarily with persons who have advanced disease (and longer treatment courses) and who therefore might not reflect the experience in persons who are uninfected (144).

Several primary side effects are associated with antiretroviral agents (Table 2). Side effects associated with many of the NRTIs are chiefly gastrointestinal (e.g., nausea or diarrhea); however, ddI has been associated with cases of fatal and nonfatal pancreatitis among HIV-infected patients treated for >4 weeks. The use of PIs has been associated with new onset diabetes mellitus, hyperglycemia, diabetic ketoacidosis, exacerbation of preexisting diabetes mellitus, and dyslipidemia (145–147). Nephrolithiasis has been associated with IDV use; however, the incidence of this potential complication might be limited by drinking at least 48 ounces (1.5 L) of fluid per 24-hour period (e.g., six 8- ounce glasses of water throughout the day) (148). NFV has been associated with the development of diarrhea; however, this side effect might respond to treatment with antimotility agents that can be prescribed for use, if necessary, at the time the drug is recommended for PEP. The NNRTIs have been associated with severe skin reactions, including life-threatening cases of Stevens-Johnson syndrome and toxic epidermal necrolysis. Hepatotoxicity, including fatal hepatic necrosis, has occurred in patients treated with nevirapine (NVP); some episodes began during the first few weeks of therapy (FDA, unpublished data, 2000). EFV has been associated with central nervous system side effects, including dizziness, somnolence, insomnia, and abnormal dreaming.

All of the approved antiretroviral agents might have potentially serious drug interactions when used with certain other drugs (Appendix C). Careful evaluation of concomitant medications used by an exposed person is required before PEP is prescribed, and close monitoring for toxicity is also needed. Further information about potential drug interactions can be found in the manufacturer's package insert.

Toxicity Associated with PEP. Information from the National Surveillance System for Health Care Workers (NaSH) and the HIV Postexposure Registry indicates that nearly 50% of HCP experience adverse symptoms (e.g., nausea, malaise, headache, anorexia, and headache) while taking PEP and that approximately 33% stop taking PEP because of adverse signs and symptoms (6,7,10,11). Some studies have demonstrated that side effects and discontinuation of PEP are more common among HCP taking three-drug

TABLE 2. Primary side effects associated with antiretroviral agents

Antiretroviral class/agent	Primary side effects and toxicities
Nucleoside reverse transcriptase inhibitors (NRTIs)	
Zidovudine (Retrovir™; ZDV; AZT)	anemia, neutropenia, nausea, headache, insomnia, muscle pain, and weakness
Lamivudine (Epivir™; 3TC)	abdominal pain, nausea, diarrhea, rash, and pancreatitis
Stavudine (Zerit™; d4T)	peripheral neuropathy, headache, diarrhea, nausea, insomnia, anorexia, pancreatitis, increased liver function tests (LFTs), anemia, and neutropenia
Didanosine (Videx™; ddI)	pancreatitis, lactic acidosis, neuropathy, diarrhea, abdominal pain, and nausea
Abacavir (Ziagen™; ABC)	nausea, diarrhea, anorexia, abdominal pain, fatigue, headache, insomnia, and hypersensitivity reactions
Nonnucleoside reverse transcriptase inhibitors (NNRTIs)	
Nevirapine (Viramune™; NVP)	rash (including cases of Stevens-Johnson syndrome), fever, nausea, headache, hepatitis, and increased LFTs
Delavirdine (Rescriptor™; DLV)	rash (including cases of Stevens-Johnson syndrome), nausea, diarrhea, headache, fatigue, and increased LFTs
Efavirenz (Sustiva™; EFV)	rash (including cases of Stevens-Johnson syndrome), insomnia, somnolence, dizziness, trouble concentrating, and abnormal dreaming
Protease inhibitors (PIs)	
Indinavir (Crixivan™; IDV)	nausea, abdominal pain, nephrolithiasis, and indirect hyperbilirubinemia
Nelfinavir (Viracept™; NFV)	diarrhea, nausea, abdominal pain, weakness, and rash
Ritonavir (Norvir™; RTV)	weakness, diarrhea, nausea, circumoral paresthesia, taste alteration, and increased cholesterol and triglycerides
Saquinavir (Fortovase™; SQV)	diarrhea, abdominal pain, nausea, hyperglycemia, and increased LFTs
Amprenavir (Agenerase™; AMP)	nausea, diarrhea, rash, circumoral paresthesia, taste alteration, and depression
Lopinavir/Ritonavir (Kaletra™)	diarrhea, fatigue, headache, nausea, and increased cholesterol and triglycerides

combination regimens for PEP compared with HCP taking two-drug combination regimens (7,10). Although similar rates of side effects were observed among persons who took PEP after sexual or drug use exposures to HIV in the San Francisco Post-Exposure Prevention Project, 80% completed 4 weeks of therapy (149). Participants in the San Francisco Project were followed at 1, 2, 4, 26, and 52 weeks postexposure and received medication adherence counseling; most participants took only two drugs for PEP.

Serious side effects, including nephrolithiasis, hepatitis, and pancytopenia have been reported with the use of combination drugs for PEP (6,7,150,151). One case of NVP-associated fulminant liver failure requiring liver transplantation and one case of hypersensitivity syndrome have been reported in HCP taking NVP for HIV PEP (152). Including these two cases, from March 1997 through September 2000, FDA received reports of 22 cases of serious adverse events related to NVP taken for PEP (153). These events included 12 cases of hepatotoxicity, 14 cases of skin reaction (including one documented and two possible cases of Stevens-Johnson syndrome), and one case of rhabdomyolysis; four cases involved both hepatotoxicty and skin reaction, and one case involved both rhabdomyolysis and skin reaction.

Resistance to Antiretroviral Agents. Known or suspected resistance of the source virus to antiretroviral agents, particularly to agents that might be included in a PEP regimen, is a concern for persons making decisions about PEP. Resistance to HIV infection occurs with all of the available antiretroviral agents, and cross-resistance within drug classes is frequent (154). Recent studies have demonstrated an emergence of drug-resistant HIV among source persons for occupational exposures (143,155). A study conducted at seven U.S. sites during 1998–1999 found that 16 (39%) of 41 source persons whose virus was sequenced had primary genetic mutations associated with resistance to RTIs, and 4 (10%) had primary mutations associated with resistance to PIs (143). In addition, occupational transmission of resistant HIV strains, despite PEP with combination drug regimens, has been reported (137,139). In one case, a hospital worker became infected after an HIV exposure despite a PEP regimen that included ddI, d4T, and NVP (139). The transmitted HIV contained two primary genetic mutations associated with resistance to NNRTIs (the source person was taking EFV at the time of the exposure). Despite recent studies and case reports, the relevance of exposure to a resistant virus is still not well understood.

Empiric decisions about the presence of antiretroviral drug resistance are often difficult to make because patients generally take more than one antiretroviral agent. Resistance should be suspected in source persons when they are experiencing clinical progression of disease or a persistently increasing viral load, and/or decline in CD4 T-cell count, despite therapy or a lack of virologic response to therapy. However, resistance testing of the source virus at the time of an exposure is not practical because the results will not be available in time to influence the choice of the initial PEP regimen. Furthermore, in this situation, whether modification of the PEP regimen is necessary or will influence the outcome of an occupational exposure is unknown. No data exist to suggest that modification of a PEP regimen after receiving results from resistance testing (usually a minimum of 1–2 weeks) improves efficacy of PEP.

Antiretroviral Drugs During Pregnancy. Data are limited on the potential effects of antiretroviral drugs on the developing fetus or neonate (156). Carcinogenicity and/or mutagenicity is evident in several in vitro screening tests for ZDV and all other FDA-licensed NRTIs. The relevance of animal data to humans is unknown; however, because teratogenic effects were observed in primates at drug exposures similar to those representing human therapeutic exposure, the use of EFV should be avoided in pregnant women (*140*). IDV is associated with infrequent side effects in adults (i.e., hyperbilirubinemia and renal stones) that could be problematic for a newborn. Because the half-life of IDV in adults is short, these concerns might be relevant only if the drug is administered shortly before delivery.

In a recent study in France of perinatal HIV transmission, two cases of progressive neurologic disease and death were reported in uninfected infants exposed to ZDV and 3TC (*157*). Laboratory studies of these children suggested mitochondrial dysfunction. In a careful review of deaths in children followed in U.S. perinatal HIV cohorts, no deaths attributable to mitochondrial disease have been found (*158*).

Recent reports of fatal and nonfatal lactic acidosis in pregnant women treated throughout gestation with a combination of d4T and ddI have prompted warnings about use of these drugs during pregnancy (*159*). Although the case-patients were HIV-infected women taking the drugs for >4 weeks, pregnant women and their providers should be advised to consider d4T and ddI only when the benefits of their use outweigh the risks.

PEP Use in Hospitals in the United States. Analysis of data from NaSH provides information on the use of PEP following occupational exposures in 47 hospitals in the United States. A total of 11,784 exposures to blood and body fluids was reported from June 1996 through November 2000 (CDC, unpublished data, 2001). For all exposures with known sources, 6% were to HIV-positive sources, 74% to HIV-negative sources, and 20% to sources with an unknown HIV status. Sixty-three percent of HCP exposed to a known HIV-positive source started PEP, and 54% of HCP took it for at least 20 days, whereas 14% of HCP exposed to a source person subsequently found to be HIV-negative initiated PEP, and 3% of those took it for at least 20 days. Information recorded about HIV exposures in NaSH indicates that 46% of exposures involving an HIV-positive source warranted only a two-drug PEP regimen (i.e., the exposure was to mucous membranes or skin or was a superficial percutaneous injury and the source person did not have end-stage AIDS or acute HIV illness); however, 53% of these exposed HCP took ≥3 drugs (CDC, unpublished data, 2000). Similarly, the National Clinicians' Post-Exposure Prophylaxis Hotline (PEPline) reported that PEPline staff recommended stopping or not starting PEP for approximately one half of the HCP who consulted them about exposures (D. Bangsberg, San Francisco General Hospital, unpublished data, September 1999). The observation that some HCP exposed to HIV-negative source persons take PEP from several days to weeks following their exposures suggests that strategies be employed such as the use of a rapid HIV antibody assay, which could minimize exposure to unnecessary PEP (*11*). A recent study demonstrated that use of a rapid HIV test for evaluation of source persons after occupational exposures not only resulted in decreased use of PEP, but also was cost-effective compared with use of the standard enzyme immunoassay (EIA) test for source persons subsequently found to be HIV-negative (*160*).

RECOMMENDATIONS FOR THE MANAGEMENT OF HCP POTENTIALLY EXPOSED TO HBV, HCV, or HIV

Exposure prevention remains the primary strategy for reducing occupational bloodborne pathogen infections; however, occupational exposures will continue to occur. Health-care organizations should make available to their personnel a system that includes written protocols for prompt reporting, evaluation, counseling, treatment, and follow-up of occupational exposures that might place HCP at risk for acquiring a bloodborne infection. HCP should be educated concerning the risk for and prevention of bloodborne infections, including the need to be vaccinated against hepatitis B (*17,21,161–163*). Employers are required to establish exposure-control plans that include postexposure follow-up for their employees and to comply with incident reporting requirements mandated by the 1992 OSHA bloodborne pathogen standard (*2*). Access to clinicians who can provide postexposure care should be available during all working hours, including nights and weekends. HBIG, hepatitis B vaccine, and antiretroviral agents for HIV PEP should be available for timely administration (i.e., either by providing access on-site or by creating linkages with other facilities or providers to make them available off-site). Persons responsible for providing postexposure management should be familiar with evaluation and treatment protocols and the facility's plans for accessing HBIG, hepatitis B vaccine, and antiretroviral drugs for HIV PEP.

HCP should be educated to report occupational exposures immediately after they occur, particularly because HBIG, hepatitis B vaccine, and HIV PEP are most likely to be effective if administered as soon after the exposure as possible. HCP who are at risk for occupational exposure to bloodborne pathogens should be familiarized with the principles of postexposure management as part of job orientation and ongoing job training.

Hepatitis B Vaccination

Any person who performs tasks involving contact with blood, blood-contaminated body fluids, other body fluids, or sharps should be vaccinated against hepatitis B (*2,21*). Prevaccination serologic screening for previous infection is not indicated for persons being vaccinated because of occupational risk, unless the hospital or health-care organization considers screening cost-effective.

Hepatitis B vaccine should always be administered by the intramuscular route in the deltoid muscle with a needle 1–1.5 inches long. Hepatitis B vaccine can be administered at the same time as other vaccines with no interference with antibody response to the other vaccines (*164*). If the vaccination series is interrupted after the first dose, the second dose should be administered as soon as possible. The second and third doses should be separated by an interval of at least 2 months. If only the third dose is delayed, it should be administered when convenient. HCP who have contact with patients or blood and are at ongoing risk for percutaneous injuries should be tested 1–2 months after completion of the 3-dose vaccination series for anti-HBs (*21*). Persons who do not respond to the primary vaccine series (i.e., anti-HBs <10 mIU/mL) should complete a second 3-dose vaccine series or be evaluated to determine if they are HBsAg-positive. Revaccinated persons should be retested at the completion of the second vaccine series. Persons who do not respond to an initial 3-dose vaccine series have a 30%–50% chance of responding to a second 3-dose series (*165*). Persons who prove to be HBsAg-positive should be counseled regarding how to prevent HBV transmission to others and regarding the need for medical evaluation (*12,163,166*). Nonresponders to vaccination who are HBsAg-negative should be considered susceptible to HBV infection and should be counseled regarding precautions to prevent HBV infection and the need to obtain HBIG prophylaxis for any known or probable parenteral exposure to HBsAg-positive blood. Booster doses of hepatitis B vaccine are not necessary, and periodic serologic testing to monitor antibody concentrations after completion of the vaccine series is not recommended. Any blood or body fluid exposure sustained by an unvaccinated, susceptible person should lead to the initiation of the hepatitis B vaccine series.

Treatment of an Exposure Site

Wounds and skin sites that have been in contact with blood or body fluids should be washed with soap and water; mucous membranes should be flushed with water. No evidence exists that using antiseptics for wound care or expressing fluid by squeezing the wound further reduces the risk of bloodborne pathogen transmission; however, the use of antiseptics is not contraindicated. The application of caustic agents (e.g., bleach) or the injection of antiseptics or disinfectants into the wound is not recommended.

Exposure Report

If an occupational exposure occurs, the circumstances and postexposure management should be recorded in the exposed person's confidential medical record (usually on a form the facility designates for this purpose) (Box 1). In addition, employers should follow all federal (including OSHA) and state requirements for recording and reporting occupational injuries and exposures.

BOX 1. Recommendations for the contents of the occupational exposure report

- date and time of exposure;
- details of the procedure being performed, including where and how the exposure occurred; if related to a sharp device, the type and brand of device and how and when in the course of handling the device the exposure occurred;
- details of the exposure, including the type and amount of fluid or material and the severity of the exposure (e.g., for a percutaneous exposure, depth of injury and whether fluid was injected; for a skin or mucous membrane exposure, the estimated volume of material and the condition of the skin [e.g., chapped, abraded, intact]);
- details about the exposure source (e.g., whether the source material contained HBV, HCV, or HIV; if the source is HIV-infected, the stage of disease, history of antiretroviral therapy, viral load, and antiretroviral resistance information, if known);
- details about the exposed person (e.g., hepatitis B vaccination and vaccine-response status); and
- details about counseling, postexposure management, and follow-up.

Evaluation of the Exposure and the Exposure Source

Evaluation of the Exposure

The exposure should be evaluated for the potential to transmit HBV, HCV, and HIV based on the type of body substance involved and the route and severity of the exposure (Box 2). Blood, fluid containing visible blood, or other potentially infectious fluid (including semen; vaginal secretions; and cerebrospinal, synovial, pleural, peritoneal, pericardial, and amniotic fluids) or tissue can be infectious for bloodborne viruses. Exposures to these fluids or tissue through a percutaneous injury (i.e., needlestick or other penetrating sharps-related event) or through contact with a mucous membrane are situations that pose a risk for bloodborne virus transmission and require further evaluation. For HCV and HIV, exposure to a blood-filled hollow needle or visibly bloody device suggests a higher risk exposure than exposure to a needle that was most likely used for giving an injection. In addition, any direct contact (i.e, personal protective equipment either was not present or was ineffective in protecting skin or mucous membranes) with concentrated virus in a research laboratory or production facility is considered an exposure that requires clinical evaluation.

For skin exposure, follow-up is indicated only if it involves exposure to a body fluid previously listed and evidence exists of compromised skin integrity (e.g., dermatitis, abrasion, or open wound). In the clinical evaluation for human bites, possible exposure of both the person bitten and the person who inflicted the bite must be considered. If a bite results in blood exposure to either person involved, postexposure follow-up should be provided.

BOX 2. Factors to consider in assessing the need for follow-up of occupational exposures

- **Type of exposure**
  - Percutaneous injury
  - Mucous membrane exposure
  - Nonintact skin exposure
  - Bites resulting in blood exposure to either person involved

- **Type and amount of fluid/tissue**
  - Blood
  - Fluids containing blood
  - Potentially infectious fluid or tissue (semen; vaginal secretions; and cerebrospinal, synovial, pleural, peritoneal, pericardial, and amniotic fluids)
  - Direct contact with concentrated virus

- **Infectious status of source**
  - Presence of HBsAg
  - Presence of HCV antibody
  - Presence of HIV antibody

- **Susceptibility of exposed person**
  - Hepatitis B vaccine and vaccine response status
  - HBV, HCV, and HIV immune status

Evaluation of the Exposure Source

The person whose blood or body fluid is the source of an occupational exposure should be evaluated for HBV, HCV, and HIV infection (Box 3). Information available in the medical record at the time of exposure (e.g., laboratory test results, admitting diagnosis, or previous medical history) or from the source person, might confirm or exclude bloodborne virus infection.

If the HBV, HCV, and/or HIV infection status of the source is unknown, the source person should be informed of the incident and tested for serologic evidence of bloodborne virus infection. Procedures should be followed for testing source persons, including obtaining informed consent, in accordance with applicable state and local laws. Any persons determined to be infected with HBV, HCV, or HIV should be referred for appropriate counseling and treatment. Confidentiality of the source person should be maintained at all times.

Testing to determine the HBV, HCV, and HIV infection status of an exposure source should be performed as soon as possible. Hospitals, clinics and other sites that manage exposed HCP should consult their laboratories regarding the most appropriate test to use to expedite obtaining these results. An FDA-approved rapid HIV-antibody test kit should be considered for use in this situation, particularly if testing by EIA cannot be completed within 24–48 hours. Repeatedly reactive results by EIA or rapid HIV-antibody tests are considered to be highly suggestive of infection, whereas a negative result is an excellent indicator of the absence of HIV antibody. Confirmation of a reactive result by Western blot or immunofluorescent antibody is not necessary to make initial decisions about postexposure management but should be done to complete the testing process and before informing the source person. Repeatedly reactive results by EIA for anti-HCV should be confirmed by a supplemental test (i.e., recombinant immunoblot assay [RIBA™] or HCV PCR). Direct virus assays (e.g., HIV p24 antigen EIA or tests for HIV RNA or HCV RNA) for routine HIV or HCV screening of source persons are not recommended.

If the exposure source is unknown or cannot be tested, information about where and under what circumstances the exposure occurred should be assessed epidemiologically for the likelihood of transmission of HBV, HCV, or HIV. Certain situations as well as the type of exposure might suggest an increased or decreased risk; an important consideration is the prevalence of HBV, HCV, or HIV in the population group (i.e., institution or community) from which the contaminated source material is derived. For example, an exposure that occurs in a geographic area where injection-drug use is prevalent or involves a needle discarded in a drug-treatment facility would be considered epidemiologically to have a higher risk for transmission than an exposure that occurs in a nursing home for the elderly.

Testing of needles or other sharp instruments implicated in an exposure, regardless of whether the source is known or unknown, is not recommended. The reliability and interpretation of findings in such circumstances are unknown, and testing might be hazardous to persons handling the sharp instrument.

Examples of information to consider when evaluating an exposure source for possible HBV, HCV, or HIV infection include laboratory information (e.g., previous HBV, HCV, or HIV test results or results of immunologic testing [e.g., CD4+ T-cell count]) or liver enzymes (e.g., ALT), clinical symptoms (e.g., acute syndrome suggestive of primary HIV infection or undiagnosed immunodeficiency disease), and history of recent (i.e., within 3 months) possible HBV, HCV, or HIV exposures (e.g., injection-drug use or sexual contact with a known positive partner). Health-care providers should be aware of local and state laws governing the collection and release of HIV serostatus information on a source person, following an occupational exposure.

If the source person is known to have HIV infection, available information about this person's stage of infection (i.e., asymptomatic, symptomatic, or AIDS), CD4+ T-cell count, results of viral load testing, current and previous antiretroviral therapy, and results of any genotypic or phenotypic viral resistance testing should be gathered for consideration in choosing an appropriate PEP regimen. If this information is not immediately available, initiation of PEP, if indicated, should not be delayed; changes in the PEP regimen can be made after PEP has been started, as appropriate. Reevaluation of exposed HCP should be considered within 72 hours postexposure, especially as additional information about the exposure or source person becomes available.

If the source person is HIV seronegative and has no clinical evidence of AIDS or symptoms of HIV infection, no further testing of the person for HIV infection is indicated. The likelihood of the source person being in the "window period" of HIV infection in the absence of symptoms of acute retroviral syndrome is extremely small.

BOX 3. Evaluation of occupational exposure sources

Known sources
- Test known sources for HBsAg, anti-HCV, and HIV antibody
  - Direct virus assays for routine screening of source patients are **not** recommended
  - Consider using a rapid HIV-antibody test
  - If the source person is **not** infected with a bloodborne pathogen, baseline testing or further follow-up of the exposed person is **not** necessary
- For sources whose infection status remains unknown (e.g., the source person refuses testing), consider medical diagnoses, clinical symptoms, and history of risk behaviors
- Do not test discarded needles for bloodborne pathogens

Unknown sources
- For unknown sources, evaluate the likelihood of exposure to a source at high risk for infection
  - Consider likelihood of bloodborne pathogen infection among patients in the exposure setting

---

Management of Exposures to HBV

For percutaneous or mucosal exposures to blood, several factors must be considered when making a decision to provide prophylaxis, including the HBsAg status of the source and the hepatitis B vaccination and vaccine-response status of the exposed person. Such exposures usually involve persons for whom hepatitis B vaccination is recommended.

Any blood or body fluid exposure to an unvaccinated person should lead to initiation of the hepatitis B vaccine series.

The hepatitis B vaccination status and the vaccine-response status (if known) of the exposed person should be reviewed. A summary of prophylaxis recommendations for percutaneous or mucosal exposure to blood according to the HBsAg status of the exposure source and the vaccination and vaccine-response status of the exposed person is included in this report (Table 3).

When HBIG is indicated, it should be administered as soon as possible after exposure (preferably within 24 hours). The effectiveness of HBIG when administered >7 days after exposure is unknown. When hepatitis B vaccine is indicated, it should also be administered as soon as possible (preferably within 24 hours) and can be administered simultaneously with HBIG at a separate site (vaccine should always be administered in the deltoid muscle).

For exposed persons who are in the process of being vaccinated but have not completed the vaccination series, vaccination should be completed as scheduled, and HBIG should be added as indicated (Table 3). Persons exposed to HBsAg-positive blood or body fluids who are known not to have responded to a primary vaccine series should receive a single dose of HBIG and reinitiate the hepatitis B vaccine series with the first dose of the hepatitis B vaccine as soon as possible after exposure. Alternatively, they should receive two doses of HBIG, one dose as soon as possible after exposure, and the second dose 1 month later. The option of administering one dose of HBIG and reinitiating the vaccine series is preferred for nonresponders who did not complete a second 3-dose vaccine series. For persons who previously completed a second vaccine series but failed to respond, two doses of HBIG are preferred.

Management of Exposures to HCV

Individual institutions should establish policies and procedures for testing HCP for HCV after percutaneous or mucosal exposures to blood and ensure that all personnel are familiar with these policies and procedures. The following are recommendations for follow-up of occupational HCV exposures:

- For the source, perform testing for anti-HCV.

- For the person exposed to an HCV-positive source

  — perform baseline testing for anti-HCV and ALT activity; and

  — perform follow-up testing (e.g., at 4–6 months) for anti-HCV and ALT activity (if earlier diagnosis of HCV infection is desired, testing for HCV RNA may be performed at 4–6 weeks).

- Confirm all anti-HCV results reported positive by enzyme immunoassay using supplemental anti-HCV testing (e.g., recombinant immunoblot assay [RIBA™]) (13).

Health-care professionals who provide care to persons exposed to HCV in the occupational setting should be knowledgeable regarding the risk for HCV infection and appropriate counseling, testing, and medical follow-up.

IG and antiviral agents are not recommended for PEP after exposure to HCV-positive blood. In addition, no guidelines exist for administration of therapy during the acute

TABLE 3. Recommended postexposure prophylaxis for exposure to hepatitis B virus

Vaccination and antibody response status of exposed workers*	Treatment		
	Source HBsAg[†] positive	Source HBsAg[†] negative	Source unknown or not available for testing
Unvaccinated	HBIG[§] x 1 and initiate HB vaccine series[¶]	Initiate HB vaccine series	Initiate HB vaccine series
Previously vaccinated			
Known responder**	No treatment	No treatment	No treatment
Known nonresponder[††]	HBIG x 1 and initiate revaccination or HBIG x 2[§§]	No treatment	If known high risk source, treat as if source were HBsAg positive
Antibody response unknown	Test exposed person for anti-HBs[¶¶] 1. If adequate,** no treatment is necessary 2. If inadequate,[††] administer HBIG x 1 and vaccine booster	No treatment	Test exposed person for anti-HBs 1. If adequate,[¶] no treatment is necessary 2. If inadequate,[¶] administer vaccine booster and recheck titer in 1–2 months

* Persons who have previously been infected with HBV are immune to reinfection and do not require postexposure prophylaxis.

[†] Hepatitis B surface antigen.

[§] Hepatitis B immune globulin; dose is 0.06 mL/kg intramuscularly.

[¶] Hepatitis B vaccine.

** A responder is a person with adequate levels of serum antibody to HBsAg (i.e., anti-HBs $\geq$10 mIU/mL).

[††] A nonresponder is a person with inadequate response to vaccination (i.e., serum anti-HBs < 10 mIU/mL).

[§§] The option of giving one dose of HBIG and reinitiating the vaccine series is preferred for nonresponders who have not completed a second 3-dose vaccine series. For persons who previously completed a second vaccine series but failed to respond, two doses of HBIG are preferred.

[¶] Antibody to HBsAg.

phase of HCV infection. However, limited data indicate that antiviral therapy might be beneficial when started early in the course of HCV infection. When HCV infection is identified early, the person should be referred for medical management to a specialist knowledgeable in this area.

Counseling for HCP Exposed to Viral Hepatitis

HCP exposed to HBV- or HCV-infected blood do not need to take any special precautions to prevent secondary transmission during the follow-up period (12,13); however, they should refrain from donating blood, plasma, organs, tissue, or semen. The exposed person does not need to modify sexual practices or refrain from becoming pregnant. If an exposed woman is breast feeding, she does not need to discontinue.

No modifications to an exposed person's patient-care responsibilities are necessary to prevent transmission to patients based solely on exposure to HBV- or HCV-positive blood. If an exposed person becomes acutely infected with HBV, the person should be evaluated according to published recommendations for infected HCP (165). No recommendations exist regarding restricting the professional activities of HCP with HCV infection (13). As recommended for all HCP, those who are chronically infected with HBV or HCV should follow all recommended infection-control practices, including standard precautions and appropriate use of hand washing, protective barriers, and care in the use and disposal of needles and other sharp instruments (162).

Management of Exposures to HIV

Clinical Evaluation and Baseline Testing of Exposed HCP

HCP exposed to HIV should be evaluated within hours (rather than days) after their exposure and should be tested for HIV at baseline (i.e., to establish infection status at the time of exposure). If the source person is seronegative for HIV, baseline testing or further follow-up of the exposed person normally is not necessary. Serologic testing should be made available to all HCP who are concerned that they might have been occupationally infected with HIV. For purposes of considering HIV PEP, the evaluation also should include information about medications the exposed person might be taking and any current or underlying medical conditions or circumstances (i.e., pregnancy, breast feeding, or renal or hepatic disease) that might influence drug selection.

PEP for HIV

The following recommendations (Tables 4 and 5) apply to situations when a person has been exposed to a source person with HIV infection or when information suggests the likelihood that the source person is HIV-infected. These recommendations are based on the risk for HIV infection after different types of exposure and on limited data regarding efficacy and toxicity of PEP. Because most occupational HIV exposures do not result in the transmission of HIV, potential toxicity must be carefully considered when prescribing PEP. To assist with the initial management of an HIV exposure, health-care facilities should have drugs for an initial PEP regimen selected and available for use. When possible, these recommendations should be implemented in consultation with persons who have expertise in antiretroviral therapy and HIV transmission (Box 4).

TABLE 4. Recommended HIV postexposure prophylaxis for percutaneous injuries

Exposure type	Infection status of source				
	HIV-Positive Class 1*	HIV-Positive Class 2*	Source of unknown HIV status†	Unknown source§	HIV-Negative
Less severe¶	Recommend basic 2-drug PEP	Recommend expanded 3-drug PEP	Generally, no PEP warranted; however, consider basic 2-drug PEP** for source with HIV risk factors††	Generally, no PEP warranted; however, consider basic 2-drug PEP** in settings where exposure to HIV-infected persons is likely	No PEP warranted
More severe§§	Recommend expanded 3-drug PEP	Recommend expanded 3-drug PEP	Generally, no PEP warranted; however, consider basic 2-drug PEP** for source with HIV risk factors††	Generally, no PEP warranted; however, consider basic 2-drug PEP** in settings where exposure to HIV-infected persons is likely	No PEP warranted

* HIV-Positive, Class 1 — asymptomatic HIV infection or known low viral load (e.g., <1,500 RNA copies/mL). HIV-Positive, Class 2 — symptomatic HIV infection, AIDS, acute seroconversion, or known high viral load. If drug resistance is a concern, obtain expert consultation. Initiation of postexposure prophylaxis (PEP) should not be delayed pending expert consultation, and, because expert consultation alone cannot substitute for face-to-face counseling, resources should be available to provide immediate evaluation and follow-up care for all exposures.

† Source of unknown HIV status (e.g., deceased source person with no samples available for HIV testing).

§ Unknown source (e.g., a needle from a sharps disposal container).

¶ Less severe (e.g., solid needle and superficial injury).

** The designation "consider PEP" indicates that PEP is optional and should be based on an individualized decision between the exposed person and the treating clinician.

†† If PEP is offered and taken and the source is later determined to be HIV-negative, PEP should be discontinued.

§§ More severe (e.g., large-bore hollow needle, deep puncture, visible blood on device, or needle used in patient's artery or vein).

TABLE 5. Recommended HIV postexposure prophylaxis for mucous membrane exposures and nonintact skin* exposures

	Infection status of source				
Exposure type	HIV-Positive Class 1†	HIV-Positive Class 2†	Source of unknown HIV status§	Unknown source¶	HIV-Negative
Small volume**	Consider basic 2-drug PEP††	Recommend basic 2-drug PEP	Generally, no PEP warranted; however, consider basic 2-drug PEP†† for source with HIV risk factors§§	Generally, no PEP warranted; however, consider basic 2-drug PEP†† in settings where exposure to HIV-infected persons is likely	No PEP warranted
Large volume¶¶	Recommend basic 2-drug PEP	Recommend expanded 3-drug PEP	Generally, no PEP warranted; however, consider basic 2-drug PEP†† for source with HIV risk factors§§	Generally, no PEP warranted; however, consider basic 2-drug PEP†† in settings where exposure to HIV-infected persons is likely	No PEP warranted

* For skin exposures, follow-up is indicated only if there is evidence of compromised skin integrity (e.g., dermatitis, abrasion, or open wound).

† HIV-Positive, Class 1 — asymptomatic HIV infection or known low viral load (e.g., <1,500 RNA copies/mL). HIV-Positive, Class 2 — symptomatic HIV infection, AIDS, acute seroconversion, or known high viral load. If drug resistance is a concern, obtain expert consultation. Initiation of postexposure prophylaxis (PEP) should not be delayed pending expert consultation, and, because expert consultation alone cannot substitute for face-to-face counseling, resources should be available to provide immediate evaluation and follow-up care for all exposures.

§ Source of unknown HIV status (e.g., deceased source person with no samples available for HIV testing).

¶ Unknown source (e.g., splash from inappropriately disposed blood).

** Small volume (i.e., a few drops).

†† The designation, "consider PEP," indicates that PEP is optional and should be based on an individualized decision between the exposed person and the treating clinician.

§§ If PEP is offered and taken and the source is later determined to be HIV-negative, PEP should be discontinued.

¶¶ Large volume (i.e., major blood splash).

Timing and Duration of PEP. PEP should be initiated as soon as possible. The interval within which PEP should be initiated for optimal efficacy is not known. Animal studies have demonstrated the importance of starting PEP soon after an exposure (*111,112,118*). If questions exist about which antiretroviral drugs to use or whether to use a basic or expanded regimen, starting the basic regimen immediately rather than delaying PEP administration is probably better. Although animal studies suggest that PEP probably is substantially less effective when started more than 24–36 hours postexposure (*112,119,122*), the interval after which no benefit is gained from PEP for humans is undefined. Therefore, if appropriate for the exposure, PEP should be started even when the interval since exposure exceeds 36 hours. Initiating therapy after a longer interval (e.g., 1 week) might be considered for exposures that represent an increased risk for transmission. The optimal duration of PEP is unknown. Because 4 weeks of ZDV appeared protective in occupational and animal studies (*100,123*), PEP probably should be administered for 4 weeks, if tolerated.

Use of PEP When HIV Infection Status of Source Person is Unknown. If the source person's HIV infection status is unknown at the time of exposure, use of PEP should be decided on a case-by-case basis, after considering the type of exposure and the clinical and/or epidemiologic likelihood of HIV infection in the source (Tables 4 and 5). If these considerations suggest a possibility for HIV transmission and HIV testing of the source person is pending, initiating a two-drug PEP regimen until laboratory results have been obtained and later modifying or discontinuing the regimen accordingly is reasonable. The following are recommendations regarding HIV postexposure prophylaxis:

- If indicated, start PEP as soon as possible after an exposure.

- Reevaluation of the exposed person should be considered within 72 hours postexposure, especially as additional information about the exposure or source person becomes available.

- Administer PEP for 4 weeks, if tolerated.

- If a source person is determined to be HIV-negative, PEP should be discontinued.

PEP for Pregnant HCP. If the exposed person is pregnant, the evaluation of risk of infection and need for PEP should be approached as with any other person who has had an HIV exposure. However, the decision to use any antiretroviral drug during pregnancy should involve discussion between the woman and her health-care provider(s) regarding the potential benefits and risks to her and her fetus.

Certain drugs should be avoided in pregnant women. Because teratogenic effects were observed in primate studies, EFV is not recommended during pregnancy. Reports of fatal lactic acidosis in pregnant women treated with a combination of d4T and ddI have prompted warnings about these drugs during pregnancy. Because of the risk of hyperbilirubinemia in newborns, IDV should not be administered to pregnant women shortly before delivery.

Recommendations for the Selection of Drugs for HIV PEP

Health-care providers must strive to balance the risk for infection against the potential toxicity of the agent(s) used when selecting a drug regimen for HIV PEP. Because PEP is potentially toxic, its use is not justified for exposures that pose a negligible risk for transmission (Tables 4 and 5). Also, insufficient evidence exists to support recommending a three-drug regimen for all HIV exposures. Therefore, two regimens for PEP are provided (Appendix C): a "basic" two-drug regimen that should be appropriate for most HIV exposures and an "expanded" three-drug regimen that should be used for exposures that pose an increased risk for transmission (Tables 4 and 5). When possible, the regimens should be implemented in consultation with persons who have expertise in antiretroviral treatment and HIV transmission.

Most HIV exposures will warrant a two-drug regimen using two nucleoside analogues (e.g., ZDV and 3TC; or 3TC and d4T; or d4T and ddI). The addition of a third drug should be considered for exposures that pose an increased risk for transmission. Selection of the PEP regimen should consider the comparative risk represented by the exposure and information about the exposure source, including history of and response to antiretroviral therapy based on clinical response, CD4+ T-cell counts, viral load measurements, and current disease stage. When the source person's virus is known or suspected to be resistant to one or more of the drugs considered for the PEP regimen, the selection of drugs to which the source person's virus is unlikely to be resistant is recommended; expert consultation is advised. If this information is not immediately available, initiation of PEP, if indicated, should not be delayed; changes in the PEP regimen can be made after PEP has been started, as appropriate. Reevaluation of the exposed person should be considered within 72 hours postexposure, especially as additional information about the exposure or source person becomes available.

Follow-up of HCP Exposed to HIV

Postexposure Testing. HCP with occupational exposure to HIV should receive follow-up counseling, postexposure testing, and medical evaluation, regardless of whether they receive PEP. HIV-antibody testing should be performed for at least 6 months postexposure (e.g., at 6 weeks, 12 weeks, and 6 months). Extended HIV follow-up (e.g., for 12 months) is recommended for HCP who become infected with HCV following exposure to a source coinfected with HIV and HCV. Whether extended follow-up is indicated in other circumstances (e.g., exposure to a source coinfected with HIV and HCV in the absence of HCV seroconversion or for exposed persons with a medical history suggesting an impaired ability to develop an antibody response to acute infection) is unclear. Although rare instances of delayed HIV seroconversion have been reported (*167,168*), the infrequency of this occurrence does not warrant adding to the anxiety level of the exposed persons by routinely extending the duration of postexposure follow-up. However, this recommendation should not preclude a decision to extend follow-up in an individual situation based on the clinical judgement of the exposed person's health-care provider. HIV testing should be performed on any exposed person who has an illness that is compatible with an acute retroviral syndrome, regardless of the interval since exposure. When HIV infection is identified, the person should be referred to a specialist knowledgeable in the area of HIV treatment and counseling for medical management.

HIV-antibody testing with EIA should be used to monitor for seroconversion. The routine use of direct virus assays (e.g., HIV p24 antigen EIA or tests for HIV RNA) to detect infection in exposed HCP generally is not recommended (*169*). The high rate of false-positive results of these tests in this setting could lead to unnecessary anxiety and/or treatment (*170,171*). Despite the ability of direct virus assays to detect HIV infection a few days earlier than EIA, the infrequency of occupational seroconversion and increased costs of these tests do not warrant their routine use in this setting.

- HIV-antibody testing should be performed for at least 6 months postexposure.

- Direct virus assays for routine follow-up of HCP are not recommended.

- HIV testing should be performed on any exposed person who has an illness compatible with an acute retroviral syndrome.

Monitoring and Management of PEP Toxicity. If PEP is used, HCP should be monitored for drug toxicity by testing at baseline and again 2 weeks after starting PEP. The scope of testing should be based on medical conditions in the exposed person and the toxicity of drugs included in the PEP regimen. Minimally, lab monitoring for toxicity should include a complete blood count and renal and hepatic function tests. Monitoring for evidence of hyperglycemia should be included for HCP whose regimens include any PI; if the exposed person is receiving IDV, monitoring for crystalluria, hematuria, hemolytic anemia, and hepatitis also should be included. If toxicity is noted, modification of the regimen should be considered after expert consultation; further diagnostic studies may be indicated.

Exposed HCP who choose to take PEP should be advised of the importance of completing the prescribed regimen. Information should be provided to HCP about potential drug interactions and the drugs that should not be taken with PEP, the side effects of the drugs that have been prescribed, measures to minimize these effects, and the methods of clinical monitoring for toxicity during the follow-up period. HCP should be advised that the evaluation of certain symptoms should not be delayed (e.g., rash, fever, back or abdominal pain, pain on urination or blood in the urine, or symptoms of hyperglycemia [increased thirst and/or frequent urination]).

HCP who fail to complete the recommended regimen often do so because of the side effects they experience (e.g., nausea and diarrhea). These symptoms often can be managed with antimotility and antiemetic agents or other medications that target the specific symptoms without changing the regimen. In other situations, modifying the dose interval (i.e., administering a lower dose of drug more frequently throughout the day, as recommended by the manufacturer), might facilitate adherence to the regimen. Serious adverse events should be reported to FDA's MedWatch Program.

Counseling and Education. Although HIV infection following an occupational exposure occurs infrequently, the emotional effect of an exposure often is substantial (172–174). In addition, HCP are given seemingly conflicting information. Although HCP are told that a low risk exists for HIV transmission, a 4-week regimen of PEP might be recommended, and they are asked to commit to behavioral measures (e.g., sexual abstinence or condom use) to prevent secondary transmission, all of which influence their lives for several weeks to months (172). Therefore, access to persons who are knowledgeable about occupational HIV transmission and who can deal with the many concerns an HIV exposure might generate for the exposed person is an important element of postexposure management. HIV-exposed HCP should be advised to use the following measures to prevent secondary transmission during the follow-up period, especially the first 6–12 weeks after the exposure when most HIV-infected persons are expected to seroconvert: exercise sexual abstinence or use condoms to prevent sexual transmission and to avoid pregnancy; and refrain from donating blood, plasma, organs, tissue, or semen. If an exposed woman is breast feeding, she should be counseled about the risk of HIV transmission through breast milk, and discontinuation of breast feeding should be considered, especially for high-risk exposures. Additionally, NRTIs are known to pass into breast milk, as is NVP; whether this also is true for the other approved antiretroviral drugs is unknown.

The patient-care responsibilities of an exposed person do not need to be modified, based solely on an HIV exposure, to prevent transmission to patients. If HIV seroconversion is detected, the person should be evaluated according to published recommendations for infected HCP (*175*).

Exposed HCP should be advised to seek medical evaluation for any acute illness that occurs during the follow-up period. Such an illness, particularly if characterized by fever, rash, myalgia, fatigue, malaise, or lymphadenopathy, might be indicative of acute HIV infection but also might be indicative of a drug reaction or another medical condition.

For exposures for which PEP is considered appropriate, HCP should be informed that a) knowledge about the efficacy of drugs used for PEP is limited; b) experts recommend combination drug regimens because of increased potency and concerns about drug-resistant virus; c) data regarding toxicity of antiretroviral drugs in persons without HIV infection or in pregnant women are limited; d) although the short-term toxicity of antiretroviral drugs is usually limited, serious adverse events have occurred in persons taking PEP; and e) any or all drugs for PEP may be declined or stopped by the exposed person. HCP who experience HIV occupational exposures for which PEP is not recommended should be informed that the potential side effects and toxicity of taking PEP outweigh the negligible risk of transmission posed by the type of exposure.

Guidelines for counseling and educating HCP with HIV exposure include

- Exposed HCP should be advised to use precautions to prevent secondary transmission during the follow-up period.

- For exposures for which PEP is prescribed, HCP should be informed about possible drug toxicities and the need for monitoring, and possible drug interactions.

Occupational Exposure Management Resources

Several resources are available that provide guidance to HCP regarding the management of occupational exposures. These resources include PEPline; the Needlestick! website; the Hepatitis Hotline; CDC (receives reports of occupationally acquired HIV infections and failures of PEP); the HIV Antiretroviral Pregnancy Registry; FDA (receives reports of unusual or severe toxicity to antiretroviral agents); and the HIV/AIDS Treatment Information Service (Box 5).

BOX 4. Situations for which expert* consultation for HIV postexposure prophylaxis is advised

- Delayed (i.e., later than 24–36 hours) exposure report
  — the interval after which there is no benefit from postexposure prophylaxis (PEP) is undefined

- Unknown source (e.g., needle in sharps disposal container or laundry)
  — decide use of PEP on a case-by-case basis
  — consider the severity of the exposure and the epidemiologic likelihood of HIV exposure
  — do not test needles or other sharp instruments for HIV

- Known or suspected pregnancy in the exposed person
  — does not preclude the use of optimal PEP regimens
  — do not deny PEP solely on the basis of pregnancy

- Resistance of the source virus to antiretroviral agents
  — influence of drug resistance on transmission risk is unknown
  — selection of drugs to which the source person's virus is unlikely to be resistant is recommended, if the source person's virus is known or suspected to be resistant to ≥ 1 of the drugs considered for the PEP regimen
  — resistance testing of the source person's virus at the time of the exposure is not recommended

- Toxicity of the initial PEP regimen
  — adverse symptoms, such as nausea and diarrhea are common with PEP
  — symptoms often can be managed without changing the PEP regimen by prescribing antimotility and/or antiemetic agents
  — modification of dose intervals (i.e., administering a lower dose of drug more frequently throughout the day, as recommended by the manufacturer), in other situations, might help alleviate symptoms

*Local experts and/or the National Clinicians' Post-Exposure Prophylaxis Hotline (PEPline [1-888-448-4911]).

BOX 5. Occupational exposure management resources

National Clinicians' Postexposure Prophylaxis Hotline (PEPline) Run by University of California–San Francisco/San Francisco General Hospital staff; supported by the Health Resources and Services Administration Ryan White CARE Act, HIV/AIDS Bureau, AIDS Education and Training Centers, and CDC.	Phone: (888) 448-4911 Internet: <http://www.ucsf.edu/hivcntr>
Needlestick! A website to help clinicians manage and document occupational blood and body fluid exposures. Developed and maintained by the University of California, Los Angeles (UCLA), Emergency Medicine Center, UCLA School of Medicine, and funded in party by CDC and the Agency for Healthcare Research and Quality.	Internet: <http:// www.needlestick.mednet.ucla.edu>
Hepatitis Hotline.	Phone: (888) 443-7232 Internet: <http://www.cdc.gov/hepatitis>
Reporting to CDC: Occupationally acquired HIV infections and failures of PEP.	Phone: (800) 893-0485
HIV Antiretroviral Pregnancy Registry.	Phone:(800) 258-4263 Fax: (800) 800-1052 Address: 1410 Commonwealth Drive Suite 215 Wilmington, NC 28405 Internet: <http://www.glaxowellcome.com/ preg_reg/antiretroviral>

BOX 5. (*Continued*) Occupational exposure management resources

Food and Drug Administration
Report unusual or severe toxicity
to antiretroviral agents.
	Phone: (800) 332-1088
	Address:
	   MedWatch
	   HF-2, FDA
	   5600 Fishers Lane
	   Rockville, MD 20857
	Internet:
	     <http://www.fda.gov/medwatch>

HIV/AIDS Treatment Information Service.	Internet: <http://www.hivatis.org>

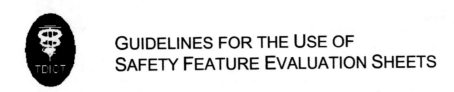

GUIDELINES FOR THE USE OF
SAFETY FEATURE EVALUATION SHEETS

Coordinators:

Determine which products are to be evaluated and provide at least four or more test samples for each individual evaluating the product. (Each evaluator should have enough samples to disassemble and examine the design thoroughly.)

Set up a testing station for each type of device which allows testers to evaluate products in a simulated patient procedure. Provide training dummies (injection pads, oranges, etc.) as necessary.

Provide visual instructions and demonstrate proper use of each device.

Review the instructions and rating system with each evaluator.

Encourage each evaluator to comment on the sheets and prioritize the questions at the end of the evaluation. This will provide a useful decision making tool and will help alert you to specific areas of concern which may not have been covered by the questionnaire.

Evaluators:

Re-enact all steps of intended or possible procedures performed with the device being tested.

Attempt to misuse the device and circumvent or disable the safety feature.

Answer each question, including the short answer section at the end. If you do not understand a question, please write comments directly on the sheets.

NOTE: The utility of these criteria is for initial screening of devices and **NOT** for clinical assessment/pilot testing. Certain assumptions have been made in the development of these forms based on information about currently available products. We recognize the likelihood that the ideal product may not exist. TDICT welcomes your comments on the use of these tools.

Source: Reprinted with permission of Training for Development of Innovative Control Technology Project
June Fisher, M.D.
© June1993, revised August 1998
Trauma Foundation, Bldg #1, Room #300
San Francisco General Hospital
1001 Potrero Avenue
San Francisco, CA 94110

SAFETY FEATURE EVALUATION FORM
SAFETY SYRINGES

Date: _____ Department: _____ Occupation: _____

Product: _____ Number of times used: _____

Please **circle** the most appropriate answer for each question. Not applicable (N/A) may be used if the question does not apply to this particular product.

agree............disagree

DURING USE:

1. The safety feature can be activated using a one-handed technique .... 1 2 3 4 5 N/A
2. The safety feature **does not** obstruct vision of the tip of the sharp .... 1 2 3 4 5 N/A
3. Use of this product requires you to use the safety feature .... 1 2 3 4 5 N/A
4. This product does not require more time to use than a non-safety device .... 1 2 3 4 5 N/A
5. The safety feature works well with a wide variety of hand sizes .... 1 2 3 4 5 N/A
6. The device is easy to handle while wearing gloves .... 1 2 3 4 5 N/A
7. This device **does not** interfere with uses that do not require a needle .... 1 2 3 4 5 N/A
8. This device offers a good view of any aspirated fluid .... 1 2 3 4 5 N/A
9. This device will work with all required syringe and needle sizes .... 1 2 3 4 5 N/A
10. This device provides a better alternative to traditional recapping .... 1 2 3 4 5 N/A

AFTER USE:

11. There is a clear and unmistakable change (audible or visible) that occurs
    when the safety feature is activated .... 1 2 3 4 5 N/A
12. The safety feature operates reliably .... 1 2 3 4 5 N/A
13. The exposed sharp is permanently blunted or covered after use and prior to disposal . 1 2 3 4 5 N/A
14. This device is no more difficult to process after use than non-safety devices .... 1 2 3 4 5 N/A

TRAINING:

15. The user **does not** need extensive training for correct operation .... 1 2 3 4 5 N/A
16. The design of the device suggests proper use .... 1 2 3 4 5 N/A
17. It is **not** easy to skip a crucial step in proper use of the device .... 1 2 3 4 5 N/A

Of the above questions, which three are the most important to **your** safety when using this product?

Are there other questions which you feel should be asked regarding the safety/utility of this product?

Source: Reprinted with permission of Training for Development of Innovative Control Technology Project
June Fisher, M.D.
© June 1993, revised August 1998

SAFETY FEATURE EVALUATION FORM
I.V. ACCESS DEVICES

Date: _____ Department: _____ Occupation: _____

Product: _____ Number of times used: _____

Please **circle** the most appropriate answer for each question. Not applicable (N/A) may be used if the question does not apply to this particular product.

	agree...........disagree
1. The safety feature can be activated using a one-handed technique	1 2 3 4 5 N/A
2. The safety feature **does not** interfere with normal use of this product	1 2 3 4 5 N/A
3. Use of this product requires you to use the safety feature	1 2 3 4 5 N/A
4. This product **does not** require more time to use than a non-safety device	1 2 3 4 5 N/A
5. The safety feature works well with a wide variety of hand sizes	1 2 3 4 5 N/A
6. The device allows for rapid visualization of flashback in the catheter or chamber ...	1 2 3 4 5 N/A
7. Use of this product **does not** increase the number of sticks to the patient	1 2 3 4 5 N/A
8. The product stops the flow of blood after the needle is removed from the catheter (or after the butterfly is inserted) and just prior to line connections or hep-lock capping	1 2 3 4 5 N/A
9. A clear and unmistakable change (either audible or visible) occurs when the safety feature is activated	1 2 3 4 5 N/A
10. The safety feature operates reliably	1 2 3 4 5 N/A
11. The exposed sharp is blunted or covered after use and prior to disposal	1 2 3 4 5 N/A
12. The product **does not** need extensive training to be operated correctly	1 2 3 4 5 N/A

Of the above questions, which three are the most important to **your** safety when using this product?

Are there other questions which you feel should be asked regarding the safety/utility of this product?

Source: Reprinted with permission of Training for Development of Innovative Control Technology Project
June Fisher, M.D.
© June1993, revised August 1998

SAFETY FEATURE EVALUATION FORM
SHARPS DISPOSAL CONTAINERS

Date: _____ Department: _____ Occupation: _____

Product: _____ Number of times used: _____

Please **circle** the most appropriate answer for each question. Not applicable (N/A) may be used if the question does not apply to this particular product.

agree...........disagree

1. The container's shape, its markings, or its color, imply danger .... 1 2 3 4 5 N/A
2. The implied warning of danger can be seen from the angle at which people commonly view it (very short people, people in wheel chairs, children, etc) .... 1 2 3 4 5 N/A
3. The implied warning can be universally understood by visitors, children, and patients .. 1 2 3 4 5 N/A
4. The container's purpose is self-explanatory and easily understood by a worker who may be pressed for time or unfamiliar with the hospital setting .... 1 2 3 4 5 N/A
5. The container can accept sharps from any direction desired .... 1 2 3 4 5 N/A
6. The container can accept all sizes and shapes of sharps .... 1 2 3 4 5 N/A
7. The container allows single handed operation. (Only the hand holding the sharp should be near the container opening) .... 1 2 3 4 5 N/A
8. It is difficult to reach in and remove a sharp .... 1 2 3 4 5 N/A
9. Sharps can go into the container without getting caught on the opening .... 1 2 3 4 5 N/A
10. Sharps can go into the container without getting caught on any molded shapes in the interior .... 1 2 3 4 5 N/A
11. The container is puncture resistant .... 1 2 3 4 5 N/A
12. When the container is dropped or turned upside down (even before it is permanently closed) sharps stay inside .... 1 2 3 4 5 N/A
13. The user can determine easily, from various viewing angles, when the container is full .... 1 2 3 4 5 N/A
14. When the container is to be used free-standing (no mounting bracket), it is stable and unlikely to tip over .... 1 2 3 4 5 N/A
15. It is safe to close the container. (Sharps should not protrude into the path of hands attempting to close the container) .... 1 2 3 4 5 N/A
16. The container closes securely. (e.g. if the closure requires glue, it may not work if the surfaces are soiled or wet.) .... 1 2 3 4 5 N/A
17. The product has handles which allow you to safely transport a full container .... 1 2 3 4 5 N/A
18. The product **does not** require extensive training to operate correctly .... 1 2 3 4 5 N/A

Of the above questions, which three are the most important to **your** safety when using this product?

Are there other questions which you feel should be asked regarding the safety/utility of this product?

Source: Reprinted with permission of Training for Development of Innovative Control Technology Project
June Fisher, M.D.
© June1993, revised August

SAFETY FEATURE EVALUATION FORM
I.V. CONNECTORS

Date: _____ Department: _____ Occupation: _____

Product: _____ Number of times used: _____

Please **circle** the most appropriate answer for each question. Not applicable (N/A) may be used if the question does not apply to this particular product.

agree..........disagree

1. Use of this connector eliminates the need for exposed needles in connections . . . . 1 2 3 4 5 N/A
2. The safety feature **does not** interfere with normal use of this product . . . . 1 2 3 4 5 N/A
3. Use of this product requires you to use the safety feature . . . . 1 2 3 4 5 N/A
4. This product **does not** require more time to use than a non-safety device . . . . 1 2 3 4 5 N/A
5. The safety feature works well with a wide variety of hand sizes . . . . 1 2 3 4 5 N/A
6. The safety feature allows you to collect blood directly into a vacuum tube,
   eliminating the need for needles . . . . 1 2 3 4 5 N/A
7. The connector can be secured (locked) to Y-sites, hep-locks, and central lines . . . . 1 2 3 4 5 N/A
8. A clear and unmistakable change (either audible or visible) occurs when the
   safety feature is activated . . . . 1 2 3 4 5 N/A
9. The safety feature operates reliably . . . . 1 2 3 4 5 N/A
10. The exposed sharp is blunted or covered after use and prior to disposal . . . . 1 2 3 4 5 N/A
11. The product **does not** need extensive training to be operated correctly . . . . 1 2 3 4 5 N/A

Of the above questions, which three are the most important to **your** safety when using this product?

Are there other questions which you feel should be asked regarding the safety/utility of this product?

Source: Reprinted with permission of Training for Development of Innovative Control Technology Project
June Fisher, M.D.
© June 1993, revised August 1998

SAFETY FEATURE EVALUATION FORM
VACUUM TUBE BLOOD COLLECTION SYSTEMS

Date: _____ Department: _____ Occupation: _____

Product: _____ Number of times used: _____

Please **circle** the most appropriate answer for each question. Not applicable (N/A) may be used if the question does not apply to this particular product.

agree............disagree

1. The safety feature can be activated using a one-handed technique .... 1 2 3 4 5 N/A
2. The safety feature **does not** interfere with normal use of this product .... 1 2 3 4 5 N/A
3. Use of this product requires you to use the safety feature .... 1 2 3 4 5 N/A
4. This product **does not** require more time to use than a non-safety device .... 1 2 3 4 5 N/A
5. The safety feature works well with a wide variety of hand sizes .... 1 2 3 4 5 N/A
6. The safety feature works with a butterfly .... 1 2 3 4 5 N/A
7. A clear and unmistakable change (either audible or visible) occurs when the
   safety feature is activated .... 1 2 3 4 5 N/A
8. The safety feature operates reliably .... 1 2 3 4 5 N/A
9. The exposed sharp is blunted or covered after use and prior to disposal .... 1 2 3 4 5 N/A
10. The inner vacuum tube needle (rubber sleeved needle) **does not** present a
    danger of exposure .... 1 2 3 4 5 N/A
11. The **product does** not need extensive training to be operated correctly .... 1 2 3 4 5 N/A

Of the above questions, which three are the most important to **your** safety when using this product?

Are there other questions which you feel should be asked regarding the safety/utility of this product?

Source: Reprinted with permission of Training for Development of Innovative Control Technology Project
June Fisher, M.D.
© June1993, revised August 1998

SAFETY FEATURE EVALUATION FORM
E. R. SHARPS DISPOSAL CONTAINERS

Date: _____ Department: _____ Occupation: _____

Product: _____ Number of times used: _____

Please **circle** the most appropriate answer for each question. Not applicable (N/A) may be used if the question does not apply to this particular product.

agree............disagree

1. The container's shape, its markings, or its color, imply danger which can be understood by visitors, children, and patients . . . . 1 2 3 4 5 N/A

2. The implied warning of danger can be seen from the angle at which people commonly view it. (very short people, people in wheel chairs, children, etc) . . . . 1 2 3 4 5 N/A

3. The container can be placed in a location that is easily accessible during emergency procedures . . . . 1 2 3 4 5 N/A

4. The container's purpose is self-explanatory and easily understood by a worker who may be pressed for time or unfamiliar with the hospital setting . . . . 1 2 3 4 5 N/A

5. The container can accept sharps from any direction desired . . . . 1 2 3 4 5 N/A

6. The container can accept all sizes and shapes of sharps . . . . 1 2 3 4 5 N/A

7. The container is temporarily closable, and will not spill contents (even after being dropped down a flight of stairs) . . . . 1 2 3 4 5 N/A

8. The container allows single handed operation. (Only the hand holding the sharp should be near the container opening) . . . . 1 2 3 4 5 N/A

9. It is difficult to reach in and remove a sharp . . . . 1 2 3 4 5 N/A

10. Sharps can go into the container without getting caught on the opening or any molded shapes in the interior . . . . 1 2 3 4 5 N/A

11. The container can be placed within arm's reach . . . . 1 2 3 4 5 N/A

12. The container is puncture resistant . . . . 1 2 3 4 5 N/A

13. When the container is dropped or turned upside down (even before it is permanently closed) sharps stay inside . . . . 1 2 3 4 5 N/A

14. The user can determine easily, from various viewing angles, when the container is full . 1 2 3 4 5 N/A

15. When the container is to be used free-standing (no mounting bracket), it is stable and unlikely to tip over . . . . 1 2 3 4 5 N/A

16. The container is large enough to accept all sizes and shapes of sharps, including 50 ml preloaded syringes . . . . 1 2 3 4 5 N/A

17. It is safe to close the container. (Sharps should not protrude into the path of hands attempting to close the container) . . . . 1 2 3 4 5 N/A

18. The container closes securely under all circumstances . . . . 1 2 3 4 5 N/A

19. The product has handles which allow you to safely transport a full container . . . . 1 2 3 4 5 N/A

20. The product **does not** require extensive training to operate correctly . . . . 1 2 3 4 5 N/A

Of the above questions, which three are the most important to **your** safety when using this product?

Are there other questions which you feel should be asked regarding the safety/ utility of this product?

Source: Reprinted with permission of Training for Development of Innovative Control Technology Project
June Fisher, M.D.
© June1993, revised August 1998

SAFETY FEATURE EVALUATION FORM
HOME USE SHARPS DISPOSAL CONTAINER

Date: _____ Department: _____ Occupation: _____

Product: _____ Number of times used: _____

Please **circle** the most appropriate answer for each question. Not applicable (N/A) may be used if the question does not apply to this particular product.

	agree............disagree
The container is puncture resistant	1 2 3 4 5 N/A
The container is stable	1 2 3 4 5 N/A
There is a handle which is robust, comfortable to carry, and compact	1 2 3 4 5 N/A
The container allows single handed use	1 2 3 4 5 N/A
The user can access the container from any direction	1 2 3 4 5 N/A
It is possible to drop sharps into the container vertically	1 2 3 4 5 N/A
Minimal or no force is required to put sharps into the container	1 2 3 4 5 N/A
The container opens and closes easily	1 2 3 4 5 N/A
Container closure maintains integrity after repeated use	1 2 3 4 5 N/A
The box accommodates a range of sharps, including 12 cc syringe, butterfly, and lancet	1 2 3 4 5 N/A
The size of the container is appropriate to its use	1 2 3 4 5 N/A
No one (including a child) can access the contents of the container to retrieve a sharp	1 2 3 4 5 N/A
Needles/tubing do not get caught on the opening or interior shape	1 2 3 4 5 N/A
There is a temporary lock for transport which is secure but reversible	1 2 3 4 5 N/A
There is a permanent lock for final disposal which is not reversible	1 2 3 4 5 N/A
There is an absorbent lining to collect excess fluid	1 2 3 4 5 N/A
The user can determine the fill level visually	1 2 3 4 5 N/A
There is a signal when the box is 2/3 full	1 2 3 4 5 N/A
The container is appropriately labeled	1 2 3 4 5 N/A
Biohazard of container contents is apparent	1 2 3 4 5 N/A
The box is not threatening to patients	1 2 3 4 5 N/A
Use of this container in no way compromises infection control practices	1 2 3 4 5 N/A

Of the above questions, which three are the most important to **your** safety when using this product?

Are there other questions which you feel should be asked regarding the safety/ utility of this product?

Source: Reprinted with permission of Training for Development of Innovative Control Technology Project
June Fisher, M.D.
© June1993, revised August 1998

EMERGING INFECTIOUS DISEASES   Volume 4 Number 1

| Past Issues | | Current Issue | Upcoming Issue | Past Issues | Search | Home | **January – March 1998** |
| Download | | ASCII Text | Adobe PDF | Postscript | |

Suggested Citation

Perspectives

Outbreak Investigations—A Perspective

Arthur L. Reingold
University of California, Berkeley, California, USA

Outbreak investigations, an important and challenging component of epidemiology and public health, can help identify the source of ongoing outbreaks and prevent additional cases. Even when an outbreak is over, a thorough epidemiologic and environmental investigation often can increase our knowledge of a given disease and prevent future outbreaks. Finally, outbreak investigations provide epidemiologic training and foster cooperation between the clinical and public health communities.

Investigations of acute infectious disease outbreaks are very common, and the results of such investigations are often published; however, surprisingly little has been written about the actual procedures followed during such investigations (1,2). Most epidemiologists and public health officials learn the procedures by conducting investigations with the initial assistance of more experienced colleagues. This article outlines the general approach to conducting an outbreak investigation. The approach applies not only to infectious disease outbreaks but also to outbreaks due to noninfectious causes (e.g., toxic exposure).

How Outbreaks Are Recognized

Possible outbreaks of disease come to the attention of public health officials in various ways. Often, an astute clinician, infection control nurse, or clinical laboratory worker first notices an unusual disease or an unusual number of cases of a disease and alerts public health officials. For example, staphylococcal toxic shock syndrome and eosinophilia myalgia syndrome were first noted by clinicians (3,4). Frequently, it is the patient (or someone close to the patient) who first suspects a problem, as is often the case in foodborne outbreaks after a shared meal and as was the case in the investigation of a cluster of cases of apparent juvenile rheumatoid arthritis near Lyme, Connecticut, which led to the discovery of Lyme disease (5). Review of routinely collected surveillance data can also detect outbreaks of known diseases, as in the case of hepatitis B infection among the patients of an oral surgeon in Connecticut and patients at a weight reduction clinic (6,7). The former outbreak was first suspected when routinely submitted communicable disease report forms for several patients from one small town indicated that all of the patients had recently had oral surgery. However, it is relatively uncommon for outbreaks to be detected in this way and even more uncommon for them to be detected in this way while they are still in progress. Finally, sometimes public health officials learn about outbreaks of disease from the local newspaper or television news.

Reasons for Investigating Outbreaks

The most compelling reason to investigate a recognized outbreak of disease is that exposure to the source(s) of infection may be continuing; by identifying and eliminating the source of infection, we can prevent additional cases. For example, if cans of mushrooms containing botulinum toxin are still on store shelves or in homes or restaurants, their recall and destruction can prevent further cases of botulism.

However, even if an outbreak is essentially over by the time the epidemiologic investigation begins—that is, if no one is being further exposed to the source of infection—investigating the outbreak may still be indicated for many reasons. Foremost is that the results of the investigation may lead to recommendations or strategies for preventing similar future outbreaks. For example, a Legionnaires' disease outbreak investigation may produce recommendations for grocery store misting machine use that may prevent other outbreaks (8). Other reasons for investigating outbreaks are the opportunity to 1) describe new diseases and learn more about known diseases; 2) evaluate existing prevention strategies, e.g., vaccines; 3) teach (and learn) epidemiology; and 4) address public concern about the outbreak.

Once a decision is made to investigate an outbreak, three types of activities are generally involved—the epidemiologic investigation; the environmental investigation; and the interaction with the public, the press, and, in many instances, the legal system. While these activities often occur simultaneously throughout the investigation, it is conceptually easier to consider each of them separately.

Epidemiologic Investigation

Outbreak investigations are, in theory, indistinguishable from other epidemiologic investigations; however, outbreak investigations encounter more constraints. 1) If the outbreak is ongoing at the time of the investigation, there is great urgency to find the source and prevent additional cases. 2) Because outbreak investigations frequently are public, there is substantial pressure to conclude them rapidly, particularly if the outbreak is ongoing. 3) In many outbreaks, the number of cases available for study is limited; therefore, the statistical power of the investigation is limited. 4) Early media reports concerning the outbreak may bias the responses of persons subsequently interviewed. 5) Because of legal liability and the financial interests of persons and institutions involved, there is pressure to conclude the investigation quickly, which may lead to hasty decisions regarding the source of the outbreak. 6) If detection of the outbreak is delayed, useful clinical and environmental samples may be very difficult or impossible to obtain.

Outbreak investigations have essential components as follows: 1) establish case definition(s); 2) confirm that cases are "real"; 3) establish the background rate of disease; 4) find cases, decide if there is an outbreak, define scope of the outbreak; 5) examine the descriptive epidemiologic features of the cases; 6) generate hypotheses; 7) test hypotheses; 8) collect and test environmental samples; 9) implement control measures; and 10) interact with the press, inform the public. While the first seven components are listed in logical order, in most outbreak investigations, many occur more or less simultaneously. The importance of these components may vary depending on the circumstances of a specific outbreak.

Case Definition

In some outbreaks, formulating the case definition(s) and exclusion criteria is straightforward; for example, in an outbreak of gastroenteritis caused by Salmonella infection, a laboratory-confirmed case would be defined as a culture-confirmed infection with Salmonella or perhaps with Salmonella of the particular serotype causing the outbreak, while a clinical case definition might be new onset of diarrhea. In other outbreaks, the case definition and exclusion criteria are complex, particularly if the disease is new and the range of clinical manifestations is unknown (e.g., in a putative outbreak of chronic fatigue syndrome). In many outbreak investigations, multiple case definitions are used (e.g., laboratory-confirmed case vs. clinical case; definite vs. probable vs. possible case; outbreak-associated case vs. nonoutbreak-associated case, primary case vs. secondary case) and the resulting data are analyzed by using different case definitions. When the number of cases available for study is not a limiting factor and a case-control study is being used to examine risk factors for becoming a case, a strict case definition is often preferable to increase specificity and reduce misclassification of disease status (i.e., reduce the chance of including cases of unrelated illness or no illness as outbreak-related cases).

334

Case Confirmation

In certain outbreaks, clinical findings in reported cases should be reviewed closely, either directly, by examining the patients, or indirectly, by detailed review of the medical records and discussion with the attending health-care provider(s), especially when a new disease appears to be emerging (e.g., in the early investigations of Legionnaires' disease, AIDS, eosinophilia myalgia syndrome, and hantavirus pulmonary syndrome) (4,9-11). Clinical findings should also be examined closely when some or all of the observed cases may be factitious, perhaps because of laboratory error (12); a discrepancy between the clinical and laboratory findings generally exists, which may be discernible only by a detailed review of the clinical findings.

Establishing the Background Rate of Disease and Finding Cases

Once it is clear that a suspected outbreak is not the result of laboratory error, a set of activities should be undertaken to establish the background rate of the disease in the affected population and to find all the cases in a given population in a certain period. This set of activities should prove that the observed number of cases truly is in excess of the "usual" number (i.e., that an outbreak has occurred), define the scope of the outbreak geographically and temporally, find cases to describe the epidemiologic features of those affected and to include them in analytic epidemiologic studies (see below) or, most often, accomplish a combination of these goals.

When hundreds of acute onset diarrhea cases are suddenly seen daily in a single outpatient setting (10), an outbreak is clearly occurring. On the other hand, when too many hospitalized patients are dying unexpectedly of cardiac arrest (13) or the number of cases of listeriosis in a given county in recent months is moderately elevated, it may be necessary to establish the background rates in the population to determine whether an outbreak is occurring. In such situations, the period and geographic areas involved would provide the most useful baseline data, keeping in mind that the labor and time required to collect such information is often directly proportional to the length of the period and the size of the geographic area selected. Because disease incidence normally fluctuates by season, data from comparable seasons in earlier years should be included.

Establishing the background rate of a disease is generally more straightforward if confirmatory tests are available than if laboratory tests are unavailable or infrequently used. The rate of certain invasive bacterial infections (e.g., listeriosis and meningococcal infections) in a given area can be easily documented by reviewing the records of hospital clinical microbiology laboratories; however, cases for which specimens were not submitted to these laboratories for testing will go undetected. When a disease is less frequently laboratory-confirmed because health-care providers may not have considered the diagnosis or ordered the appropriate laboratory tests (e.g., for Legionnaires' disease), establishing the background rate of disease in a community or a hospital suspected of having an outbreak generally requires alternative case-finding strategies and is almost invariably more labor intensive. In an outbreak of a new disease, substantial effort is often necessary to determine whether or not cases of that disease had been occurring but had gone unrecognized.

Once data concerning the background rate of a disease (including case-finding for the current period) have been collected, it is generally possible to determine whether or not an outbreak is occurring or has occurred, although in some situations it may remain unclear whether or not the number of cases observed exceeds the background rate. In part, the problem may relate to how an outbreak is defined. To paraphrase a U.S. Supreme Court justice speaking about pornography, "I can't define an outbreak, but I know one when I see one." Thus, it may be difficult to detect and prove the existence of small outbreaks, but large ones are self-evident.

An outbreak can also be difficult to identify when during the period under study changes occur in the care-seeking behavior and access to care of patients; the level of suspicion, referral patterns, and test-ordering practices of health-care providers; the diagnostic tests and other procedures used by laboratories; and the prevalence of underlying immunosuppressive conditions or other host factors in the population. All these factors, which can affect the apparent incidence of a disease and produce artifactual changes perceived as increases (or decreases) in the actual incidence, need to be considered when interpreting the findings.

Descriptive Epidemiology

By collecting patient data, the case-finding activities provide extremely important information concerning the descriptive epidemiologic features of the outbreak. By reviewing and plotting on an "epidemic curve" the times of onset of the cases and by examining the characteristics (e.g., age, sex, race/ethnicity, residence, occupation, recent travel, or attendance at events) of the ill persons, investigators can often generate hypotheses concerning the cause(s)/source(s) of the outbreak. While linking the sudden onset of gastroenteritis among scores of persons who attended a church supper to the single common meal they shared is generally not a challenge, an otherwise cryptic source can be at least hinted at by the descriptive epidemiologic features of the cases involved. For example, in a particularly perplexing outbreak of *Salmonella* Muenchen infections ultimately traced to contaminated marijuana, the age distribution of the affected persons and of their households was markedly different from that typically seen for salmonellosis (14). Or, similarly, in the outbreak of legionellosis due to contaminated misting machines in the produce section of a grocery store, before the link to this exposure was even suspected, it was noted that women constituted a substantially higher proportion of the cases usually seen with this disease (5). The shape of the epidemic curve can also be very instructive, suggesting a point-source epidemic, ongoing transmission, or a combination of the two.

Generating a Hypothesis

The source(s) and route(s) of exposure must be determined to understand why an outbreak occurred, how to prevent similar outbreaks in the future, and, if the outbreak is ongoing, how to prevent others from being exposed to the source(s) of infection. In some outbreaks, the source and route are obvious to those involved in the outbreak and to the investigators. However, even when the source of exposure appears obvious at the outset, a modicum of skepticism should be retained because the obvious answer is not invariably correct. For example, in an outbreak of nosocomial legionellosis in Rhode Island, the results of an earlier investigation into a small number of hospital-acquired cases at the same hospital had demonstrated that *Legionella pneumophila* was in the hospital potable water supply, and a sudden increase in new cases was strongly believed to be related to the potable water (15). However, a detailed epidemiologic investigation implicated a new cooling tower at the hospital as the source of the second outbreak.

While the true source of exposure, or at least a relatively short list of possibilities, is apparent in many outbreaks, this is not the case in the more challenging outbreaks. In these instances, hypotheses concerning the source/route of exposure can be generated in a number of ways beyond a detailed review of the descriptive epidemiologic findings. A review of existing epidemiologic, microbiologic, and veterinary data is very useful for learning about known and suspected sources of previous outbreaks or sporadic cases of a given infection or disease, as well as the ecologic niche of an infectious agent. Thus, in an outbreak of invasive *Streptococcus zooepidemicus* infections in New Mexico due to consumption of soft cheese made from contaminated raw milk, the investigation focused on exposure to dairy products and animals because of previous microbiologic and veterinary studies (16).

A review of existing data generally only helps confirm what is already known about a particular disease and is far less helpful in identifying totally new and unsuspected sources or routes of infection (i.e., marijuana as a source of Salmonella). When neither review of the descriptive epidemiologic features of the cases nor review of existing scientific information yields the correct hypothesis, other methods can be used to generate hypotheses about what the patients have in common. Open-ended interviews of those infected (or their surrogates) are one such method in which investigators try to identify all possibly relevant exposures (e.g., a list of all foods consumed) during a given period. For example, in an investigation of *Yersinia enterocolitica* infections in young children in Belgium, open-ended interviews of the mothers of some of the ill children showed that many gave their children raw pork sausage as a weaning food, providing the first clue as to the source of these infections (17). Similarly, in two outbreaks of foodborne listeriosis, a variant of this process led to the identification of the source of the outbreak. In one of these outbreaks, a search of the refrigerator of one of the case-patients who, as a visitor to the area, had had very limited exposure to foods there, suggested cole slaw as a possible vehicle of infection (18). In the other outbreak, an initial case-control study found no differences between cases and controls regarding exposure to a number of specific food items but showed that case households were more likely than control households to buy their food at a particular foodstore chain. To generate a list of other possible food sources of infection, investigators shopped with persons who did the shopping for case households and compiled a list of foods purchased at that foodstore chain that had not been reported in the previous study. This approach implicated pasteurized milk from that chain as the source of the outbreak (19).

In some particularly perplexing outbreaks, bringing together a subset of the patients to discuss their experiences and exposures in a way that may reveal unidentified links can be useful.

Testing the Hypothesis

Whether a hypothesis explaining the occurrence of an outbreak is easy or difficult to generate, an analytic epidemiologic study to test the proposed hypothesis should be considered. While in many instances a case-control study is used, other designs, including retrospective cohort and cross-sectional studies, can be equally or more appropriate. The goal of all these studies is to assess the relationship between a given exposure and the disease under study. Thus, each exposure of interest (e.g., each of the meals eaten together by passengers on a cruise ship and each of the foods and beverages served at those meals) constitutes a separate hypothesis to be tested in the analytic study. In outbreaks where generating the correct hypothesis is difficult, multiple analytic studies, with additional hypothesis-generating activities in between, are sometimes needed before the correct hypothesis is formed and tested (19).

In interpreting the results of such analytic studies, one must consider the possibility that "statistically significant" associations between one or more exposures and the disease may be chance findings, not indicative of a true relationship. By definition, any "statistically significant" association may have occurred by chance. (When the standard cut point of $p < 0.05$ is used, this occurs 5% of the time.) Because many analytic epidemiologic studies of outbreaks involve testing many hypotheses, the problem of "multiple comparisons" arises often.

While there are statistical methods for adjusting for multiple comparisons, when and even whether to use them is controversial. At a minimum, it is important to go beyond the statistical tests and examine the magnitude of the effect observed between exposure and disease (e.g., the odds ratio, relative risk) and the 95% confidence intervals, as well as biologic plausibility in deciding whether or not a given "statistically significant" relationship is likely to be biologically meaningful. Evidence of a dose-response effect between a given exposure and illness (i.e., the greater the exposure, the greater the risk for illness) makes a causal relationship between exposure and disease more likely. Whether the time interval between a given exposure and onset of illness is consistent with what is known about the incubation period of the disease under study must also be assessed. When illness is "statistically significantly" related to more than one exposure (e.g., to eating each of several foods at a common meal), it is important to determine whether multiple sources of infection (perhaps due to cross-contamination) are plausible and whether some of the noted associations are due to confounding (e.g., exposure to one potential source is linked to exposure to other sources) or to chance.

When trying to decide if a "statistically significant" exposure is the source of an outbreak, it is important to consider what proportion of the cases can be accounted for by that exposure. One or more of the patients may be classified as "nonexposed" for various reasons: incorrect information concerning exposure status (due to poor memory, language barriers); multiple sources of exposure or routes of transmission (perhaps due to cross-contamination); secondary person-to-person transmission that followed a common source exposure; or patients without the suspected exposure, representing background cases of the disease unrelated to the outbreak. The plausibility of each of these explanations varies by outbreak. While there is no cutoff point above or below which the proportion of exposed case-patients should fall before an exposure is thought to account for an outbreak, the lower this proportion, the less likely the exposure is, by itself, the source.

Other possibilities need to be considered when the analytic epidemiologic study finds no association between the hypothesized exposures and risk for disease. The most obvious possibility is that the real exposure was not among those examined, and additional hypotheses should be generated. However, other possibilities should also be considered, particularly when the setting of the outbreak makes this first explanation unlikely (e.g., when it is known that those involved in the outbreak shared only a single exposure or set of exposures, such as eating a single common meal). Two other explanations for failing to find a "statistically significant" link between one or more exposures and risk for illness also need to be considered—the number of persons available for study and the accuracy of the available information concerning the exposures. Thus, if the outbreak involves only a small number of cases (and non-ill persons), the statistical power of the analytic study to find a true difference in exposure between the ill and the non-ill (or a difference in the rate of disease among the exposed and the unexposed) is very limited. If the persons involved in the outbreak do not provide accurate information about their exposure to suspected sources or vehicles of infection because of lack of knowledge, poor memory, language difficulty, mental impairment, or other reasons, the resulting misclassification of exposure status also can prevent the epidemiologic study from implicating the source of infection. Studies have documented that even under ideal circumstances, memory concerning such exposures is faulty (20). However, given the usually enormous differences in rates of disease between those exposed and those not exposed to the source of the outbreak, even small studies or studies with substantial misclassification of exposure can still correctly identify the source.

Environmental Investigation

Samples of foods and beverages served at a common meal believed to be the source of an outbreak of gastroenteritis or samples of the water or drift from a cooling tower believed to be the source of an outbreak of Legionnaires' disease can support epidemiologic findings. In the best scenario, the findings of the epidemiologic investigation would guide the collection and testing of environmental samples. However, environmental specimens often need to be obtained as soon as possible, either before they are no longer available, as in the case of residual food from a common meal, or before environmental interventions are implemented, as in the case of treating a cooling tower to eradicate Legionella. Because laboratory testing of environmental samples is often expensive and labor-intensive, it is sometimes reasonable to collect and store many samples but test only a limited number. Collaborating with a sanitarian, environmental engineer, or other professional during an environmental inspection or collection of specimens is always beneficial.

While finding or not finding the causative organism in environmental samples is often perceived by the public, the media, and the courts as powerful evidence implicating or exonerating an environmental source, either positive or negative findings can be misleading for several reasons. For example, finding Legionella in a hospital potable water system does not prove that the potable water (rather than a cooling tower or some other source) is responsible for an outbreak of Legionnaires' disease (21). Similarly, not finding the causative organism in an environmental sample does not conclusively rule out a source as the cause of the problem, in part because the samples obtained and tested may not represent the source (e.g., because of error in collecting the specimens, intervening changes in the environmental source) and in part because the samples may have been mishandled. Furthermore, in some outbreaks caused by well-characterized etiologic agents, laboratory methods of detecting the agent in environmental samples are insensitive, technically difficult, or not available, as in the case of recent outbreaks of *Cyclospora* infections associated with eating imported berries (22,23).

Control Measures

Central to any outbreak investigation is the timely implementation of appropriate control measures to minimize further illness and death. At best, the implementation of control measures would be guided by the results of the epidemiologic investigation and possibly (when appropriate) the testing of environmental specimens. However, this approach may delay prevention of further exposure to a suspected source of the outbreak and is, therefore, unacceptable from a public health perspective. Because the recall of a food product, the closing of a restaurant, or similar interventions can have profound economic and legal implications for an institution, a manufacturer or owner, and the employees of the establishments involved, acting precipitously can also have substantial negative effects. The recent attribution of an outbreak of *Cyclospora* infections to strawberries from California demonstrates the economic impact that can result from releasing and acting on incorrect information (22,23). Thus, the timing and nature of control measures are difficult. Balancing the responsibility to prevent further disease with the need to protect the credibility and reputation of an institution is very challenging.

Interactions with the Public and Press

While the public and the press are not aware of most outbreak investigations, media attention and public concern become part of some investigations. Throughout the course of an outbreak investigation, the need to share information with public officials, the press, the public, and the population affected by the outbreak must be assessed. While press, radio, and television reports can at times be inaccurate, overall the media can be a powerful means of sharing information about an investigation with the public and disseminating timely information about product recalls.

Dr. Reingold worked as an epidemiologist at the Centers for Disease Control and Prevention for 8 years before joining the faculty of the School of Public Health at the University of California, Berkeley. He is currently professor of epidemiology and head of the Division of Public Health Biology and Epidemiology.

Address for correspondence: Arthur L. Reingold, Division of Public Health Biology and Epidemiology, School of Public Health, University of California, Berkeley, 140 Warren Hall, Berkeley, CA 94720-7360, USA; fax: 510-643-5163; e-mail: reingold@uclink3.berkeley.edu.

References

1. Goodman RA, Buehler JW, Koplan JP. The epidemiologic field investigation: science and judgment in public health practice. Am J Epidemiol 1990;132:9-16.
2. MacKenzie WR, Goodman RA. The public health response to an outbreak. Current Issues in Public Health1996;2:1-4.
3. Chesney PJ, Chesney RW, Purdy W, Nelson D, McPherson T, Wand P, et al. Epidemiologic notes and reports: toxic-shock syndrome—United States. MMWR Morb Mortal Wkly Rep 1980;29:229-30.
4. Hertzman PA, Blevins WL, Mayer J, Greenfield B, Ting M, Gleich GJ, et al. Association of eosinophilia-myalgia syndrome with the ingestion of tryptophan. N Engl J Med 1980;322:871.
5. Steere AC, Malawista SE, Syndman DR, Shope RF, Andman WA, Ross MR, Steele FM. Lyme arthritis: an epidemic of oligoarticular arthritis in children and adults in three Connecticut communities. Arthritis Rheum 1977;20:7.
6. Reingold AL, Kane MA, Murphy BL, Checko P, Francis DP, Maynard JE. Transmission of Hepatitis B by an oral surgeon. J Infect Dis 1982;145:262.
7. Canter J, Mackey K, Good LS, Roberto RR, Chin J, Bond WW, et al. An outbreak of hepatitis B associated with jet injections in a weight reduction clinic. Arch Intern Med 1990;150:1923-7.
8. Mahoney FJ, Hoge CW, Farley TA, Barbaree JM, Breiman RF, Benson RF, McFarland LM. Communitywide outbreak of Legionnaires' disease associated with a grocery store mist machine. J Infect Dis 1992;165:736.
9. Fraser DW, Tsai TR, Orenstein W, Parkin WE, Beecham HJ, Sharrar RG, et al. Legionnaires' disease: description of an epidemic of pneumonia. N Engl J Med 1977;297:1189-97.

1. This section provides quick information for over 150 various communicable diseases throughout the world. The following information will be provided concerning;
    - symptoms
    - the specific infectious agent (virus, bacteria, fungus)
    - where the disease is (predominately) found,
    - the reservoir (where the organism normally lives and multiplies, and depends on for survival),
    - the mode of transmission (airborne, fecal-oral, sexual, bloodborne)
    - incubation period (time from initial exposed to symptoms)
    - treatments
    - preventive measures (handwashing, insect control, immunization, etc)
    - period of communicability (how long the infectious agent can be transmitted from person to person, or animal to person, etc).

2. Also, provides information about the most common nosocomial infection, concerning;

    - Recommended treatments
    - Proper precautions
    - Sites of Infection

3. Information on which laboratory tests to diagnosis the most common infectious diseases.

4. Last, a quick reference for immunization and medication needs for international travelers.

Acanthamebiasis and Naegleriasis:

Symptoms:
Meningoencephalitis (primary amebic meningoencephalitis PAM), sore throat, severe frontal headache, nuchal rigidity, nausea vomiting, high fever.

Infectious Agent:
Amebia, naegleria fowleri

Where is it found?
Rare in continental USA; common in Mexico, North Africa, Sudan, mostly tropical climates.

Reservoir:
In water and soil

Mode of transmission:
Naegleria: Nasal passages exposed to contaminated water, usually found near the bottom of fresh water lakes or river, particularly stagnant ponds. Usually attacks young, healthily persons
Acanthamoeba: Hematogenous spread probably from skin lesion mostly attacks immunosuppressed persons.
No transmission from person to person

Incubation:
3 to 7 days, or longer with Acanthameoba

Treatment:
Amphotericin B, usually high fatality rate

Prevention Measures:
Do not swim in ponds in hot summer months with high bacterial counts

How long communicable:
Do transmitted from person to person

Adenovirus:

Symptoms:
Conjunctivitis, upper respiratory syndrome

Infectious Agent:
Adenovirus, many types 1-25

Where is it found?
Worldwide

Reservoir:
Humans

Mode of transmission:
Contact with eye, nasal secretions, directly or indirectly, contaminated surfaces, which have sectional material

Incubation:
3-12 days

Treatment:
None

Prevention measures:
Good handwashing, Standard precautions, disinfection of medical equipment after each patient.

How long communicable:
One to two days before symptoms and two to three days after onset of symptoms.

African Sleeping Sickness:

(Tryanosomiasis, Chagas disease)

Symptoms:
Acute disease occurs more in children, many people have no acute illness. May have splenomegaly. Usually chronic problems occur such as, cardiac dilatation and other abnormalities, intestinal abnormalities, etc

Infectious Agent:
Tryanosoma cruzi, a protozoan parasite. Uses bugs as vector for transmission

Where is it found?
Confined to western hemisphere, Mexico, South and Central America

Reservoir:
Humans, over 150 species of domestic and wild animals, including dogs, cats, rats, mice, etc.,

Mode of transmission:
Infected vectors, blood-sucking species of cone-nosed bugs or kissing bugs (Triatoma, Rhodnius and panstrongylus). Found in feces of animals and some humans. Infection occurs when the excreted bug feces contaminate conjunctive, mucous membranes, abrasions or skin wounds. Has occurred with blood transfusions under developed countries.

Incubation:
5-14 days, blood transfusion may be 30-40 days

Treatment:
Nifurtimox

Prevention Measures:
Usually insect control measures

How long communicable:
Not transmitted from person to person

AIDS/HIV:

Symptoms:
This disease is usually fatal Acute symptoms such a flu-like, viral meningitis, fever, headache, occur within one to two months of infection. Usually acute symptoms abate after acute infection. Chronic symptoms on average occur 10 years after acute infection. My experience chronic symptoms, fever, night sweats, lymphadenopathy, thrust, malaise, etc,

342

Opportunistic infections may occurs such as,
Pneumocystic pneumonia, Toxoplasmosis,
Kaposi's Sarcoma, wasting syndrome, etc.,
Infectious Agent:
Human immunodeficiency virus (HIV), a
retrovirus. Types one and two
Where is it found?
Worldwide
Reservoir:
Humans
Origin of HIV was from chimpanzee in east
central Africa
Mode of transmission:
Sexual, needle sharing, blood transfusions risk
from 1977-1985, occupational needle exposure,
prenatal.
Incubation:
Acute HIV infection 6 weeks to 6 months
Chronic symptoms may occur with one to two
months after infection or 10 years or longer.
About half infected will develop AIDS in 10
years
Treatment:
Highly active anti-retroviral therapy (HAART),
treatment and prophylaxis of opportunistic
infections, nutritional support, etc.,
Prevention Measures:
Cleaning-disinfection of "works" between IV
drug users or new syringe each time when
injecting. Safe sex practices, monogamy, and
abstinence. Prevent needle exposure
occupationally, prophylaxis with HAART after
needle-significant exposure.
How long communicable:
Shortly after infection, then for life. Probably
most transmittable shortly after acute infection
and during AIDS syndrome.

Amebiasis (Entamoeba histolytica)
Symptoms:
May present with diarrhea containing blood,
fever, chills to very mild abdominal pain
Infectious Agent:
Entamoeba histolytica, a parasitic
Where is it found?
Ubitious-worldwide
Reservoir:
Humans' usually a chronically ill or
asymptomatic cyst passer
Mode of transmission:
Ingestion of fecally contaminated food or water
containing amebic cysts, which are resistant to
chlorine. Sexual transmission often occurs
Incubation:
Variable from a few days to several months or
years; commonly 2-4 weeks.

Treatment:
Flagyl®
Prevention Measures:
Avoid contact with fecal matter, handwashing
after using restroom
How long communicable:
During period of passing cysts of E. histolytica,
which may continue for years if not treated

Angiostrongyliasis: (Eosinophilic meningitis)
Symptoms:
Meningitis type symptoms, headache, fever, stiff
neck, paresthesias. Symptoms last one to two
weeks. Deaths are very rare
Infectious Agent:
Paraastrongylus (Angiostrongyliasis)-nematode
(lung worm of rats)
Where is it found?
Hawaii, Tahiti, may other Pacific islands,
Vietnam, Thailand, Malaysia, China
Reservoir:
Rats
Mode of transmission:
Ingestion of raw or insufficiently cooked snails,
slugs or land planarians, which are intermediate
or transport hosts harboring infective larvae.
Seafood that has ingested above (crabs, shrimp,
etc.,).
Incubation:
Usually one to three weeks
Treatment:
None
Prevention Measures:
Thoroughly cook above food items, rat control,
avoid eating raw foods that may have been
contaminated
How long communicable:
Not transmitted from person to person

Anisakiasis:
Symptoms:
Abdominal cramping, vomiting, coughing,
nausea and epigastria pain
Infectious Agent:
Larval nematodes of the subfamily Anisakinae
genera Aniskis and Pseudoterranova
Where is it found?
Widely distributed in nature, but only certain of
those that are parasitic in sea mammals constitute
a mohor threat to humans
Reservoir:
Widely distributed in nature, but only certain of
those that are parasitic in sea mammals constitute
a major threat to humans. The natural live cycle

involves transmission of larvae by predation through small crustaceans to squid, octopus or fish, then to sea mammals, with people as incidental hosts

Mode of transmission:
The infected larvae live in abdominal mesenteries of fish; often after death of their host they invade the body muscle of fish. When ingested by people and liberated by digestion in the stomach.

Incubation:
Few days to weeks
Treatment:
Gastroscopic removal of larvae; excision of lesions
Prevention Measures:
Thoroughly cooking and storing (freezing) of sea foods.
How long communicable:
Not transmitted from person to person

Anthrax:

Symptoms:
Cutaneous: a skin lesion, with eschar, which may be moderate to severe, usually is painless
Inhalation: Respiratory distress, mild and nonspecific, fever and shock follow 3 to 5 days later
Infectious Agent:
Bacillus Anthrax-a gram positive, encapsulated, spore forming bacteria
Where is it found?
Cutaneous: South Central America, southern and Eastern Europe
Inhalation: Rare
Reservoir:
Animals, normally herbivores, both livestock and wildlife, shed the bacilli in terminal hemorrhages or spilt blood at death. On exposure to air, the vegetative forms sporulate, and the spores are very resistant to adverse environmental conditions and disinfection.
Mode of transmission:
Cutaneous: infection is by contact with tissues of animals (livestock usually) dying of disease; possibly by biting flies that had partially fed on such animals
Inhalation: In 1979 an outbreak of largely pulmonary anthrax occurred in Russia, in which 66 individuals died and 11 infected persons survived, probably many other died. This outbreak was related to an accidental aerosol generated for biological warfare.
There are concerns terrorist may try a use Anthrax as a biological warfare agent.

Incubation:
Few hours to seven days
Treatment:
Penicillin, TTC, erythromycin during acute illness for 5 to 7 days
Prevention Measures:
Immunization for military and other high-risk individuals. Also immunize livestock animals. Proper handling of animal carcass. Good skin care practices.
How long communicable:
Not transmitted from person to person

Ascariasis: (Roundworm infection)

Symptoms:
A helmenthic infection of the small intestine generally associated with little to no symptoms. Live worm found in stool, are the first recognized sign of infection
Infectious Agent:
Ascaris lumbricoides, the large intestinal roundworm of humans
Where is it found?
Common worldwide
Reservoir:
Humans; ascarid eggs in soil
Mode of transmission:
Ingestion of infected eggs from soil contaminated with human feces or from uncooked produce contaminated with soil containing effective eggs, but no directly from person to person or from fresh feces
Incubation:
4-8 weeks
Treatment:
Mebendazole
Prevention Measures:
Thoroughly cook eggs and other produce
How long communicable:
As long as mature fertilized female worms live in the intestine. Could be from 12 to 24 months, if not treated.

Aspergillosis:

Symptoms:
A fungal infection that present with a variety of symptoms produced by several of the Aspergillus species. Patient the chronic obstructive pulmonary disease or cystic fibrosis and allergy to aspergilli may develop bronchial damage and intermittent bronchial plugging.
Infectious Agent:
Aspergillus fumigatus and A. flavus, a fungus
Where is it found?
Worldwide

Reservoir:
Found to be ubiquitous in nature
Mode of transmission:
Inhalation of airborne canidia
Incubation:
Few days to weeks
Treatment:
Amphotericin B
Prevention Measures:
None, which are practical. In hospital setting separation of patients from contaminated air when construction is occurring is very important.
How long communicable:
Not transmitted from person to person

Babesia:

Symptoms:
Potentially severe and sometime fatal disease, a protozoan parasitic of Red Blood cells. Fever, chills, myalgia, fatigue and jaundice secondary to hemolytic anemia and may last days to months.
Infectious Agent:
Babesia microtic
Where is it found?
USA, particularly the northeast
Reservoir:
Rodents and cattle
Mode of transmission:
By the tick bite, specifically from Ixodes ticks
Incubation:
1 week to 12 months
Treatment:
Clindamycin+quinine or Pentamidine+TMP-SMX
Prevention Measures:
Tick control measures
How long communicable:
Not transmitted from person to person

Balantidiasis:

Symptoms:
A protozoan infection of the colon, characteristically producing diarrhea and dysentery, abdominal colic, nausea and vomiting
Infectious Agent:
Balantidium coli, a large protozoan
Where is it found?
Worldwide
Reservoir:
Swine and possibly other animals, such as rats and nonhuman primates
Mode of transmission:
Ingestion of cysts from feces of infected hosts
Incubation:

Unknown, maybe a few days
Treatment:
Penicillin, streptomycin, chloramphenicol, and TTC
Prevention Measures:
Unknown
How long communicable:
Not transmitted from person to person

Blastomycosis

Symptoms:
A fungal disease of the lungs and skin. Acute infection may present with fever, cough, and pulmonary infiltrate on X-ray exam.
Infectious Agent:
Blastomyces dermatitidis, a fungal that grows as a yeast in tissue
Where is it found?
Uncommon, however seen in USA, Canada, Africa, India, Israel and Saudi Arabia. Rare in children. Dogs and cats.
Reservoir:
Moist soil, particularly wooded areas along waterways.
Mode of transmission:
Inhaled in spore-laden dust
Incubation:
Indefinite; probably a few weeks or less to months
Treatment:
Ketraconazole, Amphotercin B
Prevention Measures:
Unknown
How long communicable:
Not transmitted directly from people or animals to people

Botulism:

Symptoms:
Foodborne: a severe intoxication resulting from ingestion of preformed toxin present in contaminated food. Illness present with acute bilateral cranial nerve impairment and descending weakness of paralysis. Visual difficulties, dysphagia and dry mouth are often the first complaints. Vomiting and constipation or diarrhea may be present. Fever is usually absent.
Infant: this is the most common Botulism in the United States. Results from spore ingestion and subsequent outgrowth and in vivo toxin production in the intestine by C. botulinum. Usually effect children <1 year. Symptoms may be constipation followed by lethargy,

listlessness, poor feeding, difficult swallowing, and loss of head control.

There is concern Botulism could be used a biological warfare agent.

Infectious Agent:
Caused by a toxin produced by clostridium botulinum, a sore forming anerobic bacteria
Where is it found?
Worldwide, although sporadic
Reservoir:
Spores are ubiquitous in soil worldwide; they are frequently recovered from agricultural products, including honey. Spores are also found in marine sediment and in the intestinal tract of animals including fish
Mode of Transmission:
Foodborne: acquired by ingestion of food in which toxin has been formed, predominantly after inadequate heating during canning and with subsequent adequate cooking.

Infant: acquired by ingestion of botulinum spores that then germinated in the intestinal tract, rather than by ingestion of preformed toxin. Possible sources of spores for infants are multiple, including foods and dust. Honey, a food item fed previously to infants, often contains C. botulinum spores. Corn syrup may also be a source of spores.
Incubation:
12-36 hours to several days
Treatment:
IV administration ASAP with trivalent botulinum antitoxin. Available at the CDC in Atlanta, GA.

Infant: supportive care is essential; antibiotics may make the situation worse.
Preventive Measures:
Proper food preparation is essential. Educate about risks of home canning food items
How long communicable:
Apparently, not transmitted from person to person

Bovine Spongiform Encephalopathy:
(Mad Cows Disease)
See Page 14

Brucellosis:
Symptoms:
A systemic bacterial disease with acute or insidious onset, characterized by continued, intermittent or irregular fever of variable duration, headache, weakness, profuse sweating, chills, arthralgia, depression, weight loss and generalized aching

Infectious Agent:
Brucella bortus-bacteria
Where is it found?
World wide, especially in Mediterranean countries of Europe and North and East Africa
Reservoir:
Cattle, swine, goats and sheep
Mode of Transmission:
Contact with tissues, blood, urine, vaginal discharges, aborted fetuses and especially placentas. Also, ingestion of raw dairy products.
Incubation:
5-60 days, 1-2 months commonplace
Treatment:
Rifampin or streptomycin and doxycylcline.
Preventive Measures:
Care in handling above animal secretions and excretions. Do not drink or ingest raw dairy products. Hunter should use barrier precautions (gloves, clothing) in dressing feral swine and to bury the remains.
How long communicable:
Not transmitted from person to person.

Campylobacter:
Symptoms:
Characteristic with diarrhea, abdominal pain, malaise, fever, nausea and vomiting. Symptoms may be rather severe to mild.

Probably a common cause of Guillian-Barre syndrome.
Infectious Agent:
Campylobacter jejuni-bacteria
Where is it found?
The most common form of diarrhea illness in all parts of the world and all age groups, causing 5-14% of diarrhea worldside
Reservoir:
Animals, most common poultry and cattle. Puppies, kittens, other pets, swine, sheep, rodents and birds. Most raw meat is contaminated with campylobacter.
Mode of Transmission:
Ingestion of any above, which is usually undercooked or cross-contamination, occurs
Incubation:
Two to five days, with a range of 1-10 days depending on dose ingested.
Treatment:
Usually rehydration, occasionally Erythromycin
Preventive Measures:
Cooking food thoroughly with good handwashing. Avoid pet fecal matter.
How long communicable:

Unlikely to be transmitted from person to person

Candidasis:
(Moniliasis, Thrush)
Symptoms:
Usually confined to the superficial layers of skin or mucous membranes, presenting as oral thrush, intertrigo, vulvovanginitis or onychomycosis. Ulcers or pseudomembranes may be formed in the esophagus, stomach or intestine. Can be a severe and even life-threating problem for patients who are severely immuno-compromised.
Infectious Agent:
Candida albicans, C. tropicalis and other species
Where is it found?
Worldwide
Reservoir:
Humans
Mode of Transmission:
Contact with secretions or excretions of mouth, skin, vagina and feces, from patients or carriers; by passage from mother to neonate during childbirth; and by endogenous spread. Prior administration of antibiotics may predispose patient to candidasis.
Incubation:
Variable, 2-5 days
Treatment:
Dependent on site of infection: ketoconazole, clotrimaxole, miconazole, fluconazole.
Preventive Measures:
Detect yearly and treat
How long communicable:
While lesions are present

Capillariasis:
Symptoms:
Clinically, an entero-pathogen with massive protein loss and a malabsorption syndrome that lead to progressive weight loss and extreme emaciation.
May also cause a fatal hepatitis.
Infectious Agent:
Capillaria philippinensis-parasite (nemtodes)
Where is it found?
Mostly Philippine Islands, however also found in Thailand, Japan, Korea, Taiwan and Eypt
Reservoir:
Unknown, maybe aquatic birds and fish?
Mode of Transmission:
A history of ingestion of raw or under cooked small fish, eaten whole.
Incubation:

Unknown in humans, in animals about one month
Treatment:
Mebendazole
Preventive Measures:
Thoroughly cook at risk foods
How long communicable:
Not transmitted from person to person

Chagas Disease:
(See American Trypanosomiasis)

Cat-Scratch Fever:
(Bartonella)
Symptoms:
Subacute, usually self-limited bacterial disease characterized by malaise, granulomatious lympthadenitis and variable pattern of fever. It is often preceded by a cat scratch, lick or bite that produces a red popular lesion in about 50-90% of cases
Infectious Agent:
Bartonella-bacteria
Where is it found?
Worldwide; but uncommon. 4/100,000
Reservoir:
Domestic cats are vectors and reservoirs for Bartonella
Mode of Transmission:
Most patients give a history of scratch, bite, lick or other exposure to a health, usually young, cat, (often a kitten)
Incubation:
Usually 3-14 days but may vary from 5- 50 days
Treatment:
Effectiveness of antibiotics, currently unclear. Antibiotics such as cipro, TMP-SMX, rifampin, gentamycin and doxycycline have been used with varying success
Preventive Measures:
Thoroughly cleaning of cat bite, lick or scratch.
How long communicable:
Not transmitted from person to person

Chanroids:
Symptoms:
Found in genital area and characterized with single or multiple painful, necrotizing ulcers at the site of infection, frequently with painful swelling and suppuration of regional lymph nodes. At increase risk for HIV.
Infectious Agent:
Haemophiulus durceyi-bacteria
Where is it found?

Mostly found in men and prostitutes. Mostly found in subtropical and tropical climates. In USA, outbreaks and some endemic transmission have occurred among migrant farm workers and poor inner-city residents

Reservoir:
Humans

Mode of Transmission:
Direct sexual contact

Incubation:
3 to 5 days, up to 14 days

Treatment:
Ceftriaxone, erythromycin or azithromycin

Preventive Measures:
Abstinence and monogamony, safe sex practices. Prompt treatment, prophylaxis of sexual contacts within window exposures

How long communicable:
Until lesions are healed, or as long lesions are present or discharge from lymphnodes.

Chicken Pox:

(Varicella/Shingles)

Symptoms:
Acute generalized viral disease with sudden onset of fever, mild constitutional symptoms and skin eruption that is maculopapular for a few hours, vesicular for 3-4 days and leaves a granular scab. Lesions may appear almost on any part of the body. Fatality rate in the USA is 2/100,000 but rises to 30/100,000 in adults. Death is more common with individuals, who are immuno-compromised.

Shingles: is a reactivation of chickenpox (mostly in elderly or immunocompromised) in the dorsal root ganglia. Lesions usually appear in crops along nerve paths.

Infectious Agent:
Human herpesvirus 3

Where is it found?
Worldwide, may be more in the Western Hemisphere. In urban communities at least 90% of population

Reservoir:
Humans

Mode of Transmission:
Person to person, by direct contact with droplet or airborne spread of vesicle fluid or secretion of the respiratory tract. Also, probably transmission through articles freshly soiled by discharges from vesicles and mucous membranes of infected persons.

Incubation:
2 to 3 weeks; commonly 13-17 days. Those who receive passive immunization (VZIG) and immunodifficient may have increased incubation, 3-4 weeks

Treatment:
Adenine arabinoside and Acyclovir are effective in treating for shortening the duration of symptoms and pain of zoster in the patient

Preventive Measures:
VZIG may codify or prevent disease if given within 96 hours of exposure. Varivax® vaccine. Exclude individuals with active lesion from work, school. Health care workers without prior immunization or history of chickenpox probably need to be dismissed from work from the 10-21 day after exposure.

How long communicable:
As long as 5 days but usually 1-2 days before onset of rash, and not more than 5 days after the appearance of the first crop of vesicles. Contagiousness may be prolonged in patients with altered immunity. The secondary attack rate among sibling is 70-90%. Patients with zoster may be sources of infection for a week after the appearance of their vesiculopustular lesions. Susceptible person should be considered to be infectious 10-21 days following exposure

Chlamydia:

Symptoms:
(Women)
Approximately 70% of infected women have few if any symptoms; asymptomatic infection in women can persist for up to 15 months. When symptoms occur they may present with: Mucopurulent endocervical discharge, with edema, erythema and easily induced cervical bleeding. Infection can progress to involve the upper reproductive tract and may result in serious complications and sequelae such as salpingitis with subsequent risk of ectopic pregnancy.
(Men):Opaque discharge of moderate or scanty quantity, urethral itching, and burning on urination. Asymptomatic infections occur in men 1 to 10% of sexual active men.
(Infants):Conjunctivitis, papillary hypertrophy particularly on the tarsal conjunctiva lining of the upper eyelid.

Infectious Agent:
Chlamydia trachomatis-bacteria

Where is it found?
Very common worldwide

Reservoir:
Humans

Mode of Transmission:
Sexual contact

Incubation:

Probably 7-14 days
Treatment:
Doxycycline, TTC, Erythromycin
Preventive Measures:
Same as Syphilis and Chanroids
How long communicable:
Until treatment occurs, if no treatment; unknown

Cholera:

(Vibrio cholerae)
Symptoms:
An acute enteric disease characterized its severe form with sudden onset with profuse painless watery diarrhea, occasional vomiting and in untreated cases rapid dehydration, acidosis, circulatory collapse, hypoglycemia in children and renal failure.
Infectious Agent:
Vibrio cholera serotype 01 which includes tow biotypes El Tor-each includes organisms of Inaba, Ogawa and Hikohima serotypes-bacteria
Where is it found?
Mostly confined to Asia; rare in the United States
Reservoir:
Humans, recently observation in the USA, Bangladesh and Australia have shown environmental reservoirs exist, apparently in association with copepods or other zoophankton in brackish water or estuaries.
Mode of Transmission:
Through ingestion of contaminated food or water; directly contaminated with feces or vomitus of infected persons
Incubation:
A few hours to 5 days
Treatment:
Rehydration; antibiotics (TTC) probably shorten diarrhea and dehydration
Preventive Measures:
Proper water and food management, handwashing, contact precautions. Immunization is available for travel to endemic countries
How long communicable:
While diarrhea is present, or if bacteria present in stool. Antibiotics will shorten communicability.

Chronic Fatigue Syndrome:
Symptoms:

Chronic fatigue syndrome, or CFS, is a debilitating and complex disorder characterized by profound fatigue that is not improved by bed rest and that may be worsened by physical or mental activity. Persons with CFS must often function at a substantially lower level of activity than they were capable of before the onset of illness. In addition to these key defining characteristics, patients report various nonspecific symptoms, including weakness, muscle pain, impaired memory and/or mental concentration, insomnia, and post-exertional fatigue lasting more than 24 hours. In some cases, CFS can persist for years. The cause or causes of CFS have not been identified and no specific diagnostic tests are available. Moreover, since many illnesses have incapacitating fatigue as a symptom, care must be taken to exclude other known and often treatable conditions before a diagnosis of CFS is made.

a. Definition of CFS

A great deal of debate has surrounded the issue of how best to define CFS. In an effort to resolve these issues, an international panel of CFS research experts convened in 1994 to draft a definition of CFS that would be useful both to researchers studying the illness and to clinicians diagnosing it. In essence, in order to receive a diagnosis of chronic fatigue syndrome, a patient must satisfy two criteria:

- have severe chronic fatigue of 6 months or longer duration with other known medical conditions excluded by clinical diagnosis; and

- concurrently have four or more of the following symptoms: substantial impairment in short-term memory or concentration; sore throat; tender lymph nodes; muscle pain; multi-joint pain without swelling or redness; headaches of a new type, pattern or severity; unrefreshing sleep; and post-exertional malaise lasting more than 24 hours. The symptoms must have persisted or recurred during 6 or more consecutive months of illness and must not have predated the fatigue.

b. Similar Medical Conditions

A number of illnesses have been described that have a similar spectrum of symptoms to CFS. These include fibromyalgia syndrome, myalgic encephalomyelitis, neurasthenia, multiple chemical sensitivities, and chronic mononucleosis. Although these illnesses may present with a primary symptom other than fatigue, chronic fatigue is commonly associated with all of them.

c. Other Conditions That May Cause Similar Symptoms

In addition, there are a large number of clinically defined, frequently treatable illnesses that can result in fatigue. Diagnosis of any of these conditions would exclude a definition of CFS unless the condition has been treated sufficiently and no longer explains the fatigue and other symptoms. These include hypothyroidism, sleep apnea and narcolepsy, major depressive disorders, chronic mononucleosis, bipolar affective disorders, schizophrenia, eating disorders, cancer, autoimmune disease, hormonal disorders*, subacute infections, obesity, alcohol or substance abuse, and reactions to prescribed medications.

d. Other Commonly Observed Symptoms in CFS

In addition to the eight primary defining symptoms of CFS, a number of other symptoms have been reported by some CFS patients. The frequencies of occurrence of these symptoms vary from 20 to 50% among CFS patients. They include abdominal pain, alcohol intolerance, bloating, chest pain, chronic cough, diarrhea, dizziness, dry eyes or mouth, earaches, irregular heartbeat, jaw pain, morning stiffness, nausea, night sweats, psychological problems (depression, irritability, anxiety, panic attacks), shortness of breath, skin sensations, tingling sensations, and weight loss.

Infectious Agent:

Due in part to its similarity to chronic mononucleosis, CFS was initially thought to be caused by a virus infection, most probably Epstein-Barr virus (EBV). It now seems clear that CFS cannot be caused exclusively by EBV or by any single recognized infectious disease agent. No firm association between infection with any known human pathogen and CFS has been established. CDC's four-city surveillance study found no association between CFS and infection by a wide variety of human pathogens, including EBV, human retroviruses, human herpesvirus 6, enteroviruses, rubella, Candida albicans, and more recently bornaviruses and Mycoplasma. Taken together, these studies suggest that among identified human pathogens, there appears to be no causal relationship for CFS. However, the possibility remains that CFS may have multiple causes leading to a common endpoint, in which case some viruses or other infectious agents might have a contributory role for a subset of CFS cases.

Where is it found?

One of the earliest attempts to estimate the prevalence of CFS was conducted by the Centers for Disease Control and Prevention (CDC) from 1989 to 1993. Physicians in four U.S. cities were asked to refer possible CFS patients for clinical evaluation by medical personnel participating in the study. The study estimated that between 4.0 and 8.7 per 100,000 persons 18 years of age or older have CFS and are under medical care. However, these projections were underestimates and could not be generalized to the U.S. population since the study did not randomly select its sites. A more recent study of the Seattle area has estimated that CFS affects between 75 and 265 people per 100,000 population. This estimate is similar to the prevalence observed in another CDC study conducted in San Francisco, which put the occurrence of CFS-like disease (not clinically diagnosed) at approximately 200 per 100,000 persons. In general, it is estimated that perhaps as many as half a million persons in the United States have a CFS-like condition.

Reservoir:
Unknown
Mode of Transmission:
Unknown
Incubation:
Unknown
Treatment:
None shown to be effective
Preventive Measures:
None identified
How long communicable:
Not transmitted from person to person

Coccidioidomycosis:
(Valley fever, Desert fever, San Joaquin fever)
Symptoms:
A deep fungal infection that generally begins as a respiratory infection. May be asymptomatic at first or resemble flu-like illness with fever chills, cough and (rarely) pleuritic pain. 10 to 15 5 develop erythema nodosum, most frequently in Caucasian females.
Disseminated coccidioidomycosis is frequently fatal, may present with lung lesion on X-Ray. Abscesses throughout the body can occur. Increased morbidity occurred after the California earthquakes of 1995.
Infectious Agent:
Coccidioides immitis-fungus

Where is it found?

In arid and semiarid areas of the western hemisphere: in the USA from California to southern Texas; and in western South American countries.

Reservoir:

Soil; especially in the around Indian middens and rodent burrows.

Mode of Transmission:

Inhalation of the infected arthroconidia from soil and in lab accidents from cultures.

Incubation:

One to four weeks. Dissemination may develop insidiously, without recognized symptoms of primary pulmonary infection and years after the primary infection.

Treatment:

Amphotericin B, Fluconazole

Preventive Measures:

In endemic areas: plant grass, oil unpaved airfields and use dust control measures

How long communicable:

No evidence of transmission from person to person.

Conjunctivitis, Acute Bacterial:

(Sticky eye, pink eye)

Symptoms:

Begins with lacrimation, irritation and hyperemia of the palpebral and bulbar conjunctivae of one or both eyes, followed by edema and lids and mucopurulent discharge. Photophobia may also occur.

On rare occasion a systemic disease have occurred among children in several communities in Brazil, 1-3 weeks after conjunctivitis due to a unique invasive clone of Haemophilus influenzae. This from may be fatal up to 70% of afflicted.

Infectious Agent:

Haemophilus influenzae, aegyptius and Streptococcus pneumoniae, Neisseria meningitides and Corynebacterium diptheriae, Pseudomonas aeruginosa,

Where is it found?

Worldwide, mostly in warmer climates

Reservoir:

Humans. Carriers are common in many areas during interepidemic periods.

Mode of Transmission:

Contact with discharges from the conjunctivae or upper respiratory tract of infected people, from contaminated fingers, cloths and other articles including makeup kits. Inadequately disinfected tonometers

Incubation:

24-72 hours

Treatment:

Local application of an ointment or drops containing as sulfonamide such as sodium sulfacetamide, gentamycin, polymyxin B

Preventive Measures:

Good handwashing and isolation of infected person with contact precautions, children should not attend school and Health Care Workers should not work!

How long communicable:

During the course of active infection.

Conjunctivitis, Acute Viral:

Symptoms:

Onset is sudden, with pain, photophobia, blurred vision and occasionally low-grade fever, headache, malaise and tender preauricular lymphadenopathy

Infectious Agent:

Typically Adenovirus types 8, 19 and 37

Where is it found?

Worldwide

Reservoir:

Humans

Mode of Transmission:

See bacterial conjunctivitis-above

Incubation:

Typically 5-12 days

Treatment:

None during the acute phase. If the residual opacities interfere with the patient's ability to work topically corticosteroids may be administered by a qualified ophthalmologist.

Preventive Measures:

Good handwashing, minimize hand to eye contact. Avoid communal eyedroppers, medicines, eye makeup, and towels

How long communicable:

From late in the incubation period to 14 days after onset

Coxsackievirus:

Symptoms:

Vesicular pharyngitis (herpangina): Sudden onset of fever, sore throat and 1-2mm discrete grayish papulovesicular pharyngeal lesions on an erythematous base.

Vesicular stomatitis (hand, foot and mouth disease): Oral lesions are more disffuse and may occur on the buccal surfaces of cheeks and gums and on the sides of the tongue.

Acute Lymphonodular pharyngitis: Lesions are usually firm, raised, discrete whites to yellow nodules surrounded by a 3-6mm zone of erthema

Infectious Agent:
Vesicular pharyngitis (herpangina):
Cossackievirus Group A 1-10, 16, and 22.
Vesicular stomatitis (hand, foot and mouth
disease): Coxsackievirus Group A: A16 and
types 4,5,9 and 10. Group B types 2 and 5
Acute Lymphonodular pharyngitis: Group A 10
Where is it found?
Worldwide
Reservoir:
Humans
Mode of Transmission:
Direct contact with nose and throat discharges
and feces of infected people.
Incubation:
Usually 3-5 days
Treatment:
None
Preventive Measures:
Good handwashing
How long communicable:
During acute phase of illness and perhaps longer,
since virus persist is stool for weeks.

Creutzfeldt-Jakob Disease:
See Page 14

Cryptococcus:
Symptoms:
A deep fungal usually presenting as a subacute
or chronic meningitis, infection of lungs,
kidneys, prostate, and bone may occur. Skin
lesions may occur
Infectious Agent:
Cryptococcus neoformans-fungus
Where is it found?
Sporadic cases all over the world
Reservoir:
Old pigeons nests dropping and soil
Mode of Transmission:
Inhalation
Incubation:
Unknown, months to years
Treatment:
Amphotericin B, Fluconazole
Preventive Measures:
Control pigeon dropping
How long communicable:
Not transmitted from person to person

Cryptospordiosis:
Symptoms:
Asymptomatic infections are common. Although
diarrhea is also common, which may be profuse

and watery, preceded by anorexia and vomiting
in children. Abdominal pain also occurs.
Infectious Agent:
Cryptosporidium parnum-protozoa
Where is it found?
Worldwide
Reservoir:
Humans, cattle and other domestic animals
Mode of Transmission:
Fecal oral, including person to person,
waterborne, and foodborne. The Oscysts are
highly resistant to chemical disinfectants used to
purify drinking water.
Incubation:
1-12 days is likely range
Treatment:
Rehydration, azithromycin may be helpful
Preventive Measures:
Good handwashing, municipal water control
measures.
How long communicable:
Oocysts, while in stool and may be infectious for
2-6 months in a moist environment.

Cyclospora:
Symptoms:
Watery diarrhea, abdominal cramps, fatigue and
weight loss; fever is rare. Fruits and vegetables
from under developed countries, which are not
peeled, may increase risk.
Infectious Agent:
Cyclospora cayetamemsos-protozan
Where is it found?
Under developed countries
Reservoir:
Humans, cattle and other animals
Mode of Transmission:
Fecal oral
Incubation:
9-43 days
Treatment:
TMP-SMX
Preventive Measures:
Washing and rinsing food thoroughly. Good
handwashing
How long communicable:
Unknown, probably same as cryptospordoisis

Cytomegalovirus:
(CMV)
Symptoms:
Severe form occurs in infants infected prenatally.
May exhibit lethargy, convulsions, jaundice,
petchiae, purpura, hepatosplenmegaly, hearing
loss etc.

Adults infection usually is in apparent, however for immuno compromised can be severe with retinitis, body rash, pneumonia, GI tract disorders, and hepatitis

Infectious Agent:
Human beta herpesvirus 5

Where is it found?
Worldwide

Reservoir:
Humans

Mode of Transmission:
Mostly sexual exposure or close intimate exposure by mucosal contact with infectious tissue, secretions and excretions. Most bodily fluids may contain CMV. Blood transfusion and transplant have occurred especially in other countries

Incubation:
Blood transfusion and transplant is usually 3-8 weeks. Infection acquired during birth is first demonstrable 3-12 weeks after delivery.

Treatment:
Ganciclovir, IV or PO for immuno-compromised persons.

Preventive Measures:
Handwashing, care in handling diapers

How long communicable:
Virus, persist for month to years after primary infections. Infants infected may excreted virus for 5-6 years. 3 to 5% of health adults are pharyngeal excretes. Excretions recur with immunodeficiency and immunosuppression.

Denque Fever:
(Bone Break Fever)

Symptoms:
An acute febrile viral disease with symptoms of fever, intense headache, malaise, arthralgia, retro-orbital pain, anorexia, GI disturbances with rash.

Hemorrhagic forms is endemic in much of south and Southeast Asia, the pacific and Latin America. Recognized primarily in children, shock may be common. Death can be between 40 to 50% but with good physiologic fluid replace therapy rates should be 1 to 2%.

Infectious Agent:
Flaviviruses which include serotypes 1-4

Where is it found?
Asia, Africa, South and Central America, and the Caribbean. Texas reported cases from 1980-1986 and in recent years

Reservoir:
The viruses are maintained in a human-Aedes aegypti mosquito cycle in tropical urban centers; a monkey mosquito cycle serves as a reservoir in Southeast Asia and West Africa.

Mode of Transmission:
By the bite of infective mosquito usually in morning and evening hours.

Incubation:
Three to fourteen days, commonly 5-7 days

Treatment:
None, supportive

Preventive Measures:
Control of mosquito populations, use of repellents with DEET.

How long communicable:
Not directly transmitted from person to person. Patients are usually infective for mosquitoes from shortly before to the end of the febrile period, an average of 6-7 days. The mosquito becomes infective 8-12 days after viremic blood meal and remains to for life.

Diphtheria:

Symptoms:
An acute bacteria disease involving primarily tonsils, pharynx, larynx (serious in children and infants), nose, occasional other mucous membranes of skin and sometimes the conjunctivae or genitalia. Rash patch or patches of an adherent grayish membrane with a surrounding inflammation. Throat is moderately sore, with swollen lympthnodes.

Infectious Agent:
Corynebacterium diptheriae-bacteria

Where is it found?
A disease of colder months, usually involving unimmunized children <15 years of age. Russia has had increase incidence to due lack of immunization.

Reservoir:
Humans

Mode of Transmission:
Contact with patients or carriers, more rarely, contact with articles soiled with discharges from lesions of infected people. Raw milk.

Incubation:
Usually 2-5 days

Treatment:
Diphtheria anti-toxin in conjunction with penicillin or erythromycin

Preventive Measures:
Immunization with booster every 10 years

How long communicable:
Variable, until virulent bacilli have disappeared from discharges and lesions; usually 2 weeks or less and seldom more than 4 weeks. Shedding is

completely stopped after administration of antibiotics.

Dracunculiasis:
Symptoms:
A blister appears usually on a lower extremity when the gravid, 60-100cm long, adult female worm is ready to discharge it larvae. Burning an itching of skin occurs around lesion and frequently diarrhea, fever, vomiting dyspnea, and nausea.
Infectious Agent:
Dracunculus medinensis-nematode
Where is it found?
Mostly Africa and Asia
Reservoir:
Humans; there are no other known animal reservoirs
Mode of Transmission:
Larvae discharged by the female worm into stagnant fresh water are ingested by minute crustacean copepods. In about 2 weeks, the larvae develops into the infectious stage. People swallow the infected copepods in drinking water from infested step well and ponds.
Incubation:
About 12 months
Treatment:
Tetanus toxin, yes tetanus toxin and local ointment on primary lesion.
Preventive Measures:
Don't drink the water
How long communicable:
In water from the copepods for about 5 days. After ingestion the larvae become infective for about 12-14 days after, and remain infective in the copepods for about 3 weeks.

Ebola-Marburg Viral Disease:
Symptoms:
Severe acute viral illness, usually with sudden onset of fever, malaise, myalgia and headache, followed by vomiting, diarrhea, and maculopapular rash. Accompanying hemorrhagic diathesis is often with hepatic damage, renal failure, CNS involvement and terminal shock. Marburg disease have been fatal about 25%; Ebola is fatal around 80 to 90%
Infectious Agent:
Virons are 80nm in diameter and 790 nm (Marburg) or 970nm (Ebola) in length are members of the Filoviridae. Longer, bizarre virion-related structures may be branched or coiled and each 10um in length
Where is it found?

Marburg: recognized five times in Germany, Yogoslavis, Africa (after exposure to green monkeys in Uganda), South Africa in Zimbabwe and Zenya
Ebola: Africa; the Sudan (outbreaks in 1976 and 1979) and 500 miles away in Zaire with more than 600 cases were identified. An outbreak in 1995 in Kiewit, Zaire occurred.
Reservoir:
Unknown despite extensive studies
Mode of Transmission:
Person to person transmission occurs by direct contact with infected blood, secretions, organs or semen. Nosocomial transmission occurred through exposure with contaminated syringes and needles. Transmission through semen has occurred 7 weeks after clinical recovery (sexual)
Incubation:
Marburg: 3 to 9 days
Ebola 2-21 days
Treatment:
None
Preventive Measures:
Contact/Standard precautions, safe sex practices. Good handwashing.
How long communicable:
As long as blood and secretions contain virus. Up to 30% of primary caregivers in Sudan were infected, while other household contacts remained uninfected. Ebola virus was isolated from the seminal fluid on the 61st, but not on the 76th day after onset of illness in a laboratory acquired case.

Echinococcosis:
(Alveolar Hydatid Disease)
Symptoms:
Hepatitis syndrome usually occurs, tumors usually develop with metastases. This disease is often fatal.
Infectious Agent:
Echinococcus multilocularis
Where is it found?
Northern hemisphere; central Europe; the former Soviet Union, Japan, Alaska, and Canada. Usually diagnosis in adults.
Reservoir:
Adult tapeworm found in foxes, although dogs and cats can be sources. Rodents, E. multilocularis is commonly maintained in nature in fox-rodent cycles
Mode of transmission:
By ingestion of eggs passed in the feces of Canidae and Felidae that have feed on infected rodents
Incubation:

Variable, from 12 months to many years depending on the numbers of cysts and how rapidly they grow.

Treatment:
Surgical resection of isolated cysts is most common treatment; however mebendazole (Vermox®) and albendzole (Zentel®) have been used with success

Prevention Measures:
Avoid contact with dog feces, handwashing, thoroughly cooking, treat high-risk dogs.

How long communicable:
Not transmitted from person to person

E. Coli:

(Which causes Diarrhea)
Strains of Escherichia coli that causes Diarrhea are of six major categories:
 1) enterohemorrhagic 2) enterotoxigenic (travelers diarrhea), 3) enteroinvasive (similar to Shigella) 4) enteropathogenic (summer diarrhea), 5) enteroaggregative (infant diarrhea) and 6) diffuse adherent

Enterohemorrhagic: (E.Coli 0157:H7)

Symptoms:
As been recognized since 1982 when an outbreak of hemorrhagic colitis occurred in the USA with a specific serotype E. Coli 0157:H7. Diarrhea may range from mild and non-bloody to completely bloody with no leukocytes. May cause the hemolytic uremic syndrome (HUS) and thrombotic thrombocytopenic purpura; they elaborate potent cytotoxins called Shiga-like toxins I and II.

Infectious Agent:
Escherichia coli 0157:H7(most common in USA), also 026:H11, 0111:H8 and 0104:H21

Where is it found?
An important problem in North America, Europe, South Africa, Japan Southern South America and Australia

Reservoir:
Cattle are the reservoir; humans may also serve as a reservoir for person to person transmission.

Mode of Transmission:
Ingestion of contaminated food, as with Salmonella, most often inadequately cooked beef (especially ground beef). Transmission can occur from person to person as with Shigella. Swimming pools and contaminated unchlorinated municipal water have been implicated.

Incubation:
Ranging from 3 to 8 days with a median of 3-4 days

Treatment:
Fluid and electrolyte replace is important when diarrhea is watery or signs of dehydration. TMX-SMX may precipitate complications of HUS.

Preventive Measures:
Thoroughly cooking of beef products; cooked well done with a temperature of 155 degrees and all pink is gone. Good handwashing to eliminate cross contamination

How long communicable:
The duration of excretion of the pathogen, which is typically for a week or less in adults but 3 weeks in one third of children. Prolonged carriage is uncommon.

Ehrlichiosis:

Symptoms:
Acute febrile, bacterial disease caused by a group of small pleomorphic organisms. Symptoms may have a sudden onset of fever, chills, general malaise, headache, lympthadenopathy with tender nodes. Also symptoms may be so mild as not to seek medical attention or to a severe life threatening or fatal disease

Infectious Agent:
Ehrlichia sennetsu and E. chafeenis

Where is it found?
E. sennetus seems to be confined to Japan
E. chafeenis to the southeast and south-central United States

Mode of Transmission:
E. Sennetus: unknown although patients report visiting a river or swamp in the past 3-4 weeks. E. chafeenis is probably tick-borne (Amblyomma americanum). Most patients report a tick bite.

Incubation:
14 days for senetus fever; 7-21 days for chafeenis

Treatment:
Tetracycline; chloramphenicol for pregnant females

Preventive Measures:
Reduce tick exposure

How long communicable:
Not transmitted from person to person

Enterobiasis:

(Pinworms)
Symptoms:
A common intestinal helminthic infection that is often asmptomatic. May have perianal itching, disturbed sleep irritability and sometimes secondary infection from scratched skin.

Infectious Agent:
Enterobius vermicularis; an intestinal nematode
Where is it found?
Worldwide
Reservoir:
Humans, Pinworms of horses or other animals are not transmissible to people.
Mode of Transmission:
Direct transfer of infected eggs by hands from anus to mouth of the same or other person, or indirectly through clothing, bedding, food or other articles contaminated with eggs of the parasite.
Incubation:
2-6 weeks-symptomatic disease with high burdens results from successive reinfection occurring with months after the initial exposure.
Treatment:
Mebendazole (Vermox®) Pyrantel pamoate (Antiminth®)
Preventive Measures:
Good handwashing, bathing, laundering of clothes, etc.,
How long communicable:
As long as females can discharged eggs on perianal skin. Eggs remain infective in an indoor environment for 2 weeks.

Erythema Infectiosum Humn Parvovirus Infection:

(Fifth disease)
Symptoms:
Usually a mild, nonfebrile viral disease with an erythematous eruption, occurring sporadically or in epidemics especially among children. May notice striking erythema of the checks (slapped face-appearance). Intrauterine infection has resulted in fetal anemia and bydrops fetalis and fetal death in < 10% of such infections, in the first half of pregnancy.
Infectious Agent:
Human parvovirus B19
Where is it found?
Worldwide
Reservoir:
Humans
Mode of Transmission:
Contact with respiratory secretions; also from mother to fetus.
Incubation:
Usually 4-20 days
Treatment:
None
Preventive Measures:

Good handwashing, Standard precautions. Pregnant females who work as health care workers or in school or day care center should wash hands frequently.
How long communicable:
Just before onset of rash, but not after appearance of rash.

Fasciliasis:

Symptoms:
A disease of the liver from a large trematode that is a natural parasite of sheep, cattle and other animals throughout the world. Flukes can measure 3 cm long and live in bile ducts, causing liver enlargement and liver damage.
Infectious Agent:
Fasciola hepatica
Where is it found?
Worldwide; mostly in South America, Europe Austrialia and the Middle east
Reservoir:
Sheep, cattle, and snails. Sometime humans by accident.
Mode of Transmission:
Eggs passed in the feces develop in water, and in about 2 weeks a motile ciliated larva hatches.
Incubation:
Variable
Treatment:
Bitin®; only available at the CDC
Preventive Measures:
Reduce fecal exposure
How long communicable:
As long as viable eggs are discharged in feces.

Filariasis:

Symptoms:
An infection that resides in lympthnodes of patients. Female worms produce microfilaria that can reach the bloodstream in 6-12 months. Patients remain asymptomatic, or may have lympthandenitis and retrograde lymphangitis; chronic symptoms may be hydrocele, chyluria and elephantiasis of the limbs, breast and genitalia.
Infectious Agent:
Wuchereria bancrofti-threadlike worms
Where is it found?
Most humid climates, including Latin America, Brazil, northern South America, Caribbean, Africa, Asia, and pacific islands
Reservoir:
Humans with microfilariae in blood, cats may be reservoir in Malaysia and southern Thailand
Mode of Transmission:

By bite of a mosquito harboring infective larvae. W. bancrofti is transmitted by many mosquito species; Culex, Anopheles, Aedes, etc

Incubation:
From one to 12 months

Treatment:
Diethylcarbamazine (DEC, Banocide®, Hetrazan®, Notezine®)

Preventive Measures:
Mosquito control measures

How long communicable:
Not transmitted from person to person. Humans may infect mosquitos if microfilariae are present in human's blood.

Foodborne Diseases:

(Below are the common foodborne illness. Diseases such as Salmonella, Campylobacter, and Shigella will be discussed in their appropriate order.)

Staphylococcal Food Intoxication:

Symptoms:
Duration of symptoms is usually for 1-2 days with vomiting nausea and prostration accompanied with diarrhea with subnormal temperature and lowered blood pressure

Infectious Agent:
Enterotoxin from Staphylococcus Aureus. Staph multiply in food and produce the toxins

Where is it found?
Worldwide; 25% of population carry staph aureus

Reservoir:
Humans

Mode of Transmission:
By ingestion of a food product containing staph enterotoxin. Foods involved are particularly those that come in contact with food handlers, hands.

Incubation:
3 minutes to 8 hours, usually 2-4 hours

Treatment:
Fluid replace when indicated

Preventive Measures:
Thoroughly cooking of food, good handwashing for food handlers

How long communicable:
Not applicable

Clostrudium Perfringens Food Intoxication:

Symptoms:
An intestinal disorder characterized by sudden onset of colic followed by diarrhea; nausea is common. Vomiting and fever are absent.

Infectious Agent:
Type A strains of C. perfringens caused typical food poisoning outbreaks

Where is it found?
Widespread

Reservoir:
Soil and GI tract of health people and animals (cattle, pigs, poultry and fish).

Mode of Transmission:
Ingestion food contaminated with soil or feces and then held under condition that permit multiplication of organisms. Most outbreaks are related to improper heating or reheating.

Incubation:
6 to 24 hours, usually 10-12 hours

Treatment:
Fluid replacement if indicated

Preventive Measures:
Careful food preparation, heating and reheating and good handwashing among food handlers.

How long communicable:
Not applicable

Bacillus Cereus Food Intoxication:

Symptoms:
Sudden onset of nausea and vomiting and may have colic and diarrhea. Illness rarely lasts past 24 hours.

Infectious Agent:
Bacillus cereus-bacteria, which release enterotoxins

Where is it found?
Wordlwide, somewhat rare in the USA

Reservoir:
Ubiquitous organism of soil and environment.

Mode of Transmission:
Ingestion of food that has been kept at ambient temperature after cooking, permitting multiplication of the organisms.

Incubation:
1-6 hours in cases where vomiting is the predominant symptoms; from 6 to 24 hours where diarrhea is predominant

Treatment:
Fluid replacement if needed

Preventive Measures:
Foods should not remain at ambient temperature after cooking; good handwashing, etc.

How long communicable:
Not transmitted from person to person

Vibrio Parahaemolyticus Enteritis:

Symptoms:
Watery diarrhea and abdominal cramps in majority of cases, and sometimes with nausea vomiting fever and headache. Can produce a dysentery-like illness with bloody diarrhea.

Infectious Agent:
Vibrio parahaemoyticus-bacteria
Where is it found?
Mostly in Japan and southeast United States
Reservoir:
Marine coastal environs are the natural habitat.
More prevalent in summer months.
Mode of Transmission:
Ingestion of raw or inadequately food seafood, or
in cross contamination by handling raw seafood.
Incubation:
Usually between 12-24 hours, but can range
from 4-30 hours
Treatment:
Fluids if needed
Preventive Measures:
Good food preparation techniques; risk of
ingestion of raw seafoods
How long communicable:
Not transmitted from person to person

Vibrio Vulnificus:
Symptoms:
Produces septicemia, (DICs) in person with
chronic liver disease. Death rate can reach 50%!
Infectious Agent:
Vibrio Vulnificus-bacteria
Where is it found?
In marine areas-same as vibrio parahaemolyticus
Reservoir:
In marine areas-same as vibrio parahaemolyticus
Mode of Transmission:
Same as vibrio parahaemolyticus
Incubation:
12 hours to 3 days
Treatment:
Tetracycline, fluid replacement
Preventive Measures:
As for vibro parahaemolyticus
How long communicable:
Not transmitted from person to person

Fish Poisoning:
1) Ciguatera:
Symptoms:
Neurological and GI may occur within 1 hour
after eating tropical reef fish. Diarrhea and
vomiting are the GI usual symptoms. Ice cream
may taste hot! Hypotensive, death and coma can
occur although somewhat rare.
Infectious Agent:
Fish toxin-Gambierdiscus toximus
Where is it found?
Florida, Southern coasts, Hawaii
Reservoir:

Reef fish; red fish usually implicated, over 400
fish species may be implicated
Mode of Transmission:
Ingestion of above reservoir foods
Incubation:
Within 24 hours, intermittent symptoms may last
for months to years
Treatment:
I.V. of mannitol
Preventive Measures:
Consumption of large predatory fish should be
avoided, especially in the reef area. Screening of
fish is also helpful
How long communicable:
Not transmitted from person to person

2) Scombroid:
Symptoms:
Tingling burning sensations around the mouth,
facial flushing, sweating, nausea, and vomiting,
headache, palpitation, dizzness and rash.
Infectious Agent:
A histamine found in certain fish
Where is it found?
Same as Ciguatera
Reservoir:
Tuna, skipjack, mackeral, bonita, bluefish,
salmon, and dolphin
Mode of Transmission:
Ingestion of above fish
Incubation:
Within a few hours of ingestion of fish.
Treatment:
None; symptoms seem to resolve spontaneously
Preventive Measures:
Adequate refrigeration or irradiation of caught
fish prevents spoilage
How long communicable:
Not transmitted from person to person

3) Paralytic Shellfish Poisoning:
Symptoms:
Neurological and GI symptoms. In severe cases
ataxia, dysphonia, dysphagia and total muscle
paralysis with respiratory arrest and death can
occur-rare.
Infectious Agent:
Neurotoxin in shellfish-more common during
massive algae blooms-the red tide
Where is it found?
Marine areas
Reservoir:
Molluscs
Mode of Transmission:
Eating bivalve molluscs
Incubation:

Minutes to hours
Treatment:
Unknown, most resolve spontaneously

Preventive Measures:
Sample collection of mollusks in commercially fished areas and testing them for toxin.
How long communicable:
Not transmitted from person to person

Gastroenteritis, Acute Viral:
1) Rotaviral Enteritis:
Symptoms:
A sporadic or seasonal, often severe gastroenteritis of infants and young children characterized by vomiting and fever, followed by a watery diarrhea occasionally associated with severe dehydration and death in the young age group:
Infectious Agent:
Rotavirus belong to the Reovirdae family
Where is it found?
Worldwide, responsible for 1million deaths each year.
Reservoir:
Humans
Mode of Transmission:
Probably fecal-oral with possible contact with respiratory secretions?
Incubation:
24-72 hours
Treatment:
None; rehydration if indicated
Preventive Measures:
Good handwashing, Contact and Standard Precautions. Vaccine may be available in future.
How long Communicable:
During the actual stage

2) Norwalk Virus:
Symptoms:
Nausea, vomiting, diarrhea, abdominal pain, myalgia, headache, malaise, low grade fever.
Infectious Agent:
Norwalk virus
Where is it found?
Worldwide
Reservoir:
People
Mode of Transmission:
Fecal oral, contact transmission may occur with infected articles (fomites).
Incubation:
Usually 24-48 hours, range is 10-50 hours
Treatment:
None; rehydration if indicated

Preventive Measures:
Standard/Contact precaution, good handwashing
How long Communicable:
During the acute stage of disease.

Giardia:
Symptoms:
A protozoan infection principally of the upper small intestine, while often asymptomatic, it may present with diarrhea, abdominal pain, steatorrhea, bloating, frequent loose stools and pain green stools, fatigue and weight loss
Infectious Agent:
Giardia Lambia-protozoan
Where is it found?
Worldwide
Reservoir:
Humans, beavers and other wild and domestic animals
Mode of Transmission:
Fecal oral; hand to mouth transfer of cysts from feces of an infected person or animal. Some acquire Giardia by drinking out of ponds or streams.
Incubation:
Usually 3-25 days, median 7-10 days
Treatment:
Metronidazole-Adults
Furazolidone-Children
Preventive Measures:
Do not drink water out of streams and ponds, good handwashing, Standard precautions
How long Communicable:
During the entire period of infection

Gonorrhea:
Symptoms: (Women)
A few days after exposure an initial urethritis or cervicitis occurs, frequently so mild as to pass unnoticed 70 to 80% of the time. Women may have mucopurulent cervicitis. In about 20% there is uterine invasion at first, second or later menstrual period, with symptoms of endometritis, salpingitis or pelvic peritonitis and subsequent risk of infertility. Chronic endocervical infection is common.
Symptoms: (Men)
Purulent discharge of the anterior urethra with dysuria. Infection maybe self-limited and may occasionally result in a chronic carrier state. Rectal infection is common among homosexual males, is usually asymptomic by may cause pruritis, tenesmus and discharge.
Symptoms: (Infants)

Acute redness and swelling of the conjunctiva of one or both eyes, with mucopurulent or purulent discharge. All infants born should be prophylaxis with 1% silver nitrate, EES or TTC.
Infectious Agents:
Nesseria gonorrhoeae
Where is it found:
Worldwide
Reservoir:
Only humans
Incubation:
Usually 2 to 7 days, occasionally longer
Mode of Transmission:
Sexual contact
Treatment:
Rocephin 125 mg, Azithromycin, Erythromycin, Cipro and Tetracycline
Preventive Measures:
Abstinence, monogamy, Safe sex practices
Period of Communicability:
May extend for months in untreated individuals. Effective therapy ends communicability within hours.

Granuloma Inguinale:
Symptoms:
A chronic and progressively destructive, but poorly communicable bacterial disease of the skin and mucous membranes of the genitalia, inguinal and anal regions. An indurated nodule or papule becomes a slowly spreading, nontender, excuberant, granulomatous, ulcerative, or cicatricial process. Ulcers can become infective and very pain. On occasion lesion may an area between the genitalia and anal regions.
Infectious Agent:
Donovania granulomatic
Where is it found?
Endemic in tropical and subtropical areas.
Reservoir:
Humans
Incubation:
Unknown; probably between 1 and 16 weeks
Treatment:
Erythromycin, TMP-SMX and doxycycline
Preventive Measures:
See Syphilis and other sexually transmitted diseases
Period of Communicability:
Unknown, probably for the duration of open lesions on the skin or mucous membranes.

Hantaviral Disease:
Symptoms:

Abrupt onset of fever, lower back pain and varying degrees of hemorrhagic manifestations and renal involvement. Five common clinical phases occurs: febrile, hyotension, oliguric, diuretic and convalescent. Fatality rate varies.
Infectious Agent:
Hantavirus
Where is it found?
Mostly prior to WWII was found in China, Japan, occasionally in Russia. Most cases are seen in the fall season.
Reservoir:
Field rodent's feces, urine.
Mode of Transmission:
Aerosol transmission from excreta is presumed, fecal and urine contact with rodent feces more probable.
Incubation:
Few days to two months, usually 2-4 weeks
Treatment:
Appropriate and careful treatment is critical for shock and renal failure to avoid fluid overload. Ribavirin IV as early as possible during the first few days of illness has shown benefit.
Preventive Measures:
Reduce contact to field rodents, particularly at residence.
How long Communicable:
Not transmitted from person to person

Hantavirus Pulmonary Syndrome:
Symptoms:
Fever, myalgia and GI complaints followed by the abrupt onset of respiratory distress and hypotension. Progresses rapidly to respiratory failure and cardio shock. Mortality rate is 40 to 50%.
Infectious Agent:
Hantavirus-Sin Nombre species and others
Where is it found?
Southwestern United States and Canada. Sporadic cases in Florida, Rhode Island, New York.
Reservoir:
Deer mouse
Mode of Transmission:
Probably contact with deer mouse excreta, aerosol and feces, urine transmission
Incubation:
Few days to 6 weeks
Treatment:
Possibility-Ribarvin; provide respiratory intensive care management
Preventive Measures:
Reduce contact with deer mouse, particularly at residence, caves.

How long Communicable:
Not transmitted from person to person

Helicobacter Pylori:

Symptoms:
A bacterial infection causing chronic gastritis, usually in the antrum of the stomach, and may contribute to duodenal ulcer disease. Gastric adenocarcinoma and gastric ulcer disease are epidemiologically associated with H. pylori.

Infectious Agent:
Helicobacter pylori-bacteria

Where is it found?
Worldwide

Reservoir:
Humans are the only know reservoir.

Mode of Transmission:
Probably through ingestion of organisms by fecal oral route. H. pylori has been transmitted through incompletely decontaminated gastroscopes and pH electrodes.

Incubation:
After ingestion of bacteria usually 5-10 days

Treatment:
Combination of antibiotic for 2-4 weeks (Metronidazole and either ampicillin or tetracycline)

Preventive Measures:
Persons living in uncrowded and clean environments are less like to acquire H. pylori. Appropriate disinfection of gastoscopes

How long Communicable:
Unknown, patients with low stomach acid may be more infectious.

Hepatitis, Viral:

1) Hepatitis A: (Infectious Hepatitis)

Symptoms:
Onset is usually abrupt with fever, malaise, anorexia, nausea and abdominal pain. Jaundice is somewhat common among adults; rare in children. Symptoms may be rather mild to a severely disabling disease lasting for several months. Death is somewhat rare. Chronic disease is rare, if non-existent.

Infectious Agent:
Hepatitis A virus

Where is it found?
Worldwide: sporadic and endemic. More common in western United States.

Reservoir:
Humans and rarely chimpanzees

Mode of Transmission:

Fecal oral, sexual

Incubation:
15 to 50 days, usually 28-30 days

Treatment:
None; supportive

Preventive Measures:
Good handwashing, Standard precautions. Immunization for children, day care workers, teachers in western states

How long Communicable:
During the latter half of incubation period to a few days after onset of illness. Most cases are probably noninfectious after the first week of jaundice, although infants may excrete virus up to six months

2) Hepatitis B: (Serum Hepatitis)

Symptoms:
Onset of disease is usually insidious with anorexia, vague abdominal discomfort, nausea and vomiting, sometimes with rash and arthralgias. 30 to 50% of adults exhibit jaundice and <10 become chronic carriers (HBsAG + > 6 months), less than 10% of children exhibit jaundice and > 90% become chronic carriers.

Infectious Agent:
Hepatitis B virus

Where is it found?
Worldwide; endemic in China, Southeast Asia, Africa (>10% of population are chronic carriers.

Reservoir:
Humans, chimpanzees are susceptible

Mode of Transmission:
Sexual, blood, prenatal (major transmission in world), occupational exposure with Health care workers (needle sticks)

Incubation:
45-180 days, usually 60-90 days

Treatment:
Chronic treatment: Interferon or Epivir

Preventive Measures:
Safe sex practices prevent needle exposure, although the surest way is to be immunized for HBV. Standard Precautions

How long Communicable:
All individuals who are HBsAG + are communicable. Some patients are infectious for life.

3) Hepatitis C: (Non A Non B Hepatitis)

Symptoms:
Acute symptoms are rare, some 10-30% may have anorexia, vague abdominal discomfort, nausea, vomiting and therefore not seek medical assistance. Many only notice symptoms have complication occur such as ascites, prolonged

fatigue and mylagia. Some individuals initialed found to be HCV infected where exposed on average 10-20 years prior. 85% of individuals infected will be chronic carriers for life.

Infectious Agent:
Hepatitis C-RNA virus

Where is it found?
Worldwide

Reservoir:
Humans

Mode of Transmission:
Usually percutaneous exposure; needle and syringe sharing among IV drug users are at great risk for HCV. Contaminated blood products or transplant before 1992 in the United Stated. Health care workers who obtain needle and blood exposure occupationally.

Incubation:
2 weeks to 6 months, average 6-9 weeks

Treatment:
Rebetron®: combination of Interferon + Ribarvin for 6 months to 1 year for appropriate candidates.

Preventive Measures:
Blood, body fluid precautions, Standard precautions.

How long Communicable:
Persist in most persons indefinitely.

4) Hepatitis D: (Delta Hepatitis)
Symptoms:
Onset is usually abrupt with signs and symptoms resembling those of hepatitis B; may be severe and is always associated with a coexistent hepatitis B virus infection. Chronicity is more likely with superinfection with Hepatitis B (25-50%) than co-infection with Hepatitis B. Fatality rare for Hepatitis D may be 20-30%.

Infectious Agent:
Hepatitis D (Delta) virus

Where is it found?
Worldwide, endemic in those countries with endemic Hepatitis B.

Reservoir:
Humans

Mode of Transmission:
Similar to Hepatitis B

Incubation:
2-8 weeks

Treatment:
Interferon?

Preventive Measures:
Same as Hepatitis B

How long Communicable:

During acute phase, peaks just before onset of illness. Then ever-viral particles are detected in the blood.

5) Hepatitis E:
Symptoms:
Similar to Hepatitis A. No chronic form.

Infectious Agent:
Hepatitis E virus

Where is it found?
Most in countries with inadequate sanitation.

Reservoir:
Unknown; possible rodents?

Mode of Transmission:
Fecal oral

Incubation:
15 to 64 days

Treatment:
None

Preventive Measures:
Same as Hepatitis A, no immunization available

How long Communicable:
Unknown

6) Hepatitis G:
Symptoms:
Usually no acute symptoms or chronic condition.

Infectious Agent:
Hepatitis G virus

Where is it found?
Worldwide

Reservoir:
Humans

Mode of Transmission:
Bloodborne Pathogen

Incubation:
Unknown

Treatment:
 Not needed

Preventive Measures:
Screening of blood supply, other blood exposure risks.

How long Communicable:
Unknown

7) Sin-V Hepatitis:
Symptoms:
Newly identified hepatitis. Has acute and chronic conditions. 300,000 acute infections probably occur each year worldwide.

Infectious Agent:
Sin-V virus

Where is it found?
Worldwide; probably rare in the United States

Reservoir:
Humans

Mode of Transmission:
Mostly parenterally, IV drug usage and blood transfusion
Incubation:
Unknown
Treatment:
None
Preventive Measures:
Screen blood products; this is not available at present. Do not share needles and prevent needle exposure.
How long Communicable:
Not known at this time.

Herpes Simplex Type 1:

(Fever blister, cold sores)
Symptoms:
A localized primary lesion, latency and a tendency to localized recurrence. Illness may greatly vary from severity, marked fever and malaise lasting a week or more, or gingivostomatitis to meningoencephalitis, or some fatal generalized infections in newborns. It causes about 2% of acute pharyngotonsillitis, a primary infection. Re-activation is very common.
Infectious Agent:
Herpes Simplex Type 1
Where is it found?
Worldwide; 60 to 90% of adults possess circulating antibodies for HSV 1.
Reservoir:
Humans
Mode of Transmission:
Contact with saliva carriers and active lesions of HSV 1
Incubation:
Two-twelve days
Treatment:
Herpetic keratitis-adenine arabinoside or trifluridine. Oral Acyclovir may be helpful in severe stomatitis if administered when lesions are first noticed. IV Acyclovir for severe cases of encephalitis, etc.
Preventive Measures:
Good person hygiene, Standard Precautions; Contact Precaution of neonatal.
How long Communicable:
Asymptomatic oral infections with vial shedding are common. Virus has been detected up to 7 weeks after recovery from stomatitis.

Herpes Simples Type II:

Symptoms:
Genital Herpes is a viral disease that may be recurrent and has no cure. Two sero-types of

HSV have been identified: HSV-1 and HSV-2; most cases of genital herpes are caused by HSV-2. On basis of serologic studies, approximately 30 million person in the United States may have HSV infection. Most infected persons never recognize signs suggestive of genital herpes; some will have symptoms shortly have infection and never again. A minority of the total infected U.S. population will have recurrent episodes of genital lesions. Some cases of first clinical episode are manifested by extensive disease that requires hospitalization. Many cases are acquired person to person who do not know that they have a genital infection with HSV or who are asymptomatic at the time of sexual contact.
Symptoms: (Women)
When symptoms occur may be ulcerative painful lesion on cervix, or vulva.
Symptoms: (Men)
Ulcerative painful lesion of the glans penis or prepuce, and in the anus and rectum of homosexual men. Other areas maybe involved depending on site of sexual encounter.
Symptoms: (Infants)
Risk of transmission occurs highest among women with first episode of genital herpes near time of delivery, and is low <3% with recurrent episodes. Vaginal delivery in pregnant women with active herpes (particularly if primary) carries high risk of infection to fetus or newborn, causing disseminated visceral infection, encephalitis and death.
Infectious Agent:
Herpes Simplex II
Where is it found?
Worldwide
Reservoir:
Humans
Mode of Transmission:
Usually sexual contact; types I and II can be transmitted sexually
Incubation:
2-12 days
Treatment:
Acylovir orally when lesions first present
Preventive Measures:
Safe sex practices, monogamy, abstinence
How long Communicable:
Virus has been detected up to 7 weeks after recovery from stomatitis. Primary lesions are infections 7-12 days while recurrent lesions are infectious for 4 days to a week.

Histoplasmosis:
Symptoms:

A systemic mycosis of varying severity and has five clinical forms: Mostly disease of immuno compromised:

1) Asymptomatic with only hypersensitivity to histoplasma
2) Acute benign respiratory-mild to acute a temporary incapacity with flu like symptoms
3) Disseminated histoplasmosis with debilitating fever, GI symptoms, evidence of bone marrow suppression
4) Chronic disseminated disease with low-grade intermittent fever and other severe illness
5) Chronic pulmonary; may resemble TB.

Infectious Agent:
Histoplasma Capsulatum-Fungus
Where is it found?
Mostly like in America, Africa, eastern Asia and Australia; rare in Europe
Reservoir:
Soil with high organic content and undisturbed bird dropping, particularly around old chicken houses, incaves harboring bats.
Mode of Transmission:
Inhalation of airborne conidia.
Incubation Period:
3-17 days after exposure.
Treatment:
Oral Ketoconazole for immuno-suppressed.
Preventive Measures:
Minimize exposure to dust in a contaminated environment; such as chicken coops and their surrounding soil.
Period of Communicability:
Not transmitted from person to person

Hookworm Disease:

Symptoms:
A common chronic parasitic infecgtion with a variety of symptoms, usually in proportion to the degree of anemia. May lead to iron deficiency and hypochromic, microcytic anemia, the major cause of disability.
Infectious Agent:
Necator americanus and others
Where is it found?
Endemic in war tropical climates
Reservoir:
Humans; dogs and cats
Mode of Transmission:
Eggs in feces are deposited on ground and hatch, under favorable conditions, larvae develops to infectious stage in about 7-10 days. Larvae penetrates the skin
Incubation:

A few weeks to many months
Treatment:
Membendaxole, albendazole, levamisole or pyrantel pamoate
Preventive Measures:
Avoid soil contamination with feces, wer shoes
How long Communicable:
Not transmitted from person to person; however infected person can contaminate soil through feces.

Influenza:

(Flu)
Symptoms:
Acute abrupt onset of the respiratory tract with fever, headache, myalgia, prostration, coryza, sore throat and cough which is severe. Children symptoms are usually indistinguishable from other respiratory illnesses. 20,000 to 30,000 patients in the United States expire each year due to influenza. 20,000 to 200,000 are hospitalized.
Infectious Agent:
Influenza agent for a particular year. A, B, or C (rare).
Where is it found?
Worldwide
Reservoir:
Usually humans however, swine, chickens, and ducks.
Mode of Transmission:
Airborne spread predominates among crowded population in enclosed spaces; school buses. Contact with respiratory secretions.
Incubation:
1-3 days
Treatment:
Relenza®, Tamiflu®, Ribavirin, Amantadine
Preventive Measures:
Good handwashing, avoid crowed setting during fall and winter months. Contact Precautions. Above treatments can be used as a prophylaxis in nursing homes. Immunization each year is the best protection to prevent influenza or minimize symptoms.
How long Communicable:
3-5 days from clinical onset in adults; up to 7 days in young children.

Kawasaki Syndrome:

Symptoms:
Acute febrile, sel limite dsystem vasculitisof early chilhood, presumably of infectious or toxin origin. High spiking fever for 12 days, irritability and mood change, cervical adenopathy,

thrombocytosis. A lengthy convalescent phase during which clinical signs fade.

Infectious Agent:
Unknown, some postulate a superantigen bacterial toxin secreted by Staphylococcus Aureus or Group A streptococcus?

Where is it found?
Worldwide-Japan has increased incidence

Reservoir:
Unknown, perhaps humans

Mode of Transmission:
Unknown

Incubation:
Unknown

Treatment:
High does IVIG, preferably as a single dose. Given when 10 days of fever to reduce fever.

Preventive Measures:
Unknown

How long Communicable:
Unknown

Lassa Fever:
Symptoms:
Onset is gradual with malaise, fever, headache, sore throat, cough, nausea, vomiting diarrhea, myalgia, and chest and abdominal pain; fever is persistent or intermittent-spiking. Inflammation and exudation of the pharynx and conjunctivae are common. Fatality rate is about 15% among hospitalized cases.

Infectious Agent:
Lassa virus-an arenavirus

Where is it found?
Endemic in sierra Leone, Liberia, Guinea and Nigeria. Also found in Central African countries.

Reservoir:
Wild rodents: in West Africa; a mouse named Mastomys

Mode of Transmission:
Through aerosol or direct contact with excreta of infected rodents deposited on surfaces such as floors, beds or in food.

Incubation:
6-21 days

Treatment:
Ribarvin, within 6 days of onset

Preventive Measures:
Control of Rodents; Contact Precaution should be adequate in control of person to person transmission

How long Communicable:
Person to person spread may occur during the acute febrile phase when virus is present in the throat. Virus may be excreted in urine of patients for 3-9 weeks from onset of illness.

Legionellosis:
Symptoms:
Usually patients notice anorexia, malaise, myalgia and headache. Within a day there is usually rapid rise in fever associated with chills. A nonproductive cough, abdominal pain and diarrhea are common.

Infectious Agent:
Legionella-bacteria: species usually pnemophila, Pontiac, micdadei and others

Where is it found?
Mostly recognized in North America, but is probably in other areas of the globe.

Reservoir:
Water: ponds and soil-hot water systems (showers), air conditioning cooling towers, whirlpool spas, and respiratory therapy devices have been implicated.

Mode of Transmission:
Airborne

Incubation:
2-10 days, most often 5-6 days; Pontiac fever 5-66 hours most often 24-48 hours

Treatment:
Erythromycin

Preventive Measures:
Cooling towers should be drained when not in use and disinfected periodically to remove scale and sediment.

How long Communicable:
No evidence of person to person transmission

Leishmaniasis:
Symptoms:
A disease of skin and mucous membranes. Starts with a papule that enlarges and usually becomes an ulcer. Lesion may be single or multiple and diffuse. Lesion may heal rather fast or last for years.

Infectious Agent:
Leishman tropica and other species -Protozan

Where is it found?
Pakistan, India and recently China, the Middle East, Iran and Afghanistan; southern regions of Russia.

Reservoir:
Humans, wild rodents, sloths, marsupials and carnivores, domestic dogs.

Mode of Transmission:
Bite of a female sand flea. Multiply in the macrophage of humans. Ruptures macrophage and more is spread to other macrophages.

Incubation:
A week to many months

Treatment:
Sodium stiboguconate, Amphotericin B may be helpful?
Preventive Measures:
Insect control measures, good hygiene measures
How long Communicable:
Not typically transmitted from person to person.

Leprosy:
(Hansen disease)
Symptoms:
A chronic bacterial disease of the skin, peripheral nerves and the upper airway. Two types of leprosy:
1) lepromatous: nodeles , papules, macules and diffuse infiltration are bilaterally symmetrical and usually numerous and extensive; involvement of the nasal mucuos may lead to crusting, obstructed breathing and epistaxis; ocular involvemet lead to iritis and keratitis.
2) tuberculoid leprosy: skin lesions are single or few, sharly demarcatd, anesthetic or hypesthetic, and bilaterally asymmetrical; peripheral nerve involvement tends to be severe.
Infectious Agent:
Mycobacterium leprae
Where is it found?
World prevalence is about 2.5 million!
Epidemic areas are in South Asia and South East Asia. Some rare cases occur in Hawaii, California, Florida, Louisiana, Texas and New York City.
Reservoir:
Humans are the only proven reservoir; Feral armadillos is Texas and Louisiana are questionable.
Mode of Transmission:
Not completely understood, although prolonged close (families) contact appears to be important. The organism can be found in untreated nasal discharges and in skin ulcers.
Incubation:
9 months to 20 years, average is probably 4 years
Treatment:
Rifampin+dapsone+clofazimine with Direct Observed Therapy!
Preventive Measures:
Treatment and prophylactic BCG (more helpful in preventing leprosy than TB)
How long Communicable:
Infectiouness is usually lost within 3 months of continuous and regular treatment with dapsone or clofazimine, or 3 days with rifampin.

Leptospirosis:

Symptoms:
/Common features are fever with sudden onset, headache, chills, severe myalgia (calves and thighs) and conjunctival suffusion, meningitis, rash, hemolytic anemia, hemorrhage into skin and mucous membranes. Heptorenal failure, jaundice, mental confusion/depression, myocarditis and pulmonary involvement with or without hemoptisis. In endemic areas the infection may be inapparent.
Infectious Agent:
Leptrospira-bacteria
Where is it found?
Worldwide; found in rural and urban areas alike. Developed and non developed countries. Can be occupation hazard for sugarcane worker, farmers, sewer workers, miners, veterinarians, dairymen, abattoir workers, fish workers and military troops.
Reservoir:
Wild and domestic animals. Notable are rats, seine, cattle, dogs and raccoons. In the United States swine a major reservoir.
Mode of Transmission:
Contact of skin if abraded or of mucous membranes with water, most soil or vegetation, especially sugarcane contaminated with urine of infected animals, as in swimming.
Incubation:
Usually 10 days, rage is 4-19 days
Treatment:
Penicillin's, cephalosporins, lincomycin and erythromycin
Preventive Measures:
Good hygiene measures; handwashing, avoid swimming in contaminated areas. Immunization of farm and pet animals prevents illness. Standard precautions.
How long Communicable:
Person to person transmission is very rare.

Listeriosis:
Symptoms:
Usually manifested as meningocencephalitis and /or septicemia in newborns an adults and abortion in pregnant. Those at increased risk are newborns, elderly, immunocompromised, and pregnant women. Onset may be sudden with fever, intense headache, nausea, vomiting and signs of meningeal irritation or may be subacute, particularly in the imunocompromised or elderly host. Asymptomatic infection occurs with all ages.
Infectious Agent:
Listeria monocytogenes-bactria
Where is it found?

United States with an incidence of about 1/200,000. Usually occurs sporadically, but may be related to outbreaks usually contaminated water, food, milk, soft cheese, vegetables, and ready to eat meats.

Reservoir:
Soil, forage, water, mud and silage. Animals become exposed during use of silage as fodder. 10% of all adults and animals may care listeria in fecal matter.

Mode of Transmission:
See above-where is it found and reservoir

Incubation:
3-70 days, usually 3 weeks

Treatment:
Penicillin and Ampicillin alone or together with aminoglycosides. Also TMP-SMX for those allergic to penicillins

Preventive Measures:
Thoroughly cook food items, pasteurize all dairy products. Irradiate soft cheeses: good handwashing. Standard Precautions

How long Communicable:
Infected individuals may shed the organisms in their stools for several months without treatment.

Loiasis:

Symptoms:
Migration of an adult worm through subcutaneous or deeper tissues of the body causing, transient swelling several centimeters in diameter.

Infectious Agent:
Loa loa-a filarial nematode

Where is it found?
Africa

Reservoir:
Humans

Mode of Transmission:
Transmitted by deer fly which ingest blood containing microfilariae, larvae develops into infectious stage within 10-12 days in the fly. Fly bites human=infection.

Incubation:
4 months to several years

Treatment:
Diethylcarbamazine

Preventive Measures:
Insect control measures

How long Communicable:
Humans can carry microfilariae for 17 years. Fly can only be communicable from 10-12 days after its infection until all infective larvae have been released, or till fly dies.

Lyme Disease:

Symptoms:
Early symptoms are intermittent and changing. The illness begins in the summer, and the first manifestation in about 60% of patients appears as a red macule or papule that expands slowly in an annular manner. Sometimes with multiple lesions. This lesion is called "erythema migrans". To be significant the lesion would reach a size of 5 cm in diameter. With or without lesion other symptoms include malaise, fatigue, fever, headache, stiff neck, myalgia, migratory arthralgias and/or lympthadenopathy usually for several weeks. Within one week of acute symptoms neurological abnormalities may occur (aseptic meningitis, facial palsy, chorea, ataxia, myelitis and encephalitis).

Infectious Agent:
Borrelia burgdorferi-spirochete bacteria

Where is it found?
Mostly from Massachusetts to Maryland, and Wisconsin and Minnesota, Illinois, to the west coast; Oregon and California.

Reservoir:
Tick-Ixodes scapularis or I. pacificus

Mode of Transmission:
Tickborne-some believe that transfer of infection only if tick is attached for 24 hours

Incubation:
3-32 days; some individuals may have subclinical or no symptoms but may present with late manifestation.

Treatment:
Early stages are effectively treated with doxycycline; 2-4 weeks

Preventive Measures:
Avoid tick infested areas, wear long sleeve shirts and long pants while in wooded, grassy areas. Used insect repellant with DEET®.
Immunization with Lymrix® for those between ages of 15-70 who reside in endemic areas in engage in activities (hiking, living in wooded area, camping, etc.,) or who have prior infection with Lyme disease.

How long Communicable:
Not transmitted from person to person.

Lymphocytic Choriomeningitis:

Symptoms:
Symptoms vary, at times flu like symptoms, with myalgia, retro-orbital headache, leukopenia and thrombocytopenia, followed by complete recovery.

Infectious Agent:
Lymphocytic Choriomeningitis virus

Where is it found?
Not uncommon in Europe and the Americas.
Reservoir:
The infected house mice, hamsters
Mode of Transmission:
Virus is excreted in urine, saliva and feces of infected animals, usually mice. Transmission is through oral or respiratory contact with virus-contaminated excreta, food or dust, or by contamination of skin lesions or cuts.
Incubation:
8-13 days
Treatment:
None
Preventive Measures:
Rodent control measures; good handwashing when handling rodents such as hamsters. Use closed food containers for hamsters.
How long Communicable:
Not transmitted from person to person.

Lymphogranuloma Venereum:
Symptoms:
A chlamydial infection beginning with a small, painless, evanescent erosion, papule, nodule or herpes-like lesion on the penis or vulva, frequently unnoticed. Lympthadenopathy is common. Can cause a severe proctitis in males. Elephantiasis of the genitalia may occur in either gender. Fever, chills, headache, joint pain and anorexia re usually present. This disease is rarely fatal.
Infectious Agent:
Chlamydia trachomatis
Where is it found?
Worldwide; especially in tropical climates
Reservoir:
Humans, often, asymptomatic females
Mode of Transmission:
Usually during sexual intercourse.
Incubation:
3-30 days, if bubo is first manifestation 10-30 days.
Treatment:
Tetracycline or doxycycline
Preventive Measures:
Safe sex practices, monogamy, abstinence
How long Communicable:
Variable from weeks to years, during presence of active lesions.

Malaria:
Symptoms:
Four human malarias can be sufficiently similar in their symptoms to make species differentiation generally impossible with lab studies. Symptoms may vary greatly, but may include fever, chills, sweats, cough, diarrhea, respiratory distress and headache, and may progress to icterus, coagulation defects, shock, renal and liver failure, acute encephalopathy, pulmonary and other CNS symptoms (such as disorientation and delerium).
Infectious Agent:
Plasmodium vivax, P. malariae, P. falciparum and P. ovale-sporozoan parasite. Mixed infections are not uncommon.
Where is it found?
Major cause of ill health in tropical and sub-tropical climates (3 million deaths each year). Most cases occur from South East Asia, South and Central America, Africa.
Reservoir:
Humans
Mode of Transmission:
The bite of an infective female Anopheles mosquito. After ingestion by the mosquito, the parasite migrates to the salivary gland of mosquito and is infective when injected into a person as the insect takes a blood meal.
Incubation:
The time between the infective bite and the appearance of clinical symptoms is approximately 7-14 days for P. falciparum, 8-14 days for vivax and ovale, and 7-30 days for malariae. Some strain of vivax may be 8-10 months.
Treatment:
Chloroquine; if sensitive. Vivax: mefloquine. Consult and Infectious Disease specialist: Treatment can be complex and prolonged, good compliance is imperative.
Preventive Measures:
Mosquito control measures, prophylaxis for individuals who may travel into endemic areas; consult with your local Health Department for visit the Travelers Information wide site at: www.cdc.gov/
How long Communicable:
As long as infective gametocytes are present in the blood of female mosquito's. This varies with species and strain of parasite. Humans who are not treated or inadequately treated could be s source of infection for 3 years, maybe longer.

Measles:
(Hard measles, Rubeola, Red measles, Morbilli)
Symptoms:
An acute highly communicable viral disease with propromal fever, conjunctivitis, coryza, cough and Koplik spots on the buccal mucosa. A red

blotchy rash appears on the 3-7 day, beginning on the face, becoming generalized, lasting 4-7 days, and sometimes ending in branny desquamation. More severe complication are not uncommon such as pneumonia, encephalitis, croup and diarrhea.

Infectious Agent:
Measles virus

Where is it found?
>90 of adults had measles before immunization in the late 1950's

Reservoir:
Humans

Mode of Transmission:
Airborne droplet spread; direct contact with nasal or throat secretions of infected persons and less commonly by articles freshly soiled with nose and throat secretions. One of the most communicable infectious diseases.

Incubation:
About 10 days, varying from 7 to 18 days from exposure to onset of fever.

Treatment:
None

Preventive Measures:
Only immunization is effective, with live attenuated vaccine.

How long Communicable:
From slightly before the beginning of the prodromal period to 4 days after appearance of rash; minimal after the second day of rash. The vaccine has *not* been shown to be communicable.

Meningitis:

1) Viral Meningitis:
Symptoms:
A common but rarely serious clinical syndrome with multiple viral etiologies, characterized with onset of febrile illness of signs and symptoms of meningeal involvement. If diarrhea or other gastrointestional symptoms occurs this usually is related to echo or coxsackie viruses.

Infectious Agent:
Most common are echo virus, coxsackievirus, arbovirus, measles, herpes, varicella

Where is it found?
Worldwide

Reservoir:
Usually humans

Mode of Transmission:
Dependant of viral etiology

Incubation:
Usually 1-10 days, again dependent on viral etiology

Treatment:
None

Preventive Measures:
Good handwashing, reduce contact with respiratory and fecal material. Standard Precautions.

How long Communicable:
Vary with infectious agent.

2) Meningococcal Meningitis:
Symptoms:
An acute bacterial disease, characterized by sudden onset with fever, intense headache, nausea and often vomiting, stiff neck and frequently a petechial rash with pink macules or very rarely vesicles. Delirium and coma often appear. Fatality rates can be > 50%, but with early diagnosis, modern therapy and supportive measures, case fatality rate is between 5-15%.

Infectious Agent:
Neisseria meningitides-bacteria

Where is it found?
Worldwide; organism is ubiquitous. Most cases occur during the winter and spring seasons. More common among children < 2years, however it can attack any age.

Reservoir:
Humans

Mode of Transmission:
By direct contact with respiratory droplets from nose and throat of infected people. Sharing same items, such as eating utensils, cigarettes, kissing, intubation or extubation can efficient transmit this organism. 20% of population may be naso-pharyngeal carriers of N. meningitidis

Incubation:
2-10 days, commonly 3-4 days

Treatment:
Rocephin® is antibiotic of choice

Preventive Measures:
Vaccines containing groups A, C, Y and W-135 may be effect in military groups or college dormitories. Prophylaxis for those with close secret ional contact before treatment of source case. Rifampin for children and usually Ciproflaxin for adults can greatly reduce risk of Meningococcal disease. Prophylaxis should be administered to those contacts two weeks back from diagnoses of source case. Contact Precautions.

How long Communicable:
N. meningitides is usually not present after 24 hours of effect therapy in naso pharyngeal tract.

3) Haemophilus Meningitis:
Symptoms:

This was the most common bacterial meningitis in children < 5 years of age, before the conjugate vaccine become available. Symptoms may include fever, vomiting, lethargy and meningeal irritation, with bulging fontanelle in infants or stiff neck and back in children.

Infectious Agent:
Haemophilus influenzae type B
Where is it found?
Worldwide
Reservoir:
Humans
Mode of Transmission:
By droplet infection and discharges form nose and throat during the infectious period. The portal of entry is most commonly the nasopharynx.
Incubation:
2-4 days
Treatment:
Parenteral Ampicillin
Preventive Measures:
Immunization of children is the most effect measure. Those with close secret ional contact may be prophylaxis with Rifampin, before treatment of source case. Contact Precautions.
How long Communicable:
Non-communicable within 24-48 hours after starting effective antibiotic therapy.

4) **Pneumococcal Meningitis:**
Symptoms:
Has a high fatality rate, with sudden onset of fever, lethargy or coma, and signs of meningeal irritation.
Infectious Agent:
Streptococcus pneumoniae
Where is it found?
Worldwide
Reservoir:
Humans
Mode of Transmission:
Probably same as H. influenza and N. meningitides.
Incubation:
Probably 1-3 days
Treatment:
Vancomycin, Chloroamphenicol. If sensitive to penicillin; use penicillin
Preventive Measures:
Immunization is available for those at increased risk ≥ 65 years of age and those immuno compromised. Also good handwashing. Standard Precautions
How long Communicable:

Effect therapy will render patient not infectious after 24-48 hours of effective therapy.

Molluscum Contagiosum:
Symptoms:
A viral disease of the skin that results in a smooth surfaced, firm and spherical papule with unblication of the vertex. May be flesh colored, white, yellow or translucent.
Infectious Agent:
Mollusipox virus
Where is it found?
Worldwide
Reservoir:
Humans
Mode of Transmission:
Usually sexual and nonsexual
Incubation:
7 days to 6 months
Treatment:
Curettage of lesions, possibility of liquid nitrogen.
Preventive Measures:
Safe sex practices, abstinence, monogamy.
How long Communicable:
Unknown, probably as long as lesion persist.

Mononucleosis, Infectious:
(Epstein Barr Disease)
Symptoms:
An acute viral syndrome characterized clinically by fever, sore throat (often with exudative phargyngotonsillitis), lymphadenopathy (especially posterior cervical), splenomegaly, characterized hematologically by mononucleosis and lympocytosis of ≥ 50% including ≥ 10% atypical cells and characterized serologically by the presence of heterophile and Epstein Barr antibodies. Many individuals infected may have rather mild symptoms or may be asymptomatic. In young children the disease is generally mild and more difficult to recognize. 4% of children have jaundice; however up to 95% have abnormal liver function tests.
Infectious Agent:
Epstein Barr (herpes) virus
Where is it found?
Worldwide
Reservoir:
Humans
Mode of Transmission:
Person to person spread by the oropharyngeal route, via saliva. Toys, hands of health care workers and other family members may spread Mononucleosis. Kissing facilitates spread among

young adults. Infection has also occurred with blood transfusion.

Incubation:
4-6 weeks

Treatment:
None

Preventive Measures:
Good handwashing; Standard precautions.

How long Communicable:
Prolonged, pharyngeal excretion may persist in cell-free form for a year or more after infection; ≥ 15-20% of EBV antibody positive healthy adults are long-term orophargyngeal carriers.

Mumps:

Symptoms:
An acute viral illness characterized by fever, swelling and tenderness of one or more salivary glands, usually the parotid and sometimes the sublingual or submaxillary glands. Orchitis, usually unilateral occurs in 20-30% of post puberty males and opphoritis is about 5% of post puberty females; sterility is an extremely rare risk.

Infectious Agent:
Mumps virus

Where is it found?
Very common among children worldwide without immunization

Reservoir:
Humans

Mode of Transmission:
By droplet spread and by direct contact with the saliva of an infected person.

Incubation:
12-25 days, commonly 18 days

Treatment:
None

Preventive Measures:
Immunization is the only effect control measure

How long Communicable:
6-7 days before parotitis to 9 days after exposed nonimmune people should be considered infectious from the 12th through the 25th day after exposure. Maximum infectiousness occurs 48 hours before onset of illness.

Myalgia, Epidemic:

Symptoms:
An acute viral disease characterized by paroxysmal spasmodic pain localized in the chest or abdomen, which may be intensified by movement, usually fever and headache occur.

Infectious Agent:
Group B coxcackievirus

Where is it found?
An uncommon disease, mostly occurs in the summer, autumn, months; ages 5-15 years

Reservoir:
Humans

Mode of Transmission:
Directly by fecal oral route

Incubation:
3-5 days

Treatment:
None

Preventive Measures:
Good handwashing; Standard Precautions

How long Communicable:
During the acute stage of disease; stools may contain virus for several weeks.

Mycetoma-Actinomycetoma-Eumycetoma: (Madura foot)

Symptoms:
Swelling and suppuration of subcutaneous tissues, and formation of sinus tracts with visible granules in the pus draining from the sinus tracts. Lesions are usually on the foot or lower leg, sometimes on the hand, shoulder and back and rarely other sites

Infectious Agent:
A combination of bacteria and fungi

Where is it found?
Rare in USA, common in Mexico.

Reservoir:
Soil and decaying vegetation

Mode of Transmission:
Subcutaneous implantation of conidia or hyhal elements from fungal source by penetrating wounds (thorns, splinters).

Incubation:
Usually months

Treatment:
Dependant on whether fungal (itraconazole) or bacterial (clindamycin).

Preventive Measures:
Good hygiene measures

How long Communicable:
Not transmitted from person to person.

Orf Virus Disease:

Symptoms:
Cutaneous disease with lesion that are solitary and located usually on hands, arms or face; is a red to violet appearance and may be pustule, progressing to weeping nodule with central umbilication.

Infectious Agent:
Orf virus-DNA virus
Where is it found?
Worldwide; and occupational disease of milk farmers, shepherds, veterinarians and abattoir workers. Important occupational disease in New Zealand.
Reservoir:
Sheep's, goats, reindeer and musk oxen. Virus can survive in the environment readily.
Mode of Transmission:
Contact with mucous membranes of animals
Incubation:
3-6 days
Treatment:
None
Preventive Measures:
Good personal hygiene
How long Communicable:
Unknown-although unlikely to be transmitted from person to person.

Paragonimiasis:

Symptoms:
A trematode disease that usually involves the lungs. Symptoms include cough, hemoptysis and pleuritic chest pain. X-ray finding may include diffuse and/or segmental infiltrates, nodules, cavities, ring cyst and pleural effusions.
Infectious Agent:
Paragonimus westemani-fluke
Where is it found?
Endemic in China with over 10 million are infected. Also found in the Americans, Far East, southwest Asia, India, and Africa.
Reservoir:
Humans, dogs, cats, pigs and wild carnivores
Mode of Transmission:
Usually when raw, salted, marinated or partially cooked flesh of freshwater crabs or crayfish is eaten.
Incubation:
Flukes mature and begin to lay eggs approximately 6-10 weeks after a person ingests in the infective larvae. The interval until symptoms is usually long and poorly defined.
Treatment:
Praziquantel and Bithionol
Preventive Measures:
Thoroughly cooking of crustacea
How long Communicable:
Not directly transmitted from person to person

Pediculosis:
Symptoms:

Infestation by head lice occurs on the hair, eyebrows; body lice are of the clothing especially along the seams of inner surfaces. Crab lice usually in present in the pubic area, axillae and body surfaces.
Infectious Agent:
Pediculus humanus capitis-head lice
P. humanus corporis-body lice
Phthirus pubis-crab louse
Where is it found?
Worldwide
Reservoir:
Humans
Mode of Transmission:
Head lice: direct contact with an infested person and object used by them
Body lice: indirect contact with their personal belongings, especially shared clothing and headgear. Head and body lice can survive for a week with food source (blood).
Crab lice: are mostly transmitted from sexual contact.
Incubation:
The life cycle is composed of three stages: eggs, nymphs and adults. The most suitable temperature for the life cycle is 89.6 °. Eggs of head lice do not hatch at temperatures < 71.6 °. Under optimal conditions the eggs of lice hatch in 7-10 days. The nymph stage last about 7-13 days depending on temperature. The egg-to-egg cycle is about 3 weeks.
Treatment:
Head and body lice: premethrin, NIX®, Pyrinate®, Lindane
Preventive Measures:
Good hygiene measures. Machine wash cloths in hot water
How long Communicable:
As long as lice or eggs remain alive on the infested person or on fomites.

Pertussis and Parapertussis:
(Whooping cough)
Symptoms:
A bacterial disease involving the respiratory tract. The initial catarrhal stage has an insidious onset with an irritating cough that gradually becomes paroxysmal, usually within 1-2 weeks, and last for 1-2 months or longer. Paroxysms are characterized by repeated violent coughs; each series of paroxysms has man cough without intervening inhalation and can be followed with a crowing or high-pitched whoop.
Infectious Agent:
Bordetella pertussis-bacteria

Where is it found?
Endemic with unimmunized children;
Worldwide
Reservoir:
Humans
Mode of Transmission:
Direct contact with discharges from respiratory
mucous membranes of infected person by the
airborne route.
Incubation:
6-20 days
Treatment:
Erythromycin
Preventive Measures:
Immunization is the only effective control
measure. DTaP
How long Communicable:
Highly communicable before cough. Once cough
is reduced or gone communicability is greatly
reduced.

Plague:

Symptoms:
A specific zoonosis involving rodents and their
fleas, which transfer the bacterial infection to
various animals and to people. Signs and
symptoms may be nonspecific with fever, chills
malaise, myalgia, nausea, prostration, sore throat
and headache. Lymphadenopathy is common,
usually receiving drainage from the site of the
fleabite, where there may have been the initial
lesion. Bubonic plague usually occurs with
lymphadenopathy in the inguinal area (90%).
Fever is usually present. Complication of
endotoxic shock, disseminated intravascular
coagulation, pneumonia mediastinitis or pleural
effusion may develop.
Infectious Agent:
Yersinia pestis-bacteria
Where is it found?
Areas with vast areas of persistent wild rodent
infection. Many parts of Africa, western half of
the United States, Southeast Asia, some areas of
Russia, India and especially in Vietnam. Plague
is endemic in China
Reservoir:
Wild rodents (especially ground squirrels) are
the natural vertebrate reservoir of plague.
Rabbits and hares, wild carnivores and domestic
cats may be a source of infection to people
Mode of Transmission:
When humans go into rodent infested areas and
are bitten by the flea (especially the Xenopsylia
cheopis). Person to person transmission can
occur when plague invades the lungs
(pneumonia).

Incubation:
1 to 7 days
Treatment:
Streptomycin is drug of choice. Gentamycin,
tetracycline, and chloramphenicol are
alternatives.
Preventive Measures:
Insecticide of patients and their cloths and other
personal belongings. Those with close face-to-
face contact with patient with plague pneumonia
can be prophylaxis with antibiotics: TTC or
chloramphenicol.
How long Communicable:
Fleas may remain infective for months under
good conditions of temperature and humidity.
Bubonic plague is not usually transmitted from
person to person unless there is contact with pus
from suppurative buboes. Pneumonic plague
may be highly communicable under appropriate
climatic conditions; overcrowding facilitates
transmission.

Pneumonias, Common:

1.   Pneumococcal Pneumonia:
Symptoms:
Characterized with sudden onset with a shaking
chill, fever, pleural pin, dyspnea, tachypnea, a
cough productive "rusty" sputum and
leukocytosis. Case fatality rate is 5 to 10% for
hospitalized patients. However those patients
with underlying disease and alcoholism may
have fatality rates of 2- to 20%.
Infectious Agent:
Streptococcus pneumoniae-bacteria
Where is it found?
A continuing epidemic in old age and infancy
and in individuals with underlying medical
conditions and in developing countries.
Reservoir:
Humans
Mode of Transmission:
By droplet spread, by direct oral contact or
indirectly through articles freshly soiled with
respiratory secretions.
Incubation:
1-3 days
Treatment:
A delay in treatment can be fatal; due to
resistance with penicillin, vancomycin and
chloroamphenicol can be utilized.
Preventive Measures:
Avoid over crowding conditions particularly
institutions, barracks and ships. Administration
of polyvalent vaccine is the only effect

protection for individuals ≥ 65 years of age or patients with any chronic medical condition.
How long Communicable:
Until discharges of mouth and nose no longer contain virulent pneumococci is significant numbers.

2. Mycoplasma Pneumonia
Symptoms:
Predominately a febrile bacterial lower respiratory infection; less often, a pharyngitis that sometimes progresses to bronchitis or pneumonia. Onset is gradual with headache, malaise, cough (often paroxysmal), sore throat and, less often, chest discomfort that may be pleuritic.
Infectious Agent:
Mycoplasma pneumoniae
Where is it found?
Worldwide
Reservoir:
Humans
Mode of Transmission:
Probably by droplet inhalation, direct contact with an infected person (those with sub-clinical infection), or with articles freshly with discharges of nose and throat from an acutely ill and coughing patient
Incubation:
6-32 days
Treatment:
Erythromycin
Preventive Measures:
Avoid crowded living and sleeping quarters, if possible. Standard precautions
How long Communicable:
Probably < than 20 days.

3. Chlamydia Pneumonia:
Symptoms:
Usually presents with cough, frequent sore throat and hoarseness, and fever at onset. Sputum is scanty; few complain of chest pain.
Infectious Agent:
Chlamydia pneumoniae-bacteria
Where is it found?
Worldwide
Reservoir:
People; mostly in young adults
Mode of Transmission:
Not well understood; possibilities include direct contact with secretions, via fomites, and airborne?
Incubation:
Unknown, may be 10 days
Treatment:

Tetracyclines and Erythromycins
Preventive Measures:
Good handwashing, same as common cold.
How long Communicable:
Not defined but presumed to be prolonged based on military outbreaks as long as 8 months.

Polio:
Symptoms:
A viral infection most often recognized by the acute onset of flaccid paralysis. Infection occurs in the GI tract with spread to regional nodes and in a minority of cases to the nervous system. Paralysis occurs in only 1% of cases which must be distinguished from poliomyelitis or Guillain-Barre syndrome; greater than 90% of cases are inapparent or a non specific fever. Aseptic meningitis occurs in about 1% of cases.
Infection Agent:
Poliovirus (genus Enterovirus) types 1, 2, and 3.
Where is it found?
Prior to immunization, polio occurred worldwide. Polio could be eradicated in the next 5-10 years.
Reservoir:
Humans, usually from people with inapparent infections.
Mode of Transmission:
Person to person-through fecal oral route. In wild outbreaks transmission can occur pharyngeal secretions.
Incubation Period:
Commonly 7-14 days for paralytic cases with a range of 3-35 days.
Treatment:
None
Preventive Measures:
Good handwashing; however immunization is the only effect long-term measure.
Period of Communicability:
As long as virus is found in feces. Virus may be found in throat for 1 week while in feces for 3-6 weeks or longer.

Psittacosis:
(Parrot Fever)
Symptoms:
Varying clinical presentation; fever, headache, rash, myalgia, chills and upper or lower respiratory tract disease are common.
Infectious Agent:
Chlamydia Psittaci-bacteria
Where is it found?
Worldwide
Reservoir:

Parakeets, parrots and lovebirds; less likely in poultry, pigeons, canaries and sea birds. Birds that are healthy can be carriers.

Mode of Transmission:
By inhaling the agent from desiccated dropping, secretions and dust from feather of infected birds.

Incubation Period:
1-4 weeks

Treatment:
Tetracycline groups of antibiotics

Prevention Measures:
Wash hands frequently when handling birds or in cleaning bird areas

Period of Communicability:
Birds may shed the bacteria intermittently, and sometime continuously. Not transmitted from person to person.

Q Fever:

Symptoms:
An acute febrile rickettsial disease; onset may be sudden with chills, retrobulbar headache, weakness, malaise and severe sweats. There is considerable variation in severity and duration; infection may be unapparent or present as a nonspecific fever. A pneumonitis is found on x-ray in some cases when symptoms of cough and chest pain are evident.

Infectious Agent:
Coxiella burnetii-

Where is it found?
Found in all continents. More endemic in countries which reservoir animals. Animal workers may be at more risk for infection.

Reservoir:
Sheep, cattle, goats, cats, dogs, some wild animals (bandicoots and many species of feral rodents). Birds and ticks also.

Mode of Transmission:
Commonly airborne dissemination of rickettsia in dust from premises contaminated by placental tissues, birth fluids and excreta of infected animals.

Incubation Period:
Usually 2-3 weeks

Treatment:
Tetracyclines or Chloroamphenicols

Preventive Measures:
Pasteurizing of milk; immunization is available for those at increased risk for infection.

Period of Communicability:
Not transmitted from person to person

Rabies:

Symptoms:
Nearly always-fatal disease in humans with acute encephalomyelitis, sense of apprehension, fever, headache, malaise, with severe site difficulties. Site of bite has sensory changes. The disease progresses to paresis or paralysis, spasm of swallowing muscles leads to fear of water; delirium and convulsions to death.

Infectious Agent:
Rabies virus (a rhabdovirus of genus Lyssavirus).

Where is it found?
Worldwide; 35,000 to 40,000 adults die each year in the world of human rabies.

Reservoir:

Many wild and domestic animals (canidae), including dogs, cats, foxes, coyotes, wolves and jackals; also skunks, raccoon, mongooses and other biting animals. Domestic animals usually become very ill or expired within 10 days after exposure to wild animals with rabies. Raccoons and other animals may not exhibit symptoms of animal rabies.

Mode of Transmission:
Virus-laden saliva of a rabid animal is introduced by bite or scratch (or, very rarely, into a fresh break in the skin or through intact mucous membranes).

Incubation Period:
Usually 3-8 weeks, rarely as short as 9 days or as long as 7 years; depending on the severity of the would, site of wound in relation to the richness of the nerve supply and it distance from the brain, the strain and amount of virus involved.

Treatment:
None

Preventive Measures:
If bitten or scratched:
1. **Disinfect bitten or scratched area with soap and water immediately!**
2. **Thorough wounds cleansing under medical supervision**
3. **Rabies immune globulin and/or vaccine as indicated**
4. **Tetanus prophylaxis and antibacterial treatment when required**
5. **No sutures or would closure advised unless unavoidable**

See chart on next page!

Animal Species	Condition of Animal at Time of Attack	Treatment of Humans
Domestic dog and cat	Healthy and available for 10 days of observation	None, unless animal develops rabies
	Rabid or suspect rabid-Unknown (escaped)	HRIG & Vaccine (Consult public health department If treatment is indicated)
Wild carnivores, skunk, fox, bat, coyote, bobcat, woodchucks	Regard as rabid unless proven negative by laboratory tests	HRIG & Vaccine
Other livestock, rodents and lagomorphs (hares and rabbits)	Contact public health department for consultation on questions about the need for prophylaxis. Generally rodents rarely transmitted rabies unless they attack very unusual	

Period of communicability:
For dogs and cats, usually for 3-7 days before onset of clinical signs (rarely over 4 days) and throughout the course of the disease.

Relapsing Fever:
Symptoms:
A systemic spirochetal disease in which periods of fever lasting 2-9 days with afebrile periods of 2-4 days. The number of relapses varies from 1 to 10 or more. Each febrile period terminates by crisis. Fatality rate is between 2 and 10% in untreated cases.
Infectious Agent:
Borrelia recurrentis-a spirochete bacteria
Where is it found?
Asia, eastern Africa, southern and central America
Reservoir:
Humans, for tickborne relapse and wild rodents
Mode of Transmission:

Vectorborne; louseborne relapsing fever is acquired by crushing an infective louse. Pediculus humanus, so that it contaminates the bite wound or an abrasion of the skin. In tickborne disease, people are infected by the bite or coxal fluid of an argasid tick; Ornitbodoros bermis O. turicata in the USA.
Incubation:
5-15 days, usually 8 days
Treatment:
Tetracyclines
Preventive Measures:
Tick and louse control measures; also rodent control measures.
How long Communicable:
Not transmitted from person to person. Louse becomes infective 4-5 days after ingestion of blood from an infective person and remains so for life (20 to 40 days). Infected ticks can live for several years without feeding; they remain infective during this period and pass the infection transovarianly to their offspring.

Respiratory Disease, Acute Viral: (Excluding Influenza)
1. **Common Cold:**
Symptoms:
An acute catarrhal infection of the URT characterized by coryza, sneezing, lacrimation, irritated nasopharynx, chillness and malaise lasting 2-7 days. Fever is uncommon for those > 3 years of age.
Infectious Agent:
Rhinovirus (over 100 serotypes)
Where is it found?
Worldwide
Reservoir:
Humans
Mode of Transmission:
By direct contact or by inhalation of airborne droplets; more importantly; indirectly by hands and articles freshly soiled by discharges of nose and throat of an infected person. Rhinovirus and RSV are transmitted by contaminated hands carrying virus to the mucous membranes of the eye or nose.
Incubation:
Between 12 hours and 5 days, usually 48 hours
Treatment:
None
Preventive Measures:
Good handwashing, covering mouth when coughing or sneezing and sanitary disposal of oral and nasal discharges.
How long Communicable:

Usually 24 hours before onset and 5 days after onset of illness.

Acute Febrile Respiratory Disease:
(RSV, Parainfluenza, adenovirus, other rhinovirus, certain coxsackievirus and echoviruses)

Symptoms:
Viral diseases of the respiratory tract usually characterized by fever, chills or chilliness, headache, general aching, malaise and anorexia; occasionally in infants by GI disturbances. Localized signs also occur at various site of respiratory tract such as pharyngitis or tonsillitis, laryngitis, laryngotrachetis, bronchitis, and pneumonia (rare).

Infectious Agent:
Respiratory Syncytial virus (common in children and infants), adenovirus, other rhinovirus, certain coronavirus, coxsackivirus Group A and B, and some echoviruses.

Where is it found?
Worldwide

Reservoir:
Humans

Mode of Transmission:
Same as common cold. Virus discharges in feces, including enterovirus and adenoviruses, may be transmitted by the fecal-oral rout. Outbreaks of illness due to adenovirus types 3,4 and 7 have been related to swimming pools.

Incubation:
1 to 10 days

Treatment:
None

Preventive Measures:
Same as common cold

How long Communicable:
Usually prior to and for the duration of active disease.

Rocky Mountain Spotted Fever:
Symptoms:
A rickettsiae is characterized by sudden onset of moderate to high fever, which persist for 2-3 weeks in the untreated cases, significant malaise, deep muscle pain, severe headache, chills and conjunctival injection. In about 50% of cases a maculopapular rash appears on the extremities on about the third day; this soon includes the palms and soles and spreads to the rest of the body. Death is uncommon if treated.

Infectious Agent:
Rickettsia rickettsii-tickborne

Where is it found?

Throughout the USA, usually from April to September. 50% are reported in south Atlantic states. Few cases are reported in the Rocky Mountain region!

Reservoir:
Maintained in nature in ticks by transovarian and transstadial passage. Can be transmitted to dogs, various rodents and other animals; animal infection are usually sub-clinical, but disease in rodents and dogs has been observed.

Mode of Transmission:
By tick bite of an infected tick. At least 4-6 hours of tick attachment and blood feeding is needed before the parasite become reactivated and infectious for people.

Incubation:
3-14 days

Treatment:
Tetracyclines

Preventive Measures:
Tick repellent collars for dogs and other tick control measures.

How long Communicable:
Not transmitted from person to person. Tick remains infectious for life.

Rubella:
(German Measles)

Symptoms:
Usually a mild febrile viral disease with a diffuse maculopapular rash sometimes resembling measles or scarlet fever. Children usually present few or no constitutional symptoms, but adults may experience a 1-5 day prodromal of low grade fever, headache, malaise, mild coryza and conjunctivitis. Postacuricular, occipital and posterior cervical lympthadenopathy is a common feature and precedes the rash by 5-10 days. Rash is only present in about half the cases.
Rubella usually causes anomalies in the developing fetus; up to 90% of pregnancies during the first trimester. Risk for congenital defects drops to 10 to 20% after the 16th week of pregnancy.

Infectious Agent:
Rubella virus

Where is it found?
Worldwide

Reservoir:
Humans

Mode of Transmission:
Contact with nasopharyngeal secretions of infected persons. Infection is by droplet spread or direct contact with patients.

Incubation:

16 to 18 days, with a range of 14-23 days.
Treatment:
None
Preventive Measures:
Immunization is the only reliable measure.
How long Communicable:
For about 1 week or 4 days after onset of rash;
highly communicable.

Salmonella:
Symptoms:
A bacterial disease, which manifests by sudden
onset of headache, abdominal pain, diarrhea,
nausea and sometimes vomiting. Dehydration,
especially among infants and the elderly. Fever
is very common. Anorexia and diarrhea often
persist for several days. Septicemia or focal
infection may occur in rare incidences (mostly
among immuno-compromised). Other
complication such as pericarditis, pneumonia or
pyelonephritis and death may occur in rare
incidences.
Infectious Agent:
Salmonella; species enteritidis and typhimurium
are the most commonly reported in the USA.
Where is it found?
Worldwide, more extensively in North America
and Europe due to better reporting.
Reservoir:
A wide range of wild or domestic animals,
including poultry, swine, cattle, rodents and pets
such as iguanas, tortoises, turtles, terrapins
chicks, dogs and cats. Humans can also be a
reservoir. Contact with reptile-like animals
contributes to 30,000 cases annually in the USA.
Mode of Transmission:
By ingestion of organism in food derived from
infected food-animals or contaminated by feces
of an infected animal or person.
Incubation:
6 to 72 hours, usually 12-36 hours
Treatment:
Usually none: except rehydration if indicated.
Antibiotics can be used for those most at risk for
complications (infants, elderly, immunocompromised). However, in those immunocompetent antibiotics may prolong the carrier
state.
Preventive Measures:
Good handwashing, proper food preparation and
prevent cross-contamination during food
preparation.
How long Communicable:
Person to person transmission is somewhat
uncommon in the USA. However,
transmissibility could occur whenever diarrhea is
present. Some individual could excrete the
organism for > 1 year.

Scabies:
Symptoms:
A parasitic disease of the skin caused by a mite,
whose penetration is visible as papules, vesicles,
or tiny linear burrows containing the mites and
their eggs. Lesions are prominent amount finger
webs; writs and elbows, under arms, belt portion
of buttock are frequently affected in women.
Infection Agent:
Sarcoptes scabiei-mite
Where is it found?
Widespread-Worldwide
Reservoir:
Humans
Mode of Transmission:
Usually sexual. Cloths may transfer organism,
only if contaminated by infested people
immediately before hand. Mites can burrow
under skin in 2-3 minutes! Norwegian scabies
can be highly contagious because of the large
number of mites that are present in scales.
Incubation Period:
2-6 weeks before onset of itching without
previous exposure. Those with previous
exposure 1-4 weeks.
Treatment:
Children: 5% permethrin. Alternateively; apply
1% benaene hexachloride (lindane, Kwell® ,
contraindicated in premature neonates and used
with caution in infants < 1 year of age and in
pregnant women). See Sexual Transmitted
Disease Treatment Guidelines: 1998.
Preventive Measures:
Safe sexual practices; good hygiene measures.
Period of Communicability:
Until mites and eggs are destroyed by treatment,
usually after 1 or occasionally 2 course of
treatment, a week apart.

Schistomsomiasis:
Symptoms:
A blood fluke that with adult male and female
worms living within mescenteric or vesical veins
of the host over many years. Eggs produce
minute granulomata and scars in organs where
they are lodged or deposited. Symptoms are
related to number of worms within the host.
Symptoms may include diarrhea, abdominal
pain, hepatosplenomegaly to urinary
manifestations, including dysuria, frequency and
hematuria.
Infectious Agent:

Schistosoma mansoni, S. haematobuim and others.

Where is it Found?
Usually in Africa and Madagascar

Reservoir:
Humans usually; other domestic and wild animals may be potential reservoirs.

Mode of Transmission:
Usually a water-borne illness. Humans may shed organism and then penetrate and develops into freshwater snails. The organisms usually leave the body through the urine and sometimes feces. Usually invades not intact skin areas exposed to contaminated water.

Incubation Period:
Usually 2-6 weeks after exposure.

Treatment:
Biltricide®

Preventive Measures:
In Africa; not to swim, work in freshwater areas with non-intact skin.

Period of Communicability:
Not directly transmitted from person to person.

Shigella:

Symptoms:
A bacterial disease which may present to mild, non-specific symptoms to bloody diarrhea, fever, vomiting. Sometimes toxemia, convulsions and dehydration. A hemo-uremic syndrome (HUS) may occasionally occur. Diarrhea usually last from 4-8 days.

Infectious Agent:
Shigella sonnie-most common in USA
Shigella dysentriae, S. flexnerii-in developing countries. Dynentriae is usually associated with increase risk for death and other complications.

Where is it Found?
Worldwide: Florida has been experiencing many community outbreaks in the past several years, although other areas in United States have also experienced outbreaks.

Reservoir:
Humans

Mode of Transmission:
Fecal Oral: ingestion between 10-100 organisms which usually result in infection

Incubation Period:
12-96 hours, usually 1-3 days

Treatment:
TMP-SMX, Cipro, Ampicillin

Preventive Measures:
Good Handwashing is the most effective measure. Proper disinfection of soiled items. Children with diarrhea should not be at school or day care, until treatment 48-72 hours after

treatment or if symptoms have completely resolved. Food handlers should not work with diarrhea.

Period of Communicability:
During acute infection and until the infectious agent is no longer present in feces, which is usually within 4 weeks after illness. Treatment with appropriate antibiotic will effectively reduce shedding in 48 to 72 hours. Carriers states are rare.

Smallpox:

This disease is eradicated worldwide: Concerns now are the potential use of smallpox as a Biological Weapon.

Symptoms:
Febrile onset with fever, and severe aching pains and prostration. 2 to 3 days later a rash develops over the face and spread to the extremities. The rash soon becomes vesicular and later, pustular. Patient will remain febrile throughout the rash evolution of rash, with pain as pustules grow and expand. Gradually, scabs form, which eventually separate, leaving pitted scars. Death usually occurs during the 2nd week.

Infectious Agent:
Smallpox virus

Where is it Found?
Where might the virus come from? At one time, it was believed that the smallpox virus was restricted to only two high-security laboratories, one at the Centers for Disease Control and Prevention in Atlanta, Georgia, and one at the Russian State Center for Research on Virology and Biotechnology, Koltsovo, Novosibirsk Region. By resolution of the 1996 World Health Assembly (WHA), those stocks were slated to be destroyed at the end of June 1999. The desirability of such an action was reaffirmed by a World Health Organization Expert Committee in January 1999. On May 22, 1999, WHA, however, passed a resolution postponing destruction until 2002, by which time any promise of the variola virus stocks for public health research could be determined. Destruction of the virus would be at least one step to limit the risk for the reemergence of smallpox. However, despite widespread acceptance of the 1972 Bioweapons Convention Treaty, which called for all countries to destroy their stocks of bioweapons and to cease all research on offensive weapons, other laboratories in Russia and perhaps in other countries maintain the virus. Iraq and the Soviet Union were signatories to the convention, as was the United States. However, as reported by the former deputy director of the

Russian Bioweapons Program, officials of the former Soviet Union took notice of the world's decision in 1980 to cease smallpox vaccination, and in the atmosphere of the cold war, they embarked on an ambitious plan to produce smallpox virus in large quantities and use it as a weapon. At least two other laboratories in the former Soviet Union are now reported to maintain smallpox virus, and one may have the capacity to produce the virus in tons at least monthly. Moreover, Russian biologists, like physicists and chemists, may have left Russia to sell their services to rogue governments. Smallpox is rated among the most dangerous of all potential biological weapons, with far-reaching ramifications.

Reservoir:
Humans
Mode of Transmission:
The virus must sustain itself must pas from person to person in a continuing chain of infection and is spread by inhalation of air droplets or aerosols.

Incubation Period:
10-15 days
Treatment:
None
Prevention Measures:
Only vaccination is effective control. Those exposed may be administered vaccine within 2 to 3 days will be protect.
Period of Communicability:
As long as patient is febrile. Only when fever is not evident and all lesions have scabbed over is patient no longer communicable.

Staphylococcal Disease:

Methicillin Resistant Staphylococcus Aureus (MRSA)
Symptoms:
A common bacterial skin lesions are impetigo, folliculitis, furuncles, carbuncles, abscesses and infected lacerations. Staphylococcus aureus may release an epidermolytic toxin. If lesions are widespread or disseminated fever, malaise, headache and anorexia may develop. Should lesions feed staph aureus in the blood stream pneumonia, lung abscess, osteomyeltitis, sepsis, endocarditis, meningitis and brain abscesses may occur.
Toxic Shock Syndrome has/had been associated with vaginal tampon use in 55% of cases. Now other risk factors are contraceptive diaphragms

and vaginal sponges, and infection following childbirth or abortion.
Infectious Agent:
Staphylococcus Aureus
Where is it Found?
Worldwide
Reservoir:
Humans
Mode of Transmission:
Colonization of anterior nares; 20 to 30% of population are nasal carriers. Auto infection is responsible for at least 1/3 of infections. Transmission is contact with person with draining lesions or asymptomatic carriers (nasal) of a pathogenic strain. *The role of objects is over stress and this is not airborne.*
Incubation Period:
Usually 4-10 days
Treatment:
Localized lesions usually need cleaning and keeping dry. Local antibiotic ointments are beneficial. Abscess should be incised to permit drainage of pus. For severe infection clindamycin, vancomycin (MRSA)is effective.
Prevention Measures:
Good handwashing, and treatment of lesions. Treatment of nasal carriers is rarely effective
Period of Communicability:
As long as purulent lesions continue to drain.

Streptococcal Disease:
Symptoms: Six common diseases
Sore Throat: Sudden onset of fever, sore throat, exudative tonsillitis or pharyngitis and tender, enlarged cervical lymph nodes. Symptoms can be minimal or absent. Otitis Media may occur as coincident or subsequent or pertonsilar abscess may occur; after 1-5 weeks acute glomerulonephritis (mean=10days) mean rheumatic fever (mean=19 days).
Skin Infection: Usually is superficial and may proceed through vesicular, pustular and encruste states. Scarlatiniform rash is unusual and rheumatic fever is not sequel; however, glomerrulonephritis may occur later, usually 3 weeks after the skin infection.
Scarlet Fever: Characterized by skin rash; it occurs when the infecting stain of strep produces a pyrogen exotoxin and the patient is sensitized by not immune to the toxin. Clinical characteristics are sore throat, or wound, skin puerperal infection as well as enanthem, strawberry tongue and exanthem. The rash is usually fine erythema, blanching on pressure, may feel like sand paper.

Erysipelas: Acute cellulites characterized by fever, constitutional symptoms, leukocytosis and red, tender edematous spreading lesion of the skin often with a definitive raised border. The central point seems to be clear as the periphery extends.

Puerperal Fever: Acute disease, usually febrile, accompanied by local general symptoms and signs of bacterial invasion of the genital tract and sometimes the bloodstream.

Toxic Shock Syndrome: In people with invasive Group A streptococcal infections has been increasingly recognized in the USA since 1987. Clinical features include hypotension and any of the; renal failure, thromboctopenis, disseminated intravascular coagulation (DIC), respiratory distress syndrome, macular rash or soft tissue necrosis (necrotizing fascitis).

Infectious Agent:
Streptoccocus pyogenes, Group A. Skin type is usually a different serologic type than throat infections.

Where is it Found?
Usually in temperate zones, well recognized in tropical climates. Usually more common in children 2-3 years of age

Reservoir:
Humans

Mode of Transmission:
Large respiratory droplets or more commonly direct contact with patients or carriers. Rarely through indirect contact with objects.

Incubation Period:
1-3 days

Treatment:
Penicillin, recurrent strep throat: clindamycin

Prevention Measures:
Good handwashing, treatment of skin lesions or other infected sites

Period of Communicability:
In untreated, uncomplicated cases, 10-21 days, in treated conditions with purulent discharges, weeks or months. With appropriate antiobiotic treatment, transmissibility is terminated in 24 hours.

Strongyloidiasis:

Symptoms:
Often an asymptomatic helminthic infection of the duodenum and upper jejunum. A transient dermatitis when larvre of the parasite penetrate the skin on initial infection may occur; cough, rales and sometimes pneumonia when passing through the lungs can also occur. Symptoms may be mild to severe, depending on the intensity of the infection.

Infectious Agent:
Strongyloides stercoralis-nematodes

Where is it Found?
Mostly in temperate and tropical areas

Reservoir:
Humans; occasionally dogs and cats

Mode of Transmission:
Infective larvae, which develop in feces or moist soil, penetrate the skin, enter the venous circulation and carried to the lungs.

Incubation Period:
Usually 2-4 weeks

Treatment:
Thiabendazole, albendazole

Prevention Measures:
Good hygiene measures, proper disposal of feces

Period of Communicability:
As long as living worms remain the intestine; up to 35 years in cases of autoinfection.

Syphilis:

Symptoms:
First stage begins with a primary lesion (chancre), which is usually painless, and lymphadenopathy in the pubic area usually occurs. Then a secondary eruption involving skin and mucous membranes, then long periods of latency (5-20 years), and late lesions of skin, bone, viscera, the CNS and the cardiovascular system.

Fetal infections occurs with high frequency in untreated early infections of pregnant women and with lower frequency later in latency. It frequency results in abortion or stillbirth.

Infectious Agent:
Treponema pallidum-a spirochete bacteria

Where is it Found?
Worldwide among sexually active individuals

Reservoir:
Humans

Mode of Transmission:
A sexually transmitted disease

Incubation Period:
10 days to 3 months, usually 3 weeks

Treatment:
Bicillin 2.4 million units, tetracycline or erythromycin

Prevention Measures:
Safe sex practices, abstinence, monogamy. Prophylaxis of contact within critical window period.

Period of Communicability:
Usually when lesions are present: first and secondary stages. Congenital transmission is

most probable during early maternal syphilis but can occur throughout the latent period. Appropriate treatment ends infectivity within 24-48 hours.

Taeniasis:

Symptoms:
An intestinal infection with the adult stage of large tapeworms; cysticercosis is a tissue infection with the larval stage of one species, Taenia solium. Clinical manifestations vary, may include nervousness, insomnia, anorexia, weight loss, abdominal pain and digestive disorders. Except for having worms emerging from the anus, many infection are asymptomatic. This disease is usually non-fatal, but the larval of T. solium may cause fatal outcome.

Infectious Agent:
Taenia solium, the pork tape worm.
T. saginata, the beef tapeworm

Where is it Found?
Worldwide; more common where beef or pork is ingested raw; Latin America, Asia, Africa and Eastern Europe.

Reservoir:
Humans

Mode of Transmission:
Follows ingestion of raw or undercooked infected pork or beef with development of tapeworm

Incubation Period:
Days to ≥ 10 years

Treatment:
Nicolcide®, Yomesan®

Prevention Measures:
Through cooking of pork and beef

Period of Communicability:
Not directly transmitted from person to person, but T. solium may be.

Tetanus:

Symptoms:
An acute disease induced by an exotoxin of the tetanus bacillus, which grows anaerobically of the site of an injury. Characterized by painful muscular contractions, primarily of the neck, secondarily of trunk muscles, abdominal rigidity in children, spasms. Fatality rate can range from 10 to 90%.

Infectious Agent:
Clostridium tetani-bacteria

Where is it Found?
Worldwide; rare in developed countries. Cases more common in elderly than children.

Reservoir:

Intestine of horses and other animals, including humans, which the organism is a harmless normal inhabitant. Soil or fomites contaminated the human or animal feces.

Mode of Transmission:
Tetanus spores are introduced in the body, usually through a type of puncture wound with soil, street dust or animal or human feces; through lacerations, burns and trivial or unnoticed wounds, and I.V. drug injection.

Incubation Period:
3-21 days

Treatment:
Possible prophylaxis with tetanus toxoid on same day of injury, if injury occurred and > than 5 years since immunization.
TIG, Im in does of 3,000 to 6,000 IU or tetanus antitoxin (equine origin). IV metronidazole in large doses should be give for 7 to 14 days. Supportive respiratory therapy.

Summary Guide for Tetanus Prophylaxis in Routine Wound Management

Hx of tetanus immunization doses	Clean, minor wounds		All other wounds	
	Td[2]	TIG	Td[2]	TIG
Uncertain or <3	Yes	No	Yes	No
3 or more	No[3]	No	No4	No

2 For children <7 years old DTaP is preferred to tetanus toxoid alone. For person ≥7 years old.
Td is preferred to tetanus alone
3 Yes if >10 years since last dose
4 Yes if >5 years since last dose

Prevention Measures:
Complete immunization is the only reliable measure. Always wash/clean wounds with soap and water!

Period of Communicability:
Not transmitted from person to person.

Toxocariasis:

Symptoms:
A chronic and usually mild disease, predominantly of young children, but increasing in adults, caused by migration of larval form of Toxocara species in the organs and tissues. Characterized by eosinophilia of variable duration, hepatomegaly, hyperglobulinemia, pulmonary symptoms, fever, abdominal pain, and rash may occur. If enters eye may cause endophthalmitis.

Infectious Agent:
Toxocara canis

Where is it found?
Probably worldwide.
Reservoir:
Dogs and cats
Mode of Transmission:
Mostly occurs with children, usually by direct transmission of infective eggs from contaminated soil to the mouth. From contaminated soil or fruits and vegetables, which are not washed.
Incubation Period:
In children weeks to months dependant on intensity of infection, reinfection and sensitivity of patient. Ocular may occur as late as 4-10 years.
Treatment:
Mebendazole or albendazole
Prevention Measures:
Proper food preparation, do not ingest soil.
Period of Communicability:
Not transmitted from person to person.

Toxoplasmosis:
Symptoms:
A protozoan disease; infection are frequently asymptomatic or present as an acute disease with only lympthadenopathy, may resemble mononucleosis, with fever, lymphocytosis for days to weeks. Many individuals have been exposed, but Toxoplasma lies dormant and usually will only re-activiate with immuno-suppression (HIV/AIDS)
Infectious Agent:
Toxoplasma gondii
Where is it found?
Worldwide; in animals and birds. Infection in humans is common
Reservoir:
Cats and other felines, most individuals in the world acquire by ingestion of raw infected mammals (especially rodents).
Mode of Transmission:
Transplacental infection in humans occurs when a pregnant women has rapidly dividing tachyzoites circulation in the bloodstream, usually in primary infection. Children may acquire from contact with cat feces in sandbox or litter box. Ingestion of raw mammals, rodents.
Incubation Period:
10-23 days from ingested raw meats.
5-20 from cats.
Treatment:
Healthy carriers; no treatment is indicated.
Immuno compromised: TMP/SMX, Daraprim®
Prevention Measures:

Food should be thoroughly cooked, Good handwashing after any contact with animal feces.
Period of Communicability:
Not transmitted from person to person.

Trachoma:
Symptoms:
A chamydial conjunctivitis of insidious or abrupt onset, the infection may persist for a few years if untreated, but the characteristic lifetime duration of active disease in hyperendemic areas is the result of frequent reinfection. Cause scarring in turned eyelashes and lid deformities, that in turn cause chronic abrasion of the cornea with visual impairment and blindness later in adult life. Early trachoma in some developing countries is an endemic childhood disease in families or communities.
Infectious Agent:
Chamylia trachomatis-bacteria
Where is it found?
Worldwide; endemic in some underdeveloped countries
Reservoir:
Humans
Mode of Transmission:
Usually through direct contact with infectious ocular or nasopharyngeal discharges on fingers or indirect contact with fomites; towels, cloths, other soiled materials.
Incubation Period:
5 to 12 days
Treatment:
5 to 6 days of TTC or EES ointments
Prevention Measures:
Good personal hygiene; handwashing. Mass treatments of all infants with TTC or EES ointments
Period of Communicability:
As long as active lesion are present in the conjunctivae and adnexal mucous membranes. Infectivity is eliminated in 2-3 days after appropriate treatment.

Trench Fever:
Symptoms:
A nonfatal, febrile, bacterial disease varying in manifestation and severity. May be characterized with headache, malaise, pain and tenderness (in spine) or on the shins; onset is sudden or slow with or without fever.
Infectious Agent:
Bartonella quintana-bacteria
Where is it found?

Epidemics occurred in Europe during WWI and II

Reservoir:
Humans

Mode of Transmission:
Infection occurs by inoculation of organism in louse feces through a break in skin, either from bite or other means.

Incubation Period:
7-30 days

Treatment:
TTC and chloramphenicol

Prevention Measures:
Delousing and rodent control

Period of Communicability:
Not transmitted from person to person. Lice may be infectious for years.

Trichinellosis:

Symptoms:
Round worm whose larvae migrate to and become encapsulated in the muscles. Illness is variable from inapparent to fatal. Muscle soreness and pain with edema of eyelids are early signs.

Infectious Agent:
Trichinella spiralis-roundworm

Where is it found?
Worldwide; more prevalence in countries that may ingest raw beef or pork

Reservoir:
Swine, dogs, cats, horses, rats and many wild animals

Mode of Transmission:
Eating raw or inadequately prepared beef or pork

Incubation Period:
5-45 days

Treatment:
Mebendazole

Prevention Measures:
Thoroughly cooking of beef and pork.

Period of Communicability:
Not transmitted from person to person.

Trichomoniasis:

Symptoms:
A common and persistent protozoal disease of the genitourinary tract, characterized in women by vaginitis with small petechial or sometime red strawberry spots and profuse, thin, foamy, greenish-yellow discharge with foul order. Co exists with gonorrhea in 40% in some studies.

Infectious Agent:
Trichomonas vaginalis-protozoan

Reservoir:
Humans

Mode of Transmission:
Sexual

Incubation Period:
4-20 days, usually 7days

Treatment:
Flagyl®

Preventive Measures:
Safe sex practices, abstinence, monogamy

Period of Communicability:
For duration of persistent infection, which may last for years.

Trichuriasis:

Symptoms:
A nematode infection of the large intestine, usually asymptomatic. Heavy infection may cause bloody, mucoid stools and diarrhea. Rectal prolapse, clubbing of the fingers, hypoproteninemia anemia and growth retardation.

Infectious Agent:
Trichuris trichiura-human whipworm

Where is it Found?
Worldwide; mostly warm moist regions

Reservoir:
Humans

Mode of Transmission:
Indirect, particularly through pica or ingestion o contaminated vegetables.

Incubation Period:
Indefinite

Treatment:
Mebendazole

Prevention Measures:
Proper handling of fecal matter, restrooms.

Period of Communicability:
Several years in untreated cases

Tuberculosis: (TB)

Symptoms:
A mycobacterial disease important as a major cause of disability and death in many parts of the world (8 million-cases and 3 million deaths each year worldwide). The initial infection usually goes unnoticed; tuberculin skin test sensitivity within a few weeks. Early lung lesions commonly heal, leaving no residual changes except occasional pulmonary or tracheobronchial lymph node calcificaion. Approximately 90 to 95% of those initially infected enter this latent phase from which there is lifelong risk of reactivation. In approximately 5% of apparently normal hosts and as many as 50% of HIV patients, the initial infection may progress directly to pulmonary, milary, meningeal or other dissemination of tuberculosis. Serious

outcome of the initial infection is more frequent in infants, adolescents, young adults and the immunosuppressed.

Pulmonary TB comprises 85% of all TB cases. Although TB can affect any organ in the body; from the skin to kidneys, bones, intestines, etc. Extrapulmonary TB occurs more commonly among HIV+ individuals, however pulmonary TB commonly also among HV+ individuals than extrapulmonary.

Progressive pulmonary TB arises from exogenous reinfection or endogenous reactivation of a latent focus remaining from the initial infection. If untreated, about 50% of patients will expire within 5 years and most within 18 months. Completion of appropriate therapy has a very high cure rate in immunocompetent and immunosuppressed patients.

Acid fast bacilli in the sputum, PPD+ (5-15mm), typical symptoms (productive cough 2-3 weeks), hemotypsis, fever, chills, night sweats, etc) with CXR are required to assist in diagnosis of TB. TB is only confirmed with a positive culture.

Infectious Agent:
Mycobacterium tuberculosis and M. africanum-humans
M. bovis-cattle

Where is it found?
Worldwide; endemic in some underdeveloped countries

Reservoir:
Primarily humans; rarely in other animals

Mode of Transmission:
Exposure to tubercle bacilli in airborne route through droplet nuclei produced by people with pulmonary or largyngeal TB during coughing, sneezing or singing. Prolonged exposure to infectious case may lead to infection of contacts.

Incubation Period:
Usually from 4-12 weeks from infection to primary lesion or significant tuberculin reaction. Progression to active TB is more likely in the first two years after initial infection, however latent infection may persist for a lifetime.

Treatment:
INH+Rifampin+PZA+ethambutol or streptomycin for 2 months or until culture sensitivity identify susceptibility to INH and Rifampin then treat for these to drugs for 6-9 months. Extrapulmonary TB may need treatment for an extended period (12 months).

Preventive Measures:
1. Identify individuals with suspicious signs and symptoms the isolate, diagnosis and treat

2. Report all suspect cases immediately to your county health department for treatment/follow-up and contact investigation!
3. In hospitals place patients while infectious in negative pressure rooms, wear N-95 respirators while entering room or when performing at risk procedures (Ventilation, bronchoscopy, etc)
4. Remove symptomatic-suspect patient from crowded condition; cover mouth with tissues or wear surgical mask.
5. Obtain PPD skin test on individuals with risk factors and suspicious symptoms
6. Administer prophylaxis for appropriate candidates with PPD+ results (5-15 mm)
7. Education for health care workers and the community is very helpful in the control and management of TB.

Period of Communicability:
After initiation of appropriate therapy, infectious status is greatly reduced after 2-3 weeks. Generally, individuals who are PPD+ with no symptoms are not infectious unless. An untreated pulmonary individual may infect up to 20 individuals in two years. Children with primary TB are generally not infectious.

Tularemia:
(Rabbit Fever, Deer-fly Fever)
Symptoms:
An animal bacterial disease with a variety of clinical manifestation usually related to rout of introduction and the virulence of the disease agent. Usually presents as an indolent ulcer at site of introduction of organism. There may be no apparent ulcer, but one or more painful lymph nodes. Ingestion of organism in contaminated food or water may produce painful pharyngitis, abdominal pain, diarrhea and vomiting. Inhalation may cause pneumonic involvement or septicemia with death rate of 30 to 60%. Could also be used for biological warfare!

Infectious Agent:
Francisella tularensis-bacteria

Where is it found?
Throughout North American and in Europe

Reservoir:
Usually rabbits; hares, muskrats, beavers and other wild animals

Mode of Transmission:
Through bite of insect, including wood tick, dog tick, and lone star -tick and less commonly by deer fly. Also, by ingestion of contaminated food or water. By bites of reservoir animals

Incubation Period:
1-14 days, usually 3-5 days
Treatment:
Streptomycin or gentamicin
Preventive Measures:
Insect control measures, Cook suspect food items thoroughly
Period of Communicability:
Not transmitted from person to person

Typhoid Fever:

Symptoms:
Systemic bacterial diseases characterized by insidious onset of sustained fever, severe headache, malaise, anorexia, a relative bradycardia, splenomegaly, rose spots on the trunk in 25% of white patients, nonproductive cough in the early stage of the illness and constipation more commonly than diarrhea (in adults). Many mild and atypical infections occur. Intestinal hemorrhage or perforation may occur due to ulcers in the ileum in about 1% of cases. Death rate can reach 10% but should only be < 1% with appropriate antibiotic therapy.
There is a ParaTyphoid Fever which tends to be milder, and the case fatality rate is must lower
Infectious Agent:
Salmonella typhi-bacteria
Where is it Found?
Worldwide: with about 17 million cases and 600,000 each year! USA has < 500 cases annually. Most cases are imported from under developed countries.
Reservoir:
Humans: women of middle age are more likely to be chronic carriers.
Mode of Transmission:
By food and water contaminated with feces and urine. Shellfish taken from contaminated sewage beds.
Incubation Period:
Usually 1-10 days
Treatment:
Chlorampehnicol, amoxicillin, Cipro or TMP/SMX for children
Prevention Measures:
Proper handling of sewage and proper treatment of human waste products. Immunization is available but not recommended in the United States. Good handwashing, contact precautions.
Period of Communicability:
As long as bacterial appear in the stool, usually from the first week throughout convalescence: variable thereafter (commonly 1-2 weeks for

paratyphiod). About 10% will discharge bacteria for 3 months after onset.

Typhus Fever:

Symptoms:
A rickettsial disease with variable onset; often duden and marked by headache, chills, prostration, fever and general pains. A macular eruption appears on the fifth to sixth day, initially on the upper trunk, followed by spread to the entire body, but usually not to the face, palms or soles. Toxemia is usually pronounced.
Infectious Agent:
Rickettsia prowazekii
Where is it Found?
In colder areas where people may live under unhygienic conditions and are louse infested. Found during war and famine. Endemic in regions of Mexico, South and Central America.
Reservoir:
Humans; flying squirrel are unknown in USA.
Mode of Transmission:
The body louse, Pediculus humanus corporis, is infected by feeding on human blood with acute typhus. Lice excrete rickettsia in feces and will defecate at time of feeding. Rubbing feces or crushed lice into the bite or into superficial abrasions infects people.
Incubation Period:
1-2 weeks
Treatment:
Prevention Measures:
Apply an effective residual insecticide power at appropriate intervals by hand or power blower to clothes and people.
Period of Communicability:
Not directly transmitted from person to person. Humans are reservoirs and can be infectious for 2-3 days after temperature returns to normal.

Scrub Typhus:

Symptoms:
A rickettsial disease often characterized by a primary "punched out" skin ulcer corresponding to the site of attachment of an infected mite. Clinical symptoms of fever, headache, sweating, conjunctival injection and lymphadenopathy often occur.
Infectious Agent:
Rickettsia tsutsugamushi
Where is it Found?
Central, eastern and Southeast Asia. From Siberia to Northern Japan.
Reservoir:

Infected larval stages of mites. Leptotrombidium akamushi are common vectors to humans. Infection is maintained by transovarian passage in mites.

Mode of Transmission:
By the bite of infected larval mites; nymphs and adults do not feed on vertebrate hosts.

Incubation Period:
6-21 days

Treatment:
Tetracyclines

Prevention Measures:
Use of mite repellents with DEET.

Period of Communicability:
Not directly transmitted from person to person

Warts, Viral:
(Common warts, Condyloma acuminatum, Papiloma venereum)

Symptoms:
Common Wart: A circumscribed, hyperkeratotic, rough texture, painless, varying in size from pinhead to large mass.
Filiform warts: elongated pointed, may reach 1 cm in size
Laryngeal papillomas: on vocal cords and epiglottis in children
Flat warts: smooth slightly elevated, usually multiply.
Flat papillomas: on the cervix
Plantar warts: flat hyperkeratotic lesions of the plantar surface of the feet, which are frequently painful
Venereal warts (condayloma acuminatum): caulifower like, fleshy growths, most often seen in moist areas in and around the genitalia, anus, anus canal.
Both laryngeal and genital warts have occasionally become malignant.

Infectious Agent:
HPV -Human papilloma virus

Where is it Found?
Worldwide

Reservoir:
Humans

Mode of Transmission:
Usually by direct contact, also possibility by razors in shaving. Venereal warts: sexual
Laryngeal: are probably transmitted during passage of the infant through the birth canal.

Incubation Period:
1-20 month range, usually 2-3 months

Treatment:

Prevention Measures:
Avoid contact with lesions, good handwashing. Safe sex practices

Period of Communicability:

Unknown, but probably at least as long as visible lesions persist

Yaws:
Symptoms:
A chronic, relapsing nonvenereal treponematosis, characterized by high contagious, primary and secondary cutaneious lesions, and noncontagious, tertiary/late destructive lesions. Usually a face lesion (papiloma) occurs, which is painless. May develop into a large ulcer. Congenital transmission does not occur and this disease is rarely fatal, but can be very disfiguring and disabling.

Infectious Agent:
Treponema pallidum-bacteria

Where is it Found?
Mostly in children (usually males) in warm, moist, tropical areas. Prevalence has dramatically decreased in the 1050s and 1960s, however a recent outbreak occurred West Africa with scattered problems in Southeast Asia and Latin America.

Reservoir:
Humans and possibly higher primates

Mode of Transmission:
Direct contact with exudates of lesions. Indirect contact through skin piercing, scratching can occur but probably rare.

Incubation Period:
2 weeks to 3 months

Treatment:
Penicllin

Prevention Measures:
Good hygiene, bathing and hand washing

Period of Communicability
Whenever lesions are moist and weeping.

Yellow Fever:
Symptoms:
An acute infectious viral disease of short duration and varying severity. The mildest cases are clinically indeterminate; typical attacks are characterized by sudden onset, fever, chills, headache, back pain, generalized muscle pain, prostration, nausea and vomiting. Pulse may be faint and weak. Leukopena appears early and is most pronounced about the 5th day. Most infections resolve at this stage. After a brief remission of hours to a day, some cases progress into the ominous stage of intoxication manifested by hemorrhagic symptoms including epitaxis, gingival bleeding, dark-black stools, and renal and liver failure; 20 to 50% of jaundiced cases

are fatal. The overall case fatality rate among indigenous populations in endemic regions is < 5%.

Infectious Agent:
Yellow virus-a Flavivirus

Where is it Found?
Has two transmission cycles, a sylvatic or jungle cycle that involves mosquitoes and nonhuman primates, and the urban cycle involving Aedes aegypti mosquitoes and human. Sylvatic is found in tropical areas of Africa and Latin America. Urban Yellow fever occurs in many cities of the Americas, although was recently found in Nigeria with more than 20,000 cases. Jungle from the Sahara desert south through northern Angola, Zaire and Tanzania

Reservoir:
Humans and Aedes aegypti mosquitoes in forest areas. Monkeys, possibly marsupials and forest mosquitoes. Transovarian transmission in mosquitoes may contribute to maintenance of infection.

Mode of Transmission:
Usually by the bite of infective Aedes aegypti mosquitoes. In forest of South America, by the bite of several species of forest mosquitoes of the genus Haemagogus. Other types of mosquitoes may transmit disease to humans.

Incubation Period:
3-6 days

Treatment:
None

Prevention Measures:
Active immunization and mosquito control measures. Immunization not recommended in the USA.

Period of Communicability:
Blood of patients is infective for mosquitoes shortly before onset of fever and for first 3-5 days of illness. The disease is highly communicable where many susceptible people and abundant vector mosquitoes coexist; not communicable by contact or common objects-vehicles.

Yersinoisis:

Symptoms:
An acute bacterial enteric disease typically manifested by acute febrile diarrhea (especially in young children), entercolitis, acute mesenteric lymphadenitis can mimic appendicitis (in old children and adults). Bloody diarrhea occurs in about 10 to 30% of cases. This disease may cause arthritis and systemic infection.

Infectious Agent:

Yersinia psudotuberculosis, Y. enterocolitica-bacteria

Where is it Found?
Worldwide, is primarily a zoonotic disease of wild and domestic birds and mammals, with humans as an incidental host.

Reservoir:
Animals are the principal reservoir, particularly the pig. Also birds, rodents and other small mammals

Mode of Transmission:
Fecal oral takes place by eating and drinking contaminated food or water or by contact with infected people or animals.

Incubation Period:
3-7 days

Treatment:
TMX/SMP and many other antibiotics.

Prevention Measures:
Have food cooked and prepared adequately, good handwashing, rodent control measures.

Period of Communicability:
Usually for 2-3 weeks in untreated cases, some may excrete bacteria for 2-3 months.

Zygomycosis:

Symptoms:
A fungal infection, which may affect blood vessels, causing thrombosis and infarction. The craniofacial form of the disease usually presents as nasal or paranasal sinus infection, most in poorly control diabetics. Necrosis of the turbinates, perforation of the hard palate, necrosis of the cheek.

Infectious Agent:
Species of Rhizopus, especially R. arrbizus-fungus.

Where is it Found?
Worldwide, incidence may be increasing due to increased life span of diabetics and certain blood dyscrasisis, like acute leukemia and aplastic anemia.

Reservoir:
Ubiquitous in the environment.

Mode of Transmission:
By inhalation or ingestion of spores of the fungal agents by susceptible individuals.

Incubation Period:
Unknown

Treatment:
Amphotericin B

Prevention Measures:
Control of diabetes

Period of Communicability:
Not transmitted from person to person.

The Most Common/Famous Nosocomial Bacteria Infections

Organism	Sites of Infection	Recommended Treatments	Precautions
Alcaligenes	UTI, Skin/Wound	IMP, AP Pen, ceftaz, MER	Standard[1]
Acinetobacter	UTI, Skin/Wound, LRI	IMP or MER or FQ + amikacin or ceftaz	Standard[1]
Burkholderia (Pseudomanas cepacia)	Skin/Wound, LRI	TMP/SMX	Standard[1]
Citrobacter	UTI, Skin/Wound	IMP or MER	Standard[1]
Clostridium difficile	Diarrhea	Metronidazole	Standard[1]
Clostridium Perfringens	Skin/Wound	Pen G ± clindamycin	Standard[1]
Eikenella corrodens	UTI, Skin/Wound	Penicillin G or AMP or AM/CL	Standard[1]
Enterobacter	UTI, Skin/Wound, LRI	IMP or MER or (AP Pen + APAG)	Standard[1]
Enterococcus	UTI, Skin/Wound, LRI	Penicillin G (AMP) add gentamcin for endocarditis or meningitis	Standard
Enterococcus-Resistant to Vancomycin	UTI, Skin/Wound, LRI	Syncercide?	Standard[1]/Contact
Eschericia coli	UTI, Skin/Wound, LRI	Cephalospirins, FQ, TMP/SMX, APAG, nitrofurantoin, IMP	Standard[1]
Klebsiella	UTI, Skin/Wound/LRI	P Ceph 3, FQ	Standard[1]
Nocardia asteroides	Skin/Wound, LRI	TMP/SMX, sulfonamides (high doses)	Standard
Proteus	UTI, Skin/Wound, LRI	AMP, TMP/SMX, P Ceph 3 or FQ	Standard[1]
Providencia		Amikacin or P ceph 3 or FQ	Standard
Pseudomonas aeruginosa	UTI, Skin/Wound, LRI	AP Pen, P ceph 3 AP, IMP, tobramycin	Standard[1]
Serritia marscens	UTI, Skin/Wound, LRI	P ceph 3, IMP, MER, FQ	Standard[1]
Staph aureus, methicillin susceptible	UTI, Skin/Wound, LRI	PRSP	Standard[1]
Staph aureus methicillin resistant	UTI, Skin/Wound, LRI	Vancomycin	Standard[1]/Contact

Bacteria			
Organism	**Sites of Infection**	**Recommended Treatments**	**Precautions**
Staph epidermidis	UTI, Skin/Wound, I.V. Site	Vancomycin	Standard
Streptococcus pneumoniae	UTI, Skin/Wound, LRI, URI	Penicillin G	Standard[1]
Streptococcus pyogenes	UTI, Skin/Wound, LRI, URI	Penicillin G	Standard[1]

AP Pen: antipseudomonal penicillin: P Ceph: parenteral cephalsporins 1-3: generations: FQ: Fluoroquinolones; AMP: ampicillin; PRSP: penicillinase-resistant synthetic penicillins; CIP: cipro; IMP impenem + clastatin; MER: meropenem [1]Standard precautions unless diarrhea or wound exudates are uncontrolled then contact precautions

Common Nosocomial Fungal Infections			
Organism	**Sites of Infection**	**Recommended Treatments**	**Precautions**
Aspergillosis	LRI, Bloodstream (rare)	Ampho B	Standard
Candidasis	LRI, Bloodstream, Skin/wound	Ampho B	Standard
Nocardosis	LRI, Bloodstream, lymphangtides	Sulfsoxazole	Standard
Penicillosis	Bloodstream, LRI, Skin/Wound	Ampho B	Standard

Amph O: Amphotericin B

MODEL EXPOSURE CONTROL PLAN

The Model Exposure Control Plan is intended to serve as an employer guide to the OSHA Bloodborne Pathogens standard. A central component of the requirements of the standard is the development of an exposure control plan (ECP).

The intent of this model is to provide small employers with an easy-to-use format for developing a written exposure control plan. Each employer will need to adjust or adapt the model for their specific use.

The information contained in this publication is not considered a substitute for the OSH Act or any provisions of OSHA standards. It provides general guidance on a particular standard-related topic but should not be considered as the legal authority for compliance with OSHA requirements. The reader should consult the OSHA standard in its entirety for specific compliance requirements.

POLICY

The _(Facility Name)_ is committed to providing a safe and healthful work environment for our entire staff. In pursuit of this endeavor, the following exposure control plan (ECP) is provided to eliminate or minimize occupational exposure to bloodborne pathogens in accordance with OSHA standard 29 CFR 1910.1030, "Occupational Exposure to Bloodborne Pathogens."

The ECP is a key document to assist our firm in implementing and ensuring compliance with the standard, thereby protecting our employees. This ECP includes:

* Determination of employee exposure
* Implementation of various methods of exposure control, including:
> Universal precautions
> Engineering and work practice controls
> Personal protective equipment
> Housekeeping

* Hepatitis B vaccination

* Post-exposure evaluation and follow-up

* Communication of hazards to employees and training

* Recordkeeping

* Procedures for evaluating circumstances surrounding an exposure incident

The methods of implementation of these elements of the standard are discussed in the subsequent pages of this ECP.

PROGRAM ADMINISTRATION

* _(Name of responsible person or department)_____ is (are) responsible for the implementation of the ECP. _(Name of responsible person or department)_____ will maintain, review, and update the ECP at least annually, and whenever necessary to include new or modified tasks and procedures. Contact location/phone number:_____

* Those employees who are determined to have occupational exposure to blood or other potentially infectious materials (OPIM) must comply with the procedures and work practices outlined in this ECP.

* ___(Name of responsible person or department)_____ will maintain and provide all necessary personal protective equipment (PPE), engineering controls (e.g., sharps containers), labels, and red bags as required by the standard. __(Name of responsible person or department_____ will ensure that adequate supplies of the aforementioned equipment are available in the appropriate sizes. Contact location/phone number:_____

* _(Name of responsible person or department)_____ will be responsible for ensuring that all medical actions required are performed and that appropriate employee health and OSHA records are maintained. Contact location/phone number:_____

* _(Name of responsible person or department)_____ will be responsible for training, documentation of training, and making the written ECP available to employees, OSHA, and NIOSH representatives. Contact location/phone number:_____

EMPLOYEE EXPOSURE DETERMINATION

The following is a list of all job classifications at our establishment in which **all** employees have occupational exposure:

JOB TITLE   DEPARTMENT/LOCATION

(Example: Phlebotomists)   *(Clinical Lab)*

_____   _____

The following is a list of job classifications in which **some** employees at our establishment have occupational exposure. Included is a list of tasks and procedures, or groups of closely related tasks and procedures, in which occupational exposure may occur for these individuals:

JOB TITLE   DEPARTMENT/LOCATION TASK/PROCEDURE

(Example: Housekeeper   *Environmental Services*   *Handling Regulated Waste)*

_____   _____   _____

Part-time, temporary, contract and per diem employees are covered by the standard. How the provisions of the standard will be met for these employees should be described in the ECP.

METHODS OF IMPLEMENTATION AND CONTROL

Universal Precautions

    All employees will utilize universal precautions.

Exposure Control Plan

    Employees covered by the bloodborne pathogens standard receive an explanation of this ECP during their initial training session. It will also be reviewed in their annual refresher training. All employees have an opportunity to review this plan at any time during their work shifts by contacting *(Name of responsible person or department)*_____. If requested, we will provide an employee with a copy of the ECP free of charge and within 15 days of the request.

    *(Name of responsible person or department)*_____ is responsible for reviewing and updating the ECP annually or more frequently if necessary to reflect any new or modified tasks and procedures which affect occupational exposure and to reflect new or revised employee positions with occupational exposure.

Engineering Controls and Work Practices

Engineering controls and work practice controls will be used to prevent or minimize exposure to bloodborne pathogens. The specific engineering controls and work practice controls used are listed below:

* *(For example: glass capillary tubes in the clinical laboratory, outpatient clinics, and pediatric units)*

* _____

* _____

Sharps disposal containers are inspected and maintained or replaced by ____*(Name of responsible person or department)*_____ every ____*(list frequency*_____ or whenever necessary to prevent overfilling.

This facility identifies the need for changes in engineering control and work practices through *(Examples: Review of OSHA records, employee interviews, committee activities, etc.)*____
_____

We evaluate need procedures or new products by *(Describe the process)*_____
_____
_____
____

The following staff are involved in this process: *(Describe how employees will be involved)*___
_____

*(Name of responsible person or department)*_____will ensure effective implementation of these recommendations.

Personal Protective Equipment (PPE)

PPE is provided to our employees at no cost to them. Training is provided by ___*(Name of responsible person or department)*_____ in the use of the appropriate PPE for the tasks or procedures employees will perform.

The types of PPE available to employees are as follows:

*(Ex., gloves, eye protection, etc.)*_____
_____

PPE is located _____*(List location)*_____ and may be obtained through _*(Name of responsible person or department)*_____
(Specify how employees are to obtain PPE, and who is responsible for ensuring that it is available.)

All employees using PPE must observe the following precautions:
* Wash hands immediately or as soon as feasible after removal of gloves or other PPE.
* Remove PPE after it becomes contaminated, and before leaving the work area.
* Used PPE may be disposed of in _____(List appropriate containers for storage, laundering, decontamination, or disposal.)
* Wear appropriate gloves when it can be reasonably anticipated that there may be hand contact with blood or OPIM, and when handling or touching contaminated items or surfaces; replace gloves if torn, punctured, contaminated, or if their ability to function as a barrier is compromised.
* Utility gloves may be decontaminated for reuse if their integrity is not compromised; discard utility gloves if they show signs of cracking, peeling, tearing, puncturing, or deterioration.
* Never wash or decontaminate disposable gloves for reuse.
* Wear appropriate face and eye protection when splashes, sprays, spatters, or droplets of blood or OPIM pose a hazard to the eye, nose, or mouth.
* Remove immediately or as soon as feasible any garment contaminated by blood or OPIM, in such a way as to avoid contact with the outer surface.

The procedure for handling used PPE is as follows: *(may refer to specific agency procedure by title or number and last date of review)*

_____

_____

(For example, how and where to decontaminate face shields, eye protection, resuscitation equipment)

Housekeeping

Regulated waste is placed in containers which are closable, constructed to contain all contents and prevent leakage, appropriately labeled or color-coded (see Labels), and closed prior to removal to prevent spillage or protrusion of contents during handling.

The procedure for handling **sharps disposal containers** is: *(may refer to specific agency procedure by title or number and last date of review)*

_____

_____

_____

The procedure for handling **other regulated waste** is: *(may refer to specific agency procedure by title or number and last date of review)*

_____

_____

_____

Contaminated sharps are discarded immediately or as soon as possible in containers that are closable, puncture-resistant, leakproof on sides and bottoms, and labeled or color-coded appropriately. Sharps disposal containers are available at _____ (*must be easily accessible and as close as feasible to the immediate area where sharps are used*).

Bins and pails (e.g., wash or emesis basins) are cleaned and decontaminated as soon as feasible after visible contamination.

Broken glassware which may be contaminated is picked up using mechanical means, such as a brush and dust pan.

Laundry

The following contaminated articles will be laundered by this company:

_____   _____

_____   _____

Laundering will be performed by *(Name of responsible person or department)*
_____ at *(time and/or location)* .

The following laundering requirements must be met:
  * handle contaminated laundry as little as possible, with minimal agitation
  * place wet contaminated laundry in leak-proof, labeled or color-coded containers before transport. Use _(red bags or bags marked with biohazard symbol)_____ for this purpose.
  * wear the following PPE when handling and/or sorting contaminated laundry: _(List appropriate PPE)_____

Labels

The following labeling method(s) is used in this facility:

EQUIPMENT TO BE LABELED	LABEL TYPE (size, color, etc.)
(e.g., specimens, contaminated laundry, etc.)	_(red bag, biohazard label, etc.)_
_____	_____
_____	_____

_(Name of responsible person or department)_____ will ensure warning labels are affixed or red bags are used as required if regulated waste or contaminated equipment is brought into the facility. Employees are to notify _____ if they discover regulated waste containers, refrigerators containing blood or OPIM, contaminated equipment, etc. without proper labels.

HEPATITIS B VACCINATION
_(Name of responsible person or department)_____ will provide training to employees on hepatitis B vaccinations, addressing the safety, benefits, efficacy, methods of administration, and availability.

The hepatitis B vaccination series is available at no cost after training and within 10 days of initial assignment to employees identified in the exposure determination section of this plan. Vaccination is encouraged unless: 1) documentation exists that the employee has previously received the series, 2) antibody testing reveals that the employee is immune, or 3) medical evaluation shows that vaccination is contraindicated.

However, if an employee chooses to decline vaccination, the employee must sign a declination form. Employees who decline may request and obtain the vaccination at a later date at no cost. Documentation of refusal of the vaccination is kept at _____ _(List location or person responsible for this recordkeeping)._

Vaccination will be *provided by* _____ *(List Health care Professional who is responsible for this part of the plan)*_____ at _____ *(location)*_____.

Following hepatitis B vaccinations, the health care professional's Written Opinion will be limited to whether the employee requires the hepatitis vaccine, and whether the vaccine was administered.

POST-EXPOSURE EVALUATION AND FOLLOW-UP

Should an exposure incident occur, contact _____*(Name of responsible person)* at the following number:_____.

An immediately available confidential medical evaluation and follow-up will be conducted by __ *(Licenced health care professional)* . Following the initial first aid (clean the wound, flush eyes or other mucous membrane, etc.), the following activities will be performed:

* Document the routes of exposure and how the exposure occurred.
* Identify and document the source individual (unless the employer can establish that identification is infeasible or prohibited by state or local law).
* Obtain consent and make arrangements to have the source individual tested as soon as possible to determine HIV, HCV, and HBV infectivity; document that the source individual's test results were conveyed to the employee's health care provider.
* If the source individual is already known to be HIV, HCV and/or HBV positive, new testing need not be performed.
* Assure that the exposed employee is provided with the source individual's test results and with information about applicable disclosure laws and regulations concerning the identity and infectious status of the source individual (e.g., laws protecting confidentiality).
* After obtaining consent, collect exposed employee's blood as soon as feasible after exposure incident, and test blood for HBV and HIV serological status
* If the employee does not give consent for HIV serological testing during collection of blood for baseline testing, preserve the baseline blood sample for at least 90 days; if the exposed employee elects to have the baseline sample tested during this waiting period, perform testing as soon as feasible.

ADMINISTRATION OF POST-EXPOSURE EVALUATION AND FOLLOW-UP

(Name of responsible person or department) _____ ensures that health care professional(s) responsible for employee's hepatitis B vaccination and post-exposure evaluation and follow-up are given a copy of OSHA's bloodborne pathogens standard.

(Name of responsible person or department) _____ ensures that the health care professional evaluating an employee after an exposure incident receives the following:

* a description of the employee's job duties relevant to the exposure incident
* route(s) of exposure
* circumstances of exposure
* if possible, results of the source individual's blood test
* relevant employee medical records, including vaccination status

(Name of responsible person or department) _____ provides the employee with a copy of the evaluating health care professional's written opinion within 15 days after completion of the evaluation.

PROCEDURES FOR EVALUATING THE CIRCUMSTANCES SURROUNDING AN EXPOSURE INCIDENT

(Name of responsible person or department) _____ will review the circumstances of all exposure incidents to determine:
* engineering controls in use at the time
* work practices followed
* a description of the device being used
* protective equipment or clothing that was used at the time of the exposure incident (_gloves, eye shields, etc._)
* location of the incident (_O.R., E.R., patient room, etc._)
* procedure being performed when the incident occurred
* employee's training

If it is determined that revisions need to be made, _(Responsible person or department)_ _____ will ensure that appropriate changes are made to this ECP. (_Changes may include an evaluation of safer devices, adding employees to the exposure determination list, etc._)

EMPLOYEE TRAINING

All employees who have occupational exposure to bloodborne pathogens receive training conducted by _____ _(Name of responsible person or department)_ _____. (_Attach a brief description of their qualifications._)

All employees who have occupational exposure to bloodborne pathogens receive training on the epidemiology, symptoms, and transmission of bloodborne pathogen diseases. In addition, the training program covers, at a minimum, the following elements:

* a copy and explanation of the standard
* an explanation of our ECP and how to obtain a copy
* an explanation of methods to recognize tasks and other activities that may involve exposure to blood and OPIM, including what constitutes an exposure incident
* an explanation of the use and limitations of engineering controls, work practices, and PPE
* an explanation of the types, uses, location, removal, handling, decontamination, and disposal of PPE
* an explanation of the basis for PPE selection
* information on the hepatitis B vaccine, including information on its efficacy, safety, method of administration, the benefits of being vaccinated, and that the vaccine will be offered free of charge
* information on the appropriate actions to take and persons to contact in an emergency involving blood or OPIM
* an explanation of the procedure to follow if an exposure incident occurs, including the method of reporting the incident and the medical follow-up that will be made available
* information on the post-exposure evaluation and follow-up that the employer is required to provide for the employee following an exposure incident
* an explanation of the signs and labels and/or color coding required by the standard and used at this facility
* an opportunity for interactive questions and answers with the person conducting the training session.

Training materials for this facility are available at _____.

RECORDKEEPING

Training Records

Training records are completed for each employee upon completion of training. These documents will be kept for at least **three years** at __*(Name of responsible person or location of records)*_____.

The training records include:

* the dates of the training sessions
* the contents or a summary of the training sessions
* the names and qualifications of persons conducting the training
* the names and job titles of all persons attending the training sessions

Employee training records are provided upon request to the employee or the employee's authorized representative within 15 working days. Such requests should be addressed to _____ *(Name of Responsible person or department)* _____.

Medical Records

Medical records are maintained for each employee with occupational exposure in accordance with 29 CFR 1910.20, "Access to Employee Exposure and Medical **Records.**"

_____ *(Name of Responsible person or department)* _____ is responsible for maintenance of the required medical records. These **confidential** records are kept at _____ *(List location)* _____ for at least the **duration of employment plus 30 years**.

Employee medical records are provided upon request of the employee or to anyone having written consent of the employee within 15 working days. Such requests should be sent to _____ *(Name of responsible person or department and address)* _____

OSHA Recordkeeping

An exposure incident is evaluated to determine if the case meets OSHA's Recordkeeping Requirements (29 CFR 1904). This determination and the recording activities are done by _____ *(Name of responsible person or department)* _____.

ENGINEERING CONTROL EVALUATION FORMS

The following pages contain sample forms that may be used in evaluating safer engineering controls. These forms are only applicable to certain groups of devices. Safer engineering controls are not limited to the devices contained in the following pages. None of these forms are specifically required by the bloodborne pathogens standard, but they may be useful as guidance documents. Employers are responsible for setting the evaluation criteria for the devices used in their facilities in accordance with the standard.

Sample Forms:

NIOSH

Questionnaire for Evaluating Sharps Disposal Container Performance

ECRI©

ECRI's Needlestick-Prevention Device Evaluation Form

NPD Cost Calculation Worksheet

Training for Development of Innovative Control Technologies Project (TDICT)©
SAFETY FEATURE EVALUATION FORMS

SAFETY SYRINGES

I.V. ACCESS DEVICES

SHARPS DISPOSAL CONTAINERS

I.V. CONNECTORS

VACUUM TUBE BLOOD COLLECTION SYSTEMS

E. R. SHARPS DISPOSAL CONTAINERS

SAFETY DENTAL SYRINGES

HOME USE SHARPS DISPOSAL CONTAINER

QUESTIONNAIRE FOR EVALUATING SHARPS
DISPOSAL CONTAINER PERFORMANCE

INSTRUCTIONS: Product evaluators should inspect and operate containers to be evaluated in side-by-side comparisons. Representative sharps (syringes, IV sets, blades, biopsy needles, pipettes, etc.) should be used to test candidate products. Actual use conditions should be simulated, if possible. Prior to inserting test sharps, attempt to reopen sealed containers and attempt to spill or remove contents from unsealed containers if this is a functional requirement. Evaluation facilitators should provide product manufacturer literature and visual instructions and should demonstrate proper operation of each of the containers. Use of this guideline requires knowledge that the ideal product may not exist and that this evaluation tool was based on common product designs available at the time.

PLEASE CIRCLE YOUR RESPONSE

FUNCTIONALITY

agree . . . . . disagree

Container is stable when placed on horizontal surface and when used as described in the product labeling for use in trays, holders, or enclosures	1	2	3	4	5
Container provides for puncture, leak, and impact resistance	1	2	3	4	5
Container, labels, warning devices, and brackets are durable	1	2	3	4	5
Container is autoclavable, if necessary	1	2	3	4	5
Container is available in various sizes and capacities	1	2	3	4	5
Container is available with auxiliary safety features (e.g., restricted access to sharps in the container), if required	1	2	3	4	5
Closure mechanism will not allow needlestick injury	1	2	3	4	5
Closure mechanism provides secure seal	1	2	3	4	5
Design minimizes needle-tip flipback	1	2	3	4	5
Design promotes clinical performance (e.g., will not compromise sterile field or increase injury or infection control hazards)	1	2	3	4	5
Design resists easy reopening after sealing for final disposal or autoclaving	1	2	3	4	5
Inlet design defeats waste removal when open	1	2	3	4	5
Inlet design prevents spillage of contents (physical or liquid) while sharps disposal container is in use in the intended upright position	1	2	3	4	5
Containers designed to be reopenable have removable lids design with tight closure that facilitates ease of removal with grip safety and comfort	1	2	3	4	5
Mounting brackets are rugged and designed for ease of service and decontamination	1	2	3	4	5

ACCESSIBILITY

agree . . . . . disagree

Container available in various opening sizes and shapes	1	2	3	4	5
Containers are supplied in sufficient quantity	1	2	3	4	5
Container has an entanglement-free opening/access way	1	2	3	4	5
Container opening/access way and current fill status visible to user prior to placing sharps into container	1	2	3	4	5
Internal design/molding of container does not impede ease of use	1	2	3	4	5
Handles, if present, located above full-fill level	1	2	3	4	5
Handles, if present, facilitate safe vertical transport and are located away from opening/access way and potentially soiled surfaces	1	2	3	4	5
Fixed locations place container within arm's reach of point of waste generation	1	2	3	4	5
Fixed locations allow for installation of the container below horizontal vision level	1	2	3	4	5
If necessary, in high patient or visitor traffic areas, container should provide for security against tampering	1	2	3	4	5

VISIBILITY

agree . . . . . disagree

Color or warning label implies danger. 1   2   3   4   5

A warning indicator (i.e., color or warning label) is readily visible to the user
   prior to user placing sharps into container 1   2   3   4   5

Overfill level provided and current fill status is readily visible to the user
   prior to use placing sharps into container 1   2   3   4   5

Sharps disposal container complies with OSHA requirements 1   2   3   4   5

Disposal opening/access way is visible prior to user placing sharps into container 1   2   3   4   5

Security, mounting, aesthetic, and safety features do not distort visibility of the
   opening/access way or fill status indicator 1   2   3   4   5

ACCOMMODATION

agree . . . . . disagree

No sharp edges in construction or materials 1   2   3   4   5

Safety features do not impede free access 1   2   3   4   5

Promotes patient and user satisfaction (i.e., aesthetic to extent possible) 1   2   3   4   5

Is simple to operate 1   2   3   4   5

Any emissions from final disposal comply with pollution regulations 1   2   3   4   5

Easy to assemble, if required 1   2   3   4   5

Components of containers that require assembly are easy to store prior to use 1   2   3   4   5

Use allows onehanded disposal 1   2   3   4   5

Product available in special designs for environments with specific needs
   (e.g., laboratories, emergency rooms, emergency medical services, pediatrics,
   correctional facilities) 1   2   3   4   5

Mounting system durable, secure, safe, cleanable, and, where appropriate, lockable 1   2   3   4   5

Mounting systems allow height adjustments 1   2   3   4   5

Design promotes task confidence 1   2   3   4   5

Cost effectiveness 1   2   3   4   5

OTHER COMMENTS

What design or performance requirements are missing from the product you evaluated that are really needed to safely or more comfortably conduct your job or sharps related task?

Additional Evaluator Concerns and Comments:

This product selection questionnaire was developed by the Centers for Disease Control and Prevention's National Institute for Occupational Safety and Health in conjunction with NIOSH Educational Resource Centers; The Johns Hopkins University, Baltimore; the University of Texas, Houston; the University of California, Berkeley; and the Mount Sinai School of Medicine, New York City.

ECRI's Needlestick-Prevention Device Evaluation Form

Device: _____

Supplies/Trade Name _____

Applications: _____

Reviewer: _____ Date: _____

For each question circle the appropriate response for the needlestick-prevention (NPD) device being evaluated.

Healthcare Worker Safety

1.   A. Does the NPD prevent needlesticks during use (i.e., before disposal)? .... Yes   No

    B. Does it do so after use(i.e., does the safety mechanism remain activated through disposal of the NPD)? .... Yes   No

2.   A. Does NPD provide protection one of the following ways: Either intrinsically or automatically? (Answer "No" if a specific action by the user is required to activate the safety mechanism.) .... Yes   No

    B. If "No," is the mechanism activated in one of the following ways: either by one-handed technique or by a two-handed technique accomplished as part of the usual procedure? .... Yes   No

3.   During the use of NPD do user's hands remain behind the needle until activation of the safety mechanism is complete? .... Yes   No

4.   Is the safety mechanism reliable when activated properly? .... Yes   No

5.   Does the NPD minimize the risk of user exposure to the patient's blood? .... Yes   No

Patient Safety and Comfort

6.   Does the NPD minimize the risk of infection to the patient (e.g., through cross-contamination)? .... Yes   No

7.   Can the NPD be used without causing more patient discomfort than a conventional device? .... Yes   No

8.   *For IV NPDs* : Does the NPD attach comfortably (i.e., without causing patient discomfort at the catheter port or IV tubing? .... Yes   No

Ease of use and Training

9.   Is NPD Operation obvious? That is can the device be used properly without extensive training? .... Yes   No

10.   Can the NPD be used by a left-handed person as easily as by a right handed person? .... Yes   No

11.   Is the technique required for using the NPD the same as that for using a conventional device? .... Yes   No

12.   Is it easy to identify the type and size of the product from the packaging? .... Yes   No

13.   *For intravenous (IV) catheters and blood collection needle sets*: Does the NPD provide a visible blood flashback during initial insertion? .... Yes   No

14.   Please rate the ease of using this NPD .... Exc.   Good   Fair   Poor

15.   Please rate the quality of the in-service training .... Exc.   Good   Fair   Poor

Compatibility

16.   Is the NPD compatible with devices (e.g., blood collection tubes) from a variety of suppliers? .... Yes   No

17.   *For IV NPDs*:

    A. Is the NPD compatible with intralipid solutions? .... Yes   No

    B. Does the NPD attach securely at the catheter port? .... Yes   No

    C. Doe the NPD attach securely or lock at a Y-site (e.g. for piggybacking)? .... Yes   No

18.   Is the NPD easy to dispose of in sharps containers of all sizes (if required)? .... Yes   No

19   Does using the NPD instead of a conventional device result in only a modest (if any) increase in sharps container waste volume? (Answer "No" if the NPD will increase waste volume significantly.) .... Yes   No

Overall

20   Would you recommend using this device? .... Yes   No

Comments (e.g., describe problems, list incompatibilities)

_____   _____

Source: Reprinted with permission of ECRI, Plymouth Meeting, Pennsylvania © 1998 ECRI

NPD Cost Calculation Worksheet*

WORKSHEET			SAMPLE DATA

PROTECTIVE SYSTEM _____

NPD (supplier/trade name) _____			**Protective blood collection tube holder**
			XYZ Medical Pro Hold
A. Price per device	A=	$ _____	A= $4.00
B. Uses per year	B=	_____	B= 130,000
C. Uses per device	C=	_____	C= 300
D. Quantity used per year (B ÷ C)	D=	_____	D= 433
E. NPD cost per year (A × D)	E=	$ _____	E= $ 1,732
Additional component _____			XYZ Medical ProHold Companion 1 Qt Sharps Container
F. Price per device	F=	$ _____	F= $3.50
G. Uses per year	G=	_____	G= Dispose of 130,000 needles
H. Uses per device	H=	_____	H= NA (see next entry)
I. Quantity used per year (G ÷ H)	I=	_____	I= 32**
J. Additional component cost per year (F × I)	J=	$ _____	J= $112
K. Annual protective system cost (E ÷ J)	K=	$ _____	K= $1,844

CONVENTIONAL SYSTEM _____

Conventional device _____			**Blood collection tube holder**
			XYZ Medical Tube Holder
L. Price per device	L=	$ _____	L= $0.15
M. Uses per year	M=	_____	M= 130,000
N. Uses per device	N=	_____	N= 300
O. Quantity used per year (M ÷ N)	O=	_____	O= 433
P. Conventional device cost per year (L × O)	P=	$ _____	P= $65
Additional component _____			**Conventional 1qt sharps container**
Q. Price per device	Q=	$ _____	Q= $2.13
R. Uses per year	R=	_____	R= Dispose of 130,000 needles
S. Uses per device	S=	_____	S= NA (see next entry)
T. Quantity used per year (R ÷ S)	T=	_____	T= 32**
U. Additional component cost per year (Q × T)	U=	$ _____	U= $68.16
V. Annual conventional system cost (P + U)	V=	$ _____	V= $133.16

RELATED DISPOSAL COSTS

Additional sharps containers			
W. Disposal volume of each NPD	W=	_____	W= 14 cm³ (tube holder only)
X. Disposal volume of each conventional device	X=	_____	X= 12 cm³ (tube holder only)
Y. Sharps container volume	Y=	_____	Y= 1 qt (943cm³)
Z. Number of additional sharps containers per year ([[W ×		_____	Z= 1 (assumes 100% packing efficiency)
AA. Price per sharps container	AA=	$ _____	AA= $3.50
AB. Annual additional sharps containers cost (Z ×AA)	AB=	$ _____	AB= $3.50
AC. Other additional disposal costs	AC=	$ _____	AC= None
AD. Total annual increase in disposal costs (AB + AC)	AD=	$ _____	AD= $3.50

NSI COST

AE. Number of NSIs per year with conventional device	AE=	_____	AE= 6
AF. Projected NSIs per year with NPD (50% × AE)	AF=	_____	AF= 3
AG. Cost of each NSI	AG=	$ _____	AG= $540
AH. Annual NSI cost savings (AG × [AE - AF])	AH=	$ _____	AH= $1,620
AI. MISCELLANEOUS COSTS	AI=	$ _____	AI= None
AJ. NET PROTECTIVE SYSTEM COSTS (K+AD+AI -AH)	AJ=	$ _____	AJ= $227.50
AK. ANNUAL INCREASE IN EXPENDITURES (AJ - V)	AK=	$ _____	**Annual increase in expenditures: $94.34**

*The figures obtained by completing this worksheet should be used for comparison purposes only. These figures will not reflect the actual costs and cost savings- associated with implementing the alternative under consideration, and they cannot reflect the true value of using an NPD in terms of staff safety and the economic impact on NSIs that result in seroconversion.

**Calculated by multiplying the estimated volume of one needle (0.23 cm) by the number of needles per year (130,000) and then dividing by the volume of one sharps container (1 qt = 943 cm). Note that this analysis assume 100% packing efficiency.

Source: Reprinted with permission of ECRI, Plymouth Meeting, Pennsylvania © 1998 ECRI

SAFETY FEATURE EVALUATION FORM
SAFETY SYRINGES

Date: _____ Department: _____ Occupation: _____

Product: _____ Number of times used: _____

Please **circle** the most appropriate answer for each question. Not applicable (N/A) may be used if the question does not apply to this particular product.

agree...........disagree

DURING USE:

1. The safety feature can be activated using a one-handed technique . . . . 1 2 3 4 5 N/A
2. The safety feature **does not** obstruct vision of the tip of the sharp . . . . 1 2 3 4 5 N/A
3. Use of this product requires you to use the safety feature . . . . 1 2 3 4 5 N/A
4. This product does not require more time to use than a non-safety device . . . . 1 2 3 4 5 N/A
5. The safety feature works well with a wide variety of hand sizes . . . . 1 2 3 4 5 N/A
6. The device is easy to handle while wearing gloves . . . . 1 2 3 4 5 N/A
7. This device **does not** interfere with uses that do not require a needle . . . . 1 2 3 4 5 N/A
8. This device offers a good view of any aspirated fluid . . . . 1 2 3 4 5 N/A
9. This device will work with all required syringe and needle sizes . . . . 1 2 3 4 5 N/A
10. This device provides a better alternative to traditional recapping . . . . 1 2 3 4 5 N/A

AFTER USE:

11. There is a clear and unmistakable change (audible or visible) that occurs
    when the safety feature is activated . . . . 1 2 3 4 5 N/A
12. The safety feature operates reliably . . . . 1 2 3 4 5 N/A
13. The exposed sharp is permanently blunted or covered after use and prior to disposal . . . 1 2 3 4 5 N/A
14. This device is no more difficult to process after use than non-safety devices . . . . 1 2 3 4 5 N/A

TRAINING:

15. The user **does not** need extensive training for correct operation . . . . 1 2 3 4 5 N/A
16. The design of the device suggests proper use . . . . 1 2 3 4 5 N/A
17. It is **not** easy to skip a crucial step in proper use of the device . . . . 1 2 3 4 5 N/A

Of the above questions, which three are the most important to **your** safety when using this product?

Are there other questions which you feel should be asked regarding the safety/utility of this product?

GUIDELINES FOR THE USE OF
SAFETY FEATURE EVALUATION SHEETS

Coordinators:

Determine which products are to be evaluated and provide at least four or more test samples for each individual evaluating the product. (Each evaluator should have enough samples to disassemble and examine the design thoroughly.)

Set up a testing station for each type of device which allows testers to evaluate products in a simulated patient procedure. Provide training dummies (injection pads, oranges, etc.) as necessary.

Provide visual instructions and demonstrate proper use of each device.

Review the instructions and rating system with each evaluator.

Encourage each evaluator to comment on the sheets and prioritize the questions at the end of the evaluation. This will provide a useful decision making tool and will help alert you to specific areas of concern which may not have been covered by the questionnaire.

Evaluators:

Re-enact all steps of intended or possible procedures performed with the device being tested.

Attempt to misuse the device and circumvent or disable the safety feature.

Answer each question, including the short answer section at the end. If you do not understand a question, please write comments directly on the sheets.

NOTE: Certain assumptions have been made in the development of these forms based on information about currently available products. We recognize the likelihood that the ideal product may not exist. TDICT welcomes your comments on the use of these tools.

Source: Reprinted with permission of Training for Development of Innovative Control Technology Project
June Fisher, M.D.
© June 1993, revised August 1998
Trauma Foundation, Bldg #1, Room #300
San Francisco General Hospital
1001 Potrero Avenue
San Francisco, CA 94110

SAFETY FEATURE EVALUATION FORM
I.V. ACCESS DEVICES

Date: _____ Department: _____ Occupation: _____

Product: _____ Number of times used: _____

Please **circle** the most appropriate answer for each question. Not applicable (N/A) may be used if the question does not apply to this particular product.

<table>
<tr><td></td><td align="right">agree............disagree</td></tr>
</table>

	agree..........disagree
1. The safety feature can be activated using a one-handed technique	1 2 3 4 5 N/A
2. The safety feature **does not** interfere with normal use of this product	1 2 3 4 5 N/A
3. Use of this product requires you to use the safety feature	1 2 3 4 5 N/A
4. This product **does not** require more time to use than a non-safety device	1 2 3 4 5 N/A
5. The safety feature works well with a wide variety of hand sizes	1 2 3 4 5 N/A
6. The device allows for rapid visualization of flashback in the catheter or chamber	1 2 3 4 5 N/A
7. Use of this product **does not** increase the number of sticks to the patient	1 2 3 4 5 N/A
8. The product stops the flow of blood after the needle is removed from the catheter (or after the butterfly is inserted) and just prior to line connections or hep-lock capping	1 2 3 4 5 N/A
9. A clear and unmistakable change (either audible or visible) occurs when the safety feature is activated	1 2 3 4 5 N/A
10. The safety feature operates reliably	1 2 3 4 5 N/A
11. The exposed sharp is blunted or covered after use and prior to disposal	1 2 3 4 5 N/A
12. The product **does not** need extensive training to be operated correctly	1 2 3 4 5 N/A

Of the above questions, which three are the most important to **your** safety when using this product?

Are there other questions which you feel should be asked regarding the safety/utility of this product?

Source: Reprinted with permission of Training for Development of Innovative Control Technology Project
June Fisher, M.D.
© June 1993, revised August 1998

SAFETY FEATURE EVALUATION FORM
SHARPS DISPOSAL CONTAINERS

Date: _____ Department: _____ Occupation: _____

Product: _____ Number of times used: _____

Please **circle** the most appropriate answer for each question. Not applicable (N/A) may be used if the question does not apply to this particular product.

agree...........disagree

1. The container's shape, its markings, or its color, imply danger . . . . 1 2 3 4 5 N/A
2. The implied warning of danger can be seen from the angle at which people
   commonly view it (very short people, people in wheel chairs, children, etc) . . . . 1 2 3 4 5 N/A
3. The implied warning can be universally understood by visitors, children, and patients . . . . 1 2 3 4 5 N/A
4. The container's purpose is self-explanatory and easily understood by a worker
   who may be pressed for time or unfamiliar with the hospital setting . . . . 1 2 3 4 5 N/A
5. The container can accept sharps from any direction desired . . . . 1 2 3 4 5 N/A
6. The container can accept all sizes and shapes of sharps . . . . 1 2 3 4 5 N/A
7. The container allows single handed operation. (Only the hand holding the
   sharp should be near the container opening) . . . . 1 2 3 4 5 N/A
8. It is difficult to reach in and remove a sharp . . . . 1 2 3 4 5 N/A
9. Sharps can go into the container without getting caught on the opening . . . . 1 2 3 4 5 N/A
10. Sharps can go into the container without getting caught on any molded
    shapes in the interior . . . . 1 2 3 4 5 N/A
11. The container is puncture resistant . . . . 1 2 3 4 5 N/A
12. When the container is dropped or turned upside down (even before it is
    permanently closed) sharps stay inside . . . . 1 2 3 4 5 N/A
13. The user can determine easily, from various viewing angles, when the
    container is full . . . . 1 2 3 4 5 N/A
14. When the container is to be used free-standing (no mounting bracket), it is stable
    and unlikely to tip over . . . . 1 2 3 4 5 N/A
15. It is safe to close the container. (Sharps should not protrude into the path of
    hands attempting to close the container) . . . . 1 2 3 4 5 N/A
16. The container closes securely. (e.g. if the closure requires glue, it may not
    work if the surfaces are soiled or wet.) . . . . 1 2 3 4 5 N/A
17. The product has handles which allow you to safely transport a full container . . . . 1 2 3 4 5 N/A
18. The product **does not** require extensive training to operate correctly . . . . 1 2 3 4 5 N/A

Of the above questions, which three are the most important to **your** safety when using this product?

Are there other questions which you feel should be asked regarding the safety/utility of this product?

411

SAFETY FEATURE EVALUATION FORM
I.V. CONNECTORS

Date: _____ Department: _____ Occupation: _____
_____

Product: _____ Number of times used: _____
_____

Please **circle** the most appropriate answer for each question. Not applicable (N/A) may be used if the question does not apply to this particular product.

agree..........disagree

1. Use of this connector eliminates the need for exposed needles in connections . . . . 1 2 3 4 5 N/A
2. The safety feature **does not** interfere with normal use of this product . . . . 1 2 3 4 5 N/A
3. Use of this product requires you to use the safety feature . . . . 1 2 3 4 5 N/A
4. This product **does not** require more time to use than a non-safety device . . . . 1 2 3 4 5 N/A
5. The safety feature works well with a wide variety of hand sizes . . . . 1 2 3 4 5 N/A
6. The safety feature allows you to collect blood directly into a vacuum tube,
   eliminating the need for needles . . . . 1 2 3 4 5 N/A
7. The connector can be secured (locked) to Y-sites, hep-locks, and central lines . . . . 1 2 3 4 5 N/A
8. A clear and unmistakable change (either audible or visible) occurs when the
   safety feature is activated . . . . 1 2 3 4 5 N/A
9. The safety feature operates reliably . . . . 1 2 3 4 5 N/A
10. The exposed sharp is blunted or covered after use and prior to disposal . . . . 1 2 3 4 5 N/A
11. The product **does not** need extensive training to be operated correctly . . . . 1 2 3 4 5 N/A

Of the above questions, which three are the most important to **your** safety when using this product?

Are there other questions which you feel should be asked regarding the safety/utility of this product?

412

SAFETY FEATURE EVALUATION FORM
VACUUM TUBE BLOOD COLLECTION SYSTEMS

Date: _____ Department: _____ Occupation: _____

Product: _____ Number of times used: _____

Please **circle** the most appropriate answer for each question. Not applicable (N/A) may be used if the question does not apply to this particular product.

agree...........disagree

1. The safety feature can be activated using a one-handed technique . . . . 1 2 3 4 5 N/A
2. The safety feature **does not** interfere with normal use of this product . . . . 1 2 3 4 5 N/A
3. Use of this product requires you to use the safety feature . . . . 1 2 3 4 5 N/A
4. This product **does not** require more time to use than a non-safety device . . . . 1 2 3 4 5 N/A
5. The safety feature works well with a wide variety of hand sizes . . . . 1 2 3 4 5 N/A
6. The safety feature works with a butterfly . . . . 1 2 3 4 5 N/A
7. A clear and unmistakable change (either audible or visible) occurs when the
   safety feature is activated . . . . 1 2 3 4 5 N/A
8. The safety feature operates reliably . . . . 1 2 3 4 5 N/A
9. The exposed sharp is blunted or covered after use and prior to disposal . . . . 1 2 3 4 5 N/A
10. The inner vacuum tube needle (rubber sleeved needle) **does not** present a
    danger of exposure . . . . 1 2 3 4 5 N/A
11. The **product does** not need extensive training to be operated correctly . . . . 1 2 3 4 5 N/A

Of the above questions, which three are the most important to **your** safety when using this product?

Are there other questions which you feel should be asked regarding the safety/utility of this product?

413

Safety Feature Evaluation Form
E. R. SHARPS DISPOSAL CONTAINERS

Date: _____ Department: _____ Occupation: _____
_____

Product: _____ Number of times used: _____

Please **circle** the most appropriate answer for each question. Not applicable (N/A) may be used if the question does not apply to this particular product.

agree............disagree

1. The container's shape, its markings, or its color, imply danger which can be
   understood by visitors, children, and patients . . . . 1 2 3 4 5 N/A
2. The implied warning of danger can be seen from the angle at which people
   commonly view it. (very short people, people in wheel chairs, children, etc) . . . . 1 2 3 4 5 N/A
3. The container can be placed in a location that is easily accessible during
   emergency procedures . . . . 1 2 3 4 5 N/A
4. The container's purpose is self-explanatory and easily understood by a worker
   who may be pressed for time or unfamiliar with the hospital setting . . . . 1 2 3 4 5 N/A
5. The container can accept sharps from any direction desired . . . . 1 2 3 4 5 N/A
6. The container can accept all sizes and shapes of sharps . . . . 1 2 3 4 5 N/A
7. The container is temporarily closable, and will not spill contents (even after
   being dropped down a flight of stairs) . . . . 1 2 3 4 5 N/A
8. The container allows single handed operation. (Only the hand holding the sharp
   should be near the container opening) . . . . 1 2 3 4 5 N/A
9. It is difficult to reach in and remove a sharp . . . . 1 2 3 4 5 N/A
10. Sharps can go into the container without getting caught on the opening or any
    molded shapes in the interior . . . . 1 2 3 4 5 N/A
11. The container can be placed within arm's reach . . . . 1 2 3 4 5 N/A
12. The container is puncture resistant . . . . 1 2 3 4 5 N/A
13. When the container is dropped or turned upside down (even before it is permanently
    closed) sharps stay inside . . . . 1 2 3 4 5 N/A
14. The user can determine easily, from various viewing angles, when the container is full . . . 1 2 3 4 5 N/A
15. When the container is to be used free-standing (no mounting bracket), it is stable
    and unlikely to tip over . . . . 1 2 3 4 5 N/A
16. The container is large enough to accept all sizes and shapes of sharps, including
    50 ml preloaded syringes . . . . 1 2 3 4 5 N/A
17. It is safe to close the container. (Sharps should not protrude into the path of hands
    attempting to close the container) . . . . 1 2 3 4 5 N/A
18. The container closes securely under all circumstances . . . . 1 2 3 4 5 N/A
19. The product has handles which allow you to safely transport a full container . . . . 1 2 3 4 5 N/A
20. The product **does not** require extensive training to operate correctly . . . . 1 2 3 4 5 N/A

Of the above questions, which three are the most important to **your** safety when using this product?

Are there other questions which you feel should be asked regarding the safety/ utility of this product?

414

SAFETY FEATURE EVALUATION FORM
SAFETY DENTAL SYRINGES

Date: _____ Department: _____ Occupation: _____

Product: _____ Number of times used: _____

Please **circle** the most appropriate answer for each question. Not applicable (N/A) may be used if the question does not apply to this particular product.

agree...........disagree

1. The safety feature can be activated using a one-handed technique . . . . 1 2 3 4 5 N/A

2. The safety feature **does not** obstruct vision of the tip of the sharp and the intraoral injection site. . . . . 1 2 3 4 5 N/A

3. Use of this product requires you to use the safety feature . . . . 1 2 3 4 5 N/A

4. This product **does not** require more time to use than a non-safety device . . . . 1 2 3 4 5 N/A

5. The safety feature works well with a wide variety of hand sizes . . . . 1 2 3 4 5 N/A

6. The device is easy to handle while wearing gloves . . . . 1 2 3 4 5 N/A

7. The device is easy to handle when wet . . . . 1 2 3 4 5 N/A

8. This device accepts standard anesthetic carpules and does not hinder carpule changing . . . . 1 2 3 4 5 N/A

9. The safety feature **does not** restrict visibility of carpule contents intraorally . . . . 1 2 3 4 5 N/A

10. This device accepts standard dental needles of all common lengths and gauges, and does not interfere with needle changing . . . . 1 2 3 4 5 N/A

11. The device provides a better alternative to traditional recapping . . . . 1 2 3 4 5 N/A

12. Sterilization of this device is as easy as a standard dental syringe . . . . 1 2 3 4 5 N/A

13. For syringes with integral needles only: The needle on this syringe **will not** break while bending and repositioning in the tissue . . . . 1 2 3 4 5 N/A

14. This device is no more difficult to break down after use for sterilization than a standard dental syringe . . . . 1 2 3 4 5 N/A

15. The safety feature operates reliably . . . . 1 2 3 4 5 N/A

16. The exposed sharp is permanently blunted or covered after use and prior to disposal . . . . 1 2 3 4 5 N/A

17. There is a clear and unmistakable change (either visible or audible) that occurs when the safety feature is activated . . . . 1 2 3 4 5 N/A

18. The user **does not** need extensive training to operate the product correctly . . . . 1 2 3 4 5 N/A

19. The design of the device allows for easy removal of the needle from the syringe . . . . 1 2 3 4 5 N/A

20. The design of the device allows for easy removal of the carpule from the syringe . . . . 1 2 3 4 5 N/A

Safety Feature Evaluation Form
Home Use Sharps Disposal Container

Date: _____ Department: _____ Occupation: _____
____

Product: _____ Number of times used: _____
____

Please **circle** the most appropriate answer for each question. Not applicable (N/A) may be used if the question does not apply to this particular product.

agree............disagree

The container is puncture resistant . . . . 1 2 3 4 5 N/A
The container is stable . . . . 1 2 3 4 5 N/A
There is a handle which is robust, comfortable to carry, and compact . . . . 1 2 3 4 5 N/A
The container allows single handed use . . . . 1 2 3 4 5 N/A
The user can access the container from any direction . . . . 1 2 3 4 5 N/A
It is possible to drop sharps into the container vertically . . . . 1 2 3 4 5 N/A
Minimal or no force is required to put sharps into the container . . . . 1 2 3 4 5 N/A
The container opens and closes easily . . . . 1 2 3 4 5 N/A
Container closure maintains integrity after repeated use . . . . 1 2 3 4 5 N/A
The box accommodates a range of sharps, including 12 cc syringe, butterfly,
      and lancet . . . . 1 2 3 4 5 N/A
The size of the container is appropriate to its use . . . . 1 2 3 4 5 N/A
No one (including a child) can access the contents of the container to retrieve a
      sharp . . . . 1 2 3 4 5 N/A
Needles/tubing do not get caught on the opening or interior shape . . . . 1 2 3 4 5 N/A
There is a temporary lock for transport which is secure but reversible . . . . 1 2 3 4 5 N/A
There is a permanent lock for final disposal which is not reversible . . . . 1 2 3 4 5 N/A
There is an absorbent lining to collect excess fluid . . . . 1 2 3 4 5 N/A
The user can determine the fill level visually . . . . 1 2 3 4 5 N/A
There is a signal when the box is 2/3 full . . . . 1 2 3 4 5 N/A
The container is appropriately labeled . . . . 1 2 3 4 5 N/A
Biohazard of container contents is apparent . . . . 1 2 3 4 5 N/A
The box is not threatening to patients . . . . 1 2 3 4 5 N/A
Use of this container in no way compromises infection control practices . . . . 1 2 3 4 5 N/A

Of the above questions, which three are the most important to **your** safety when using this product?

Are there other questions which you feel should be asked regarding the safety/ utility of this product?

WATCH FOR THESE SYMPTOMS

Disease	Signs & Symptoms	Incubation Time (Range)	Person-to-Person Transmission	Isolation	Diagnosis	Postexposure Prophylaxis for Adults	Treatment for Adults
Anthrax *Bacillus anthracis* **A. Inhalation**	Flu-like symptoms (fever, fatigue, muscle aches, dyspnea, nonproductive cough, headache), chest pain, possible 1-2 day improvement then rapid respiratory failure and shock. Meningitis may develop.	1 to 6 days (up to 6 wks)	None	Standard Precautions	Chest x-ray evidence of widening mediastinum; obtain sputum and blood culture. Sensitivity and specificity of nasal swabs unknown - do not rely on for diagnosis.	Prophylaxis for 60 days: Ciprofloxacin* 500 mg PO q 12h Or Doxycycline 100 mg PO q 12h Alternative (if strain susceptible and above contraindicated): Amoxicillin 500 mg PO q 8h *In vitro studies suggest that Levofloxacin 500 mg PO q 24h Or Gatifloxacin 400 mg PO q 24h Or Moxifloxacin 400 mg PO q 24h could be substituted	Inhalation anthrax Combined IV/PO therapy for 60d Ciprofloxacin 500 mg q 12h Or Doxycycline 100 mg q 12h, AND 1 or 2 additional drugs (vancomycin, rifampin, imipenem clindamycin, chloramphenicol, clarithromycin, and if susceptible penicillin or ampicillin
B. Cutaneous	Intense itching followed by painless papular lesions, then vesicular lesions, developing into eschar surrounded by edema.	1 to 12 days	Direct contact with skin lesions may result in cutane-ous infection.	Contact Precautions	Peripheral blood smear may demonstrate gram positive bacilli on unspun smear with sepsis.		Cutaneous anthrax Ciprofloxacin 500 mg PO q 12h Or Doxycycline 100 mg PO q 12h Recommendations same for pregnant women and immunocompromised persons
C. Gastrointestinal (GI)	Abdominal pain, nausea and vomiting, severe diarrhea, GI bleeding, and fever.	1 to 7 days	None	Standard Precautions	Culture blood and stool.	Recommendations same for pregnant women and immunocompromised persons	
Botulism botulinum toxin	Afebrile, excess mucus in throat, dysphagia, dry mouth and throat, dizziness, then difficulty moving eyes, mild pupillary dilation and nystagmus, intermittent ptosis, indistinct speech, unsteady gait, extreme symmetric descending weakness, flaccid paralysis; generally normal mental status.	Inhalation: 12-80 hours Foodborne: 12-72 hours (2-8 days)	None	Standard Precautions	Laboratory tests available from CDC or Public Health Dept; obtain serum, stool, gastric aspirate and suspect foods prior to administering antitoxin. Differential diagnosis includes polio, Guillain Barre, myasthenia, tick paralysis, CVA, meningococcal meningitis.	Pentavalent toxoid (types A, B, C, D, E) 0.5 ml SQ may be available as investigational product from USAMRIID.	Botulism antitoxins from public health authorities. Supportive care and ventillatory support. Avoid clindamycin and aminoglycosides.
Pneumonic Plague *Yersinia pestis*	High fever, cough, hemoptysis, chest pain, nausea and vomiting, headache. Advanced disease: purpuric skin lesions, copious watery or purulent sputum production; respiratory failure in 1 to 6 days.	2-3 days (2-6 days)	Yes, droplet aerosols	Droplet Precautions until 48 hrs of effective antibiotic therapy	A presumptive diagnosis may be made by Gram, Wayson or Wright stain of lymph node aspirates, sputum, or cerebrospinal fluid with gram negative bacilli with bipolar (safety pin) staining.	Doxycycline 100 mg PO q 12h Or Ciprofloxacin 500 mg PO q 12h	Streptomycin 1 gm IM q 12h; Or Gentamicin 2 mg/kg, then 1.0 to 1.7 mg/kg IV q 8h Alternatives: Doxycycline 200 mg PO load, then 100 PO mg q 12h Or Ciprofloxacin 400 mg IV q 12h
Smallpox variola virus	Prodromal period: malaise, fever, rigors, vomiting, headache, and backache. After 2-4 days, skin lesions appear and progress uniformly from macules to papules to vesicles and pustules, mostly on face, neck, palms, soles, and subsequently progress to trunk.	12-14 days (7-17 days)	Yes, airborne droplet nuclei or direct contact with skin lesions or secretions until all scabs separate and fall off (3 to 4 weeks)	Airborne (includes N95 mask) and Contact Precautions	Swab culture of vesicular fluid or scab, send to BL-4 laboratory. All lesions similar in appearance and develop synchronously as opposed to chickenpox. Electron microscopy can differentiate *variola virus* from *varicella*.	Early vaccine critical (in less than 4 days). Call CDC for vaccinia. Vaccinia immune globulin in special cases - call USAMRIID 301-619-2833.	Supportive care. Previous vaccination against smallpox does not confer lifelong immunity. Potential role for Cidofovir.

Photo Credits: Anthrax A and C - JAMA 1999;281:1737-8 ; Anthrax B - CDC; Botulism - JAMA 2001;285:1062 Copyrighted 2001 American Medical Association; Plague - JAMA 2000;283:2283; Smallpox - CDC

References:

- Arnon SS, Schechter R, Inglesby TV, et al. for the Working Group on Civilian Biodefense. Botulinum toxin as a biological weapon: medical and public health management. JAMA 2001;285:1059-1070.
- Centers for Disease Control and Prevention. Chemical/Biological Survival Cards for Civilians. 2000.
- Chin J, ed. Control of Communicable Diseases Manual. 17th edition. Washington, DC: American Public Health Association. 2000.
- Henderson DA, Inglesby TV, Bartlett JG, et al. for the Working Group on Civilian Biodefense. Smallpox as a biological weapon; medical and public health management. JAMA 1999;281:2127-2137.
- Inglesby TV, Henderson DA, Bartlett JG, et al. for the Working Group on Civilian Biodefense. Anthrax as a biological weapon: medical and public health management. JAMA 2002;287:2236-2252.
- Inglesby TV, Dennis DT, Henderson DA, et al. for the Working Group on Civilian Biodefense. Plague as a biological weapon: medical and public health management. JAMA 2000;283:2281-2290.
- U.S. Army Medical Research Institute of Infectious Diseases. USAMRIID's Medical Management of Biological Casualties Handbook. 4th ed. Fort Detrick, Frederick, Maryland. 2001.
- Update: Investigation of Bioterrorism-Related Anthrax and Interim Guidelines for Clinical Evaluation of Persons with Possible Anthrax. MMWR 2001;50:941-948.

DECONTAMINATION FOR ALL OF THESE AGENTS

1. Place clothing from suspected victims in airtight impervious (e.g., plastic) bags and save for law authorities (e.g., FBI, SBI).
2. Use soap and water for washing victim.
3. For environmental disinfection for all of the above, use bleach (standard 6.0% - 6.15% sodium hypochlorite) in a 0.6% concentration (1 part bleach to 9 parts water). For botulism, plague and smallpox an alternative is to use an EPA-approved germicidal detergent.
4. For smallpox, all bedding and clothing must be autoclaved or laundered in hot water and bleach.
5. Healthcare worker should wear PPE (gowns, gloves and mask) during decontamination of anthrax, plague, and smallpox.

DETECTION OF OUTBREAKS

Epidemiologic Strategies

- A rapidly increasing disease incidence
- An unusual increase in the number of people seeking care, especially with fever, respiratory, or gastrointestinal symptoms
- An endemic disease rapidly emerging at an uncharacteristic time or in an unusual pattern
- Lower attack rate among persons who had been indoors
- Clusters of patients arriving from a single locale
- Large numbers of rapidly fatal cases
- Any patient presenting with a disease that is relatively uncommon and has bioterrorism potential

NOTIFICATION PROCEDURES IN THE EVENT OF A BIOTERRORIST INCIDENT

1. **First call the Public Health Officer at your local health department; after hours contact local Health Director via 911.**
2. **If criminal activity is suspected, call your local law enforcement and the FBI in your state.**

FOR MORE INFORMATION ON BIOTERRORISM:

CDC - Centers for Disease Control and Prevention
www.bt.cdc.gov/

APIC - Association for Professionals in Infection Control & Epidemiology
www.apic.org/bioterror/

SPICE - North Carolina Statewide Program for Infection Control and Epidemiology
www.unc.edu/depts/spice/
919-966-3242

USAMRIID's Medical Management of Biological Casualties Handbook
www.usamriid.army.mil/education/bluebook.html

Chart developed by:

North Carolina Statewide Program for Infection Control and Epidemiology (SPICE)   email: spice@unc.edu
KK Hoffmann, DJ Weber, EP Clontz, WA Rutala

Support provided by:

The North Carolina Institute for Public Health and The North Carolina Center for Public Health Preparedness, in the School of Public Health at The University of North Carolina at Chapel Hill

In view of the possibility of human error or changes in medical sciences, neither the authors, nor the publisher, nor any other party who has been involved in the preparation or publication of this work warrants that the information contained herein is in every respect accurate or complete. Readers are encouraged to confirm the information contained herein with other sources and check drug package insert for warnings and contraindications.

418

NOTES

NOTES

NOTES

NOTES